Ruqiya Shama Tareen, Donald E. Greydanus, Mohammad Jafferany,
Dilip R. Patel and Joav Merrick (eds.)
Pediatric Psychodermatology

Health, Medicine and Human Development

Edited by
Joav Merrick

Health is a key component of human development, growth and quality of life. The *Health, Medicine and Human Development* book series aim to provide a public forum for book publications from a multidisciplinary group of researchers, practitioners and clinicians for an international professional forum interested in the broad spectrum of health, medicine and human development. We welcome research on a wide variety of substantive areas that will promote and impact healthy human development including prevention, intervention and care also among people in vulnerable conditions.

Bricker JT, Omar HA, Merrick J, eds.
Adults with Childhood Illnesses: Considerations for Practice.
Berlin: De Gruyter, 2011.
ISBN 978-3-11-025521-8
e-ISBN 978-3-11-025568-3

Derevensky JL, Shek D, Merrick J, eds.
Youth Gambling: The Hidden Addiction.
Berlin: De Gruyter, 2011.
ISBN 978-3-11-025520-1
e-ISBN 978-3-11-025569-0

Greydanus DE, Patel DR, Omar HA, Feucht C, Merrick J, eds.
Adolescent Medicine: Pharmacotherapeutics in General, Mental and Sexual Health.
Berlin: De Gruyter, 2012.
ISBN 978-3-11-025522-5
e-ISBN 978-3-11-025570

Greydanus DE, Patel DR, Omar HA, Feucht C, Merrick J, eds.
Adolescent Medicine: Pharmacotherapeutics in Medical Disorders.
Berlin: De Gruyter, 2012.
ISBN 978-3-11-027580-3
e-ISBN 978-3-11-027636-7

Pediatric Psychodermatology

A Clinical Manual of Child and Adolescent Psychocutaneous Disorders

Edited by
Ruqiya Shama Tareen, Donald E. Greydanus,
Mohammad Jafferany, Dilip R. Patel and Joav Merrick

DE GRUYTER

Editors
Ruqiya Shama Tareen, MD, MBBS, DDSc
Western Michigan University
School of Medicine
Kalamazoo, MI
United States
shama.tareen@med.wmich.edu

Donald E. Greydanus, MD, Dr. HC (ATHENS), FAAP, FSAM (Emeritus), FIAP (HON)
Western Michigan University
School of Medicine
Kalamazoo, MI
United States
donald.greydanus@med.wmich.edu

Mohammad Jafferany, MD
Michigan State University
College of Human Medicine and Osteopathic Medicine
East Lansing, MI
United States
mjafferany@yahoo.com

Dilip R. Patel, MD, FAAP, FSAM, FAACPDM, FACSM
Western Michigan University
School of Medicine
Kalamazoo, MI
United States
dilip.patel@med.wmich.edu

Joav Merrick, MD, MMedSc, DMSc
Ministry of Social Affairs and Social Services
National Institute of Child Health and Human Development
Jerusalem
Israel
jmerrick@zahav.net.il

ISBN 978-3-11-027387-8
e-ISBN 978-3-11-027393-9

Library of Congress Cataloging-in-Publication Data
A CIP Catalog record for this book has been applied for at the Library of Congress.

Bibliographic information published by the Deutsche Nationalbibliothek
The Deutsche Nationalbibliothek lists this publication in the Deutsche Nationalbibliografie; detailed bibliographic data are available in the Internet at http://dnb.d-nb.de.

Typesetting: Apex CoVantage
Printing: Hubert & Co. GmbH & Co. KG, Göttingen
Cover image: iStockphoto/Thinkstock

∞ Printed on acid-free paper
Printed in Germany
www.degruyter.com

Dedication

Ruqiya Shama Tareen. I dedicate this book to my late father, Dr. A. Qadir Tareen, who very early on kindled the passion of learning in me; my mother, Khairunisa Tareen, who lovingly guided this passion in the right direction; my mentor, Dr. David C. Dunstone, who quietly sculpted my passion into academic pursuit; my wonderful husband, Nisar Tareen, who was the force behind me so I could pursue my passion; and my beautiful daughters, Anam, Kinza, and Salwa, who taught me the fine act of balance between my passion and just being a mother.

Donald E. Greydanus. I dedicate this book to Allan Ellis, MD—a man for all seasons and times. Thank you for helping me and teaching me that *nam et ipsa scientia potestas est. Requiescat in pace cum Deo.*

Mohammad Jafferany. I dedicate this book to my pediatric psychodermatological patients who continue to teach me so much.

Dilip R. Patel. I dedicate this work to my lovely wife, Ranjan, and wonderful son, Neil, for their years of love and support.

Joav Merrick. I dedicate this book to my wife and children for their support.

Contents

Andrew Y. Finlay

Foreword I

The importance of psychodermatology to all dermatologists is at last being recognized. This book is a major step forward in enhancing understanding of psychodermatology issues in children and adolescents. Professor Tareen has an unusual strength for a psychiatrist – namely, background training in dermatology – and, therefore, has been ideally placed to orchestrate this book.

Psychodermatology research has mainly been focused on adults, with the exception of atopic dermatitis, where complex psychological issues impact both the affected child and the parents. However, it is clear that there are great differences in the issues that are of importance for children and for adolescents. The bringing together of detailed reviews of these areas in this book will be very useful not only for dermatologists and psychologists, but also for paediatricians, psychiatrists, and for trainees in all these professions. This book also highlights the many areas where more research is needed.

In the first section the interrelationship between diseases of the skin and mind are explored, including the ways that skin disease may affect the quality of life of those who are psychologically affected. All of the common skin diseases, such as acne, may have a secondary psychological impact and are reviewed in the second section.

Although only a small number of people develop skin diseases that are primarily psychiatric, these conditions are among the most challenging and interesting in clinical dermatology and are well described in the third section. Body dysmorphic disorder or delusions of parasitosis, for example, are devastating conditions for those affected and remain in need of further research.

There are some skin conditions that, although relatively uncommon, are so devastating to the lives of those affected that there is a high chance that sufferers may develop psychiatric disorders, in particular depression. Severe alopecia, vitiligo, and hidradenitis suppurativa are good examples, and are covered in the fourth section. Another association occurs in the context of systemic disease that may have both skin disease and psychiatric aspects. The two are not necessarily causally related, but occur together, and so later become intertwined in a negative feedback loop that provides huge challenges in untangling, especially in adolescents. These issues are explored in the fifth section.

Finally, there are a variety of special aspects to the management of children and adolescents that may not be at first obvious. Despite the successful growth of the speciality of pediatric dermatology, currently worldwide most children and teenagers with skin disease are under the care of general dermatologists, primarily trained and experienced in adult dermatology. The sixth section addresses some of the additional broader aspects of psychodermatology in the young and very young.

Where is this book placed in relation to the development of psychodermatology as a recognized skill or discipline? There has been a complex history to the understanding of the relationship between psychological matters and skin disease. In the 19th century the lack of understanding of the cause of many skin diseases led physicians to assume a major role for psychological issues or psychiatric disease in the pathogenesis of skin disease: many conditions were considered to be of "nervous" or "neurotic" origin. Over the last century, however, the many advances in understanding of cellular or immunological mechanisms in skin disease pathogenesis, for example, in psoriasis, led to a rejection of the concept of psychological causation. This was replaced by the view that psychological issues were an important secondary result of skin disease. This century we are starting another phase of understanding as it becomes clear that psychological states may have a direct impact on disease activity. In addition, both the role of psychological support and the treatment of psychological disease in parallel with treatment aimed at the skin are now beginning to be subjected to proper scientific scrutiny. There are already many lessons arising from this that have clinical relevance for every practitioner. This book brings these areas together succinctly.

But why, despite the long history of awareness of psychological issues inherent in clinical dermatology, is there still so little training in psychodermatology and so little provision of specialist psychodermatology services? Time devoted to this aspect of dermatology in national and international clinical dermatology meetings is small in proportion to the all-pervasive nature of the issues involved. Scientific societies, such as the European Society of Dermatology and Psychiatry, have been set up to promote the understanding of psychodermatology but they reach relatively few dermatologists, and mainly those who are already especially interested.

One of the reasons for the subject being relatively ignored may be the limited use of validated assessment tools. In medicine, subjects that cannot or are not measured tend to be ignored in the face of the constant avalanche of publications dependant on hard facts and their offspring, statistics and analysis. Over the last two decades the impact of skin disease on quality of life has become widely appreciated, thanks to the availability of simple measurement techniques that can be applied in the clinic.

The challenge for psychodermatology research is to use measurement methods, or create new ones that are more appropriate to clinical needs. Large properly controlled studies designed to correctly evaluate different types of therapeutic intervention are essential, using validated and relevant outcome measures. It is only in this way that psychodermatology will develop into a more scientifically respected aspect of dermatology. The many unanswered questions that this book raises will only be resolved by this approach. The difficulties to achieve this in the future should not be underestimated; for example, rare diseases will have to be studied in the context of multicenter clinical trial networks. Also, carrying out such studies in children and adolescents poses major ethical, funding, and recruitment challenges.

This book is an important landmark in the development of psychodermatology, broadening our narrow adult-focussed framework of thinking about the subject. The publication of this book is a call to arms for those who wish to see the special issues of children and adolescents given more attention. In the meantime it successfully brings together a wealth of practical information that is of direct help to a wide range of clinicians.

Andrew Y. Finlay, MBBS, FRCP, CBE
Cardiff University School of Medicine
Department of Dermatology and Wound Healing
Cardiff, Wales
United Kingdom
finlayay@cardiff.ac.uk

Elizabeth A. Burns

Foreword II

I am honored to contribute a foreword to this unique textbook *Pediatric Psychodermatology: A Clinical Manual of Child and Adolescent Psychocutaneous Disorders*. The authors address not only the etiology of skin disorders and psychological component of dermatopathology but also the stigmatizing consequences of skin disease and the importance of addressing this as part of the treatment plan. The breadth of the chapters, addressing both common and rare disorders, makes this text particularly useful.

As a family physician, I was often confronted by the pathology described in this text. When a child is involved, the impact goes beyond the patient to the family. What parent does not suffer when their young child is in distress with atopic dermatitis? I have seen parents question everything from the food they are preparing and the soap they are using to their parenting skills. Extended families can contribute more opinions regarding etiology and treatment. It is no wonder that some parents are overwhelmed when trying to manage this disease. Mohammad Khurshid Azam Basra, in Chapter 4 on quality-of-life issues, specifically addresses the quality of life of both the patient and the family. As a primary care physician, the holistic approach in patient assessment throughout this text provides practical information that can be applied within a busy office setting. This is apparent in Ruqiya Shama Tareen's Chapter 5 on atopic dermatitis, where the multiple causes of atopy are reviewed. Treatment of both skin and psyche is addressed.

As the Associate Dean, Faculty and Clinical Affairs, Western Michigan University School of Medicine, I am in awe of the collaborative work of our faculty. Our small educational institution brings together faculty from many disciplines. This milieu has resulted in interdisciplinary work that benefits our learners and our patients. International collaboration adds perspective and depth. I congratulate the authors on their work.

Elizabeth A. Burns, MD, MA
Associate Dean
Faculty & Clinical Affairs
Western Michigan University
School of Medicine
Kalamazoo, Michigan
United States
elizabeth.burns@med.umich.edu

Donald E. Greydanus and Ruqiya Shama Tareen

Preface

> "My body is clothed with worms and scabs, my skin is broken and festering.
> My days are swifter than a weaver's shuttle and they come to an end without hope." (Job 7:5,6)

The skin has evolved over millions of years from a simple envelope to cover microscopic organisms to a complex organ system that has marvellously protected complex life from a harsh environment. The skin and central nervous system (CNS) develop together in utero and remain intricately connected throughout the life of *Homo sapiens*. Diseases of the skin have led to considerable medical as well as psychological morbidity, caustic contumely, and even Stygian mortality over the hundreds of years of the hominoid existence. When the skin is diseased, significant psychosomatic, behavioral, and psychiatric factors can result in a gallimaufry of primary and/or secondary disorders.

This monumental dance between the body's largest organ and the CNS (sympathetic and parasympathetic nervous systems) can be seen as far back as recorded history. The Ebers Papyrus is an Egyptian medical papyrus that contains medical advice from one of the oldest recorded pharmacopoeia. It was written around 1500 BCE but is based on earlier texts that date back to 3400 BCE (1). It revealed recommendations for various medical problems including dermatological. For example, it provided practical advice on treatment for Dracunculiasis (Guinea worm) in which the end of the worm was wrapped around a stick and slowly pulled out; over 4000 years later, this is still the basic treatment!

This 110-page scroll provided advice on treatment of dermatological conditions based on application of *henna* (Kupros or Cyperus). There were seven forms of henna based on where it was collected, the age of the plant, and what part was used. Henna was one of 400 plants, minerals, and animal parts used to develop remedies found in the Ebers Papyrus pharmacopoeia. Henna was mixed with various other ingredients such as goose oil, semen, red grain, onion meal, incense, wild date juice, and others. Such concoctions were used to treat what was called "scabs in every limb," "itching from all limbs," and others that were very disturbing to the sufferer (1). This document used the term "Aku-t," which referred to "boils, blains, sores, pustules, or any inflamed skin." Pharaohs were known to have acne, and this document notes various treatments, including sulphur.

An early reference to the stigmatization of skin disease can be found in the Genesis 4:15 reference to the mark of Cain who was given this dermatological disfigurement for the murder of his brother, Abel, which some scholars concluded was the red face of acne rosacea (2). Perhaps Cain had exfoliative dermatitis or the so-called red man syndrome. We, of course, do not know today what this mark was. However, such an account goes back to the very beginning of *Homo sapiens,* although the account of Genesis was probably written around the same time as the Ebers Papyrus in 1400–1500 BCE. Another early reference to potential negative effects of skin disease is found in the plague of boils that afflicted ancient Egyptians in 1440 BCE as told in the Exodus 9:6–17 account of the exodus by the Israelites from Egypt.

When individuals in the Bible had a severe skin disease, the term "leprosy" was often the translation in English that was used. In the Hebrew text, the word was *tzaraath*; this term was used for various dermatological conditions, especially if the skin disease involved sores or eruptions (3,4). The English word *leprosy* comes from the Greek work *lepros*, or *lepra* (λεπρα), which was used in translation in Greek for the Hebrew word *tzaraath*. Since there were no trained histopathologists and dermatologists around, one can only speculate on what these various diseases were and were not.

It is clear that many skin disorders evoked considerable horror on the part of the victim and those around him or her. Leviticus 13 and 14 (1400 BCE) discuss a disfiguring skin disease that prompted isolation of the victim in hopes it would clear up. Sometimes the noun *tzaraath* referred to a skin disease with scales, but it also referred to mildew on houses and clothes. In Leviticus 13:18–28 *tzaraath* (or leprosy) could be a skin disease with boils and burns, while in Leviticus 13:39–44 it referred to bald patches or scalp/beard lesions. Skin patches were called *tzaraath* if at least two hairs in a skin patch turned white, if normal skin appeared in a patch, or if the patch had enlarged since the original examinations.

Those who were called lepers lived a wretched life outside of civilized areas and their skin disease was often felt by others to be God's punishment for their sins. In Leviticus 14 Moses was commanded to take the leprous person to the priest (someone from the lineage of Aaron) who would examine this person and decide what was to be done based on his exam as well as other techniques such as the killing of a bird. Those with severe skin diseases were frightening to others and strict laws were developed, partly to prevent the afflicted person from spreading this potentially contagious disease to others.

In Leviticus 13 (1400 BCE) the handling of someone with leprosy was detailed:

> The *Lord* spoke to Moses and Aaron, saying, "When a person has on the skin of his body a swelling or an eruption or a spot, and it turns into a case of leprous disease on the skin of his body, then he shall be brought to Aaron the priest or to one of his sons the priests, and the priest shall examine the diseased area on the skin of his body. And if the hair in the diseased area has turned white and the disease appears to be deeper than the skin of his body, it is a case of leprous disease. When the priest has examined him, he shall pronounce him unclean. But if the spot is white in the skin of his body and appears no deeper than the skin, and the hair in it has not turned white, the priest shall shut up the diseased person for seven days. And the priest shall examine him on the seventh day, and if in his eyes the disease is checked and the disease has not spread in the skin, then the priest shall shut him up for another seven days. . . . The leprous person who has the disease shall wear torn clothes and let the hair of his head hang loose, and he shall cover his upper lip and cry out, 'Unclean, unclean.' He shall remain unclean as long as he has the disease. He is unclean. He shall live alone. His dwelling shall be outside the camp."

Skin diseases have imposed a terrible price of misery on these sufferers for thousands of years. Certainly part of the suffering was the isolation that lepers had to accept. Numbers 5: 1–3 (1430 BCE) notes: "Command the Israelites to send away from the camp anyone who has an infectious skin disease or a discharge of any kind . . . Send away male and female alike; send them outside the camp." The misery of those with these skin diseases was reflected in 2 Kings 7:3 (860 BCE) by one who noted: "why are we sitting here until we die?"

Perhaps one of the most famous persons in the Old Testament with leprosy was Naaman (commander of the army of the king of Syria and described as a "great" man) who was actually healed from his skin condition as described in 2 Kings 5:1–27. Even Kings were not excluded from skin disease and isolation. In 2 Chronicles 26:21–23: "King Uzziah had leprosy until the day he died. He lived in a separate house—leprous, and excluded from the temple of the Lord. Jotham his son had charge of the palace and governed the people of his land . . . Uzziah rested with his fathers and was buried with them in a field for burial that belonged to the kings, for people said, 'He had leprosy.' "

Perhaps one of the earliest and most poignant accounts of the severe medical and psychological distress that dermatological disorders can render is found in the story of Job in the Old Testament. It is unclear if Job was a real person and when this classic story was written. However, this well-known story movingly expresses the misery and agony that severe skin conditions have given to countless millions of *Homo sapiens* over the past millennia.

In Job 2:7,8 the story notes: "So Satan . . . afflicted Job with painful sores from the soles of his feet to the top of his head. Then Job took a piece of broken pottery and scraped himself with it as he sat among the ashes." It is unclear what condition Job had, whether true leprosy, syphilis, acne fulminans, psoriasis, SAPHO syndrome (combination of synovitis, acne, pustulosis, hyperostosis, and osteitis), hidradenitis suppurativa, neurocutaneous syndrome, systemic lupus erythematosus, or other conditions. Job describes his skin condition in various versus:

> "My body is clothed with worms and scabs, my skin is broken and festering.
> My days are swifter than a weaver's shuttle and they come to an end without hope." (Job 7:5,6)

> "Even if I washed myself with soap and my hands with washing soda,
> You would plunge me into a slime pit so that even my clothes detest me." (Job 9:30)

> "My skin grows black and peels; my body burns with fever." (Job 30:30)

It is the psychological impact on Job that perhaps was worse than the medical effects due to the depression and ostracism that severe skin disease had caused. Job, however, became an archetype of dignity despite his suffering and retained his izzat despite the jactations and accipitrine attacks of his peers. The threnody of Job is illustrated by these various verses:

> "If only my anguish could be weighed and all my misery be placed on the scales! It would surely outweigh the sand of the seas." (Job 6:1–2)

> "I loathe my life, therefore I will give free rein to my complaint and speak out in the bitterness of my soul." (Job 10:1)
>
> "Why then did you bring me out of the womb? I wish I had died before any eye saw me." (Job 10:18)
>
> "I have become a laughingstock to my friends." (Job 12:4)
>
> "I have sewed sackcloth over my skin and buried my brow in the dust. My face is red with weeping, deep shadows ring my eyes." (Job 16:15,16)
>
> "Even little boys scorn me; when I appear they ridicule me. All my intimate friends detest me, those I love have turned against me." (Job 19:18,19)
>
> "And now their sons mock me; I have become a byword among them. They detest me and keep their distance; they do not hesitate to spit in my face." (Job 30:9,10)

The ancient Greeks also sought to help their fellow humans deal with the ravages of skin disorders. They used the term *psora* to describe itchy skin conditions; this was a term that led to *psoriasis* as a skin disease known for many centuries. The term *eczema* also comes from the Greek (ἔκζεμα [*ēkzema*], "to boil over"). In some ancient languages eczema was also called dermatitis, acute in some languages and chronic in others (5). The ancient Greeks coined the term *acne* and were aware that many people had this disorder whether rich or poor. Aristole (384–322 BCE) described this condition in some detail. In 400 BC Hippocrates, the so-called Father of Western Medicine, associated acne with puberty (5). Hippocrates (460–370 BCE) also noted that mucus from the land snail was helpful in treating dry skin by hydration. Hippocrates, in his famous *Corpus Hippocraticum* first used the term *alopecia*, which is literally translated as "fox's disease." Theocritus (300–260 BCE), the creator of Greek pastoral poetry, described rosacea but described no treatment for it.

The emperor Octavius Augustus (63 BC–AD 14), considered by historians as the first emperor of the Roman Empire, was documented as one with atopy that included very itchy, dry skin, seasonal rhinitis, and chest tightness (6). Examination of persons in Israel with skin disease (leprosy) by priests was still the rule in this early part of the first century as noted in the New Testament (Luke 17:14). Around AD 30 Jesus of Nazareth cured a "leprous" person by touching this person (Luke 5:13) and then, as described in Luke 17:12–14, Jesus cured ten lepers at a distance and then told them to go to the priests to show that they were "clean."

Aulus Cornelius Celsus (25 BC–AD 50) was a Roman scholar who lived in Rome and is credited with writing *De Medicina*, which was an encyclopedia that provided medical knowledge in the first-century Roman world. It detailed medical treatments based on diet, pharmacy, surgery, and other healing disciplines. Celsus described human disease and developed such terms as inflammation, calor (warmth), dolor (pain), tumor (swelling), rubor (redness), and others. Celsus advocated the use of hot baths with mineral water and sulphur for treatment of a various skin problems including acne (5). Also, Celsus advanced on the Hippocratic concept of alopecia and described two forms: alopecia totalis and ophiasis (translated as "snake");

ophiasis described hair loss in the form of a snake and was felt to occur only in children (7). In honor of Celsus, an archetype of medicine and science for many centuries, alopecia areata was called "area celsi" until the 18th century.

Soranus was a Greek physician from Ephesus who lived at the first and second century interface, practiced in Alexandria, and eventually lived in Rome. He is credited by history as the first pediatrician for his work "On Acute and Chronic Diseases," in which he wrote about infant care in addition to women's diseases and pregnancy (8). Claudius Galen (AD 130–210) was the famous physician and surgeon to the Roman emperor and gladiators of ancient Rome whose recommendation for skin diseases (such as acne) in adolescents and young adult males included the admonition that they stop masturbating (9,10).

Such medical knowledge, both correct and false, was lost for centuries with the fall of Rome in AD 475 and the appearance of the so-called Dark Ages in Western civilization from AD 475 to 800. Concepts of medicine were kept alive by the great Persian physician and scholar Abu al-Hasan Ali ibn Sahl Rabban al-Tabari (AD 865–925), who produced an encyclopedia of medicine and work on child development that was reviewed in his book "Firdous al-Hikmah" (Paradise of Wisdom) (11). His student was the famous Persian physician Rhazes (Muhammad ibn Zakariya Razi [865–925]), who wrote the first known book on diseases of children (10).

The West began to awake very slowly from its Dark Ages slumber. For example, an unknown Anglo Saxon poet between the 8th and 11th centuries wrote the classic *Beowulf,* while Trotula Platearius (Salerno, Italy) wrote a book on children and women called *De Mylierum Passionibus* in AD 1050. The Renaissance in Europe allowed humans to focus on discoveries in art, science, medicine, law, and much more. Europe reveled in Dante's *Divine Comedy* in 1302, Chaucer's *Canterbury Tales* in 1386, Michaelangelo's *Pieta* in 1500, Leonardi da Vinci's *Mona Lisa* in 1505, Raphael's *Sistine Madonna (La Madonna di San Sisto)* in 1514, and perhaps the essence of the Renaissance period ended with the death of Michelangelo in 1564.

In Chaucer's "Prologue" to the *Canterbury Tales,* he gives us a Job-like glimpse into emotional sequelae of skin diseases in which he describes one of his characters (Somnour) with probable acne rosacea; Chaucer describes Somnour: "that had a fyrreed cherubbines face . . . of his visage children were afraid" (Prologue 23–35) (2,12). Indeed, the red face has historically been used by novelists and others down through the ages to denote negative traits of those with rosacea.

However, the seeds of progress were sown and discoveries in medicine followed, including human anatomy with the famous Flemish physician Andreas Vesalius's *De Humani Corporis Fabrica* that was published in 1543. Science began to blossom with the work of such giants as Francis Bacon (1561–1626), Galileo Galilei (1564–1642), Rene Descartes (1596–1650), Robert Hooke (1635–1703), and others. Antony van Leeuwenhoek (1632–1723) was a poorly educated nonscientist from Delft, The Netherlands, whose work with the microscope and his description of "little animals" revolutionized medicine forever (13).

Thomas Phaer (1510–1560) was an English pediatrician, lawyer, and author who wrote the first textbook in the English language on pediatrics called *The Boke of Chyldren,* which was published in 1545 (14). Physicians were finally focusing on children and their disorders in contrast to only dealing with adults. The term *adolescence* can be traced to the 15th century in Europe and is derived from the Latin word, *adolescere,* which means "to grow into maturity." The idea of studying diseases of children and adolescents was thousands of years in the making. In 1776 a famous book of its time in Europe linked diseases of children to that idea that "the nerves of children are very irritable" (in contrast to adults), "much the more softened, and also covered with very thin membranes" (15). The term *biology* was used in the early 19th century in attempts to identify scientific etiologies versus theories derived from ancient philosophical theories.

Psoriasis was called *Willan's lepra* in the late 18th century when dermatologists Robert Willan and Thomas Bateman separated out this disorder from other skin diseases (such as leprosy). The Viennese dermatologist Ferdinand von Hebra coined the term *psoriasis* from the Greek *psora* meaning "to itch." Gradually the science of dermatology was advancing as the scientific method was utilized around the world. G. A. Hansen discovered that leprosy was caused by a bacterium called *Mycobacterium leprae* and the disease was then called Hansen's disease.

Various skin diseases, previous called leprosy, were now being specifically categorized into specific disorders. Though physicians knew that skin diseases could induce considerable psychological distress (as per the quotes from Job), the complex interplay between the skin (ectoderm) and the central nervous system (sympathetic and parasympathetic nervous systems) was not yet appreciated. In the era of bacteriology in the 19th century, *Corynebacterium acnes* (now called *Propionibacterium acnes*) was identified as being etiologically linked in acne in 1896.

The 20th century revealed various dermatological treatments. Sulphur, which had been used for thousands of years to ameliorate unknown skin diseases, gave way to more modern treatments. For acne, benzoyl peroxide was identified in the 1920s, tretinoin in the 1970s, and oral isotretinoin in the 1980s.

Perhaps the link between the ectoderm and the CNS became more evident with the description of delusional infestations, reviewed in Chapter 10 of this book. The Swedish neurologist Karl Axel Ekbom (1907–1977) published reports of this condition in the late 1930s (16). Also called Ekbom's syndrome, people become convinced they have an infestation with an object (i.e., insect, worm, bacteria, virus, others) though there is no medical evidence of this infestation. It is a *delusional* infestation and must be treated psychiatrically. The object changed over time as science evolved, as for example, bacteria in the 19th century (when bacteria were being identified), and then to viruses as well as parasites in the 20th century (17). The 21st century has already seen an additional Lilliputian delusional object, that of "Morgellons," which is seeking an academic aura of its own thanks to bureaucratic interdiction (18).

This book is developed with this historical perspective in mind and seeks to summarize current knowledge regarding complex links between the skin and psychiatric illnesses as detailed in these pages. Indeed, we have learned that our skin, being our most visible aspect of ourselves, becomes the first interface with our world around us. Since antiquity we have paid tremendous attention to how we looked by enhancing the appearance of our skin. The human race in the early ages learned to distinguish individuals from one another by painting their bare skin with natural pigments. They learned to pierce skin in various places, decorating it with bones, rocks, feathers, and other natural elements to gain and display certain social hierarchy. The tradition of paying attention to skin has continued through our journey through time and even after centuries of evolution and social development. In today's modern world, where social interaction has outgrown the usual boundaries of personal contact and has taken us to cyberspace where one can instantly connect with someone on the other side of globe via face time and Internet video chats, this emphasis on our appearance and first impression has not gone down but possibly may have increased.

We dedicate this book in an ex post facto manner to the millions of humans who, despite their velleity to improve their dermatological fate, have irrefragably suffered as a result of the complex chemistry between skin and emotional stability. Cain, Job, all the biblical lepers, Chaucer's *Somnour*, and so many more have developed lifelong anguish and agony because of these connections. In the 21st century we have learned much, although much more is still waiting to be discovered. However, all clinicians can help our patients with real and even imagined dermatological conditions. Indeed, we can help many with psychiatric co-conditions if we are willing to recognize and deal with them.

Dermatologists, primary care clinicians, psychiatrists, psychologists, and others can take this knowledge and apply it to our patients. We can be a lighthouse to the millions of *Homo sapiens* drifting in a large sea of psychiatric distress because of dermatological problems. Pediatric psychodermatology is not simply an arcane sesquipedalian term, but this clinical manual brings this discipline to practical reality in the 21st century. The editors thank the many experts who have so graciously given up their precious time to provide the readers with their vast expertise. The editors hope that this example of translational research will be of considerable benefit to the readers of this publication. We offer this "tree" of knowledge to the readers for the benefit of our patients (19).

> "Those having torches will pass them on to others."
> (Plato, 429–347 BCE)

References

1. Bryan C. Ancient Egyptian medicine. Chicago: Papyrus Ebers Ares Publishers, 1974.
2. Cribier B. The red face: art, history and medical representations. Ann Dermatol Venereol 2011;138 (Suppl 2):S116–23.

3. Jastrow M. The so-called 'leprosy' laws: An analysis of Leviticus, chapters 13 and 14. Jewish Quart Rev 1914:4(3):357–418.
4. Lewis A. Lesson from Leviticus: Leprosy. Man New Series 1987;22(4):593–612.
5. Grant RNR. The history of acne. Proc R Soc Med 1951;44(8):647–52.
6. Ring J, Pryzybilla B, Razicka T. Handbook of atopic eczema. Berlin: Springer, 2006.
7. Barber HW. Alopecia areata. Br J Dermatol Syph 1921;33:1–14.
8. Drabkin IE. Soranus and his system of medicine. Bull Hist Med 1951;25:503–18.
9. Greydanus DE, Geller B. Masturbation: Historic perspective. NY State J Med 1980;80:1892–6.
10. Park R. An epitome of the history of medicine. Philadelphia, PA: FA Davis, 1897.
11. Prioreschi P. A history of medicine: Byzantine and Islamic medicine. Omaha, NB: Horatius Press, 2001.
12. Cooper H. The Canterbury tales. Oxford: Oxford University Press, 1996.
13. Toledo-Pereyra LH. Surgical revolutions: A historical and philosophical view. London: World Scientific, 2011.
14. Greydanus DE, Calles JL Jr, Patel DR, Nazeer A, Merrick J. Introduction: Pediatric psychopharmacology. In: Greydanus DE, Calles JL Jr, Patel DR, Nazeer A, Merrick J, eds. Clinical aspects of psychopharmacology in childhood and adolescence. New York: Nova Science, 2011:xi–xiv.
15. Von Rosenstei R. The diseases of children and their remedies. London: T Cadell, 1776:31.
16. Ekbom KA. Der praesenile Dermatozoenwahn. Acta Psychiatr Neurol Scand 1938;13:227–59.
17. Leppings P, Freudenmann RW. Delusional infestation in children, adolescence, and adulthood. In: Tareen RS, Greydanus DE, Jannerany M, Patel DR, Merrick J, eds. Pediatric psychodermatology: A clinical manual of child and adolescent psychocutaneous disorders. Berlin: De Gruyter, 2012:chapter 10.
18. Fair B. Morgellons: contested illness, diagnostic compromise and medicalisation. Sociol Health Illn 2011;32(4):597–612.
19. Greydanus DE, Patel DR, Merrick J. TR:EE: Translational research for every educator. Int J Child Health Hum Dev 2012;5(4):25–7.

Author index

Mohammad Khurshid Azam Basra, MBBS, DDSc, MD
Department of Dermatology and Wound Healing
Cardiff University School of Medicine
Cardiff, Wales, United Kingdom
drkhurshid69@hotmail.com
Chapter 4

Eulalia Baselga
Dermatology Department
Hospital de la Santa Creu I Sant Pau
Barcelona, Spain
EBaselga@santpau.cat
Chapter 6

Elizabeth A. Burns, MD, MA
Western Michigan University
School of Medicine
Kalamazoo, Michigan, United States
elizabeth.burns@med.wmich.edu
Foreword II

Joseph L. Calles, MD
Western Michigan University
School of Medicine
Kalamazoo, Michigan, United States
joseph.calles@med.wmich.edu
Chapter 21

Arthur N. Feinberg, MD
Western Michigan University
School of Medicine
Kalamazoo, Michigan, United States
arthur.feinberg@med.wmich.edu
Chapters 1, 12

Andrew Y. Finlay, MBBS, FRCP, CBE
Department of Dermatology and Wound Healing
Cardiff University School of Medicine
Cardiff, Wales, United Kingdom
finlayay@cardiff.ac.uk
Foreword I

Roland W. Freudenmann
Department of Psychiatry and Psychotherapy
University of Ulm
Ulm, Germany
roland.freudenmann@uni-ulm.de
Chapter 10

Donald E. Greydanus, MD, Dr. HC (ATHENS), FAAP, FSAM (Emeritus), FIAP (HON)
Western Michigan University
School of Medicine
Kalamazoo, Michigan, United States
donald.greydanus@med.wmich.edu
Chapters 3, 7

Zeba Hasan Hafeez, MD
Department of Psychiatry
Touro University, California
Vallejo, California, United States
zebahafeez@hotmail.com
Chapter 17

Misha M. Heller, BA
Keck School of Medicine
University of Southern California
Los Angeles, California, United States
misha.max.heller@gmail.com
Chapter 22

Josephine L. Howard, MD
Departments of Dermatology and Psychiatry
University of California San Francisco Medical Center
San Francisco, California, United States
josie.howard@ucsf.edu
Chapter 22

Mohammad Jafferany, MD
College of Human Medicine and Osteopathic Medicine
Michigan State University
East Lansing, Michigan, United States
mjafferany@yahoo.com
Chapter 8

Manmohan K. Kamboj, MD
Division of Endocrinology, Metabolism, and Diabetes
The Ohio State University
Columbus, Ohio, United States
manmohan.kamboj@nationwidechildrens.com
Chapters 18, 19, 20

Peter Lepping
Betsi Cadwaladr University Health Board
Wrexham, Wales, United Kingdom
peter.lepping@wales.nhs.uk
Chapter 10

Servando E. Marron, MD
Dermatology Department
Alcañiz Hospital
Alcañiz, Spain
Chapter 9

Ladan Mostaghimi, MD
Dermatology Department
University of Wisconsin Madison
Madison, Wisconsin United States
lmostaghimi@dermatology.wisc.edu
Chapter 16

Dilip R. Patel, MD, FAAP, FSAM, FAACPDM, FACSM
Western Michigan University School of Medicine
Kalamazoo, Michigan, United States
dilip.patel@med.wmich.edu
Chapters 14, 15

Helen D. Pratt, PhD
Western Michigan University School of Medicine
Kalamazoo, Michigan, United States
helen.pratt@med.wmich.edu
Chapter 11

Adam Reich
Department of Dermatology, Venereology and Allergology
Wroclaw Medical University
Wroclaw, Poland
adi_medicalis@o2.pl
Chapter 13

Sandra Ros
Dermatology Department
Hospital de la Santa Creu I Sant Pau
Barcelona, Spain
sros@santpau.cat
Chapter 6

Philip D. Shenefelt, MD
Department of Dermatology and Cutaneous Surgey
University of South Florida
Tampa, Florida, United States
pshenefe@health.usf.edu
Chapter 23

Tor A. Shwayder, MD
Pediatric Dermatology
Henry Ford Medical Center
Detroit, Michigan, United States
tshwayd1@hfhs.org
Chapter 1

Jacek C. Szepietowski
Department of Dermatology, Venereology and Allergology
Wroclaw Medical University
Wroclaw, Poland
jszepiet@derm.am.wroc.pl
Chapter 13

Stefani Takahashi, MD
Department of Dermatology
Keck School of Medicine
University of Southern California
Los Angeles, California, United States
steftaka@usc.edu
Chapter 22

Anam Nisar Tareen
Kalamazoo Center for Medical Studies
Michigan State University
Kalamazoo, Michigan, United States
anam.tareen@gmail.com
Chapter 24

Ruqiya Shama Tareen, MD, MBBS, DDSc
Western Michigan University
School of Medicine
Kalamazoo, Michigan, United States
shama.tareen@med.wmich.edu
Chapters 1, 2, 5, 18, 19, 20, 24

Therdpong Tempark, MD
Pediatric Dermatology Fellowship
Henry Ford Hospital Detroit, Michigan, United States
Department of Pediatrics
King Chulalongkorn Memorial Hospital
Bangkok, Thailand
Chapter 1

Lucia Tomas-Aragones, PhD
Aragon Health Sciences Institute
Zaragoza, Spain
luciatomas@cop.es
Chapter 9

Abbreviations

Aapp	American Academy on Physician and Patient
ACDRs	adverse cutaneous drug reactions
ACE	angiotensin-converting enzyme
ACLE	acute cutaneous lupus erythematosus
ACR	American College of Rheumatology
ACTH	adrenocorticotropin hormone
AD	Addison disease
AD	atopic dermatitis
ADR	adverse drug reaction
AI	adrenal insufficiency
AMT	anxiety management training
AN	Acanthosis nigricans
AN	anorexia nervosa
APA	American Psychiatric Association
APT	atopic patch test
ARDS	adult respiratory distress syndrome
ASD	autism spectrum disorders
ATRA	all-trans retinoic acid
AVP	arginine vasopressin
BAN	bilateral acoustic neurofibromatosis
BCIE	Bullous congenital ichthyosiform erythroderma
BDD	body dysmorphic disorder
BED	binge eating disorder
BI	Bullous ichthyosis
BLT	Buschke-Loewenstein tumor
BMI	basal metabolic index
BN	bulimia nervosa
BPD	borderline personality disorder
BT	behavior therapy
CA	Condylomata Acuminatum
CADIS	Childhood Atopic Dermatitis Impact Scale
CAH	congenital adrenal hyperplasia
cAMP	
CA-MRSA	Community acquired methicillin-resistant Staphylococcus aureus
CBC	complete blood count
CBCL	Childhood Behavior Checklist
CBT	cognitive behavioral therapy
CCT	crude coal tar
CD	conduct disorder

CDLQI	Children's Dermatology Life Quality Index
CEP	congenital erythropoietic porphyria
CH	congenital hypothyroidism
CIE	Congenital ichthyosiform erythroderma
CLM	cutaneous larva migrans
CMN	Congenital melanocytic nevi
CMV	cytomegalovirus
CNS	central nervous system
CRH	corticotropin releasing hormone
CS	Cushing syndrome
CSD	cat scratch disease
CSHQ	Children's Sleep Habits Questionnaire
CT	computed tomography
DBPCFC	double blind placebo controlled food challenge
DBT	dialectical behavior therapy
DFI	Dermatitis Family Impact questionnaire
DHEA	dehydroepiandrosterone
DHEAS	dehydroepiandrosterone sulfate
DI	delusional infestation
DIP	distal interphalangeal
DKA	diabetic ketoacidosis
DLE	disseminated lupus erythematosus
DLJMS	diabetic limited joint mobility syndrome
DLQI	Dermatology Life Quality Index
DPCP	diphenylcyclopropenone
DM	diabetes mellitus
DS	Down syndrome
DSM-IV-R	Diagnostic and Statistical Manual of Mental Disorders (4th ed., revised)
DSH	deliberate self-harm
EB	epidermal barrier
ECT	electroconvulsive shock therapy
ED	eating disorders
ED	ectodermal dysplasias
EDNOS	eating disorders not otherwise specified
EFT	emotional freedom techniques
EHK	Epidermolytic hyperkeratosis
EIA	enzyme immunoassay
ELISA	enzyme-linked immunosobent assay
EMB	extreme male brain
EMDR	eye movement desensitization and reprocessing
EMG	electromyographic

EOPBD	early onset pediatric bipolar disorder
EPS	epidermal nevus syndrome
EPS	extrapyramidal symptoms
ERP	exposure and response prevention
ERP	exposure relapse prevention
ESDaP	European Society of Dermatology and Psychiatry
EST	empirically supported treatments
ET	epidermolytic toxin
ETFAD	European Task Force on Atopic Dermatitis
EULAR	European League against Rheumatism
FDA	United States Food and Drug Administration
FDLQI	Family Dermatology Life Quality Index
FFA	free fatty acids
FHH	familial hypercalciuric hypocalcemia
FPDG	French Psychodermatology Group
FQoL	Family Quality of Life
FTU	fingertip unit
GABHS	beta-hemolytic Streptococcus
GAD	generalized anxiety disorder
GBS	Group B streptococcus
GH	growth hormone
GHQ	general health questionnaire
GSR	galvanic skin resistance
GWBI	General Well-Being Index
HAART	highly active antiretroviral therapy
HD	Hartnup disease
HED	hypohidrotic ectodermal dysplasia
HFMD	hand-foot-and-mouth disease
HIPAA	Health Insurance Portability and Accountability Act
HPA	hypothalamic-pituitary-adrenal
HPV	human papilloma virus
HRQoL	health-related quality of life
HS	hidradenitis suppurativa
HSV	Herpes simplex virus
HZV	Herpes zoster virus
IBD	inflammatory bowel disease
ID	intellectual disabilities
IDQoL	Infant's Dermatitis Quality of Life Index
IEMs	inborn errors of metabolism
IFA	immunofluorescent antibody
IFSI	International Forum for the Study of Itch
IGF1	insulin like growth factor 1

ILVEN	Inflammatory linear verrucous epidermal nevus
INF γ	interferon γ
IPT	interpersonal behavior therapy
JIA	juvenile idiopathic arthritis
JPD	juvenile plantar dermatosis
JRA	juvenile rheumatoid arthritis
KOH	potassium hydroxide
LAM	lymphoangiomatosis
LCD	liquor carbonis detergent
LE	lupus erythematosus
LI	Lamellar ichthyosis
LN	Lichen nitidus
LP	Lichen planus
LRINEC	Laboratory Risk Indicator for necrotizing fascitis
MAOIs	monoamine oxidase inhibitors
MC2	melanocortin receptors 2
MDD	major depressive disorder
MED	minimal erythema doses
MGH-HS	Massachusetts General Hospital Hair pulling Symptom Severity Scale
MHC	major histocompatibility complex
MOSF	multi organ system failure
MR	mental retardation
MRI	magnetic resonance imaging
MRSA	methicillin-resistant Staphylococcus aureus
MSH	melanocyte stimulating hormone
NAAF	National Alopecia Areata Foundation
NBCIE	Non-bullous congenital ichthyosiform erythroderma
NBS	newborn screening programs
NB-UVB	narrow band UVB
NCM	Neurocutaneous melanosis
NF	necrotizing fasciitis
NGF	nerve growth factor
NICE	Neuro-Immuno-Cutaneous-Endocrine network
NK	natural killer
NLD	necrobiosis lipoidica diabeticorum
NPSLE	neuropsychiatric systemic lupus erythematoses
NSAIDS	non-steroidal anti-inflammatory drugs
NSSI	non-suicidal self-injurious
OCD	obsessive compulsive disorder
OCPD	obsessive compulsive personality disorder
OCPs	oral contraceptive pills
ODD	oppositional defiant disorder

OSP	outer surface protein
PABA	para-aminobenzoic acid
PBD	pediatric bipolar disorder
PBMCs	peripheral blood mononuclear cells
PCOS	polycystic ovarian syndrome
PCR	polymerase chain reaction
PCT	porphyria cutaneatarda
PDD	pervasive developmental disorders
PDs	personality disorders
PDT	photodynamic therapy
PedsQL	Pediatric Quality of life
PFI	Psoriasis Family Index
PIQoL-AD	Parents' Index of Quality of Life in Atopic Dermatitis
PKU	phenylketonuria
PLC	Pityriasis lichenoides chronica
PLEVA	Pityriasis lichenoides et varioliformis acuta
PMNs	polymorphonuclear neutrophils
PNS	peripheral nervous system
PPAR	peroxisome proliferator-activated receptor
PPE	personal protective equipment
PR	Pityriasis rosea
PTH	parathyroid hormone
PTSD	posttraumatic stress disorder
PUVA	Psoralens with Ultraviolet A
PWS	Prader-Willi syndrome
QoL	quality of life
RA	rheumatoid arthritis
RAI	radioactive iodine ablation therapy
RCT	randomized control trial
SAD	social anxiety disorder
SCLE	subacute cutaneous lupus erythematosus
SCTEs	stratum corneum tryptic enzymes
SHBG	sex hormone-binding globulin
SIB	self-injurious behavior
SJS	Stevens-Johnson syndrome
SLE	systemic lupus erythematosus
SMB	self-mutilation behavior
SNRI	serotonin-norepinephrine reuptake inhibitor
SP	skin picking
SP	substance P
SPEA	streptococcal pyrogenic exotoxins
SPT	skin prick test

SPT	supportive psychotherapy
SSPE	subacute sclerosing panencephalitis
SSR	Sleep Self-Report
SSRIs	aelective serotonin reuptake inhibitors
SSSS	Staphylococcal scalded skin syndrome
TCAs	tricyclic antidepressants
TEN	toxic epidermal necrolysis
TFTs	thyroid function tests
TLRs	Toll-like receptors
TNF α	tumor necrosis factor α
TPMT	thiopurine methyltransferase
TSH	thyroid stimulating hormone
TSI	thyroid stimulating immunoglobulins
TSS	toxic shock syndrome
T-QoL	Teenager's QoL questionnaire
TTM	trichotillomania
UVB	ultraviolet B
VZV	varicella-zoster virus

Part I: INTERFACE OF DERMATOLOGY AND PSYCHIATRY

Arthur N. Feinberg, Tor A. Shwayder, Ruqiya Shama Tareen, and Therdpong Tempark

1 Perspectives on management of pediatric dermatologic disorders

Dermatological conditions are a very important part of pediatric medicine and can have considerable influence on the patient's medical as well as psychological health. This chapter presents a brief summary of etiologic and pathogenesis of these conditions followed by a standard case management, including newer developments where pertinent. The chapter reviews these areas: skin infections and infestations (bacterial, viral, fungal, and parasitic); dermatitis (nonallergic, allergic, and idiopathic); hypersensitivity reactions (urticaria, erythema multiforme, and drug eruptions); miscellaneous skin conditions (acne, nevi, papulosquamous disorders); dermatologic manifestations of systemic disorders (pruritis without rash, inflammatory bowel disease, collagen vascular disorders, and endocrine disorders); and disorders of the hair and nails.

1.1 Introduction

The goals of this chapter are to discuss the more common skin conditions encountered in adolescents in the day-to-day practice of a primary care physician. We present a brief summary of etiology and pathogenesis of the conditions followed by a discussion of standard case management, including newer developments where pertinent. The chapter is divided into six main sections:

- Skin infections and infestations (bacterial, viral, fungal, and parasitic)
- Dermatitis (non-allergic, allergic, and idiopathic)
- Hypersensitivity reactions (urticaria, erythema multiforme, and drug eruptions)
- Miscellaneous skin conditions (acne, nevi, papulosquamous disorders)
- Dermatologic manifestations of systemic disorders (pruritis without rash, inflammatory bowel, collagen vascular disorders, and endocrine disorders)
- Disorders of the hair and nails

1.2 Skin infections and infestations

1.2.1 Bacterial infections

Bacterial infections of the skin are summarized clinically in Table 1.1 (1,2,3,4,5,6).

Table 1.1: Characteristics of common bacterial infections

Skin layers/ Structures	Disease	Common sites	Predominant organism	Secondary organism
Epidermis	Impetigo	Face	Staphylococcus Aureus	Streptococcus Pyogenes (GABHS)
	Superficial Folliculitis	Face, scalp,	Staphylococcus Aureus	
	Furunculosis	Face, scalp, axillae	Staphylococcus Aureus	
	Staphylococcal Scalded Skin Syndrome		Staphylococcus Aureus Phage group II	
	Scarlatina	Face and scalp can involve whole body	Streptococcus Pyogenes (GABHS)	
Epidermal/ Subepidermal	Toxic Shock Syndrome	Whole body	Staphylococcus Aureus	
	Ecthyma	Legs, buttocks	Pseudomonas aeruginosa	Many gram negative and some gram positive organism
Dermis	Carbuncle	Back, thighs	Staphylococcus Aureus	
	Erysipelas	Face	Streptococcus Pyogenes (GABHS)	
	Deep Folliculitis	Scalp	Staphylococcus Aureus	
	Folliculitis Deculvans	Scalp		
Dermis and upper part of subcutaneous tissues	Cellulitis	Legs	Staphylococcus aureus	Streptococcus pyogenes (GABHS)
Deeper Dermis, Subcutaneous Tissues & Fascia	Necrotizing Fasciitis Type I: Mixed aerobic & anaerobic infection	Legs Arms Less commonly; Trunk Perineum Buttocks Head Neck	Facultative Strptococci, Stphylococci, Enterococci Gram-negative bacilli, such as Escherichia coli, Klebsiella, Pseudomonas, Enterobacter, and Proteus, and Anaerobes, such as Peptostreptococcus,	

(*Continued*)

Table 1.1: Characteristics of common bacterial infections (*Continued*)

Skin layers/ Structures	Disease	Common sites	Predominant organism	Secondary organism
			Bacteroides, and Clostridium specie	
	Necrotizing Fasciitis Type II: Monomicrobial		Streptococcus pyogenes (GABHS)	Streptococcus Agalactiae and pneumoniae V vulnificus Clostridium Staphylococcus aureus [28] and Aeromonas spp

1.2.1.1 Impetigo

A common skin infection, impetigo affects about 2.8% of children under 4 years and 1.6% of those 5 to 15 years of age. Certain conditions that compromise the immune system can lead to impetigo, including burns, diabetes mellitus, B-cell immunodeficiency states, etc. Infection has a predilection for face especially around the mouth and nose area. Typical lesions can be bullous or non-bullous, as well as have a mixed presentation occurring within the same area. Previously beta-hemolytic Streptococcus (GABHS) was thought to be the main causative agent especially in the non-bullous form, but current literature suggests Staphylococcus aureus as the predominant etiology in both forms of impetigo.

Contact dermatitis presents with tiny vesicles on erythematous skin, but they are very itchy and usually occur on exposed areas with a history of contact with a sensitizing agent. Small clear fluid filled vesicles of herpes simplex infection are more common on the lips and perioral area and can be quite painful. Varicella vesicles easily rupture and encrust like impetigo but involve the whole body and occur in crops with lesions of different stages present in the same area. Ecthyma is usually a solitary ulcerative lesion surrounded by tiny vesicles that leaves a scar, unlike impetigo, which seldom does. Pemphigus foliaceus is a rare disease usually involving the face in a butterfly like fashion that also presents with vesicles and occasional bullae on an erythematous base.

Bullous impetigo

Accounting for 70% of cases, this starts as innocuous reddish papules that coalesce and form small bullae, which easily rupture, forming erosions covered with the typical honey colored thick crust.

Non-Bullous impetigo

This less common form presents with expanding honey-colored crusts leaving a raw erosive area.

Secondary impetigo

Secondary infection of minor cuts, insect bites, and excessive scratching of eczematous, scabies, and other pruritic lesions especially in diabetic or immunocompromised children can result in impetigenous lesions, usually of the non-bullous type.

Management

Prevention of infection spread is important, although topical disinfectants are not indicated. First line of treatment for small lesions confined to one or two areas is a topical antibiotic like mupirocin, bacitracin or fusidic acid. Topical antibiotics are not only superior to placebo but mupirocin and bacitracin were found to be superior to oral erythromycin. Amoxicillin/clavulanate (125/30 mg per ml) three times daily, cephalexin 30 mg/kg/day in 2 divided doses, erythromycin 40 mg/kg/day in 2–4 divided doses, and dicloxacillin 90 mg/kg in 2–4 divided doses per day, for 7–10 days resulted in satisfactory outcomes.

1.2.1.2 Cellulitis

A rapidly spreading infection of skin and subcutaneous tissues results from introduction of infecting organism through a minor cut, prick or any break in the skin. Any part of the body can be involved, but it typically occurs on lower extremities, although in young children face involvement is common. The diffuse rapidly progressive lesion with no clear margins presents with typical signs of acute inflammation, i.e. warm and tender to touch and shiny red in appearance because of swelling. Immunocompromised hosts are susceptible to cellulitis and its complications. Staphylococcus aureus, Streptococcus pyogenes, and Enterococcus sp. are common offenders. Rare infection with Hemophilus influenza especially in infants and with Clostridium difficile is possible. Cellulitis can present with signs of systemic infection like fever, malaise, pain, lymhangitis, and lymphadenitis.

Periorbital (pre-septal) and orbital (post-septal) cellulitis

These are mostly unilateral and often are due to a spread of infection from the adjacent inflamed sinuses (7). Local skin infection may also be the initiating factor. Infections can be recurrent and often present in winter months in young children with average age of presentation being 6.8 years with a 2:1 male preponderance. Most common agents involved are Staphylococcus aureus, S. epidermidis, and Streptococcus pyogenes. Orbital cellulitis is an emergency as it can lead to serious complications like cavernous sinus thrombosis, meningitis, permanent loss of vision, and diplopia.

Management

Prompt recognition and initiation of antibiotics is required for quick resolution and prevention of complications. Penicillins, cephalosporins, amoxicillin-clavulanate, and macrolides all are effective in uncomplicated cases. Adolescents with diabetes, immunocompromised status, may require hospitalization and intravenous administration of second or third generation cephalosporins with or without aminoglycosides. Attempts to isolate the organism are indicated if empiric treatment fails to show any signs of improvement. Orbital cellulitis should be treated as an emergency; intravenous antibiotics and hospitalization is necessary as well as a consultation with ophthalmology and otorhinolaryngology.

1.2.1.3 Erysipelas

This is a localized infection of skin and subcutaneous tissue caused by group A ß hemolytic streptococcus, usually affecting the face and extremities. Unlike cellulitis, lesions are sharply demarcated and may present with a prodrome of fever, chills, nausea, vomiting, and arthralgia. It responds well to oral antibiotics, but at times intravenous antibiotics are indicated. Other well localized lesions with defined margins like a drug reaction or contact dermatitis may pose a diagnostic challenge, but targeted questioning may delineate history of exposure.

1.2.1.4 Folliculitis

An infection of hair follicle, it is divided in types based on the depth of hair follicle involved, infecting agent, and area involved:

Superficial folliculitis

This is the most common form that can affect any area of the body with hair follicles, mostly in areas with poor hygiene and maceration. Staphylococcus is the usual causative organism. Small pustules with hair in center generally resolve without treatment and with no scarring. Chronic recurring infection responds to topical antibiotics such as mupirocin 2%, clindamycin, or erythromycin.

Deep folliculitis

Less commonly, infection reaches to the base of follicle resulting in painful papules and pustules, healing with scarring. Treatment with oral antibiotics targeting Staphylococcus aureus is indicated.

Gram-negative folliculitis

This is common in adolescents with acne vulgaris who are being treated with a long term antibiotic regimen, which give rise an opportunity for gram negative bacteria like Klebsiella, Enterobacter, and Proteus to over populate and infect the hair follicles. Usually the folliculitis affects the areas where acne is predominant, such as the face and chest.

Hot-tub folliculitis

Erythematous itchy papules or pustules overlying large areas of trunk, extremities, and other areas usually present after few hours to up to 3 days after exposure to a hot-tub, whirlpool, or swimming pool that has not been chlorinated properly or if the water pH was suboptimal. Outbreaks have been reported with use of community pools, whirlpools, and water slides. In cases of severe infection fever, malaise, sore throat, and lymphadenopathy may occur. Lesions are self limiting over a few days. 1% acetic acid soaks can hasten drying.

1.2.1.5 Furunculosis

A perifollicular erythematous abscess due to Staphylococcus aureus, commonly affects intertrigenous areas but also can occur on scalp and at other sites where hair follicles are abundant. Furuncles when they occur inside the auditory canal or nasal cavity can be very painful. Nasal carriage can be the primary source of infection. Hyperhidrosis can predispose to furunculosis, and maintaining good hygiene of intertriginous areas may be the key to prevent autoinoculation and recurrence. Community acquired methicillin-resistant Staphylococcus aureus (CA-MRSA) is becoming a more frequent cause of furunculosis. Children with immunocompromised status like HIV or inherited immune deficiencies are susceptible to treatment-resistant and recurrent furunculosis.

Carbuncle

These are collections of multiple inflamed furuncles in a small area. Favored sites for carbuncles are where dermis is thick such as thighs, back of the neck, and trunk. A carbuncle is a large erythematous, painful, indurated mass located within deep subcutaneous tissue. Multiple small furuncles that comprise a carbuncle connect to each other via subcutaneous tracts and ultimately drain pus to the surface (see Chapter 16).

Management

Solitary furuncles of less then 5 cm in diameters respond well to the excision and drainage only. In cases where multiple or larger lesions are present or where systemic signs of inflammation are evident, an oral antibiotic like minocycline or doxycycline (children 8 years and older) 100 mg every 12 hours is indicated. Clindamycin can be used in cases of MRSA furunculosis at a dose of 2–8 mg/kg/dose every 6–8 hours. In patients with MRSA furunculosis leading to systemic infection, hospitalization and a course of intravenous antibiotics such as vancomycin is necessary.

Incision and drainage is the treatment of choice for carbuncles. Surgical consultation may be indicated for large carbuncles to excise and drain the abscesses and to clean some of the tracts. Deep seated carbuncles are hard and fixed and feel like a malignant tumor on palpation. If they perforate they cause deep lesions that heal with scarring. Oral anti-staphylococcal antibiotics are only indicated in case of systemic involvement or when concomitant cellulitis is present.

1.2.1.6 Scarletina

Also known as scarlet fever, it is a presentation of acute systemic Streptococcus pyogenes infection. It is given this name due to its distinctive reddish punctate sandpapery skin rash and mucous membrane involvement. A patient will have high fever, sore throat, vomiting, and listlessness. The rash appears on the second day and starts on the upper trunk; it soon becomes generalized, sparing perioral area leaving a pale ring around the mouth. It soon concentrates in the axilla and groin. Mucous membranes also have a bright red hue with petechial lesions on the palate. The tongue becomes smooth and red strawberry colored. Laboratory studies reveal leukocytosis and elevated anti-streptolysin O titer. A swab culture will confirm the hemolytic Streptococcus. Empiric treatment with penicillin should be started as soon as possible to avoid the non-suppurative complication rheumatic fever.

1.2.1.7 Staphylococcal scalded skin syndrome (SSSS) and toxic shock syndrome (TSS)

SSSS is predominantly a disease of younger children; 98% of cases are under 6 years, and 62% are under 2 years of age. Inoculation of skin is usually via blood stream seeding from a distant infection from the pharynx, conjunctiva, or middle ear. The pathogenesis of SSSS is Staphylococcus aureus producing an epidermolytic toxin (ET), mostly group phage II, causing lysis of epidermis at the level of granular layer. Cleavage of the epidermis results in positive Nikolsky sign with production of bullae, which easily burst with minor pressure. Systemic signs of infection like high fever usually appear first, followed in 24–48 hours by an orange-red macular rash resembling scarlatina with sandpaper like quality to touch. The skin becomes extremely tender and peels away easily leaving large denuded areas. The rash starts from the scalp and face and descends downward, with axillae and groins commonly affected. It is important to consider other epidermolytic conditions in the differential diagnosis such as toxic epidermal necrolysis, erythroderma, and drug eruptions.

TSS

Staphylococcal TSS was first elucidated as a severe complication associated with usage of tampons during the menstrual period. Presently, about 50% of cases are menstrual-related and 50% are non-menstrual, specifically post-surgical or post-infectious. The pathogenesis is due to the TSST 1 toxin, which accounts for 90% or more of menstrual cases. Staphylococcal enterotoxins are more prevalent in non-menstrual cases. It presents with a flu-like prodrome then progresses to high fever and hypotension. The dermatologic manifestations are diffuse erythema involving the palms and soles. In non-menstrual cases the erythema may be more concentrated at the site of surgery or infection. The patient may progress to shock and/or adult respiratory distress syndrome (ARDS) and multi organ system failure (MOSF). The diagnosis is clinical as bacterial cultures are not reliably positive (only in 5% of cases).

Streptococcal TSS is due to increased virulence related to its M protein as well as presence of streptococcal pyrogenic exotoxins (SPEA). It occurs as a complication of delivery, surgery, viral infection such as varicella, or use of NSAIDs. It presents with a prodromal flu-like picture and then proceeds to a diffuse erythema (10% of the time scarletinaform), but unlike staphylococcal infection, it is followed by ecchymosis and sloughing, appearing more like necrotizing fasciitis. Complications include sepsis, ARDS, and MOSF.

Management

Blood culture may be negative in TSSS, but one should attempt to obtain culture and sensitivity to ensure the targeted antibiotic treatment. Local treatment with potassium permagnate 1:9,000 bath of the skin may provide some comfort, although excessive use may cause dryness and further dehydration. The mainstay of treatment remains the Penicillinase-resistant systemic antibiotics like naficillin, flucoxacillin, and methicillin, which can be used in severe cases by intravenous route. Re-epithelization of the skin usually occurs quickly and without any scarring. Despite the severity of the rash, the prognosis of uncomplicated SSSS is favorable with mortality rate of less than 5%.

Antibiotics of choice for staphylococcal TSS are clindamycin 600 mg IV every 8 hours and vancomycin, 30 mg/kg/day in 2 divided doses. Intensive care support is critical in cases of shock. For streptococcal TSS, studies have shown that S. pyogenes does not respond well to penicillin, though susceptible, primarily because of the status of the host. Therefore, empiric antibiotics should include clindamycin 900 mg. IV every 8 hours and imipenem 500 gm IV every 6 hours for 14 days. Antibiotics may need to continue until no additional surgical debridement is needed or there are no systemic signs.

1.2.1.8 Necrotizing fascitis

A life threatening infection invading all layers of skin and going beyond subcutaneous tissues including fat and superficial layer of fascia, necrotizing fasciitis (NF) affects younger children and neonates especially if they have another infection like pharyngitis, chicken pox, or respiratory tract or urinary tract infection (8). Children with lowered immunity and other debilitating conditions like diabetes, trauma, or surgery are more susceptible. Two types of NF are known based on the organism involved. Type I NF is caused by multiple organisms both aerobic and anaerobic. Type II NF is caused mostly by a single agent, usually Streptococcus pyogenes, but other organisms are also known to be responsible for it (Table 1.1). Infection is rapid and presents with severe systemic signs of infection. The skin becomes erythematous followed by development of severe edema and hemorrhagic bullae. The patient complains of severe unrelenting pain, which later on can be replaced by numbness in the affected area once the nerve endings are damaged. Crepitus in subcutaneous tissue signifies infection with a gas producing organism like Clostridium or Enterobacteriaceae.

Management

Prompt recognition of NF and isolation of the organism is the key to recovery. A scoring system has been used to streamline the process for early diagnosis of NF known as Laboratory Risk Indicator for necrotizing fascitis (LRINEC), which includes the basic laboratory screens, total WBC, hemoglobin, sodium, glucose, serum creatinine, and C-reactive protein. A cut off score of 6 is used for a clinician to be alert to the possibility of NF. Tissue oxygen saturation of less then 70% has been used to identify NF in lower extremities in adults. In about 13% of cases of NF subcutaneous gas can be detected by radiography. Computed tomography is superior to plain radiographs as it can also detect early soft tissue changes like fat stranding, fascial thickening, and dissection along the fascial plains. Magnetic resonance imaging (MRI) has also been shown to be highly sensitive in diagnosing NF. Recently ultrasound has been used more frequently and has shown some efficacy.

A multidimensional approach to these patients is the key to resolution of NF, including surgical and infectious disease consultation, sterile precautions, hydration, and nutritional status of patient. Emergency surgical exploration and debridement is the key component of treating NF; multiple debridements may be necessary. Hyperbaric oxygen and IV immunoglobulins with varying degrees of evidence for support have been used as adjunctive treatments to hasten the tissue healing process. Empiric treatment with broad spectrum antibiotics with coverage for MRSA as well as Streptococcus pyogenes should be started as soon as possible; change it to a more specific regimen once results of culture and sensitivity are available. Refer to treatment of streptococcal TSS above for antibiotic selection.

1.2.1.9 Ecthyma gangrenosum

This is a relatively rare infection, resulting from occlusive vasculitis usually associated with pseudomonas septicemia. It mostly affects patients who are immunocompromised. Victims of burns have a high rate of pseudomonas septicemia. It usually affects the buttocks and anogenital area but can occur anywhere. It presents as a small innocuous macule, which becomes purulent and develops into a thick walled hemorrhagic bullous lesion, which ultimately becomes a gangrenous ulcer. The pathognomonic feature is a grayish-black eschar surrounded by an erythematous ring. A localized form at the site of infection is also reported, more commonly in immune deficient hosts, especially children with hematologic cancers. Non pseudomonas ecthyma gangrenosum has also been reported. Differentiation between ecthyma gangrenosum and pyoderma gangrenosum can be difficult on clinical grounds. Histopathological features and absence of septicemia in pyoderma can distinguish between two almost similar gangrenous ulcers. In rare cases pyoderma can be complicated with superimposed ecthyma gangrenosum.

Management

Blood cultures and culture of aspirate from a lesion can confirm the Pseudomonas aeuroginosa. Biopsy and histopathology may be necessary at times. Localized smaller lesions can be treated with topical silver sulfadiazine. For larger lesions systemic antibiotics with pseudomonas the use of ß lactam penicillins including piperacillin-tazobactam, ceftazidime, cefepime, imipenem, or the aminoglycosides gentamicin, or tobramycin is efficacious.

1.2.1.10 Cat scratch disease (CSD)

CSD is caused by the gram-negative bacillus Bartonella Henselae, a common infection acquired by playing with kittens and stray cats (9). It is more commonly seen in humid climates and especially during autumn and winter season. The initial scratch is followed by the development of a reddish papule within the next 1–2 weeks, which later becomes larger and firmer with development of high grade fever in about 30% of patients. Regional adenopathy occurs most commonly in lymph nodes draining arms and legs, especially in the axillae, groins, and epitrochlear areas. The head and neck region is involved in up to 49% of cases. Lymphadenopathy may persist for weeks, and CSD is the most common cause of chronic lymphadenopathy in young children. The lesions heal completely within about two weeks with symptomatic treatments, such as warm soaks, analgesics, and antipyretics. Skin lesions can be confused with pyogenic granuloma, Kaposi's sarcoma, and epithelioid hemangoioma. Other diseases with lymphadenopathy including tuberculous adenitis, infectious mononucleosis, tularemia, and tumors can cause a diagnostic dilemma, especially in about 10% of patients where a typical CSD skin lesion was not present or noted.

Management
Immunofluorescent antibody (IFA) test or the enzyme immunoassay (EIA) test can be used to confirm diagnosis when in doubt. DNA polymerase chain reaction (PCR) assays are less commonly used but are highly sensitive. The atypical presentation Parinaud oculoglandular syndrome with high fever, regional lymphadenopathy, and ocular involvement is seen in about 5% of patients. Encephalpathy and severe systemic disease occur in about 2.5% of cases. Treatment is generally not necessary in typical CSD, but in immunocompromised patients or patients with severe systemic infection treatment with antibiotics may be effective. Macrolide antibiotics are most commonly used, such as azithromycin at doses of 10 mg/kg/day for 2–5 days and rifampin 20 mg/kg per day in divided doses for 2–3 weeks. Children over 12 years of age can be treated with ciprofloxacin 20–30 mg/kg/day for 2–3 weeks or trimethoprim (8 mg/kg/day)/sulfamethoxazole (50 mg/kg day) for 7–10 days. In severely ill patients with systemic involvement gentamicin 5 mg/kg/day IM or IV every 8 hours is efficacious.

1.2.1.11 Treponemal infections

Due to Treponema pallidum, syphilis has an incubation period of 9–90 days (average of 3 weeks). Supportive laboratory data are reviewed in Chapter 17 (10). The spirochete gains access via mucosal abrasions during sexual activity with the induction of local immune response and secondary hematogenous spread. The dermatologic manifestation of primary syphilis is classic chancre, a well-defined painless erythematous ulcer with a firm (rubbery) base; there often is associated inguinal adenopathy, unilateral or bilateral, non-tender, and non suppurative.

Secondary syphilis appears 6 weeks to 6 months after disappearance of the chancre and can present with a wide variety of findings in its role as “the great imitator” with fever, malaise, headache, arthralgia, generalized lymphadenopathy, hepatosplenomegaly, rhinitis, sore throat, alopecia (moth-eaten, patchy), and polymorphic rash usually involving the palms and soles. The rash may be macular, popular, maculopapular, morbilliform, and, on occasion, pustular, papulosquamous, annular, or nodular. Skin manifestations of secondary syphilis will resolve spontaneously over 2 or more weeks if not treated, but it would leave the patient at risk for further manifestations of syphilis.

Warts due to syphilis, known as condylomata lata are moist warty papules seen in moist areas of the body such as the perineum and intertrigenous areas. A mucous patch, usually a red papule is another manifestation of syphilis appearing in the mouth, tongue, and genital areas.

Management
Primary, secondary, and early latent stages of syphilis are treated with benzathine penicillin G (2.4 million units IM) in one dose; late latent and tertiary syphilis

are treated with a similar dose for 3 weeks. Penicillin-allergic patients may be desensitized. Alternative antibiotic treatment includes tetracycline, 500 mg orally, four times daily, or doxycycline, 100 mg orally twice daily, for 14 days.

1.2.1.12 Lyme borreliosis (Lyme disease)

This is an infection transmitted by a deer tick Ixodes damini introducing the spirochete borrelia burgdorferi (11,12,13). Lyme disease is the most common vector-borne disease in the United States with about 15,000 cases being reported annually. Initially confined to the wooded New England States, it is now considered endemic in 15 States. The hallmark lesion is erythema migrans, which develops in about 75–80% of patients at the site of tick bite in days to weeks. It can occur over any part of the body and typically leaves a central pale region that slowly expands. Low grade fever, malaise, arthralgia, myalgia regional adenopathy, and headaches are common and in the absence of a definitive erythema migrans are difficult to distinguish from a common flu-like illness.

Atypical and chronic cutaneous manifestations can occur in a subset of patients, including acrodermatitis chronica atrophicans usually affecting extensor surfaces of extremities and present as an indurated, hyperpigmented plaque. Systemic involvement can present in various forms, including about 15% of patients developing lymphocytic meningitis with signs of meningeal irritation, encephalitis, and cranial nerve involvement. Facial nerve palsy in young children living in endemic areas is common up to 34% to 65% depending on different studies from different geographic locations. Other systemic manifestations include hepatosplenomegaly, chronic fatigue, migratory pain, and cardiac and joint involvement.

Management

Prevention of tick bite should be emphasized to patients living in or traveling in endemic areas who should avoid heavily wooded areas, not sit on the ground, wear proper clothing, and apply n,n-diethyl- m-toluamide (DEET) sparingly; Permethrin can be sprayed on clothing. Prophylactic antibiotics to prevent Lyme disease after a tick bite are not recommended as up to 70–80% of deer ticks are not infective. Purified recombinant outer surface protein (OSP) vaccine has been approved for use in children 15 years of age and up, with 49% efficacy in the first year and ultimately 76% efficacy in preventing Lyme disease. Serologic testing is not useful in endemic areas as there is up to 30% chance of false results. Indirect florescent antibody and enzyme-linked immunosobent assay (ELISA) tests are available. They may be negative in the early phase of infection, later becoming more sensitive and specific.

Recommended treatment for early Lyme disease with children presenting with Bells palsy, mild carditis, and arthritis is based on age. In children less then 9 years of age, penicillin or ampicillin 25–50 mg/kg/day in divided doses for a total dose of about 1–2 g/day is effective, while children older than 9 years can be treated with tetracycline 250 mg QID or doxycycline 100 mg BID. In complicated late Lyme disease where persistent arthritis, severe carditis, meningitis, or encephalitis is present, ceftriaxone 75–100 mg/kg/day or penicillin G 300,000 U/kg/day is recommended.

1.2.2 Viral infections

Viral exanthems are summarized briefly in Table 1.2 (14).

1.2.2.1 Measles (rubeola)

This has been much a less common infection since the advent of a vaccination regimen in 1963, although in the late 1980s to early 1990s, a resurgence of measles occurred in the United States mainly because of decline in levels of antibodies and in vaccination administration in certain populations. There have been other isolated outbreaks such as in San Diego, CA, in 2008, where a single case of a non-vaccinated child who returned from a trip abroad ultimately exposed 839 people. Measles is highly contagious, is acquired by droplet infection, and starts with high fever, sore throat, rhinorrhea, conjunctivitis, photophobia, cough, and malaise. Simultaneous involvement of mucous membranes also occurs with the appearance of tiny grayish-white lesions on the buccal mucosa known as Koplik spots.

Table 1.2: Viral exanthems of childhood

Exanthems	Virus	Incubation	Hallmark
Measles	Paramyxovirus	10–12 days	Koplik's Spots
Rubella	Togaviridae/ Rubivirus	14–21 days	Cephalo-caudal progression of rash
Erythema Infectiosum	Parvovirus B19	4–15 days	Slapped cheek, lacy reticular rash on extremities
Roseola Infantum	HHV-6 and -7	5–15 days	Rosy pink rash
Chicken pox	Varicella-zoster	10–21 days	Polymorphous lesions in crops
Hand-foot-mouth	Coxsackie A16, et al.	3–7 days	Painful palmer, planter, and buccal vesicles
Mollusum contagiosum	Molluscipox virus		Pearly umblicated dome shaped papules
Verucca Vulgaris (Warts)	Human Papilloma Virus		Dome shaped/filiform/cauliflower/flat lesions

A maculopapular rash appears 3–4 days after the prodrome, starting usually on the forehead and behind the ears and then spreading to involve the face, trunk, and limbs. When rash is fully erupted fever subsides, and resolution of the rash is usually rapid without scarring. Complications that can occur during the acute phase of infection include superimposed bacterial infection leading to otitis media, gastroenteritis, pneumonia, and, rarely, encephalitis. A serious dematologic complication of measles is the appearance of purpura secondary to thrombocytopenia (black measles). The virus may persist within the CNS for months to years after initial infection and may give rise to a post infectious form of encephalitis known as subacute sclerosing panencephalitis (SSPE), which can occur in 1:100,000 patients.

Management
Supportive treatment includes rest, hydration, balanced nutrition, and protection from direct sunlight. Symptomatic treatment with antipyretics and cough suppression is helpful. In secondary bacterial infection, culture and sensitivity and targeted antibiotic therapy is indicated. Hospitalization is needed in patients with encephalitis, and corticosteroid treatment is appropriate.

1.2.2.2 Varicella (chicken pox)

This is highly contagious and quickly spread by direct contact and droplet infection. After an incubation period of 1–2 weeks, the disease starts with flu-like symptoms, fever, sore throat, and headaches. After 2–3 days of prodrome, a rash first appears on the trunk and spreads laterally. The mildly pruritic rash comes in crops; it starts as erythematous macules, which evolve into vesicles (dew-drop on a petal), and then into pustules. This eventually gives rise to a polymorphous rash with lesions in different stages of evolution and healing. Lesions rupture and become encrusted before completely healing. Usually there is no scarring or pigmentary change, though it may occur if pruritus is more severe than usual. Varicella usually runs a benign course, but there may be rare secondary infections of the lesions with group A Streptococcus or Staphylococcus aureus. More serious complications such as necrotizing fasciitis, meningitis, encephalitis, transverse myelitis, or Guillain-Bare syndrome can occur.

Management
Supportive and symptomatic treatment is all that is needed in cases of an uncomplicated varicella infection. Aspirin should be avoided because of the possibility of inducing Reye syndrome. Antibiotic treatment will be indicated in secondary bacterial infections. Varicella vaccine became available in the United States in 1995 with the indication for routine vaccination for healthy children at 12–18 months of age or for older children who have not yet had a varicella infection. Varicella vaccine is considered effective in up to 85% of cases, but it appears that protection against

varicella declines 1 year post vaccination. Children vaccinated at younger than 14 months are more susceptible to breakthrough infection. Secondary infections are treated with appropriate antibiotics for group A streptococcus and staphylococcus as discussed previously.

1.2.2.3 Rubella (German measles)

When acquired postnatally, it is a benign self-limiting disease that begins 2–3 weeks after exposure and presents with the prodromal phase comprising mild fever, sore throat, eye pain, headache, and lymphadenopathy of the head and neck. In the next 1–5 days a maculopapular rash appears on the face, which then progresses to involve the rest of the body. The rash begins to clear by day 3 without leaving any marks. Postpubertal girls are susceptible to persistent arthritis and arthralgia for several weeks. Encephalitis and thrombocytopenic purpura are rare complications.

1.2.2.4 Erythema infectiosum (fifth disease)

Due to Parvovirus B19 infection, this is usually seen in childre 4–10 years old, but it does occur in adolescents with outbreaks occurring in late spring and fall. Following a prodromal phase with low grade fever, sore throat, headache, myalgia, and arthralgia, a confluent erythematous maculopapular rash appears bilaterally on cheeks, in a butterfly fashion sparing the nasal bridge giving the slapped cheeks appearance. Mucous membrane involvement is evident with reddish punctate lesions on the buccal mucosa. The rash then spreads to the trunk and on the extensor surface of the limbs, where it persists for about 5–9 days, leaving behind a lacy or reticular pattern that fades over time. Exposure to an irritant like sunlight within the next few weeks to months may cause recurrence of the rash. Transmission of acute infection from mother to fetus results in failure of erythropoiesis, causing development of hydrops fetalis in 10% of patients. Aplastic anemia is seen in patients who are susceptible due to underlying hemoglobinopaties or hemopoetic defects.

1.2.2.5 Hand-foot-and-mouth disease (HFMD)

This enterovirus (Coxsackie A and B sp.) infection is highly contagious and spread by the oral fecal route with epidemics in the United States occurring about every 3 years. A brief prodromal phase of 12–36 hours presents with abdominal pain, anorexia, burning sensation in mouth, malaise, and low grade fever followed by development of painful erosive lesions on the hard palate and buccal mucosa. A painful vesicular rash on hands and feet appears, more pronounced on the hands especially on the palms and along the sides of the fingers. Symptomatic treatment including attention to nutrition is all that is needed, as painful oral lesions lead to avoidance of food.

1.2.2.6 Molluscum contagiosum

This common infection of school aged children, due mainly to Poxvirus 1, is highly contagious in close quarters, especially with community facilities such as shared bathtubs, swimming pools, etc. Typical dome shaped skin-colored papules are 2–8 mm in size and can occur as single or multiple lesions. They then become umblicated and turn pearly white. Common sites are face, hands, trunk, and genitalia. Secondary bacterial infections can occur, especially in the large papules, which can reach up to multiple centimeters in size.

Management

Topical application of cantharidin as 0.7% cantharone is safe when applied sparingly and is effective especially in localized lesions. Other less common therapies include use of the immunomodulatory agent tarcolimus, which, although effective, may predispose to herpetic infection. Cryotherapy with liquid nitrogen application on each lesion for 6–10 seconds is effective and may need to be repeated in 3 weeks. Imiquimod has also shown some efficacy but evidence is limited. Excision and curettage and electrodessication can be employed when lesions are fewer and localized. Oral cimetidine may show some efficacy, especially when molluscum is associated with atopic dermatitis. As this condition is benign and self-limited, albeit over 6–12 months, watchful waiting is also appropriate in relatively mild cases.

1.2.2.7 Verruca vulgaris (viral warts)

This human papilloma virus (HPV) infection is very common, affecting up to 10% of children. The most common age group affected is between 12–16 years, and it is transmitted by direct person-to-person contact and autoinoculation. Sun exposure can increase susceptibility to warts. Common warts are well circumscribed small papular lesions with a keratinized surface most commonly seen on hands, arms, and legs, especially on knees and elbows. Filiform warts have frond like projections usually found in the perioral area and on lips. Flat topped, smooth warts occur on sun exposed areas like face, neck, and on the dorsum of hands. Planter and palmer warts are more commonly surrounded by an outer keratinized ring. Anogenital warts are cauliflower like soft lesions known as condylomata acuminata.

Management

Warts are self-limiting in 30% of cases within 3 months and 78% involute in 2 years. Warts in children have higher spontaneous resolution rates. Topical therapy with keratolytic agents like salicylic acid 10–25% applied topically is effective in 67% of hand warts and 84% of planter warts within 12 weeks. Cryotherapy has a cure rate of 31% to 52% depending on the intensity of treatment. Pain and blister formation at the site of treatment has been reported. Only one study has reported use of topical immunotherapy with dinitrochlorobenzene in 40 children with an 80% cure rate. Imiquimod, an immune modifier has shown some efficacy in anogenital warts in adults, but no data are available in children and adolescents. Intra-lesional bleomycin has also shown efficacy of up to 82–94% but the number of subjects studied was small. Mosaic warts are much more resistant to treatment.

1.3 HIV/AIDS

The acute exanthem of HIV infection is an erythematous morbilliform rash on trunk and extremities that manifests itself after 2–4 weeks incubation period with a prodrome of fever, lymphadenopathy, and night sweats (15). The rash resolves within 5–7 days.

1.3.1 Non-infectious skin lesions

Sweet Syndrome is a manifestation of underlying systemic disease characterized by painful violaceous indurated plaques with neutrophilic infiltration of the dermis and has been reported in children with HIV/AIDS. Eosinophilic folliculitis is an altered immune response to the common skin antigens and is seen in advanced HIV infection, especially when CD4 lymphocyte counts decrease to <200 cells/mm^3. Also, acute urticaria can become chronic urticaria with angioedema and gives rise to indurated lesions with a peau d'orange appearance. Many common skin diseases such as atopic and seborrheic dermatitis become more extensive and difficult to treat in patients with HIV/AIDS. Psoriasis, although not more common in this population, can be very problematic.

Trimethoprim-sulfamethoxazole is the most common drug-related cause of such reactions, but other drugs can also cause eruptions, including Stevens Johnson syndrome and toxic epidermal necrolysis.

1.3.2 Bacterial infections in HIV

Many bacterial skin infections, such as impetigo, folliculitis, furuncles, etc., have a very aggressive and extensive course in the HIV/AIDS population. Bacillary angiomatosis presents with pinpoint erythematous macular lesion, which may form a larger lesion like pyoderma. It is seen more commonly in HIV/AIDs patients and may be confused with Kaposi's sarcoma. Biopsy may be the only way to distinguish between them. It does respond very well to the macrolide antibiotics doxycycline or erythromycin. Incidence of Group B streptococcus (GBS) in infants exposed to HIV infection in utero is late and more severe than in the non-exposed infants.

1.3.3 Viral infections in HIV

Herpes simplex (HSV) and Herpes zoster (HZV) infections are very common in HIV/AIDS patients. Both of these infections are much more serious, recurrent, and recalcitrant to therapy. HZV infections can be debilitating and can involve multiple dermatomes at one time. Since lesions can be extensive, necrotic, and atypical, laboratory testing with Tzanck preparation, biopsy of lesion, or viral culture is necessary. Acyclovir is the treatment of choice. Incidence of HPV infection in HIV/AIDS patients has increased not only due to increased susceptibility to this infection due to immunosuppression but also due to decreased clearance of established infections and reactivation of latent infections. Condylomata Acuminatum (CA) is the most common presentation of HPV in HIV/AIDS patients. They tend to be much larger and numerous and may spread to involve extensive areas of the body. Hypopigmented verruciform papules can spread easily in children. Common warts, including veruccae vulgaris and veruucae plantaris, are 16–17% more common in this population. Mulloscum Contagiosum occurs in 20% of HIV/AIDS patients and can become generalized, affecting large areas of the body and reaching sizes up to 1 cm.

HPV is responsible for several carcinomas in situ or premalignant lesions, including giant CA, also known as Buschke-Loewenstein tumor (BLT) and intraepithelial neoplasia of anogenital region, which can progress to become anal, vulvar, or penile carcinoma. Acute cytomegalovirus (CMV) infections are seen in up to 90% of HIV/AIDS patients. Skin manifestations of CMV are varied, ranging from vesicular, morbilliform rashes to indurated plaques to ulcerative lesions. These lesions respond well to foscarnet, ganciclovir, or cidofovir. Epstien-Barr virus can cause oral hairy leukoplakia and Burkitt's lymphoma or large cell lymphoma, which can be treated with acyclovir at a dosage of 200 to 400 mg 5 times a day and highly active antiretroviral therapy (HAART).

1.3.4 Fungal infections in HIV

The most common fungal infection in HIV patient is candidiasis, which could be the only presenting sign of HIV in early phase, with oral thrush. Other areas of involvement include the axillae, groin, vagina, and under other skin folds where maceration is likely. Systemic fungal infections are common in advanced cases of HIV/AIDS like Cryptococcus neoformans presenting with pleomorphic rash. Histoplasma capsulatum may present with skin lesions in about 17% of cases. Spirotrichosis can cause ulcerative papules or nodules along with systemic involvement.

1.3.4.1 Yeast infections

Superficial candidal infection is most common, affecting skin and mucous membranes. Candida albicans is a budding yeast, which is a commensal organism of mucous membranes and is found around the skin adjacent to mucous membranes, gut, and vaginal areas. Carriage in these areas is one other way of acquiring infection. Candidal mucocutaneous infections are common in very young and old and in debilitated populations. Any condition predisposing to defects in immunity especially of cellular immunity can predispose to candidal infections. Candida is known to have specific immunomodulatory effect, which can also dampen the host's immune response. Diabetes mellitus is often complicated with mucocutaneous candidal infections. Other situations predisposing to candidiasis include use of antibiotics or corticosteroids, malnutrition, and HIV infection. Candida favors the moist occluded areas of skin, most commonly intertriginous, perineal, and perianal areas, especially in obese patients. Diagnosis can be confirmed by identification of pseudohyphae in a microscopic KOH preparation.

1.3.4.2 Management

Attempts should be made to keep the affected areas well aerated. Use of mild soap with water with gentle cleansing is recommended. Wet wipes without the strong additives like fragrances or preservatives are also effective. In recurring infection using barrier preparations like petroleum, Titanium oxide in paraffin, and Zinc oxide cream can provide added protection against infection. Combination of corticosteroid plus antifungal preparations should be avoided. In any dermatitis where diagnoses is in doubt or which is present for more than 72 hours, use of a topical antifungal agent twice daily with continuation for a week after disappearance of the rash is appropriate. Nystatin, ketoconazole, clotrimazole, econazole, miconazole, oxiconazole, and ciclopirox are effective anti-candidal agents.

1.3.5 Fungal infections

Fungal infections are summarized in Table 1.3 (16,17).

Fungi are saprophytes, originally soil keratinophiles that have evolved to be able to infect animals and humans. They can be unicellular like Candida or multicellular like Dermatophytes. Candida sp. can infect both skin and mucous membrane, while dermatophytes can only infect keratinized areas like skin, hair, and nails. Skin infections are localized to the stratum corneum, the superficial

Table 1.3: Clinical aspects of fungal infections

Clinical presentation	Fungi	Site of infection	Other presentations
Tinea Corporis	Microsporum equinum Microsporum fulvum Microsporum gypseum Trichophyton equinum Trichophyton gallinae Trichophyton rubrum Trichophyton tonsurans Epidermophyton floccosum	Anywhere on body Except groin, hair, and nails	
Tinea Gladiatorum	Trichophyton verrucosum Trichophyton tonsurans	Highly contagious anywhere on body except groin, hair, and nails	
Tinea Facie Tinea Barbae	Trichophyton mentagrophytes	Face and beard area	
Tinea Cruris	Trichophyton rubrum	Groin, perianal, and perineal area	Tinea corporis, pedis, and manuum
	Epidermophyton floccosum		Tinea corporis and pedis
Tinea Pedis	Trichophyton interdigitale		Tinea pedis

layer of skin, and never invade the deeper layers. Dermatophytes, also known as Tinea, and commonly called ringworm, have specific predilection for different sites of the body. Dermatophytes are divided into three main groups: Trichophytons, epidermophyton, and microsporum. They spread by direct contact with soil, infected surfaces, or contact with an infected body area. The types of infections are classified based on the body area affected. Tinea capitis (head) and fungal nail infections, tinea unguum, as examples, are discussed in the following sections.

1.3.5.1 Tinea corporis

Dermatophyte infections of the body, excluding groin area, feet, scalp, facial cheeks, and nails, are known as tinea corporis. Trichophyton rubrum is the most prevalent organism. Most commonly infection is acquired via direct skin to skin contact. After invading the stratum corneum, the organism produces hyphae and grows outward, producing the typical round or annular lesions with erythematous slightly raised margins surrounding a clear center. The expanding border is scaly and when scraped can provide sample to identify hyphae microscopically.

1.3.5.2 Tinea gladiatorum

A highly contagious variant of tinea corporis, this is common in populations where physical contact with bare skin occurs. Most cases are reported in wrestlers, but other physical contact sports have been sources of reports of outbreak of such lesions. The infection is more prevalent in seasons of active competitions and intense training. Skin lesions are unlike typical tinea corporis and may appear as scaly erythematous papules and plaques. Lesions have a predilection for the head, neck, and arms and are seldom seen on legs. Spread of infection to other athletes is frequent, and covering of localized lesions during sports encounter should be practiced. In cases of extensive rash, there should be avoidance of contact sports. Resumption of such activities can occur after treatment for 1 week.

1.3.5.3 Tinea cruris

Commonly known as "jock itch," this is a superficial fungal infection of inguinal folds, perineal and perianal areas, common in adolescent males and post pubertal females. Moist, non-aerated areas of skin such as in between skin folds can give rise to maceration, which is a perfect breeding ground for dermatophytes such as Trichophyton rubrum, Mentagrophytes sp., or Epidermophyton floccosum. It is more common in summer months and in children or adolescents who are obese or who wear tight fitting under garments, especially in young girls with nylon panty hose. In children participating in team sports the co-occurrence of tinea pedis and tinea cruris is common. At times it is difficult to differentiate between other rashes affecting this area, such as erythrasma, a chronic intertriginous infection due to Corynebacterium minutissimum, which fluoresces orange under Woods lamp examination. Other fungal infection like Candida can be distinguished by presence of pinkish red smooth lesions without a definite border and satellite punctate lesions in adjacent areas. In younger children, especially those wearing diapers, contact dermatitis can present a diagnostic problem but usually a correlation to the offending agent will be clear. Psoriasis and seborrheic dermatitis are also included in the differential diagnosis.

1.3.5.4 Tinea pedis

This is a common condition in children and athletes commonly known as athlete's foot. Sometimes the term "moccasin foot" is used to describe extensive infection where the whole foot is involved in the distribution of a shoe covering the foot. Infection is usually in between toes where moist skin nurtures dermatophytes, producing itchy, macerated lesions with fissuring and often a foul odor. Common risk factors are use of community shower stalls at schools, swimming pools, and sports clubs; sharing slippers, socks, and shoes; wearing shoes for long time, especially when not wearing absorbent socks; and walking barefoot on a sandy beach or other moist grounds, which can harbor fomites. Most common organisms are the same as in tinea cruris (Table 1.4). Tinea rubrum affect the relatively dry area of the foot like heels, soles, and sides, producing somewhat thickened pink lesions covered with fine silver scales. Differential diagnosis includes contact and atopic dermatitis, psoriasis, and candidal infection between the toes.

Table 1.4: Topical steroids in treatment of atopic dermatitis

Generic Name	Brand Name
Class I	
Clobetasol proprionate	Temovate 0.05%
Betamethasone	Diprolene 0.05% cream or ointment.
dipropionate	
Class II	
Betamethasone	Diprosone 0.05% ointment
diproprionate	Elocon 0.1% ointment
Mometasone furoate	Halog 0.1%
Halcinonide	Lidex 0.05%
Flucinonide	Topicort 0.25% cream, 0.05% gel
Desoximetasone	
Class III	
Triamcinolone acetonide	Aristocort A 0.1% ointment
Betamethasone	Diprosone 0.05% cream
dipropionate	Valisone 0.1% ointment
Betamethasone valerate	
Class IV	
Triamcinolone acetonide	Aristocort 0.1% ointment
Flurandrenolide	Cordran 0.05% ointment
Mometasone furorate	Elocon 0.1% cream, lotion
Triamcinolone acetonide	Kenalog 0.1% cream or ointment
Fluocinolone	Synalar 0.025% ointment
Desoximetasone	Topicort LP 0.05% cream
Class V	
Flurandrenolide	Cordran 0.05% cream
Triamcinolone acetonide	Kenalog 0.1% lotion, 0.025% ointment
Fluocinolone	Synalar 0.025% cream
Tridesilon	Desonide 0.05% ointment
Betamethasone	Valisone 0.1% cream or lotion
Hydrocortisone valerate	Westcort 0.2% cream or lotion
Class VI	
Triamcinolone acetonide	Aristocort 0.01% cream, Kenalog 0.25% cream or ointment
Flumetasone pivalate	Locorten 0.03% cream
Tridesilon	Desonide 0.05% cream
Class VII	
Hydrocortisone	Hytone 1% or 2.5% lotion cream or ointment

Adapted from *The Harriet Lane Handbook*, 18th edition, Mosby/Elsevier 2009.

1.3.5.5 Pityriasis (tinea) versicolor

This superficial fungal infection is caused by different genus Malassezia and especially by the species Malassezia fufur. It gives rise to typical fine scaly macular lesions mostly affecting the trunk, back, and arms but can also involve other areas, especially in children where face involvement is common. It is more frequent in hot and humid climates and in those who use topical corticosteroid and oil based skin products. It presents differently according to the color of skin of the individual affected, hence the name versicolor. In light colored individuals typical leaf like macular lesions are hyperchromic or brownish, while in dark colored skin the macules are hypochromic. Lesions have fine white scale on margins and occur in large numbers. A Christmas tree distribution is seen on the back and is pathognomonic of this condition. Lesions are completely asymptomatic, and the only reason patients seek help is for cosmetic concerns. Vitligo can be confused with tinea versicolor, especially in dark skinned individuals.

1.3.5.6 Management

Most infections are diagnosed purely on clinical judgment, although a potassium hydroxide (KOH) preparation can provide a cheap, quick, and highly sensitive (88%) method of confirming the diagnosis within the office setting. Scrapings of the lesion border are placed on a slide with a drop of 10–20% of KOH, and typical septate hyphae of dermatophytes are easy to detect. Wood's light examination is not as useful in dermatophyte infections other than tinea capitis as Microsporum will fluoresce, whereas the more common Tricophyton will not.

1.3.6 Topical antifungals

These are highly effective in most cases of superficial infections except in tinea capitis and tinea unguium where systemic antifungal treatment is indicated. Commonly used topical preparations are Terbinafine, miconazole, and clotrimazole, which can be applied twice daily for 2 weeks. Butenafine has the advantage of once daily application for 2 weeks with the same effectiveness, but it is more costly. The patient should apply topical medication to about 2 cm of surrounding area past the advancing edge of the infection and should be educated to avoid risk factors predisposing to reinfection.

1.3.6.1 Combination therapy

Combination preparations, including antifungal and corticosteroids, are widely used and mostly prescribed when diagnosis is not fully established. There is a growing concern that such treatment leads to partial resolution and quick relapse of infection resulting is prolonged treatment for months. One of the common such preparations available, Clotrimazole/betamethasone, has shown a 45% failure and a 36% relapse rate. Therefore, this treatment is not recommended.

1.3.7 Infestations

1.3.7.1 Head lice

Infestation with pediculosis humanus capitis is very common all over the world with prevalence rates ranging from 2% in the United Kingdom to 13% in Australia and 100% in some remote communities of central and South America (18,19). Approximately 6–12 million people are infested with head lice each year in the United States. It usually affects children between ages of 3 to 12 years with a higher preponderance for girls and a lower predilection for African Americans. Head to head contact is the main source of transmission, but sharing combs, hats, scarves, hair bands, etc., or sleeping on the bedding of the infested person can also cause transmission. Outbreaks in preschools and elementary schools are common. In the United States, treatment cost associated with head lice infestation is estimated to be $1 billion annually. Head lice feed on the host's blood and can cause significant itching, which leads to frequent scratching, which in turn may give rise to secondary infections like impetigo. Diagnosis is best established by visualizing the live lice, which at times could be very difficult as they tend to hide in areas where the hair is thickest as in the nape of the neck. Use of a louse comb can aid is diagnosis. Diagnosis cannot be established by finding occasional eggs especially >1/4 inch far from the skull as they are most likely dead nits from previous infestation. Finding many nits within 1/4 inch of the scalp can be predictive of active infestation in about one third of cases.

Management

Prevention of spread is the most effective way of controlling the infection. Education not to share personal items like combs, hairbrush, hats, etc., can be effective in limiting spread. Once the diagnosis is established, application of 1% Permethrin, pyrethrins, or 0.5% Malathion in children older than 24 months can be effective. 1% Permethrin is very effective in the form of a crème rinse when left in the hair for 10 minutes and rinsed. The residue it leaves behind continues to kill the nymphs emerging from eggs. A second application is suggested in 7–10 days, preferably on the 9th day. Pyrethrin preparations are derivatives of chrysanthemums and should be avoided in children with allergies to ragweed or chrysanthemums. This should be applied for 10 minutes and rinsed, with a recommended second treatment on the 9th day. Alternatively, treatment on 0, 7, and between 13 to 15 days has been proposed. Efficacy has decreased due to development of resistance. Malathion 0.5% is an organophosphate and is applied to dry hair and left for 8–12 hours with good ovicidal activity. Repeat application is not necessary unless live lice are detected, in which case reapplication on day 7–9 is recommended. Benzyl Alcohol 5% is approved for use in infants older than 6 months. Lindane 1% (gamma benzene hexachloride) shampoo is contraindicated in neonates and is not recommended for children less than 50 kg in weight because of seizure risk. A single oral dose of ivermectin 200 μg/kg has shown 74% effectiveness, which increased to 95% when dose was repeated at 10 days. Prophylactic treatment of persons sharing the same bedding is recommended. All clothes, hairbrushes, combs, and linens used 2 days prior to treatment should be washed in hot water (130° F). Floor and furniture can be vacuumed with minimal risk of transmission after 1–2 days.

1.3.7.2 Scabies

Scabies affects people of all social classes and ages, but it is more commonly seen in children and adolescents (20). It is estimated that about 300 million new cases occur worldwide each year. Caused by an arthropod Sarcoptes scabiei var hominis, this mite can not only transmit by skin-to-skin contact but also by contact with contaminated material like bedding or clothing where it can survive for up to 36 hours. Scabies is more common in crowded urban areas. Children are more at risk due to their propensity of being in close contact with each other. Teenage girls tend to be the highest group affected. After an incubation period of 3–6 weeks, the female mite burrows in the epidermis where it lays eggs. The larva emerges within 2–3 days and matures in an adult mite within 15 days, increasing the population of mites thus the risk of transmission to others. The ensuing rash is highly pruritic due to a hypersensitivity reaction to the mite. Itching is worse during night when the skin is warmer. Scratching may cause excoriations and breaks in skin leading to secondary infections like impetigo. The initial lesion is a small erythematous papule, which can become a vesicle or pustule. Typical lesions are small linear brownish lesions called burrows, most commonly seen in between the finger webs, but they also can be found along the sides of fingers, on the border of the hand, and on the flexor aspects of the wrist. Other areas like, elbows, axilla, buttocks, and genitalia can be affected.

Management

Diagnosis is confirmed by clinical examination and by finding typical burrow lesions in between finger webs. Attempt should be made to extract the mite or eggs from these burrows by gently scraping and examination under light microscope. Failure to isolate mite or eggs does not rule out scabies and treatment can be started based on clinical judgment. Videodermatoscopy can provide high-resolution magnification of skin up to 600 times under incidental light and is a noninvasive and effective diagnostic tool to locate mites and eggs. Other techniques, such as epiluminescence microscopy and dermatoscopy, have also shown diagnostic accuracy. Permethrin 5% cream is effective and safe when applied to the whole body, including the head, and washed off after 8–12 hours, with reapplication recommended after 2 weeks. Transient burning and erythema can occur.

Malathion 0.5%, an organophosphate applied to body and left for 24 hours, is also effective. Lindane 1% has now become a second line treatment due to the concerns with neurotoxicity in cases of accidental ingestion and with local irritation and continued itching. With randomized controlled trials, in comparison to topical crotamiton, lindane, and oral ivermectin, permethrin has shown superior results. Permethrin was also found to be more effective in relieving itch in comparison to lindane and crotamiton. Oral ivermectin is shown to be effective treatment when topical treatment is not effective or disease is severe and widespread. Oral ivermectin is not indicated in children less then <15 kg in weight.

1.3.7.3 Cutaneous larva migrans (CLM)

Cutaneous larva migrans is a most common infestation acquired during travel. CLM is caused mostly by hookworm Ancylostoma brazilienseis and less commonly by Ancylostoma caninum. Hookworms are most commonly found in tropical and subtropical countries in Southeast Asia, South and Central America, and the southern states of the United States. Ancylostoma brazilienseis and related hookworms are also common in Australia, the Caribbean, and in some parts of Europe. The adult hookworm lives in intestines of cats and dogs; ova are shed via feces in the soil where the larvae are hatched and can survive for several weeks. The most common risk factor for CLM infestation is walking bare foot on a beach, but any contact between uncovered skin and contaminated soil or sand can cause the transmission. Upon becoming attached to bare skin the larva secretes hyaluronidase to gain entry in the superficial layers of skin. After an incubation period of up to 6 days the typical erythematous serpiginous lesion develops, known as creeping eruption or creeping dermatitis.

Vesicles and bullae also develop along the larva migration track along with local edema. Intense pruritus may also give rise to excoriation and secondary infection. Since humans are incidental hosts, once the larvae cannot penetrate deep enough to gain entry in deeper tissue their journey comes to a natural end with death of the larvae. The lesion completely resolves within 8 weeks, but in rare cases it may persist for longer. On rare occasion systemic invasion can lead to development of Loffler's syndrome characterized by transient pulmonary infiltrate, eosinophilia, and hepatomegaly.

Management

Diagnosis can be established clinically with a temporal relationship with a visit to endemic areas, and finding the typical creeping eruption about 3 mm wide, which grows in length by a few mm to a few cm daily. No specific serological markers or specific diagnostic test are available for diagnosis of CLM. Eosinophilia can be present in about 20% of cases. Ivermectin is well tolerated and very effective when used as a single dose of 200 µg /kg with a cure rate of 94%. In cases of treatment failure the same dose can be repeated in 7 days to ensure complete eradication of infection. The rash and pruritus may take a few days to resolve. Albendazole for children 6 years and older 15 mg/kg/day in divided doses with maximum daily dose of 800 mg/day for 3 days is also effective. In younger children topical albendazole 10% ointment applied twice daily for 10 days can be effective.

1.4 Dermatitis

1.4.1 Irritant dermatitis

The most common irritant dermatitis occurs in infants in diapers secondary to contact with urine and feces. In children and adolescents caustics such as acids, alkali, or hydrocarbons are the etiologic agents and usually cause an acute irritating reaction.

Management of irritant dermatitis consists mainly of identifying and ridding the patient of the offending agent.

1.4.2 Dry-skin dermatitis

This is generally due to excessive drying of the skin with agents such as soaps, alcohols, lotions, or low humidity. It may occur in patterns, an example of which is “lip-smacking” dermatitis presenting as dry erythematous irritation around the lips. Another example of dry-skin dermatitis is Juvenile plantar dermatosis (JPD, or “sweaty sock syndrome”), presenting initially as erythema of the larger toes and subsequent peeling of the weight-bearing aspects of the plantar aspect of the feet. It is often mistaken for Tinea pedis (athlete’s foot), which occurs initially at the smaller toes and more over the dorsum of the foot.

The goal of management of dry-skin dermatitis is to provide sufficient water to the skin plus a means of keeping it there, usually through liberal use of lubricants. The use of water-in-oil emulsions will also serve this purpose.

1.4.3 Seborrheic dermatitis

Seborrheic dermatitis is due to over-production of sebum from sebaceous glands and appears as a greasy accumulation of scales (21). The lesions are diffuse in infants, more over the face and scalp (cradle cap) as well as in the flexural areas. In adolescents, seborrhea is relegated mainly to the scalp (dandruff), the naso-labial folds, post-auricular area, and the chest. It may be confused with fungal lesions, eczema, contact dermatitis, or psoriasis. The etiology of this condition is unknown, although association with the yeast Pityrosporum sp. has been demonstrated. It remains unclear whether this yeast is causal or acts as an agent in the inflammatory process.

Treatment consists of low-potency topical steroids. Keratolytics (salicylic acid), inhibitors of epithelialization (selenium sulfide), and antifungal shampoos (ketoconazole) may be applied locally but should be used judiciously around the face as they can be irritating to the eyes.

1.4.4 Allergic dermatitides

1.4.4.1 Atopic dermatitis

Atopic dermatitis is a hereditary condition associated with other allergic hypersensitivity such as asthma and/or allergic rhinitis (22,23) (see Chapter 5). Often the respiratory problems are seasonal. When occurring in smaller children, the rash is more diffuse, but by early childhood and adolescence it appears primarily in the flexural creases and the dorsum of the hands. The skin is often dry. The initial lesion may be erythematous papules or, in the case of darker-skinned individuals, a follicular hyperkeratosis (chicken-skin) appearance. The skin is invariably pruritic, which then sets off the classic "itch-scratch-itch" cycle. The lesions then may start weeping, become excoriated, fissured, and eventually lichenified. There also may be post inflammatory hypo- or hyperpigmentation in the affected areas.

There may be physical findings associated with allergy such as Dennie lines under the eyes or the "allergic salute" consisting of horizontal creases on the bridge of the nose. There may be peripheral eosinophilia or elevated serum IgE levels. Lesions may flare up due to overheating, over-drying, sweating, or other contact allergens. Also, secondary bacterial infection or herpetic infection (eczema herpeticum, Kaposi's varicelliform eruption) may worsen the appearance considerably.

The etiology of atopic dermatitis remains elusive. Although there have been associations with other conditions causing dry skin, such as icthyosis, with food intake or presence of house dust mites, or with immunodeficiency, as in Wiskott-Aldrich syndrome, there are no studies that convincingly demonstrate a cause–effect link.

The management of atopic dermatitis is long term and is often fraught with relapses and much frustration on the part of both patients and physicians. If there is a family history of atopy, the patient may be more familiar with the necessary course of treatment, but it is nonetheless important for the clinician to stress the chronicity as well as the frequency of flare-ups.

1.4.4.2 Management

There are four main goals to therapy:

Dryness of skin

Emollients soften the surface of the skin, allowing for exposure of extra water-binding sites. Examples of this are a-hydroxy acids, lactic acid, salicylic acid, and urea, which remove excess scales form the skin. Lubricants will aid in retention of water either by attracting water to the skin or by containing vehicles that will prevent water from escaping the skin (occlusion). Petrolatum is a commonly used vehicle to aid in the retention of heat and moisture, but it can feel greasy to the patient with subsequent low-compliance to therapy. Substances such as cetyl or stearyl alcohol when added to petrolatum will feel more comfortable to the patient as well as increase the ability of the petrolatum to take up water.

Creams and lotions are oil-in-water emulsions and are effective in less-severe cases. They are more cosmetically pleasing to the patient and are more easily removable. Ointments contain more water-insoluble components, which does have maximal occlusive properties. As they can be disagreeable to the patient, emulsifiers added to them may increase compliance, although they may diminish water-retention. Gels are primarily useful to facilitate penetration of other topical medications. Because they have an alcoholic base, they can sting when applied.

Pruritus

Management of pruritus consists of oral sedating antihistamines used primarily at night to prevent scratching and subsequent excoriation. Examples of such medications are hydroxyzine, 1 mg/kg/dose at bedtime, or Cetirizine 2.5 mg under age 6 and 5 mg over age 6 at bedtime.

Inflammation

The mainstay of anti-inflammatory management of atopic dermatitis is the use of topical steroids. The main issues for treatment revolve about the choice of the medication and the means by which it is applied. As the treatment of atopic dermatitis is multi-pronged, it is important to combine skin moisturization with the use of topical steroids, and flexibly, with the ultimate goal of diminishing the potency of the steroids and hopefully their use altogether, until the next relapse. The art of management of atopic dermatitis lies in the juxtaposition of different modes of treatment. The choice of a steroid should begin with one of low potency, such as Hydrocortisone 2.5% or Desonide 0.05%. If not effective, mid-potency steroids such as Fluocinolone acetonide 0.025% or Triamcinolone 0.1% may be of help. Less frequently, high-potency steroids such as betamethasone dipopionate cream 0.05% may be necessary. It is important to recognize the consequences of overuse of topical steroids, particularly in areas such as the face and genital area, such as skin atrophy and striae. Table 1.4 lists topical steroid medications with their potencies.

Prior to resorting to high-potency steroid topical therapy, often moist occlusive dressings are effective, which consists of applying damp cotton gauze followed by dry cotton gauze over a moderate-potency steroid. This may be difficult in an adolescent who would be embarrassed to be seen in them during the day, so it may be employed while at home and during sleep. If is often necessary to encourage parents continuously to maintain this treatment. Patient and parental education is of foremost importance to maintain effectively the treatment plan, even in the face of many failures and frustrations along the way.

Treatment failure may necessitate a dermatologist referral. Some primary care physicians may try coal tar applications to restore normal keratinization or immunosuppressive agents such as tacrolimus or pimecrolimus. Coal tar preparations stain and have an unpleasant odor, which often are barriers to compliance. Immunosuppressive agents may be irritating to the skin when applied.

Complications (secondary infection)
Treating secondary bacterial infections is of paramount importance. The most common infecting agents are Staphylococcus aureus, Stpretococcus pyogenes, and Herpes simplex. Appropriate antibiotic therapy, local or systemic, is necessary to treat these complications.

1.4.4.3 Contact dermatitis

Contact dermatitis occurs as the result of incomplete antigens, called haptens, which penetrate the epidermis, are carried to lymph nodes where they are presented to T lymphocytes, and which then migrate back to the skin. Depending on the strength of the antigen (e.g. poison ivy or urushiol), it may take a week to process, or considerably longer for weaker allergens such as nickel. Upon a second exposure to the antigen, the inflammatory reaction occurs with the T lymphocyte releasing inflammatory mediators resulting in acute erythematous, often vesicular, pruritic dermatitis.

The hallmark of diagnosis is recognition of the distribution and pattern of the dermatitis. Typically it occurs only at the area of contact. Often a streaky appearance is the clue to the patient having brushed against the allergen while in a wooded area. If the lesions due to contact with poison ivy or poison oak appear to be diffuse, it is due to the patient having spread the oil with his hands at the time of initial contact. Often the shape of the lesion is helpful. If it is close to perfectly round, it may be secondary to a metallic contact such as clothing snaps. The location may also be helpful as in nickel in earrings causing lesions about the ear lobes. Allergens present in leather or rubber may cause sensitization of the feet and toes. Perfumes, soaps, and make-up will cause dermatitis in the regions to which they are applied.

Treatment consists of local applications of low potency corticosteroids and antihistamines to lessen the pruritic component. Generally symptoms last for 3–4 weeks with or without treatment.

1.4.5 Idiopathic dermatitides

1.4.5.1 Dyshidrotic eczema

This condition has been erroneously considered to be secondary to dysfunction of the eccrine, or sweat glands. However, histopathology demonstrates normal sweat glands. As there is a clinical association with atopy and contact irritants, a single etiology remains elusive. It presents with highly pruritic vesicles starting at the lateral aspects of the digits, which eventually progress to fissuring and cracking of the palms and soles. Treatment is similar to atopic eczema usually with low-potency corticosteroid ointments and, if necessary, moisture applications followed by covered dry dressings.

1.4.5.2 Keratosis pilaris

This common condition presents as follicular plugs of stratum corneum and appear most often on the extensor aspects of the upper and lower extremities and buttocks. It may also appear on the facial cheeks in younger children, especially during colder and dryer months. The lesions feel rough and dry and may be either flesh-colored or erythematous. Associations with atopy and icthyosis have been reported, but this condition often occurs independently. This condition may be chronic and responds to moisturizers (Urea) and keratoltics (Lactic acid or Retinoic acid).

1.4.5.3 Nummular eczema

This condition may be associated with atopic eczema but may also occur independently. It is characterized by coin-like lesions, can be intensely pruritic, and is treated similarly as atopic eczema. The duration of treatment is considerably longer than that of atopic dermatitis.

1.5 Hypersensitivity

1.5.1 Urticaria

1.5.1.1 Acute Urticaria

This condition is short-lived and more often a consequence of infection (24). Bacterial etiologies include streptococcus, and viral include EB virus, hepatitis, and others. Urticaria may be allergic in nature, with elevated IgE levels and histamine mediation of the skin reaction, although only 3–5% of cases have been reported with this etiology confirmed. Allergic agents include hymenoptera, scorpions and jellyfish stings, drug reactions, and food allergies, particularly to peanuts, tree nuts, eggs, shellfish, berries, and tomatoes. Scombroid fish with high amounts of histamine may cause this reaction. Urticaria may be a manifestation of systemic diseases, which is discussed in the following section. The hallmark lesion of urticaria is the wheal and flare, which is very pruritic. It is transitory in nature but with several relapses and remissions over a few days.

The course is generally benign and self-limited; however, there may be associated angioedema with swelling particularly of the hands and feet. During more severe local reactions there may be blistering with weeping clear fluid, often mistaken for bacterial cellulitis. Over time, urticarial lesions may appear dusky and be mistaken for ecchymoses. One must always be mindful of a more severe generalized reaction with upper airway obstruction due to oropharyngeal swelling (anaphylaxis).

Several conditions may be confused with urticaria such as hereditary angiodedma (C'1 esterase deficiency), erythema multiforme (target lesions), vasculitis, urticaria pigmentosa (mastocytosis), and viral exanthems.

1.5.1.2 Chronic urticaria

This condition is defined by symptoms lasting for more than 4–6 weeks. About 15% of them are the physical urticarias, which are secondary to heat, exercise, cold, or pressure (25). Cold urticarias may be hereditary or of immunogenic origin. Cases of severe anaphylactic reactions have been reported in patients with this condition jumping into cold water. Pressure and some cold urticarias are histamine-mediated, but others may be mediated through cholinergic nerves.

1.5.1.3 Management of urticaria

Acute urticaria that is not severe is best treated with antihistamines. Sedating antihistamines such as Hydroxyzine 1–2 mg/kg/day and Diphenhydramine 5 mg/kg/day are more effective than non-sedating antihistamines. In more severe cases, adrenergic medications may be necessary to manage angioedema. In severe cases of anaphylaxis, airway maintenance is the first priority. Epinephrine, subcutaneously 0.01ml/kg of a 1:1,000 solution acts rapidly in this situation. Albuterol inhalers may be used, as well as oral pseudoephedrine, but these may cause significant adrenergic side-effects.

Patients should be counseled that the course may last up to 6 weeks. If longer, then further studies are necessary to identify the type of chronic urticaria. Simple placement of ice on a patient's skin for several minutes will produce the wheal and flare. Similarly, heat and exercise or pressure will reproduce urticaria. Cold-agglutinins and cryoglobulins may be identified. Further studies to look for an infectious or autoimmune etiology may be necessary.

1.5.1.4 Erythema multiforme

This condition presents as fixed erythematous lesions varying in size and shape without prodrome. They follow an outbreak of Herpes labialis in about 50% of cases. The lesions last several weeks and progress to the classical "target" or "iris" lesions, occurring most commonly over extensor surfaces in an acral distribution. They may turn dusky or become encrusted over time. Oral involvement occurs rarely and is not extensive. There are few systemic symptoms, and the condition is self-limiting. Subsequent Herpes labialis infections will induce recurrences. Although formerly connected with Stevens-Johnson syndrome (SJS, see Section 1.5.2.5), it is now considered a separate entity. One should no longer use the terms "erythema multiforme minor" and "erythema multiforme major." Treatment is expectant, and occasional use of antihistamines may relieve rare instances of pruritus.

1.5.2 Drug eruptions

The most common drug eruptions are morbiliform (measles-like), urticarial, and fixed. Others include pustular, phototoxic, scarletiniform, bullous, and lichenoid (26,27,28).

1.5.2.1 Morbilliform eruptions

These rashes are diffuse maculopapular and appear about 1–3 weeks after institution of the medication. They are the most common and account for up to 50% of drug eruptions. There may or may not be pruritus. The rash usually involves the trunk and extremities and may ultimately become confluent. The most common offending agents are antibiotics, anticonvulsants, antifungals, and non-steroidal anti-inflammatory agents. It is paramount to elicit a drug history in all patients with rashes. It is also important to consider that the primary illness may be the cause of the rash (strep, EB virus). Amoxicillin may elicit a morbilliform rash in a patient with EB viral infection 50% of the time.

1.5.2.2 Urticarial drug eruptions

These IgE-mediated reactions are the second-most common drug eruptions accounting for about 25% of them. They present as a wheal and flare from hours to days after exposure and may be associated with angioedema, although rarely anaphylaxis. The intravenous or intramuscular route is more likely to cause anaphylaxis than oral dosing. Drugs most commonly associated with this condition are non-steroidal anti-inflammatory medications and antibiotics (penicillins, cephalosporins, and sulfonamides). Note that Cefaclor produces a reaction resembling serum-sickness.

1.5.2.3 Fixed drug eruptions

These present as erythematous lesions of varying size, appearing at first urticarial, but then becoming well-demarcated and eventually hyperpigmented. The main offending drugs are antibiotics (Trimethoprim, Sulfonamides, Tetracyclines, and Ciprofloxacin), anticonvulsants (Barbiturates, Carbamazepine), and oral contraceptives. They recover slowly over months and re-occur with re-introduction of the offending agent.

1.5.2.4 Less common drug eruptions

Less common drug eruptions include vasculitis, erythema nodosum, photosensitivity, lichenoid, and bullous eruptions. Offending agents for vasculitis include anticonvulsants, NSAIDS, antibiotics (penicillins, sulfonamides, and macrolides), gold, diuretics, and cimetidine. Erythema nodosum is associated with oral contraceptives, NSAIDs, sulfonamides, and opiates. Photosensitive reactions may be phototoxic, due to direct damage due to sunlight altering the drug. They occur in sun-exposed areas and are often quite painful, resembling severe sunburn. The more common offending agents are antibiotics, particularly Tetracycline, Sulfa drugs, griseofulvin, NSAIDs, diuretics (furosemide, thiazides), psoralens, and coal tar derivatives. The other photosensitive reaction is a true allergy presenting as severe urticaria in sun-exposed areas. Ultra-violet light acts directly on the drug, altering it to an allergenic form. The most common offending agents are perfumes, para-amino benzoic acid, phenothiazines, and sulfonamides. Lichenoid reactions occur months after exposure to drugs such as diuretics, beta blockers, and phenothiazines, and their violaceous plaques are often mistaken for rashes associated with collagen vascular disorders.

1.5.2.5 Life threatening eruptions

Stevens-Johnson Syndrome (SJS) and Toxic Epidermal Necrolysis (TEN) were once considered part of the spectrum of "erythema multiforme" but are now separated from that condition (29). It is difficult to distinguish SJS from TEN clinically and pathologically (separation at the dermal-epidermal junction), and therefore, some consider the two conditions a continuum with TEN being a more severe form. Some experts have defined SJS as epidermal detachment of <10% of body surface area and TEN as >30%. They present with a 1–2 week prodrome consisting of fever, headache, malaise, vomiting, and/or diarrhea. Skin involvement consists of blisters, progressing to bullae with epidermal necrosis. There is mucosal involvement, frequently occurring 1–2 days before the cutaneous lesions in at least two sites. Especially involved are the mouth and eyes with crusty hemorrhagic lesions, but involvement may extend to the lower gastrointestinal tract, kidneys, liver, heart, and genitourinary tract in more severe instances. Skin and mucosal lesions often result in severe scarring, contracture, and dyschromia, and there may be permanent damage to the nails.

Triggers are most commonly antibiotics (sulfonamides, penicillins), anticonvulsants, and NSAIDS. In rare instances Herpes simplex and Mycoplasma pneumonia have been implicated. There is evidence that there may be a genetic predisposition for these conditions. One study confirmed evidence of a gene, HLA-B1502, associated with SJS in Han Chinese population after intake of carbamazepine. Outcomes can be poor with a mortality rate of up to 30% reported.

1.5.2.6 Management of drug eruptions

The hallmark of management of drug reactions is prompt discontinuation of the offending agent. If there is any concern about anaphylaxis, airway must be maintained and subcutaneous epinephrine 1:1,000, 0.01 cc/kg up to 0.5cc should be administered immediately with intravenous fluids. Systemic steroids may also be of benefit. In the event of anaphylaxis, the patient should carry information of this allergy usually as a wrist-band. In addition, it is paramount to document all allergies on the patient's medical record.

Most other reactions (urticarial, fixed, or lichenoid) are not life-threatening and may take several weeks to months to subside. Medication is generally not necessary, although antihistamines may be of benefit for pruritus in urticarial reactions.

Treatment of SJS and TEN is challenging. The conditions manifest themselves clinically as burns, and appropriate fluid replacement is necessary. As with burns, the lesions must be kept clean and debrided with serial cultures and appropriate antibiotic therapy as warranted. The use of corticosteroids and intravenous immunoglobulin is controversial. It is important to obtain dermatologic and ophthalmologic consultation to prevent or treat keratitis, iritis, and scarring. Oral and airway hygiene is important as is support with total parenteral nutrition.

1.6 Miscellaneous skin conditions

1.6.1 Acne vulgaris

Acne vulgaris is one of the most common skin problems in primary care and dermatology offices (30,31) (see Chapter 7). It usually begins at the onset of puberty. Genetic susceptibility influences development of acne and relates to severity.

Pathogenesis of acne involves multiple factors, including abnormal keratinization, hormone and sebum production (androgen stimulation), bacterial colonization (Propionibacterium acnes), and host immune response with inflammation.

The obstruction of a pilosebaceous unit on the face, a follicular plug, is a microcomedone caused by excessive amount of sebum from desquamated epithelial cells in the follicular wall. Adrenal and gonadal androgens during the adolescent period affect sebum production. Microcomedones subsequently change to comedones in black head (opened head) and white head (closed head) forms. Propionibacterium acne, a Gram-positive anaerobic bacteria, colonizes at pilosebaceous follicles. This bacterium hydrolyzes triglycerides to free fatty acids (FFA) and produces proinflammatory mediators and chemotactic factors that are the causes of inflammation. This results in papules, pustules, and nodulocystic acne. The severity of acne correlates with stage of sexual maturity and rate of sebum production.

The proposed trigger factors of acne are stress (activation of androgen hormone), mechanical factors, topical products (obstruction pilosebaceous unit), and medications (anabolic steroid, progestin, isoniazid, phenytoin, vitamin B12).

The presentation of acne is variable and includes comedones, papules, pustules, cysts, nodules, scarring, and dyspigmentation at the face, neck, chest, and back area.

1.6.1.1 Topical therapy

Benzoyl peroxide

The mechanisms of action are antimicrobial, comedolytic, and anti-inflammatory. These actions are useful in mild inflammatory and/or comedonal acne.

There are varieties of concentration (2.5–10%) and preparation (gel, wash, foam, cream), and it also comes in combination with other medications (topical antibacterial, vitamin A). This agent is usually used as a thin coat (pea sized) to all acne prone areas once to twice daily.

The common side effects are stinging, drying, redness, peeling of the skin, and bleaching of colored clothes.

Topical antibiotics

The mechanisms of action are reduction of bacteria on the skin surface, within follicles and anti-inflammatory effects. The most common topical medications are clindamycin and erythromycin. Less commonly used are metronidazole and sulfonamide (sulfacetamide).

These medications are appropriately used in mild to moderate acne, mixed inflammatory and comedonal acne, usually once to twice daily.

Data recently show topical antibacterial resistance of P. acnes to erythromycin or clindamycin. Multiple drugs resistance is also reported. Recommendations for topical antibiotics are short-term use and avoidance of concomitant oral and topical therapy with the same medication. The combination use of topical antibiotics with topical benzoyl peroxide or topical retinoid decreases the risk of resistance. Antibiotics used in the treatment of acne are summarized in Table 1.5.

Table 1.5: Oral antibiotics for treatment of acne

Drug	Dose/Frequency	Age	Side effects	Remarks
Tetracycline Cap (250, 500 mg)	250–500 mg Twice daily	Age > 9 yrs.	-Dental staining -GI upset, esophageal irritation -Photosensitivity	-Empty stomach -Avoid taking with antacids or dairy products -Take with a large glass of water
Doxycycline Cap (50, 100 mg)	50–100 mg Twice daily	Age > 9 yrs.	-Dental staining (less) -GI upset -Photosensitivity / photo-onycholysis	-Avoid taking with dairy products
Minocycline Cap (50, 100 mg)	50–100 mg Twice daily	Age > 9 yrs.	-Dental staining (less) -GI upset, hepatitis -Blue-gray skin pigmentation -Drug induced lupus -Headache, vertigo (vestibular disturbance) -Serum sickness like reaction	-Empty stomach -Avoid taking with dairy products
Erythromycin Tab (250,500 mg)	250–500 mg Twice daily	Any age	-GI upset	-Empty stomach
Trimetroprim-sufamethoxazole Tab (80/400, 160/800 mg)	80/400, 160/800 mg Once / twice daily	Any age	-Drug hypersensitivity reaction -Bone marrow suppression -GI upset, hepatitis -Renal toxicity	-Avoid in G6PD -Use as second-line drug
Cephalexin Tab (250, 500 mg)	250–500 mg Twice daily	Any age	-GI upset	Use as second-line drug

Retinoids

The mechanisms of action are normalization of keratinization, comedolytic, and anti-inflammatory effects. There are varieties of concentration (0.01% and 0.1%) and preparations (gel, microgel, cream form, vitamin A, and Adapalene). One may combine retinoids with other products such as benzoyl peroxide or tazarotene. The combination of many products enhances therapeutic efficacy.

This agents are usually used as a thin coat (pea sized) once nightly on the dry face because of the effects of skin irritation and sun sensitivity. Post-inflammatory hypo- or hyperpigmentation may occur in darker-skinned individuals. To prevent these effects begin with a lower strength preparation. The evidence of teratogenicity from topical retinoid use is inconclusive (pregnancy category C classification, no controlled studies in women; risk to the fetus cannot be ruled out).

Azelaic acid

This medication is produced from the yeast Pityrosporum ovale. The mechanisms of action are minimal both in antibacterial and anti-comedonal effect. It may be an alternative treatment for mild inflammatory and comedonal acne. The dominantly beneficial effect is ability to ameliorate hyperpigmented lesions.

The available form is a 20% cream. The side effects are pruritus, burning, and erythema.

Dapsone

This medication has FDA approval for treatment of acne. The available form is 5% gel. The supportive evidence of efficacy is lesion reduction in number and improvement of acne severity.

1.6.1.2 Systemic therapy

Oral antibiotics

Oral antibiotics are used in cases of moderate to severe inflammatory acne. The mechanisms of action are decrease P. acnes resulting in decreased inflammation from reduction of neutrophil chemotaxis and pro-inflammatory cytokines. They are generally used to control the acne for several months, with improvement in 4–8 weeks after initiation.

The most common twice-daily antibiotics used are tetracycline, doxycycline, minocycline, and erythromycin. Table 1.4 summarizes antibiotic treatment of acne.

Isotretinoin

Isotretinoin is cis-retinoic acid, a derivative of vitamin A, usually used in recalcitrant acne with severe and nodulocystic lesions. The mechanism of action is to eradicate all types of acne pathogenesis.

This medication is usually started on dose 0.5–1 mg/kg/day up to 2 mg/kg/day. A cumulative dose of 100–150 mg/kg is associated with successful treatment. The dose and duration of therapy depends on individual response, and a repeated course maybe necessary.

The potential side effects are dry skin and mucosa, alopecia, pseudotumor cerebri (esp. taken with oral antibiotics), abnormal lipid profiles and liver function tests, exacerbation of inflammatory bowel disease, and teratogenic effects (pregnancy category X classification).

Female patients must be tested to reassure that they are not pregnant before beginning isotretinoin and be supervised to have at least two methods of contraception during the course of treatment. Signature of a consent form with risks and benefits is required before initiation of treatment.

1.6.1.3 Hormonal therapy

Hormonal therapy is an optional treatment in female patients especially in hyperandrogenic acne (hirsutism, androgenetic alopecia, menstrual irregularity, polycystic ovarian syndrome). The mechanisms of action are reduction of active free testosterone and ovarian androgen production.

Oral contraceptive pills, norgestimate, and ethinyl estradiol are approved by FDA to treat acne vulgaris.

Spironolactone, anti-androgenic agonist, is also an optional treatment in females. The side effects are breast soreness, menstrual irregularities, hyperkalemia, and fatigue.

1.6.2 Nevi

1.6.2.1 Melanocytic nevi

The melanocytic nevus is a common skin disorder and may be congenital or acquired (32). The acquired form may be due to internal factors (genetic, race, skin type, hormone, and pregnancy) or external factors (sun exposure, cutaneous surgery, systemic immunosuppression, medications).

Melanocytic nevi result from benign proliferation of melanocytes leading to accumulation of nevus cells (nevocyte) in the layers of skin. This condition is divided into junctional nevi (nevocytes in dermo-epidermal junction), compound nevi (nevocytes in the junction and dermis), and intradermal nevi (nevocytes limited to the dermis).The risk of transformation from melanocytic nevus to malignant melanoma is extremely low.

1.6.2.2 Congenital melanocytic nevi (CMN)

These lesions usually present at birth or in the first year of life. CMN is most commonly classified based on the diameter into three groups:

- Small (<1.5 cm. in diameter)
- Medium (1.5–19.9 cm. in diameter)
- Large/giant (>20 cm. in diameter)

Giant melanocytic nevi in the neonatal period are considered when the size is larger than the palm of baby (about 6 cm.). CMN usually are brown colored macules, papules, or patches on any location of the body. Giant melanocytic nevi tend to have color, size, texture, variation, and become hairy with increasing age. The posterior trunk is the most common location of giant melanocytic nevi.

CMN of all sizes carry an increased risk of malignant melanoma especially in giant melanocytic nevi. Higher malignancy risk of giant melanocytic nevus is associated with large diameter, increasing of satellite lesions, and location of the back. Malignancy risk rates range between 2% and 4% for giant congenital nevi. The malignancy risk for small congenital nevi is unknown but is probably less than 1%.

Neurocutaneous melanosis (NCM) is due to proliferation of intracerebral melanocytes, which may result in seizure, malignant melanoma of CNS, increased intracranial pressure, and spinal cord compression. NCM is mostly found in giant melanocytic nevi with satellite lesions.

The treatment of giant melanocytic nevus is complicated and controversial. The vast majority are simply followed with biopsy or removal only when worrisome lesions arise. Factors in management include location, size, neurocutaneous melanosis, cosmetic result, risk of malignant melanoma, and anesthetic issues. Multidisciplinary approach with the patients and families should be provided.

1.6.2.3 Spitz nevus

The presentation of a Spitz nevus is a well-circumscribed reddish-brown dome-shaped papules or nodule, mostly as a solitary lesion. Spitz nevi are predominant in the pediatric population and most commonly occur on the face, neck, and lower extremities.

They are usually acquired proliferations of melanocytes with histopathological features, which sometimes overlap with melanoma.

The differential diagnosis consists of atypical melanocytic nevus, melanoma, pyogenic granuloma, and early stage of juvenile xanthogranuloma.

Although the potential risk of malignant transformation is minimal, there is no definite consensus on the management of Spitz nevi. Surgical excision to confirm the diagnosis and risk of malignancy is the usual approach. Care should be taken to remove the entire lesion on the first biopsy as examination of the deep component is essential for a correct diagnosis.

1.6.2.4 Halo nevus (Sutton's nevus)

This presents as a halo or hypopigmented macule surrounding a pigmented nevus. The halo is usually symmetrical and with a regular border differing from the irregular halo of melanoma. The most common location of halo nevi is on the back. Half of the patients have multiple lesions.

Pathogenesis of this disorder is unknown. It has been proposed to be an immune-mediated attack to the nevus cells in the lesion. Autoimmune conditions such as vitiligo and thyroiditis are rarely found together with halo nevi.

The treatment of halo nevi is observational. Excision is unnecessary when the central lesion appears benign.

1.6.2.5 Nevus spilus (Speckled lentiginous nevus)

The initial lesion may reveal a large brown patch in the first few years of life and gradually develops the secondary variable darker lesion of superimposed, small-pigmented macules and/or papules. It is typically solitary. The trunk and extremities are the most common locations. The lesion varies in size.

The characteristic presentation is multiple dark brown to black macules superimposed on the larger brown patch.

Nevus spilus should be monitored because of the potential risk of malignant transformation.

1.6.2.6 Becker's nevus

Becker's nevi are acquired. The clinical presentation is a unilateral slightly thickened irregular border of brownish hyperpigmented plaque, usually found at the chest wall, upper trunk, and shoulder of adolescent males. Hypertrichosis is a common concomitant finding.

Pathogenesis of this condition is unclear. Increased androgen receptors in the lesion are presumed to relate to hypertrichosis in these nevi. Becker's nevi are associated with smooth muscle hamartomas that affect arrector pili muscle contractions.

Hyperpigmented patch and hypertrichosis tend to persist for life. Laser therapy is not recommended in most cases because of the unpleasant results.

1.6.2.7 Epidermal nevus

The epidermal nevus is a hamartoma of the top layer of skin. It presents as localized flesh to brownish verrucous surface papules or plaques, single to linear in configuration, sometimes along Blaschko's lines.

The differential diagnosis includes lichen striatus, linear lichen planus. Skin biopsy is helpful to distinguish these conditions.

Treatment of epidermal nevus includes surgical procedure (excision, liquid nitrogen, cryotherapy, dermabrasion, laser ablation) and topical treatment (tretinoin, podophyllin, keratolytic agents).

Cutaneous findings of epidermal nevus are concomitant with an array of extracutaneous abnormalities/systemic complications such as limb defect/deformity, seizures, developmental delay, macrocephaly, eye abnormalities, and skeletal abnormalities (kyphosis, scoliosis). This is known as Epidermal nevus syndrome (EPS).

The inflammation of linear epidermal nevus is termed Inflammatory linear verrucous epidermal nevus (ILVEN). This condition is a chronic and inflammatory cause of epidermal nevus variants. The symptoms are characteristically extreme pruritus and recurrent inflammation. Treatment of ILVEN is very difficult. Choices include topical or intralesional corticosteroid, topical retinoid, topical calcineurin inhibitor, topical vitamin D derivatives, CO2 laser, and surgical excision. Responses are often poor.

1.6.3 Papulosquamous disorders

1.6.3.1 Primary forms of ichthyosis (non-syndrome ichthyosis)

We discuss congenital forms of icthyosis mainly because they persist into childhood and adolescence and will require treatment (33,34,35,36).

1.6.3.2 Ichthyosis vulgaris

Ichthyosis vulgaris is the most common form of ichthyosis, which is frequently associated with atopic dermatitis. The other minor criteria of atopic dermatitis include xerosis, hyperlinearity of palm-sole, keratosis pilaris. This condition transmitted as an autosomal dominant trait. The examination of parents' skin may be helpful in diagnosis.

The presentation reveals white to gray scales on the extensor surface of extremities particularly on the lower leg. The flexor surface and groin are always spared. Scale is characterized by small, white to gray, like a fish scale, and worse in dry weather.

The diagnosis is clinical. Skin biopsy may be done only in cases of uncertainty. The treatments include hydration, then topical emollient and/or keratolytic agents such as urea and lactic acid.

1.6.3.3 Recessive X-linked ichthyosis

The mode of transmission of this condition is X-linked recessive. The affected patients are males. Females are mostly carriers. The pathogenesis is a defect of the gene encoding the enzyme steroid sulfatase. The onset of this condition usually begins in the first few months of age. It presents as generalized large dark brownish scales accentuated on the lateral side of neck, pre-auricular area, abdomen, back, feet but sparing the palm, soles, central face, and flexural areas.

Corneal opacity is usually found in affected adult males. Because of contiguous gene syndromes, hypogonadism and/or cryptochidism are sometimes present. The treatments include topical emollient and/or keratolytic agents such as urea and lactic acid.

1.6.3.4 Bullous congenital ichthyosiform erythroderma (BCIE)/Epidermolytic hyperkeratosis (EHK)/Bullous ichthyosis (BI)

The clinical presentation of BCIE is extremely variable. The classic presentation is superficial bullae and broad sheets of desquamation, generalized erythroderma in the first few days of life. The skin and bullous disease will change to hyperkeratosis in the next first few months.

The characteristic findings are thick, hyperpigmented verrucous scales on the flexural surfaces, intertriginous areas of the body, and on dorsal surfaces of the hands and feet. Palms, soles, and scalp are frequently involved. Unpleasant odor is very common due to fermented bacteria, yeast, and fungi in the hyperkeratotic skin.

The pathogenesis is a mutation of the keratin gene leading to abnormal keratin protein. Thickening skin is believed to be a compensatory mechanism for skin protection.

Emollients are the proper management. Mechanical trauma and prolonged use of keratolytic agents should be avoided because of increased skin fragility. Mild antibacterial cleanser (e.g. chlorhexidine) or bleach bath is beneficial to decrease bacterial fermentation. Oral vitamin A derivatives (isotrentinoin, aciretin, etc.) help slough the scale.

1.6.3.5 Lamellar ichthyosis (LI)

This severe condition is transmitted as an autosomal recessive trait. The pathogenesis is the TGM1 gene mutation resulting in defect of transglutaminase-1 enzyme, which is necessary to for desquamation of the top skin layer.

The diagnosis is based on clinical findings, which are large plate-like scales, ectropion, eclabium, and scarring alopecia. Ectropion is eversion of the eyelid, which exposes the palpebral conjunctiva and induces keratitis and madorosis. Eclabium is eversion of the lips. The patient usually presents at birth with a collodion membrane. There are generalized large quadrangular dark brown thick scales at the face, trunk, and flexor surface of the extremities. The classic scales are centrally attached with raised borders. Palms and soles are frequently involved with a varying degree of keratoderma and fissuring. Scarring alopecia particularly at the hairline is a common finding. The thickened skin also causes the obstruction of sweat ducts resulting in heat intolerance.

Treatments include topical emollients and/or potent keratolytic agents. Oral retinoids (e.g. acitretin) may be helpful in severe cases. Ectropion should be corrected to prevent long term visual complications.

1.6.3.6 Congenital ichthyosiform erythroderma (CIE)/Non-bullous congenital ichthyosiform erythroderma (NBCIE)

CIE is transmitted as an autosomal recessive trait. The pathogenesis is mutation of TGM1 gene, the same as in lamellar ichthyosis.

The patient initially presents with collodion membrane at birth. After being shed, the skin turns red (erythroderma) and develops fine white powdery scales on the face, scalp, and trunk. Hyperkeratosis of palm and soles with deep fissures are common. Ectropion and scarring alopecia may occur in various degrees.

The treatments include topical emollients and/or keratolytic agents such as urea, salicylic acid, alpha hydroxyl acid, propylene glycol, or a combination of them.

1.6.3.7 Harlequin ichthyosis

Harlequin ichthyosis is the most severe form of congenital ichthyosis with high morbidity and mortality. This condition is transmitted as an autosomal recessive trait. Most patients are usually born prematurely and suffer complications of prematurity (e.g. respiratory distress, sepsis, and hypothermia).

The clinical is characterized by hard, thickened armor-like skin with brownish fissures leading to polygonal, triangular plaques. Rigidity of skin results in facial deformity, ectropion, eclabium, and everted O-shaped lip (fish mouth deformity). The limbs are limited in flexion of hands and feet. Constriction of the chest wall often results in respiratory and feeding problems.

The treatment of harlequin fetus is controversial. High mortality rate is due to severe infection, poor feeding, and electrolyte imbalance. The treatment for survivors is systemic retinoid (acitretin), which may improve, ectropion, eclabium, and accelerate shedding skin. Risks and benefits of long term use of medication should be discussed before starting treatment. Supportive treatment with emollients may be adjunctive therapy.

1.6.4 Lichens

1.6.4.1 Lichen nitidus (LN)

This condition is most commonly seen in children of pre-school and school age. The exact pathogenesis is unknown. The characteristic findings are minute sharply demarcated flesh-colored flat-topped papules arranged in groups that may circumscribe the trunk, genitalia, abdomen, and forearm. Koebner's phenomenon (lesions developing at site of trauma) can be found in many patients. The condition is seen on the glans penis.

The differential diagnoses include papular eczema, flat warts, keratosis pilaris, micropapular lichen planus, and follicular psoriasis. The characteristic histopathological features are used to confirm diagnosis in uncertain cases.

The natural course of this condition varies from weeks to months and recovers spontaneously. Supportive treatment with oral antihistamines and topical corticosteroids may be helpful.

1.6.4.2 Lichen planus (LP)

Lichen planus is a common disorder, usually found in all age groups. The exact pathogensis is unknown.The characteristic findings are small flat-topped pruritic polyglonal purplish papules (the four P's). The distribution is usually seen in the flexural surface of lower legs, ankles, wrist, genitalia, lower back, face, and mucous membranes, or along Blaschko's lines. Papules may develop at the site of trauma (Koebner's phenomenon).

The polymorphic variants of lichen planus in pediatric patients consist of bullous LP, actinic LP, annular LP, atrophic LP, hypertrophic LP, linear LP, ulcerative LP, LP pemphigoid, LP lupus erythematosus, and lichen planopilaris. Linear LP is the most common variant in pediatric patients. Follicular LP on the scalp (Lichen planopilaris) can lead to scarring alopecia.

Mucous membranes of the mouth may demonstrate a characteristic reticulated delicate white line or annular-linear lacy reticulate pattern defined as "Wickham's striae." The buccal mucosa, lip, and tongue are the most commonly affected areas.

Nail involvement is uncommon in pediatric patients with lichen planus but may present with pitting, lusterless nail with thinning nail plate, longitudinal ridging, and twenty-nail-dystrophy.

The differential diagnosis depends on the variants presenting and includes lichen striatus, Lichen nitidus, lichen simplex chronicus, lichenoid drug eruption, and papular granuloma annulare.

The diagnosis of LP relies on the characteristic pattern of lesions. The typical histopathologic features from skin biopsy are helpful to confirm the diagnosis.

Treatment of choice of LP is moderate to potent topical corticosteroids and antihistamines. In cases of extensive or recalcitrant symptoms systemic corticosteroid injection (triamcinolone acetonide 5–10 mg/ml dose or 1 mg/kg/dose) is effective. Other treatments include topical tacrolimus, oral dapsone, PUVA or UVB light therapy, oral retinoid, cyclosporine, and thalidomide.

1.6.4.3 Pityriasis lichenoides

Pityriasis lichenoides is an inflammatory papulosquamous skin disorder with characteristic clinical and histopathologic features. This condition has been divided into two forms, including the acute form, Pityriasis lichenoides et varioliformis acuta (PLEVA, Mucha-Habermann disease), and the chronic form, Pityriasis lichenoides chronica (PLC).

The exact pathogenesis of pityriasis lichenoides is unknown. Recent data reveal an abnormal response to an antigenic stimulus provided by unidentified infectious agents, possibly viral. Pityriasis lichenoides is primarily a cutaneous T-cell lymphoproliferative disorder. Nevertheless, the progression of pityriasis lichenoides to cutaneous T-cell lymphoma in children has been rarely reported.

PLEVA is a polymorphous papulosquamous eruption. It presents as asymptomatic or pruritic symmetrical erythematous macules, and papules coalesce in crops and turn to vesicular, necrotic, and purpuric lesions. Lesions are most common on the trunk, proximal thighs, and upper arms. The natural course of disorder usually lasts several weeks to months.

The differential diagnosis is chicken pox, insect bite reaction, leukocytoclastic vasculitis, and vesicular pityriasis rosea.

PLC is a chronic form of pityriasis lichenoides. The course of PLC is variable from months to years. The skin lesions reveal scaling papules and plaques and usually resolve with post-inflammatory hypopigmentation, or less commonly with hyperpigmentation.

The differential diagnosis is pityriasis rosea, secondary syphilis, or guttate psoriasis.

Histopathology from skin biopsy may be helpful in cases of uncertain clinical diagnosis.

Patients and families should be reassured of the self-limited natural course of this condition. There is no specific treatment. Optional treatments include oral erythromycin, topical corticosteroid, and phototherapy. Topical corticosteroid or oral antihistamine may decrease the pruritus. Oral erythromycin, 30–50 mg/kg/day for 1–2 months, is partially effective in some cases. Ultraviolet light therapy may be helpful in cases not responding to oral erythromycin. Spontaneous recovery usually occurs in several months to years.

1.6.4.4 Pityriasis rosea (PR)

Pityriasis rosea is an acute benign self-limited papulosquamous disorder. The exact etiology of this condition is unknown. There may be a viral like prodrome and/or history of preceding upper respiratory tract infection in some cases.

The clinical manifestation is initially a single isolated lesion defined as "herald patch." The most common area of herald patch is on the trunk, upper arm, neck, or thigh. The lesion is characterized by a sharply demarcated oval shape with surrounding fine white scale "collar sign," usually seen 1–2 weeks prior to appearance of other lesions. Only about 50% of cases begin with a herald patch.

The secondary lesions reveal generalized erythematous patches, papules with fine white scale bilaterally and symmetrically discrete to the line of skin cleavage, in a "Christmas tree pattern" on the upper arm, neck, back, trunk, and upper thigh. The white scales reveal a "collarette of scale" surrounding the lesion, characteristic of pityriasis rosea. Each individual lesion is football-shaped with a raised red border, trailing scale, and darker flat interior.

The duration of secondary lesions may be days to weeks. Spontaneous recovery usually occurs within 6–12 weeks but may be prolonged over a period of 6 months. There may be residual post-inflammatory hypo-hyperpigmentation.

The diagnosis is based upon the history, distribution pattern, and the characteristic of the lesions. Histopathology of pityriasis rosea is not diagnostic because of the similarity with subacute or chronic dermatitis.

Patients and families should be reassured of the self-limited natural course of this condition. The treatment is supportive with topical or systemic antipruritic medications. Optional treatments include oral erythromycin, topical corticosteroid, and UVB light therapy. Mild to moderate corticosteroid may temporarily reduce pruritus in some patients. Oral erythromycin (dose 25–40 mg/kg/day over 2 weeks) may shorten the course of disorder. UVB light therapy over 5–10 days can significantly improve the eruption and reduce the degree of pruritus as well as hasten the resolution.

1.6.5 Psoriasis

Psoriasis is an immune-mediated papulosquamous disorder (34) (see Chapter 6). Its pathophysiology is postulated to be a combination of genetic predisposition, environmental factors, and innate and acquired immune system problems resulting in hyperproliferation and abnormal differentiation of keratinocytes.

The characteristic lesions of psoriasis are erythematous plaques with well-defined borders and papules with grayish or silvery scales. The papules may coalesce to large plaque, usually seen in a symmetrical pattern on scalp and the extensor surface of elbow, knee, lumbosacral, and anogenital areas.

The term "inverse psoriasis" may be used in a variant of flexural surface involvement of axillae, groin, perineum, central chest, and umbilical region.

The "Auspitz sign" is a characteristic phenomenon that results from removal of the white scale leading to fine punctuate bleeding points. Koebner's phenomenon may develop at sites of trauma.

Facial psoriasis especially in the periorbital area is more common in children than in adults. These often present with small round psoriatic plaques in the upper inner eyelid area.

The scalp is one of the most common sites of psoriatic involvement. The presentation is a well-defined, white scale on an erythematous base resulting in variable degree of temporary hair loss. The distribution involves the scalp, eyebrows, pre-post-auricular area and beyond the hairline. The term "tinea amiantacia" or "pityriasis amiantacia" is used for the generalized white scale pattern.

The most common manifestation of nail change in psoriasis is pitting. The others are discoloration of nail (oil drops), onycholysis and subungual hyperkeratosis.

Extra-cutaneous involvement of psoriasis may include psoriatic arthritis and symmetrical anterior uveitis in adult patients, rarely in children.

There are variable patterns of presentation.

1.6.5.1 Guttate psoriasis

This is usually the first manifestation of psoriasis in children and young adults. The lesion is characterized by drop-like (guttate), round/oval shaped, and white scale in a symmetrical distribution on the trunk and proximal aspects of the extremities. Group A Streptococcal infection is the most common trigger of this condition. The reason for this sequence of events is unknown.

1.6.5.2 Pustular psoriasis

This is the most severe variant of childhood psoriasis. The explosion of generalized sterile pustules on the erythematous skin with previous plaque psoriasis or on normal skin characterizes the lesion.

The overlying pustules may be discrete or rapidly coalesce to large plaque as "lake of pus" before drying over 3–4 days with desquamation. The repetitive explosions of pustules consequently develop over several weeks.

The trigger factors are withdrawal of systemic corticosteroids, potent topical corticosteroid, and/or respiratory tract infection.

Pustular psoriasis palmaris et plantaris is a chronic eruption usually symmetrical on both palms and soles. The lesions are characterized by deep-seated sterile pustules with white scales on top of a bright erythematous base. They finally turn to dark yellow or brown scales in several days. The crop of pustular lesions is often recurrent and sometimes is associated with secondary bacterial infection due to Staphylococcus aureus.

The diagnosis of psoriasis depends on the characteristic clinical findings. Histopathology from skin biopsy is used for confirmation.

The natural course of psoriasis is unpredictable but prolonged and chronic. The trigger factors that may aggravate psoriasis are traumatization (Koebner's phenomenon), medications (lithium, antimalarials, beta-blockers, withdrawal of systemic corticosteroids), and infection (especially Streptococcal).

1.6.5.3 Management of psoriasis

Topical therapy

Topical corticosteroids are the most commonly used therapy for children. The options depend on the site of lesion, body surface area, and duration of treatment. Risks of side effects should be considered and minimized by monitoring the amount of usage, potency, proper site, and intermittent rotational or combination therapy. The combination of topical corticosteroids with other medications e.g. topical calcipotriene is beneficial in older children.

Calcipotriene is an analogue of vitamin D3, usually combined with topical corticosteroid to facilitate the onset of action. This medication is one of the effective treatments for mild to moderate plaque type psoriasis in children and adult. The most common side effect is lesional or peri-lesional irritation especially on the face and in folds.

Tars are anti-inflammatory and anti-proliferative. There are many forms of tar preparations such as 1–10% crude coal tar (CCT), 5–10% liquor carbonis detergent (LCD), and topical corticosteroid and salicylic acid combinations. The concentration of medications is appropriately selected to age and lesion sites. Tar shampoo is used as monotherapy for scalp psoriasis or in combination with other topical therapy.

Tacrolimus ointment is a calcineurin inhibitor effective in the facial and neck area and in intertrigenous psoriasis (psoriasis inversus).

Anthralin 0.1–1% cream and ointment is primarily effective treatment for chronic plaque type psoriasis. Short contact therapy is initially applied for 5 min. and gradually increased over time as tolerated before being rinsed off. The most common side effects are irritant contact dermatitis and perilesional staining.

Phototherapy

Natural sunlight is beneficial in psoriatic patients. Phototherapy is the most frequently optional treatment in children with moderate to severe psoriasis who are recalcitrant to topical therapy.

Narrow band ultraviolet B (UVB-312 nm.) is the currently effective treatment of psoriasis. Administration three times per week is usually required until clearance occurs. The side effects of UVB therapy include skin darkening and burning.

Systemic therapy

Antibiotics are used to eradicate Streptococcal spp., which is one of the trigger factors of guttate or plaque type psoriasis. This medication should be prescribed only in case of positive throat culture, although the culture may also be positive in the carrier stage.

Methotrexate is started orally at 2.5 mg up to 15–20 mg/wk based on ideal body weight (dose 0.3–0.5 mg/kg/wk). The most common side effects are nausea, headache, and fatigue. The most common serious side effect is bone marrow suppression.

Supplementary folic acid 1–5 mg/day diminishes the risk of mucosal ulceration and macrocytic anemia. Complete blood count and liver function tests should be monitored for patients on this medication.

Retinoids (acitretin: dose 0.5–0.75 mg/kg/day) are often used in combination with topical treatment and UVB therapy. The most common side effect is dryness of skin and mucosa. Other complications are hypertriglyceridemia, teratogenic effects, premature epiphyseal closure, and hyperostosis. Complete blood count, liver function test, and lipid profiles should be monitored during administration of the medication.

Cyclosporine is effective in pediatric plaque type psoriasis at a dose of 3–3.5 mg/kg/day. The supportive data in childhood psoriasis is limited to a small case series. The side effects are hypertension, immunosuppression, and renal and hepatic toxicity.

Biologic agents: Etanercept has been systematically studied in a small number of pediatric patients with plaque type psoriasis. Infliximab has only case reports of effective treatment in childhood psoriasis.

1.7 Dermatologic manifestations of systematic disorders

The goal of this section is to demonstrate dermatologic manifestations of other conditions. This will enable the clinician to ameliorate dermatologic conditions by approaching the primary cause, often in conjunction with specialty consultation. We select disorders not uncommon in adolescents.

1.7.1 Pruritus without rash

Pruritus can be a manifestation of several conditions (see Chapter 13). There may often be no physical findings until the areas become excoriated. While malignancies such as Hodgkin and non-Hodgkin lymphoma are associated with pruritus, relatively few patients with pruritus without skin findings actually have a malignancy. Other malignancies will be associated with abnormal dermatologic findings, which may be pruritic. Examples of such are mycosis fungoides associated with leukemia and carcinoid associated with histamine flush. Renal failure patients, especially at the time of dialysis, will complain of pruritus. Cholestasis will frequently cause itching, especially in the palms and soles, primarily due to deposition of bile salts in the skin. Specific hepatic causes include primary biliary cirrhosis, sclerosing cholangitis, pregnancy, and hepatitis. Endocrine causes include hyperthyroidism and diabetes mellitus. Other conditions common in adolescence associated with pruritus include iron deficiency anemia and occasionally allergies. In patients with immunodeficiencies such as HIV, pruritus may be a complication of the primary condition (eosinophilic folliculitis in HIV), or due to a secondary infection or infestation such as scabies.

1.7.2 Inflammatory bowel disease (IBD)

Primary skin manifestations of IBD consist of mouth ulcerations and perianal fissures and fistulae, more common in Crohn's disease (37; see Chapter 23).

1.7.3 Erythema nodosum

This is the most common skin manifestation of IBD, slightly more common in Crohn's disease than in Ulcerative colitis. They are red, tender, or violaceous subcutaneous nodules most commonly on the pretibial area. They often become more manifest during exacerbations.

1.7.4 Pyoderma gangrenosum

This occurs in about 5% of patients with ulcerative colitis and 2% of patients with Crohn's disease. They present initially as a red papule and progress to central necrosis with subsequent ulceration.

1.7.5 Less common skin manifestations

Other lesions associated with IBD include psoriasis, epidermolysis bullosa, Sweet syndrome (neutrophilic infiltrates, also seen in myelogenous leukemia), and primary granulomas (metastatic Crohn's disease).

1.7.6 Management

This consists of treating the primary condition and inducing remission. This should be done in conjunction with specialty consultation from a gastroenterologist for appropriate management of corticosteroid dosages, or, in more severe cases, immunomodulators (azathioprine or 6-mercaptopurine), calcineurn inhibitors (cyclosporine), and monoclonal antibodies (infliximab). Sometimes surgical intervention in IBD will allow for remission of skin manifestations.

Regarding the specific conditions mentioned in this section, Erythema nodosum usually responds well to corticosteroid therapy. Pyoderma gangrenosum may also respond to interlesional steroids, local Chromoglycate, oral Dapsone, hyperbaric oxygen, and granulocytopheresis. Sweet syndrome is particularly sensitive to corticosteroids.

1.8 Collagen vascular disease

These conditions are not uncommon in adolescents, and identification of dermatologic manifestations is paramount to proper diagnosis and management (see Chapter 18).

1.8.1 Lupus erythematosus (SLE)

Lesions may manifest as vesicles, bullae, or ulcerations of the nasal or oral mucosa as well as the integument (38). Skin lesions may progress to atrophy or scarring. Typical lesions also consist of the malar "butterfly rash," generalized maculopapular rashes, dermatitis, frequently sun-sensitive, and vasculitis (periungual erythema, Livedo reticularis, Telangiectasia, and Raynaud phenomenon). Dermatitis often results in post-inflammatory hypo- or hyperpigmentation.

Discoid lesions may be present in 25% of patients with clinical SLE or may be its sole manifestation. They are erythematous plaques often on the face, neck, and trunk. They often heal with scarring, atrophy, telangiectasias, or hyper- and hypopigmentation. Lupus panniculitis, hypertrophic LE, and Lupus tumidus (photosensitive pink plaques or nodules) may also be a sole manifestation.

SLE may have hair and nail manifestations including alopecia, scarring and non-scarring, and pitting, ridging, and onycholysis of the nails.

1.8.2 Dermatomyositis

Classic skin manifestations include the heliotrope rash (red-purple eyelids, telangiectasia of eyelid capillaries, periorbital edema, and malar and facial erythema), Gottron's papules (red papulo-squamous lesions over knuckles and sometimes extensor surfaces), nail capillary dilatation and tortuosity, and skin ulcers. Calcinosis may occur not only in the skin, but also in muscle and fascial planes.

1.8.3 Juvenile idiopathic arthritis

The rash associated with JIA is salmon-pink in color, fleeting, and becomes more prominent with heat, both external and with fever. Skin trauma may bring out the rash (Koebner phenomenon).

1.8.4 Management

The goal of management of skin and mucous membrane lesions in LE is to prevent scarring and atrophy. An important aspect of dermatologic management in LE is preventative. Patients with photosensitivity should avoid excessive sun-exposure, use sunscreens, and select light bulbs for their homes that do not emit ultraviolet light. Patients should avoid triggers of Raynaud's phenomenon such as smoking, cold, vasoconstrictors, and caffeine.

Skin lesions in LE that are isolated often respond to topical therapy. Topical steroids are often effective, starting with low-potency medications, although it may be necessary to advance to fluorinated corticosteroids for deeper lesions. However, it is important not to overuse these medications as atrophy, striae, and telangectasia may be complications. Topical immunosuppressants such as Tacrolimus are presently under investigation and may be effective.

If systemic medications are necessary, antimalarial drugs such as Chloroquine and Quinacrine are recommended. It may take 6–12 months to see improvement. Ocular pathology is a serious side effect of these medications, and the prescribing physician should always be mindful of this. Systemic corticosteroids and immunosuppressive agents may be helpful for bullous lesions, but generally are not necessary.

1.9 Endocrinologic disorders

1.9.1 Thyroid disorders

Patients with hypo- or hyperthyroidism will present with pruritus, sometimes idiopathic, sometimes due to dry skin (see Chapter 19). In hyperthyoridism the skin is thin and diaphoretic; in hypothyroidism it may be cool, pale, and myxedmatous. There may be a yellowish hue due to carotenemia in hypothyroidism. Patients with thyroid disease have an increased incidence of vitiligo, especially in patients with auto-immune conditions. Hair may be thickened in hypothyroidism and thinned in hyperthyroidism.

1.9.2 Diabetes mellitus

Pruritus in diabetics may be secondary to neuropathy but also may be a consequence of fungal and yeast infections. Antifungals are the treatment of choice.

1.9.3 Adrenal disorders

In patients with adrenal insufficiency, the skin is hyperpigmented especially in the palmar creases and areas exposed to trauma or sunlight. Pigmentation may be exaggerated in areas that are normally darker. Mucous membranes may display spots of pigmentation. Vitiligo may be present in patients with primary immune disorders.

Dermatologic manifestations of Cushings disease are primarily skin atrophy, bruisability, and striae. Hyperpigmentation due to overproduction of adrenocorticotropic hormone (ACTH) may also occur.

1.9.4 Management

Treatment of skin manifestations of endocrinological conditions is contingent upon management of the primary disorder and should always be done with consultation from an endocrinologist.

1.10 Hair and nails

1.10.1 Alopecia areata

The sudden onset of localized alopecia is characterized by sharply demarcated round or oval patches of hair loss (see Chapter 14).

The pathogenesis of alopecia areata is proposed to be a combination of genetic susceptibility, relating to the inner root sheath and faint association with autoimmune diseases (39). The classic autoimmune disorders include thyroid diseases (Hashimoto's thyroiditis), vitiligo, lupus erythematosus, rheumatoid arthritis, pernicious anemia, and myasthenia gravis. The association with these diseases is not clear, and testing for them is directed by family history.

The skin is smooth and almost totally devoid of hair with or without scale. The areas of hair loss may be single or numerous. The rim of alopecia reveals the pathognomonic sign of "exclamation hair," The inflammatory process of hair is located at the attenuated hair bulb resulting in easy loosening. The initial hair loss may reveal an irregular border.

The typical pattern of hair loss along the bilateral parietotemporal to posterior occiput is called the "Ophiasis pattern," usually indicating a poor prognosis. The progressive terminal scalp hair loss including the eyelashes and eyebrows is "Alopecia totalis," and the total complete loss of body hair is "Alopecia universalis." This progression is more common in children than in adults.

One of the differential diagnoses is trichotillomania. Trichotillomania typically presents with irregular border of hair loss with bizarre shaped and variation in length of unplucked hair.

The diagnosis is clinical. Histopathology from skin biopsy may be helpful in cases of uncertain history and atypical presentation. Nail changes may be found, especially a fine pitting nail either in a horizontal or vertical pattern.

There is variability of the natural course of disease and treatment. Poor prognostic factors are autoimmune diseases, family history of alopecia areata, vitiligo, thyroid diseases, young age of onset, extensive hair loss, Ophiasis pattern, Down syndrome, and nail dystrophy.

1.10.1.1 Management of alopecia areata

- Topical corticosteroid is the most common therapy for alopecia areata in children (40). Mid to high potency preparations are usually prescribed with monitoring of side effects. Re-growth of hair should be assessed 6–14 weeks after starting treatment. Intradermal corticosteroid injection is mostly used in older children and in cases of failure of topical treatment. The concentration of triamcinolone acetonide varying from 2.5 to 5 mg/ml is administrated as multiple intradermal injections of 0.1–0.3 ml/site, approximately 1 cm. apart and repeated every 4–6 weeks.
- Oral prednisolone dose 0.5–1 mg/kg/day for 4 weeks or until the hair loss stops is used in selected difficult cases, but high relapse rate often occurs after dosage reduction.
- Topical Minoxidil may stimulate follicular DNA synthesis with proliferation, differentiation of follicular keratinocyte, and re-regulation of hair physiology. The concentrations of minoxidil are 2–5% and may be applied twice daily. Hair growth is usually seen after 2 months of treatment. The uncommon side effects are allergic contact dermatitis, hypertrichosis, and local irritation.
- Topical immunotherapy (Contact sensitizer)has been used in chronic and extensive alopecia areata. These agents will sensitize contacted skin inducing erythema, scaling, and pruritus. T suppressor cells are generated to contacted area that may result in a non-specific inhibitory effect on the autoimmune reaction in hair follicles and in re-growth of the hair.
- Diphenylcyclopropenone (DPCP) is the most commonly used topical sensitizer in children. The efficacy of DPCP in alopecia areata ranges from 48% to 85%. The side effects of DPCP include eczematous reaction, itching, facial or scalp edema and cervical or post-auricular lymphadenopathy.
- Anthralin (Dithranol), 0.25–1% Anthralin cream, is initially used as short contact therapy and with gradually increasing contact time as tolerated prior to rinsing. The side effects of this medication are scalp irritation, folliculitis, and staining of the skin and clothes. It can be used in combination with twice daily topical corticosteroid therapy.
- PUVA (Psoralens with Ultraviolet A). The presumed mechanism of action is photoimmunologic effect by inhibition of local immunologic attack of hair follicle. The response rate and high relapse rates vary with the dose. There is a known incidence of induced skin cancers with oral PUVA treatment.

1.10.2 Telogen effluvium

The characteristic pattern is diffuse thinning of the scalp hair. There are several anecdotal trigger factors including emotional stress, high fever, systemic illness, severe infection, surgery, nutritional deficiency, thyroid abnormalities, and systemic lupus erythematosus. Medications (Albendazole, Amphetamine, Retinoids, Beta-blockers, Anticonvulsants, ACE inhibitors) also affect this condition. These factors may interrupt the normal cycle pattern of the anagen phase and result in early telogen phase. Telogen phase with >25% of hair count is significantly abnormal.

The diagnosis of telogen effluvium is supported by the prior history of illness or stress for 6 weeks to 4 months and the percentage of telogen hairs in the scalp biopsy of more than 12–15% of terminal follicles.

In cases of telogen effluvium without evidence of historical trigger factors, complete blood count and serum iron/ferritin and thyroid function tests are useful screening tests.

The treatment of telogen effluvium is supportive. Spontaneous re-growth of the hair may appear in several months unless the trigger is repeated. Re-growth of the hair is usually complete within 6 months.

1.10.3 Androgenic alopecia

Androgenic alopecia (male-pattern baldness) with a genetic predisposition is the most common cause of hair loss in adults. Androgen hormones gradually transform large scalp hair follicles to smaller follicles and turn anagen phase to telogen phase in a faster than normal cycle.

Androgenic alopecia can occur in either gender, but males are affected more severely than females. The male pattern reveals the symmetrical frontoparietal recession of the hairline and/or vertex thinning, where as the female pattern is relatively unaffected at the hairline but seen at the vertex and/or as diffuse thinning. Some cases begin during adolescence.

The diagnosis is based on the pattern of scalp hair loss. Hair plucking of frontal area reveals the increased ratio of telogen to anagen phase, but it is usually unnecessary to do this to make the diagnosis.

Topical treatment with 2.5% Minoxidil solution is used to stimulate follicular proliferation, dermal papilla vascularization, increased anagen duration, and enlargement of miniaturized follicles. This solution should be routinely applied to maintain hair growth. It works well on vertex and frontal scalp thinning. Topical Minoxidil may cause telogen effluvium to occur 2–8 weeks after initial treatment due to releasing of telogen hair as anagen promotion begins. Irritation, erythema, and hypertrichosis are the common side effects of Minoxidil.

Oral fenasteride is a specific type II 5 alpha reductase inhibitor resulting in reduction of levels of dihydrotestosterone both in serum and scalp skin. Fenasteride 1 mg/day is effective treatment in men older than 18 years of age. Response time to this medication may occur as early as 3 months. Medication should be continued at least 24 months before reevaluation. The side effect is sexual dysfunction in 4.2% of men.

Spironolactone, an aldosterone antagonist, 50–200 mg/day is the optional treatment of androgenetic alopecia in women. Breast soreness and menstrual irregularities are side effects of this medication.

1.10.4 Trichotillomania

Trichotillomania is classified as an impulse-control disorder (see Chapter 12). The scalp is the most common area of involvement, but the eyebrows and eyelashes may be involved as well.

This condition usually occurs in adolescents or older children, predominantly in females. The characteristic hair pattern is bizarre configuration, irregular border, frequently distributing to the side of patient's handedness with varying length, and/or broken hair from traction. The affected areas are commonly found at the frontal, frontotemporal, and vertex areas of the scalp.

Direct evidence from observation hair plucking and indirect evidence of broken groups of hair in the patient's room are helpful to confirm diagnosis.

The management of trichotillomania is difficult. The patients should be reassured the cause of disease is stress and that stress reduction will improve the condition. Supportive treatment such as mild shampoo or mild topical scalp lotion (hydrocortisone) may be useful to relieve pruritus and irritation. The mainstay of treatment is psychiatric intervention and behavior therapy.

1.10.5 Traction alopecia

Traction alopecia is traumatic hair loss secondary to tensile force on the scalp hair. It presents as oval or linear areas of hair loss along the margin of the hairline depending on type of traction or trauma. This condition is common in females who pull braids, adolescents with ponytails, or who use barrettes and hair rollers.

Hair will re-grow in a few months after stopping traction. However, scarring and little re-growth may occur because of follicular destruction.

1.10.6 Hirsutism and hypertrichosis

Hirsutism is excessive hair growth in women and girls due to androgens. This may appear at the upper lip, neck, anterior chest wall, breast, abdomen, upper inner thigh, and legs. Often it is genetic, with one or both parents being hirsuite.

Hypertrichosis is excessive hair growth in male and female of non-androgen etiology without evidence of masculinization or menstrual abnormality. The excessive hair growth may occur both in generalized and localized pattern.

The ideal treatment is correction of the cause of these conditions. The simplest methods to eradicate the excessive hair are cutting with razors, scissors, or shaving. Side effects include pseudofolliculitis and irritation. Epilation includes plucking, threading, and waxing. Plucking and wax epilation are usually painful and induce folliculitis, pseudofolliculitis, and post inflammatory hyperpigmentation.

Chemical depilatory agents, 2–10% thioglycolates, mercaptans, and sulfide may be effective but cause irritation, have an unpleasant odor, and systemic absorption may occur in extensive areas of usage.

Electrolysis permanently damages hair follicles but is difficult to use in younger children. The side effects include erythema, edema, pain, and post inflammatory dyspigmentation.

Laser hair removal includes the ruby laser (694 nm.), the alexandrite laser (755 nm.), the diode laser (800–810 nm.), and Nd:YAG laser (1064 nm.).

Systemic medication to control hirsutism should be used under supervision of an endocrinologist or gynecologist.

1.10.7 Hair changes with systemic disease

1.10.7.1 Anagen effluvium

The effects of systemic treatment of radiation and chemotherapy may result in this condition. Hair loss may be prominent at the frontal, vertex, parietal area of the scalp or generalized. The severity of generalized hair loss depends on the toxicity of the causative agents.

Several manipulations may minimize hair loss such as applying ice packs or tourniquets to the scalp for 30 min. before drug administration.

The medical history, physical examination, and microscopic examination of hair are useful to diagnose this condition.

The ideal treatment is cessation of the causative agents and to wait for hair re-growth.

1.10.8 Infection

1.10.8.1 Tinea capitis

Tinea capitis is the most common hair infection of childhood (41). The characteristic pattern is localized alopecia and broken hair with scaling. The most common age groups are prepubertal children because the effect of sex hormones in adolescence may change the sebum of scalp to free fatty acid with a protective effect.

There are varieties of dermatophytes that cause tinea capitis such as Trichophyton spp., Microsporum spp., and Epidermophyton spp. The predominant species vary according to geographic location. The different pathogens may affect varieties of clinical presentation. Trichophyton tonsurans is the major cause of tinea capitis in the United States. Predisposing factors of tinea capitis are large family size, overcrowded living condition, low socioeconomic status, the postmenstrual period, and an immunocompromised host.

Transmission of diseases usually occurs by contact with infected spores in shedding scale, hair, or fomites from person-to-person or animal-to-person.

The classic manifestations vary as patchy alopecia, gray patch, scaling with or without hair loss, follicular pustules/papules, erythema, black dot, kerion, scarring, and favus:

- Gray patch is a non-inflammatory type of tinea capitis. The clinical reveals the grayish patches of spores covering the hair shaft (Ectothrix) and usually present with scaling. Microsporum spp. is the common agent causing this form.
- Black dot presents with small black dots from broken hair shafts with alopecia. The cause of this form is dermatophyte invasion of the medulla hair (Endothrix). Trichophyton tonsurans is the most common etiologic agent.
- Kerion is an inflammatory type of tinea capitis. It presents as a boggy mass, an erythematous plaque with pustules and purulent discharge. Alopecia with loosening hair is also a significant presentation. Sinus drainage may occur, and it is frequently misdiagnosed as a bacterial abscess. This form often results in scarring alopecia from permanent damage to hair follicles.
- Favus is a severe chronic condition. The characteristic pattern is scaly erythematous patches with yellow-red perifollicular papules. Yellow cup-shaped fungal mycelia called scutula are present. This lesion may result in scarring, atrophy, and permanent alopecia.

The differential diagnosis of tinea capitis includes seborrheic dermatitis, psoriasis, alopecia areata, trichotillomania, follicultis, lupus erythematosus, and lichen planopilaris.

A potassium hydroxide preparation of scaling and broken hair confirms the diagnosis. The microscopic examination reveals tiny arthrospores surrounding or within the hair shaft. However, the gold standard of diagnosis is fungal culture.

The treatment of tinea capitis is systemic therapy because of the requirement of penetration of medication to hair follicles. The drug of choice for tinea capits is griseofulvin because of its efficacy, safety profile, and cost. The dose is 20 mg/kg of the ultra-microsize form administered once daily for a month. Problems with liver function are now not thought to be as significant as they once were, and thus liver function tests should be obtained only if treatment is going to last >1 month.

Topical therapy may be an additional treatment. Shampoo containing selenium sulfide, ketoconazole, or zinc pyrithion and twice-daily usage is adjunctive therapy to eliminate contagious spores of dermatophytes.

Contaminated individual hairbrushes, pillowcases, and hats of infected patients should be cleaned and not shared with others. Symptomatic family members and contacts should be evaluated.

1.10.8.2 Herpetic whitlow

Herpetic whitlow is the localized form of HSV infection, usually seen in dentists and physicians who have contact with herpetic lesions. Autoinoculation to other sites also may occur. Clinical manifestations are a deep-seated painful group of vesicles with surrounding erythema. Ipsilateral regional lymphadenopathy may occur.

The differential diagnosis is blistering dactylytis, impetigo, burns, and friction blisters. Viral culture or direct fluorescent antibody testing are helpful to confirm the diagnosis.

The proper treatment is supportive therapy. Spontaneous recovery usually occurs over 3 weeks. However, the oral antiviral therapy may relieve pain and speed recovery.

1.10.9 Bacterial

1.10.9.1 Paronychia

Paronychia is bacterial infection surrounding the nail. Acute paronychia usually presents as painful, erythema, swelling of the proximal and lateral nail fold. The cuticle is sometimes obliterated. The most common pathogen is Staphylococcus aureus. The pathogen in ingrown toe nail is usually Pseudomonas spp. and Gram-negative organisms.

Chronic paronychia usually manifests as asymptomatic periungual erythema. The most common pathogen is Candida spp. particularly with repeated and chronic exposure to moisture at work or due to finger sucking.

Systemic candidiasis, acrodermatits enteropathica, multiple carboxylase deficiency, chronic mucocutaneous candidiasis, and immunodeficiency should be considered in cases of multiple involvements of nails in both hands and feet.

The ideal treatment of paronychia is to eradicate infectious pathogens and keep the finger dry. Either alcohol-propylene glycol vehicle or thymol concentration 4% in chloroform is applied to dry the nail fold. Topical clindamycin solution may beneficial in secondary bacterial infection.

1.10.9.2 Ingrown nail

The distal-lateral edge of the nail curves inward and penetrates the underlying tissue. The causes of this disorder are improper cutting of the nail, tearing the nail plate, and/or too tightly fitting footwear. There may be genetic predisposition.

It presents as painful erythema and swelling and may turn to granulation tissue over time. Complications of ingrown nail are paronychia and recurrent dactylitis.

Treatments are use of properly fitting footwear, special trimming, waiting for the nail to grow past the free edge, and to control infection by compression dressings, topical, and/or systemic antibiotics. Antiseptic soaks such as Hibiclens soap, Dakins solution, or potassium permanganate may be helpful. Surgical procedure such as partial/total nail avulsion is necessary in painful cases or in frequent recurrence.

1.10.10 Fungal

1.10.10.1 Onychomycosis/Tinea ungium

The term "onychomycosis" refers to a fungal infection of the nail (42,43,44). However, "tinea ungium" is a specific term for dermatophyte infection of the nail.

Onychomycosis is more common in adults than children. Toe nail onychomycosis is usually associated with tinea pedis. This condition is classified in four patterns of infection site including distal subungual, proximal subungual, lateral subungual, and superficial white onychomycosis.

Distal subungual onychomycosis is the most common form of fungal infection. The separation of nail plate and nail bed by fungal invasion leads to onycholysis and thickening of subungual nail.

Proximal subungual onychomycosis is an uncommon presentation in a normal host and is usually seen in HIV or other immunocompromised conditions. The cuticle of proximal nail fold is initially disrupted. Proximal separation of the nail plate and nail bed results in onycholysis, scaling, and discoloration.

Superficial white onychomycosis is the superficial infection of nail plate. The organisms directly invade to the dorsal nail plate. The infected nail plate is fragile and easily removed. Trichophyton spp. is the most common pathogen of the finger nails.

The common findings of onychomycosis are not usually symmetrical, and only one to three nails of one hand or foot may be involved. If all of the nails are involved, other diagnoses should be suspected, including psoriatic nail, chronic paronychia, drug induced onycholysis, trauma, lichen planus, and pachyonychia congenita.

The treatment of onychomycosis is systemic therapy because of poor topical penetration to the nail plate. However, topical therapy (such as Amorolfine, Ciclopirox) is used as adjuctive therapy in some cases. Topical usage is appropriate in superficial white onychomycosis.

Table 1.6: Systemic antifungal agents for onychomycosis in children

Antifungal agents	Dose	Remark
Gresiofulvin (tablet)	*-Continuous therapy* 15–20 mg/kg/day	*-Continuous* Toe nail 6–12 months Finger nail 3–6 months
Itraconazole (capsule, oral solution)	*-Pulse therapy* 5 mg/kg/day	*-Pulse* 1 week on, 3 weeks off Toe nail 3 pulses, follow up Finger nail 2 pulses, follow up
	-Continuous therapy 5 mg/kg/day	*-Continuous* Toe nail 12 weeks Finger nail 6 weeks
Fluconazole (tablet)	*-Intermittent therapy* 3–6 mg/kg/day (one dose/week)	*-Intermittent* Toe nail 26 weeks Finger nail 12 weeks
Terbinafine (tablet)	*-Continuous therapy* <20 kg–62.5 mg/day 20–40 kg–125 mg/day >40 kg–250 mg/day	*-Continuous* Toe nail 12 weeks Finger nail 6 weeks

Oral griseofulvin is the drug of choice for onychomycosis. Other oral antifungals such as terbinafine (Lamisil), itraconazole (Sporonox), and fluconazole (Diflucan) are increasing in usage with good supportive evidence. Table 1.6 lists systemic antifungal agents for onychomycosis.

1.10.11 Onychodystrophy

1.10.11.1 Pitting nail

This is a common problem in children. The alteration of the proximal matrix results in pitting of the nail plate surface. The characteristic pattern is punctuate depression of the nail plate, which may be small and shallow or large and deep involving few or all of the nails. It frequently occurs in normal healthy adolescents. There are many disorders associated with this condition including atopic dermatitis, alopecia areata, psoriasis, and trauma.

1.10.11.2 Beau's line/Onychomadesis

Beau's line is a transverse groove/furrow of the nail plate resulting from the interruption of nail formation. There are several causes of nail matrix interruption, such as systemic illness, high fever, or systemic maladies such as Kawasaki disease, severe bullous eruption, thyroid disease, radiation therapy, Stevens-Johnson syndrome, and chemotherapy.

The duration time of systemic illness is associated with the distance between the cuticle and the groove.

Onychomadesis is complete separation of the nail plate resulting from the arrest of nail matrix. The causes of Beau's line have also been reported to be the causes of onychomadesis. Trauma to the nail matrix can lead to this deformity.

These conditions are transient phenomena, and nails re-grow without nail plate scarring.

1.10.11.3 Trachyonychia (twenty nail dystrophy)

Trachyonychia is a deformity of nail with opaque discoloration, rough, sandpaper-like, ridging, grooves, or striations. The number of nails involved may be used in lieu of the term "twenty nail dystrophy."

This condition may occur months preceding cutaneous signs of other diseases. Commonly associated disorders are lichen planus, atopic dermatitis, psoriasis, and alopecia areata, but it may occur commonly in a normal healthy adolescent.

The exact cause of this condition is unknown. The natural course varies from 6 months to 16 years. We do not see it in adults, so it is either self-limiting or progresses to another condition.

An optional treatment is watchful waiting especially if the primary causative condition recovers. Treatment with potent topical corticosteroid at the proximal nail fold may be helpful only in some cases, but reports are anecdotal. Some practitioners use intralesional corticosteroid, triamcinolone, 0.5–1 mg/kg/month for 3–6 months.

1.10.12 Nail changes with systemic and nutritional disorders

1.10.12.1 Spoon nail/Koilonychia

Koilonychia is a common disorder of the nail plate. Physiologic koilonychia may be found in the great toenail of newborns and young infants. The nail is characterized by a central concavity with turned up distal and lateral margins.

This condition may be a secondary feature of several dermatological disorders (lichen planus, trachyonychia) or systemic diseases such as hypothyroidism, hemochromatosis, and iron deficiency anemia.

1.10.12.2 Clubbing of finger/Acropachy

Clubbing of fingers is one of the presentations of multiple systemic disorders. The most common diseases in adolescent patients include congenital cyanotic heart disease, inflammatory bowel syndrome, chronic hypoxia of pulmonary disease, and endocrinopathy.

1.10.12.3 Red lunula

This condition can be seen in several systemic diseases such as alopecia areata, lupus erythematosus, psoriasis, dermatomyositis, congestive heart failure, and carbon monoxide poisoning.

1.10.12.4 Terry's nail

This discoloration is characterized by the pink distal portion and the proximal white portion of the nail. It can be seen in cirrhosis, chronic congestive heart failure, and adult-onset diabetes.

1.10.12.5 Half-and-half nail/Lindsey's nail

This proximal nail bed is white and the distal half is red, pink, or brown; it is usually seen in renal disease with azotemia.

1.10.12.6 Yellow nail syndrome

The triad of yellow nail syndrome consists of yellow nail, lymphedema, and respiratory disease. The pathogenesis of this condition is unclear, and it is persistent.

This syndrome is associated with severe long term lymphedema, respiratory distress (especially chronic bronchitis, bronchiectasis, interstitial pneumonitis, and pleural effusion), thyroid disease, lymphoreticular malignancy, rheumatoid arthritis, lupus erythematosus, Hodgkin's lymphoma, and nephrotic syndrome. Treatment with vitamin E and/or zinc supplement may be helpful.

Acknowledgments

Modified with permission from: Feinberg AN, Schwayder TA, Tareen R, Tempark T. Adolescence and dermatology. *Int J Child Health* 2012;5(4).

References

1. Cole C, Gazewood J. Diagnosis and treatment of impetigo. *Am Fam Physician* 2007;75:859–64.
2. Rhody C. Bacterial infections of the skin. *Prim Care* 2000;27(2):459–73.
3. Stulberg DL, Penrod MA, Blatny RA. Common skin infections. *Am Fam Physician* 2002;66(1):119–24.
4. King RW, Kulkarni R. Staphylococcal scalded skin syndrome in emergency medicine. Accessed 2011 Jun 15. URL: http://emedicine.medscape.com/article/788199–overview

5. Hogan PA. Pseudomonas folliculitis. *Australas J Dermatol* 1997; 38(2):93–4.
6. Eneli I, Davies HD. Epidemiology and outcome of necrotizing fasciitis in children: An active surveillance study of the Canadian Paediatric Surveillance Program. *J Pediatr* 2007;151(1):79–84.
7. Hauser A, Fogarasi S. Periorbital and orbital cellulitis. *Pediatr Rev* 2010;31(6):242–9.
8. Stoneback JW, Hak DJ. Diagnosis and management of necrotizing fasciitis. *Orthopedics* 2011;34 (3):196.
9. Florin TA, Zaoutis TE, Zaoutis LB. Beyond cat scratch disease: Widening spectrum of Bartonella henselae infection. *Pediatrics* 2008;121(5):e1413–25.
10. Rawstron SA, Mehta S, Bromberg K. Evaluation of a Treponema pallidum-specific IgM enzyme immunoassay and Treponema pallidum western blot antibody detection in the diagnosis of maternal and congenital syphilis. *Sex Transm Dis* 2004;31(2):123–6.
11. Steere AC. Lyme disease. *N Engl J Med* 2001;345(2):115–25.
12. Murray T, Feder HM Jr. Management of tick bites and early Lyme disease: A survey of Connecticut physicians. *Pediatrics* 2001;108(6):1367–70.
13. Ilowite NT. Muscle, reticuloendothelial, and late skin manifestations of Lyme disease. *Am J Med* 1995;98(4A):63S–8.
14. Scott LA, Stone MS. Viral exanthems. *Dermatol Online J* 2003;9(3):4.
15. Aftergut K, Cockerell CJ. Update on the cutaneous manifestations of HIV infection. *Dermatol Clin* 1999;17(3):445–71.
16. Andrews MD, Burns M. Common tinea infections in children. *Am Fam Physician* 2008;77 (10):1415–20.
17. Berg D, Erickson P. Fungal skin infections in children. New developments and treatments. *Postgrad Med* 2001;110(1):83–4,87–8, 93–4.
18. Centers for Disease Control and Prevention. Accessed 2011 Jun 15. URL: http://www.cdc.gov/parasites/lice/head/diagnosis.html
19. Burkhart CN, Burkhart CG. An assessment of topical and oral prescription and over-the-counter treatments for head lice. *J Am Acad Dermatol* 1998;38(6 Pt 1):979–82.
20. Chosidow O. Scabies and pediculosis. *Lancet* 2000;355(9206):819–26.
21. Naldi L, Rebora A. Clinical practice. Seborrheic dermatitis. *N Engl J Med* 2009;360(4):387.
22. Williams HC. Clinical practice. Atopic dermatitis. *N Engl J Med* 2005;352(22):2314.
23. Leung DY. Atopic dermatitis: New insights and opportunities for therapeutic intervention. *J Allergy Clin Immunol* 2000;105(5):860.
24. Sackesen C, Sekerel BE, Orhan F, Kocabas CN, Tuncer A, Adalioglu G. The etiology of different forms of urticaria in childhood. *Pediatr Dermatol* 2004;21(2):102–8.
25. Kaplan AP. Chronic urticaria and angioedema. *N Engl J Med* 2002; 346(3):175.
26. Samel AD. Drug eruptions. Up to date. Accessed 2011 Jun 15. URL: http://www.uptodate.com/contents/drug-eruptions
27. Weston WF, Lane AT, Morelli JG. *Color textbook of pediatric dermatology,* 4th edn. Philadelphia PA: Mosby, 2007.
28. Cohen BA. *Pediatric dermatology,* 3rd edn. Philadelphia PA: Mosby, 2005.
29. Koh MJA, Tay YK. An update on Stevens-Johnson syndrome and toxic epidermal necrolysis in children. *Curr Opin Pediatr* 2009; 21:505–10.
30. Antoniou C, Dessinioti C, Stratigos AJ, Katsambas AD. Clinical and therapeutic approach to childhood acne: An update. *Pediatr Dermatol* 2009;26(4):373–80.
31. Krowchuk DP, Gelmetti C, Lucky AW. Acne. In: Schachner LA, Hansen RC, eds. *Pediatric dermatology,* 4th edn. Philadelphia, PA: Mosby, 2011:827–50.
32. Marcoux DA, Duran-McKinster C, Baselga E. Pigmentary abnormalities. In: Schachner LA, Hansen RC, eds. *Pediatric dermatology,* 4th edn. Philadelphia, PA: Mosby, 2011:700–46.

33. Paller AS, Mancini AJ. Papulosquamous and related disorders. In: Paller AS, Mancini AJ. *Hurwitz clinical pediatric dermatology: A textbook of skin disorders of childhood and adolescence,* 3rd edn. Philadelphia, PA: Elsevier Saunders; 2005:85–106.
34. Benoit S, Hamm H. Childhood psoriasis. *Clin Dermatol* 2007;25(6):555–62.
35. Shwayder T. Disorders of keratinization: Diagnosis and management. *Am J Clin Dermatol* 2004;5 (1):17–29.
36. Oji V, Traupe H. Ichthyosis: Clinical manifestations and practical treatment options. *Am J Clin Dermatol* 2009;10(6):351–64.
37. Peppercorn, MJ. Skin and eye manifestations of inflammatory bowel disease. UpToDate. Accessed 2011 Jun 15. URL: http://www.uptodate.com/contents/skin-and-eye-manifestations-of-inflammatory-bowel-disease
38. Schur PH and Moschella SL. Mucocutaneous manifestations of systemic lupus erythematosus. UpToDate. Accessed 2011 Jun 15. URL: http://www.uptodate.com/contents/mucocutaneous-manifestations-of-systemic-lupus-erythematosus
39. Paller AS, Mancini AJ. Disease of hair and nails. In: Paller AS, Mancini AJ. *Hurwitz clinical pediatric dermatology: A textbook of skin disorders of childhood and adolescence,* 3rd edn. Philadelphia, PA: Elsevier Saunders; 2005:145–83.
40. Alkhalifah A, Alsantali A, Wang E, McElwee KJ, Shapiro J. Alopecia areata update: Part II, treatment. *J Am Acad Dermatol* 2010;62(2):191–202.
41. Kakourou T, Uksal U. Guidelines for the management of tinea capitis in children. *Pediatr Dermatol* 2010;27(3):226–8.
42. Gupta AK, Skinner AR. Onychomycosis in children: A brief overview with treatment strategies. *Pediatr Dermatol* 2004; 21(1):74–9.
43. Berker D. Childhood nail diseases. *Dermatol Clin* 2006;24:355–63.
44. Holzberg M. Common nail disorders. *Dermatol Clin* 2006;24:349–54.

Ruqiya Shama Tareen

2 Psychoneuroimmunology and other interactions between skin and psyche

Psychodermatology is an emerging subspeciality of psychiatry and dermatology. A significant number of patients presenting to dermatologic practices have underlying psychiatric disorders, and many of them not only go undetected and undertreated, but also seem to have poor prognoses of their dermatologic presentations. There are intricate multidirectional interactions between skin, body, and psyche. Although our understanding of these disorders has grown significantly in the last few decades, it is still in its infancy. There are some obvious connections between skin and psyche, such as common embryologic roots and disfigurement due to skin lesions leading to psychiatric disturbances; however, there are several other interactions between skin and psyche that are lesser known. Psychoneuroimmunology is one of those phenomena that is still relatively new but offers significant insight into psychodermatologic disorders. This chapter presents a brief overview of psychodermatology including patients' perspectives of these diseases and impact on their quality of life. It also reviews the history of psychodermatology as an emerging field, psychological perspectives of skin, embyologic connections between skin and mind, and different components of psychoneuroimmunology, including neuroendocrine response to stress and interactions of central as well as peripheral nervous systems, skin, and psychiatry.

2.1 Introduction

Psychodermatology appears to be a new concept to many of us who are practicing as dermatologists, primary care clinicians, or psychiatrists, although it has been around for a long time. Physicians of the early 1930s noticed the mind–skin connection, but this connection did not gain any mainstream recognition until just a few decades ago. Figure 2.1 presents on the viscous cycle of stress, psychoneuroimmunology, psychodermatoses, and quality of life issues. Nothing can describe the multidirectional complexity of a psychodermatose with its profound impact on quality of life and low sense of general well-being better than a person who is simultaneously suffering from a debilitating skin and psychiatric condition. In a recent article about patients' perspectives, a young patient who is suffering from hidradenitis suppurativa describes it very eloquently:

> Over the years, I have become a recluse at times due to the severity of disease, and the embarrassment of draining, smelly, disgusting lesions. There are many missed days from work. Emotionally this disease can be devastating. It becomes a terrible cycle: stress leads to outbreaks,

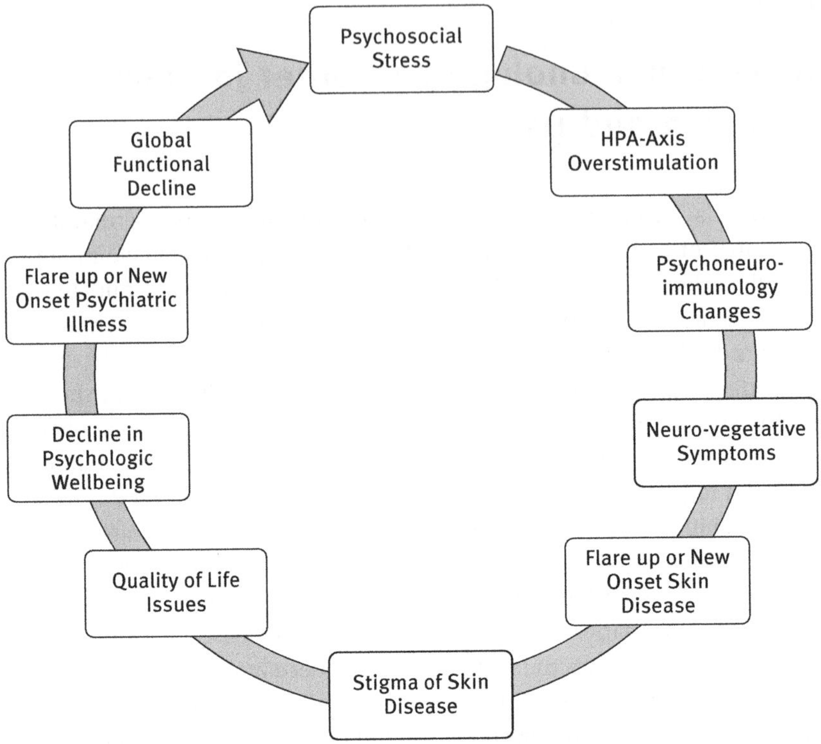

Figure 2.1: The viscious cycle of stress, psychoneuroimmunology, psychodermatoses, and quality of life issues.

> which lead to missed work, which leads to job loss, which leads to financial hardship, which leads to stress, which leads to more outbreaks, which lead to mental and emotional instability, self doubt, feelings of poor self worth, disgusting self image, and eventually severe depression, including thoughts of suicide. (1)

2.1.1 History of psychodermatology

Rodríguez-Cerdeira et al. (2) stated, "Psychodermatology has a long history but a short past." This quote has captured the history of psychodermatology very precisely. Despite that anecdotes about a skin–mind connection were found even as early as in Biblical and ancient literature, and psychoanalytical school alluded to it in various ways, it was not until 1930s and more so in the 1940s that a clearer image of psychodermatology started to emerge (2). The unitarian concept of psychosomatic medicine was that soma and psych are interconnected at many levels, leading to the expression of a disease that was initially proposed by Hippocrates, Plato, and Aesculapians around 400–500 BC (3).

It was not until 1850 when a definite description of a "cutaneous neuroses" appeared in a dermatology book written by Erasmus Wilson (2). In the earlier phase psychocutaneous connection was viewed through the prism of personality structures, and certain personalities were viewed as predisposing to psychodermatologic presentation (3). The anecdotal references and sporadic observation of a psychiatric overlay in several dermatologic disorders continued for many decades without any tangible data to support the presence of this connection until the dawn of what is termed a methodological era in psychodermatology in the mid-twentieth century (2,3).

During this phase a concerted effort was made to elucidate the concept of psychodermatology based on laying down clear definitions, collecting data from large populations of patients, and categorizing as well as developing evidence supporting the psychocutaneous connection based on data that was tangible and reliably reproducible. This gave much needed credence to this field and led more people on both sides of this discipline, i.e. dermatologist and psychiatrist, to evaluate the place of psychodermatology in their perspective fields and how to integrate it in their practice in a meaningful way. This integrative phase of the history of psychodermatology was marked by focusing on how to best address the needs of such a patient at different stages of illness. A biopsychosocial approach was proposed so that beside the dermatologic and psychiatric dual approach, the patient is also viewed in the context of their environment, family, occupation, and other social needs (2).

In the contemporary era of psychodermatology, efforts were made to delineate a clearer classification system, to propagate the field, and to increase its reach to many clinicians. A need was felt to provide common ground for fostering close relationships between dermatologists, psychiatrists, and psychologists in order to further enhance the field. The First International Congress on Psychosomatic Dermatology convened in Vienna in 1987, giving rise to the establishment of the European Society of Dermatology and Psychiatry (ESDaP) in 1993. ESDaP strives to be a unified forum where information and ideas can be exchanged to promote interdisciplinary research to ultimately improve the outcomes for patients suffering from psychodermatologic disorders (2). Figure 2.2 provides an historical outline of the history of psychodermatology (2).

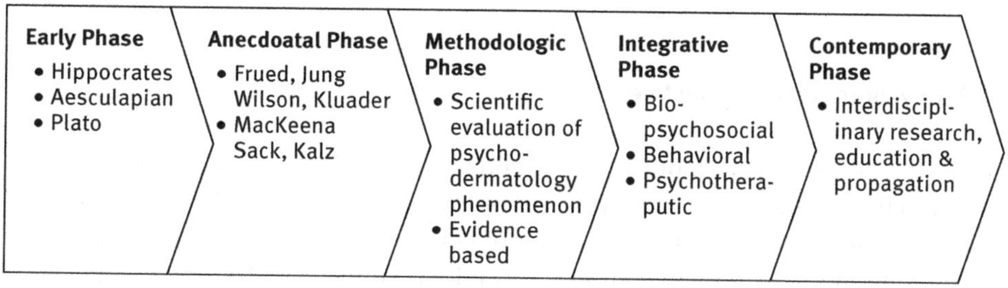

Figure 2.2: History of Psychodermatology based on Rodríguez-Cerdeira et al., Psychodermatology: Past, Present and Future. *The Open Dermatology Journal*, 2011: 5:21–27.

2.1.2 Classification of psychodermatologic disorders

Several classification systems of psychodermatologic disorders have been proposed in the last few decades. The inherent difficulty in attempting to classify these disorders lies in the fact that there is significant overlap in several disorders in terms of etiopathogenesis and factors perpetuating the disease. Examples are disorders of hair loss, such as alopecia areata, and other conditions such as acne vulgaris, psoriasis, atopic dermatitis, and vitiligo; in these conditions, there is a clear psychophysiologic origin, but all of these diseases cause disfiguring skin lesions, leading to negative body image, low self-esteem, and low self worth, culminating in secondary psychiatric disorders of mood or anxiety.

Most classifications focused on one class in some way or other, as cutaneous manifestations of a psychiatric disorder. In this class dermatologic findings are self-induced as in trichotillomania, neuroexcoriations, or dermatitis artefacta; however, other diseases under this category could be based on a specific delusional system such as delusional infestation. Self inflicted wounds can be seen in personality disorders. Then, there are other diseases where no clear primary psychiatric disease can be elicited; however, chronic psychological stressors, maladaptive behaviors, and other psychosocial factors play a predisposing and perpetuating role.

The most commonly used classification is the one proposed by Koo et al. (4), which classifies the psychodermatoses into three main groups:

- Psychophysiologic disorders: These include dermatologic diseases with a well established etiologic role of psychological stress. They include psoriasis, alopecia areata, atopic dermatitis, acne vulgaris, and others (4).
- Primary psychiatric disorders: A psychiatric disorder manifests itself with dermatologic manifestations, such as dermatitis artefacta, delusional infestation, trichotillomania, neurotic excoriations, and others (4).
- Secondary psychiatric disorders: Psychological impact of a disfiguring dermatologic condition can result in a psychiatric disease. Examples in this category include vitiligo, alopecia areata, cystic acne, ichthyosis and others (4). Figure 2.3 illustrates some of the other proposed classifications in a chronological manner (3,4,5,6,7).

2.1.3 Psychological perspective of skin

Skin is the largest organ in our body, although it is not just any organ. Indeed, it is the organ that defines our boundaries without which the self would be in dissolution with everything around it. It is our organ of communication, telling us our place in world around us – with people around us and with ourselves. Though it appears to be the most superficial organ, it can be our instantaneous connection to the deepest and most inaccessible parts of our body and soul. Our skin is our mirror into our soul

Classifications of Psychodermatologic Disease

Koblenzer 1997

- Disorders in which body image is impaired.
- Disorder in which self-esteem is impaired.
- Disorders of affect regulation (Psychophysiologic skin disease)
- The somato-psychic effects (emotional cost of skin disease)

Koo & Lebwohl 2001

- Psychophysiologic
- Primary Pschiatric disorders
- Secondary Psychiatric disorders

Folks & Warnock 2001

- Primary dermatologic disorders with secondary psychiatric sequela
- Primary dermatologic disorders significantly influenced by stress
- Primary psychiatric disorders with secondary dermatologic sequela

Harth & Gieler 2008

- Mental and psychiatric disorders accompanied by dermatologic symptoms
- Multifactorial skin diseases where mental effects play a role
- Mental disturbances as comorbidity or mental complications of skin diseases

Locala 2009

- Psychosocial factors affecting primary cutaneous disorder
- Primary psychiatric disorders manifest by cutaneous symptoms or complaints
- Secondary psychiatric disorders resulting from coping with skin disease
- Comorbid psychiatric disorders with skin disorders
- Skin diseases caused or exacerbated by psychotropic medication
- Psychiatric effects of dermatologic medications

References

- Koblennzer PJ. A brief history of psychosoamtic dermatology. Psychodermatology. Dermatlogic Clinics. 1996; 14:3: 395-97.
- Koo J, Lebwohl A. Psychodermatology: The mind and skin connection. *American Family Physician;* Dec 1, 2001; 64, 1873-8.
- Folks DG, Warnock JK. Psychocutaneous Disorders. Current Psychiatry Reports 2001, 3:219–25.
- Harth W, Gieler U. Psychosomatische.Dermatologie. Springer Medizin Verlag, Heidelberg, 2006.
- Locala JA. Current Concepts in Psychodermatology. Current Psychiatry Reports 2009, 11:211–18

Figure 2.3: Different proposed classifications of psychodermatologic disorders.

and it is the organ of expression, as it truly reflects what we are feeling, no matter how much we try to hide it from others. We blush with embarrassment, go pale with fear, appear wrinkled and haggard when stressed, sweat when anxious, and have goose bumps when afraid. It is the organ of understanding and impression; we perceive things and decide whether we like something or not based on smell, color, and aesthetic appeal of how they appear. Skin appears to merely give us a nice outer aesthetic covering, yet it gives us our identity, sense of attachment, and our very sense of belonging to others. It is our very first introduction to the outer world, starting from the very first interface with every kind of encounter from birth onward.

A neonate learns to develop trust and bonding with the mother through the tactile sensations and slowly learns to reciprocate to the mother by smiling, suckling on mother's breast, and holding her finger in the little palm, which is the first assertion of identifying an object and learning to incorporate it in a symbolic form in the psyche. The psychological experience of this earliest tactile communication between child and mother gives rise to the internal symbolization of this relationship in the child's mind, laying the foundation for all future relationships that will be encountered over the course of the entire life span. When the skin is diseased, this communication is interrupted, and the child may interpret this lack of connection as abandonment or rejection; such experiences lead to a faulty object internalization, which may predispose this child to a lifelong struggle with relationship difficulties and interpersonal maladjustments; this sets the stage for potential psychiatric problems (8). Imagine the struggles of an adolescent seeking to navigate potential problems of adolescence with a face reflective of such severe acne disease that intense shame and anger become dominant in his or her life.

2.1.4 Skin, mind, and the embryological embrace

Skin and brain both share an embryological origin from the single layer of germinal cells – the ectoderm. The ectoderm differentiates into columnar neural ectoderm and forms the neural fold in the central part; on the ends it gives rise to cells forming surface ectoderm. The neural ectoderm becomes internalized with closure of the neural fold resulting in formation of the neural tube, which will form the central nervous system. The surface ectoderm then covers the embryo from the outside. A specialized population of multi-potent cells known as neural crest cells emerge from the junction of neural and surface ectoderm; these cells gives rise to many different types of tissues including the epidermis, sympathetic nervous system, peripheral sensory neurons, and melanocytes (9). The differentiation and full individuation of different neurons interspersed within epidermal cells depend on the neurotrophins such as nerve growth factor and other chemical signals that attract or dispel certain cells, ensuring growth and expansion of the sensory peripheral nerve cells, ganglion, and interconnection between the neuronal system in the right direction (10,11).

2.2 Psychoneuroimmunology

Psychoneuroimmunology is defined as the study of behavioral-neural-endocrine-immune system interactions (12). This is an intriguing field of immunology that has intricate multidimensional relationships with the central and peripheral nervous system, stress, and the systemic response of body and mind to it as well as how it results in expression of certain diseases, including skin diseases. See Figure 2.4.

2.2.1 Neuroendocrine response to stress

Skin is very well connected with the endocrine system and plays a vital role in maintaining homeostatis when faced with internal or external stress. The intricate relationship of stress and causation of disease in different organ system is well established, but it is nowhere so transparent as in skin and psychiatric disease. The hypothalamic-pituitary-adrenal axis (HPA axis) is a multilevel endocrine system starting with the hypothalamus; there is synchronizing activation or down regulation of pituitary and adrenal glands, which is the vital system of the body to respond and adapt to all kinds of stress. Many skin diseases have a cause and effect relationship with the HPA axis due to its ability to maintain basal and stress related homeostasis when dealing with internal and external stress (13).

Corticotropin releasing hormone (CRH) not only triggers the hormonal cascade of the HPA axis from the hypothalamus in response to stressors, but it also has a wide distribution of CRH receptors in other neural circuits, including the limbic system and the sympathetic arousal system both in the brain and spinal cord. This leads to a well-coordinated chain of events in response to various stresses, including

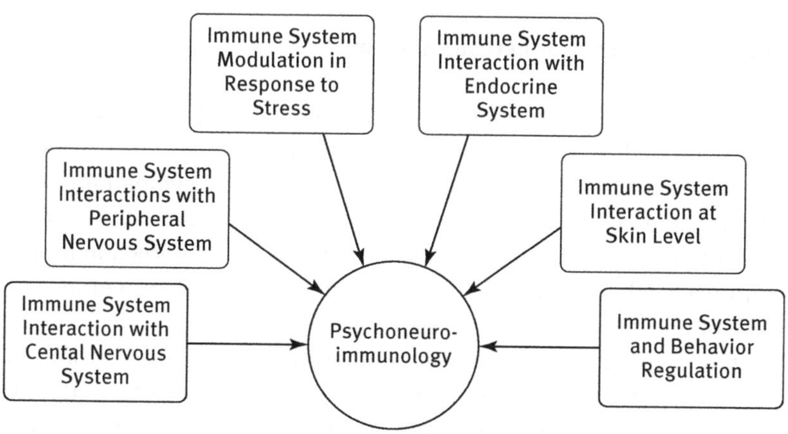

Figure 2.4: Psychoneuroimmunology: An interaction of behavioral-neural-endocrine-immune systems.

physiologic, behavioral, and arousal as well as changes in appetite and sexual and activity levels.

At the anterior pituitary gland the stress response is also co-mediated by arginine vasopressin (AVP) and other nonapeptides. CRH and AVP are secreted in near synchronized pulses, inducing the secretion of adrenocorticotropin hormone (ACTH) (13). The CRH stimulation of ACTH has a diurnal variation with highest peak between 6:00 AM to 8:00 AM and lowest trough at midnight; also, it is greatly affected by levels of stress. ACTH exerts its action by binding with melanocortin receptors 2 (MC2) found in all three layers of adrenal cortex, stimulating adenyl cyclase, and generating cyclic adenosine monophosphate (cAMP) that activates downstream enzyme pathways in steroidogenesis (13). Glucocorticoid synthesis mainly takes place in the zona fasciculata of the adrenal cortex and is responsible for activating the negative feedback loop to terminate the stress response at the level of suprahypothalamic centers, hypothalamus, and pituitary gland.

This self-regulatory and time limited cycle prevents adverse consequences of prolonged adaptive changes such as catabolism and immunosuppression (13). In cases when stress is chronic and gives rise to continual hypersecretion of CRH, this perpetuates an unrelenting activation of the HPA axis. The result is a syndromal state characterized by behavioral disturbances such as depression and various anxiety spectrum disorders, anorexia nervosa, and several systemic sequelae that include central obesity, hyperthyroidism, diabetes mellitus, metabolic syndrome, osteoporosis, atherosclerosis, immunosuppression, and increased susceptibility to certain infectious as well as neoplastic diseases (13). The role of chronic stress in the pathogenesis of skin disease has been proposed since the early era of modern medicine, although good scientific data has only emerged in the last few decades to support and consolidate this hypothesis (13).

2.2.2 Immune response and central nervous system

The central nervous system (CNS) modulates the immune response by two pathways. One is through its neuroendocrine response of the HPA axis as described in Section 2.2.1, and the second is the central activation of the autonomic sympathetic system outflow, affecting the release of norepinephrine from the adrenal cortex in response to a physiologic stimulus. Both of these pathways are bidirectional and work in-synch with each other to maintain integrity of the immune system and to modulate the level and duration of immune responses (14).

The central nervous system (CNS) also exerts other modulatory effects through specific neuroendocrine receptors located on leukocytes such as growth hormone (GH), β-endorphin, thyroid hormone, luteinizing hormone-releasing hormone, and somatostatin. Deficiency of GH can lead to decreased production of antibodies and decreased activity of natural killer (NK) cells as well as T-cell lymphocytes. Similar deficiency of prolactin can inhibit cellular and antibody response predisposing to certain infections (14,15). When there is an interruption in this neuroendocrine pathway, for example, as a result of a lesion in anterior hypothalmic region, it can lead to suppression of cellular response from the spleen and thymus and antibody production as well as impaired response of natural killer cells and anaphylactic reaction (14).

A third way the CNS participates in immune responses is more local and is via microglia, which are inactive or resting macrophages found all over the brain and spinal cord. When responding to a stimuli, these resting microglia can become active by first expressing cell-surface markers such as major histocompatibility complex (MHC) molecules, complement receptors, and CD4 cells; they then morphologically change to become active phagocytes. However, their phagocytic abilities are much lower than their peripheral counterparts, and when activated, they can release certain pro-inflammatory cytokines such as platelet-activating factor, reactive oxygen molecules, and nitric oxide that can cause neuronal injury (15).

2.2.3 Immune response and peripheral nervous system

Both primary and secondary peripheral lymphoid organs and tissues are heavily innervated by the peripheral nervous system and especially by sympathetic nerves. The function of sympathetic innervation is to modulate the innate immune response in such a way that a specific immune response is initiated and terminated accordingly to the stimulus strength and not to continue beyond what is needed. The sympathetic innervations generally follow a similar pattern in different tissues. The nerve fibers are more dense in T-cell zones as compared to the B-cell zone. The noradrenergic innervated areas are also rich with neuropeptides involved in modulation of immunologic processes; these include substance P, neuropeptide Y, calcitonin gene-related peptide, somatostatin, opiate peptides, and vasoactive intestinal peptide (14,15).

Many lymphoid cells and tissues have catecholamine receptors, especially β2-adrenergic-receptor subtype and various neuropeptide-specific receptors. When stimulated by the catecholamines and other neurotransmitters released from nerve fibers, these neuropeptides can exert their affect by binding to specific receptors to modulate the immune response by initiating a cascade of intracellular signals; this leads to alteration of particular cell line proliferation and antibody and cytotoxin production that promotes vasodilation and facilitates adhesions of leukocytes to modulate local inflammatory response as well as retention of these cells in certain lymphoid tissues (15).

2.2.4 Immune response and skin disease

The immuno-neuro-endocrine network can be compromised by stress and be unable to respond to predictable stressors such as seasonal changes or an unpredictable stressor such as a psychosocial stress. This results in what is defined as an allostatic overload, resulting in various levels of dysregulation ranging from inflammation to immunosuppression (16). Skin mast cells are crucial in maintaining an allostatic balance. Paus et al. describes them as a "central switchboard" of skin-stress-response (16). Skin mast cells are regulated by various factors; they are activated and promoted by stress mediators such as CRH, ACTH, NGF (nerve growth factor), SP (substance P), and stem-cell factor while inhibited by glucocorticoids and cathecholamines (16). Several skin diseases represent a classic model of this paradigm; these include atopic dermatitis, psoriasis, hair disorders, urticaria, angioedema, and skin infections (16).

Stress can cause new onset and relapses in psoriasis or resistance to treatment. HPA-axis dysregulation has been proposed as a pathogenic factor in psoriasis. Patients who consider their disease as stress-responsive, when exposed to an experimental acute social stressor, demonstrate lower levels of cortisol production versus those who were exposed to cognitive or emotional stress. These stress-responsive patients were also more likely to be anxious. Patients with psoriasis also seem to have an incoordinated response to stress with an overactive sympathetic adrenal-medullary axis coupled with a hyperactive HPA axis (17). Psoriatic plaques have increased sensory nerve fiber density in comparison to unaffected skin. They also show dysregulation of the HPA axis with an attenuated glucocorticoid response when exposed to a stressor (17). There is a also a higher than expected expression of T-cell migration and chemotaxis mediated by NGF. Psychosocial therapies such as meditation and relaxation techniques have been shown to be effective adjunctive measures in treating psoriasis (18).

Atopic dermatitis (AD), a chronic neurogenic inflammatory disease, provides us with a good model to understand the implication of psychoneuroimmunology in such psychophysiologic diseases (see Chapter 5). Stress plays an important role in exacerbation or initial expression of AD. In a survey of more than 1,457 patients with AD living in and around the area hit by a major earthquake in 1995, about 38% of the patients living near the epicenter reported relapse of AD compared to 7% of control group. The presence of subjective stress was reported by 63% of patients in comparison to 19% from a control group (19).

Since AD is a disease of early childhood, the early life stress has been studied in this regard. Stress due to stressful early life experiences (such as improper, neglectful, or inconsistent care by the primary care giver – in most instances the mother) can lead to a sense of abandonment and rejection, which can sensitize the immune system at such an early age leading to a dysregulated immune system. When the HPA axis is continually overactive, it leads to increased productions of catecholamines and glucocorticoids, which in turn can cause an imbalance of T lymphocyte helper T_H1 and T_H2 cells ratio by overproducing the T_{H2} cells. Atopic lesions have abnormal population of T_{H2} cells. This leads to an up-regulation of T_{H2} mediated antibody production including IL-4, IL-10, and IL-13 (20). This is coupled with release of neuropeptides such as Substance P (SP), nerve growth factor, and calcitonin gene related peptide from efferent nerve fibers; such a result is in response to stimulation by cytokines and proteases (20).

Skin mast cells also carry various neuropeptides receptors on their surface enabling them to play a pivotal role in this psycho-immuno-neuro-endocrine axis. Skin mast cells also produce various pro-inflammatory substances leading to the local effects of inflammation within the skin, initiating the classic itch–scratch cycle. Any stressful event leading to psychological stress can easily cause a flare up of AD, exacerbating this itch–scratch cycle (20). This can lead to physical disturbance of the epidermal barrier by constant trauma due to scratching, leading to worsening of AD lesions and perpetuating the itch–scratch cycle all over again. Unrelenting pruritus itself can cause significant anxiety and mood problems; psychotropic medications such as selective serotonin reuptake inhibitors have been shown to be effective in these instances (20).

A significant number of patients with urticaria report psychosocial stress as a cause of onset with exacerbation of chronic urticaria (21). Although it is not well appreciated, chronic idiopathic can impact the quality of life (QoL) in significant ways, almost as much that seen in patients with AD and even more than the QoL impairment seen in patients with psoriasis, acne, and vitiligo. Mast cell degranulation is a prominent finding in physical urticaria induced by sun or cold exposure as well as cholinergic or dermatographic urticarias. Basophils also play an important role in magnitude and duration of urticaria. Basophils show a decreased functional response to IgE receptor stimulation. In autoimmune urticaria, histamine-releasing autoantibodies activate mast cells and basophils via complement to potentiate histamine release (22).

The skin is our first interface with the environment and defends us from all sorts of toxins, infections, and other noxious agents. Psychological stress can cause dysregulation of the immune system, resulting in weakening of the skin defense system against all sorts of infecting agents, or reactivation of dormant pathogens. This phenomenon is best illustrated with an example of herpes virus (HSV-1) infection and relapses. Cellular immunity is the main defense to keep this virus within the cells in an inactive state. Yang et al has shown that the stress of taking an examination resulted in a decrease in NK cell activity, down-regulation of production of interferon-Υ, and deficiency of virus specific T-cells and antibody production (23). Once the immune system is under duress due to any kind of stress, whether it is physical or psychological, the latent virus has a chance to rejuvenate itself, resulting in disease flare up (23).

2.2.5 Immune response and psychiatric disease

Many psychiatric illnesses are known to have associated abnormalities of immune and endocrine system. Diseases that have been shown to have evidence of hyperactive

HPA-axis include depression (especially melancholic depression), anorexia nervosa, and several anxiety disorders, including obsessive compulsive disorder and panic disorders. On the other hand, atypical depression and seasonal affective disorder are associated with a hypoactive HPA axis (13). Melancholic depression is a classic example of how a chronically dysregulated HPA axis leads to a persistent overproduction of glucocorticoids that induces an attenuation of ACTH response to exogenous CRH.

Patients suffering from melancholic depression also show sequelae of an over-stimulated HPA axis, such as the metabolic syndrome with central obesity, insulin resistance, increased blood pressure, a high blood sugar level, and abnormal cholesterol levels. There is also evidence of innate and T-call mediated immune suppression. The life expectancy of patients with melancholic depression is decreased by 15–20 years because of an over-stimulated HPA axis and also due to the fact that this hyperactive state predisposes patients to atherosclerosis, certain infections, and neoplastic conditions (13). Alcohol dependence and narcotic withdrawal can also cause an overactive HPA axis.

Other abnormalities of the immune system have been reported in patients suffering from chronic depression; these include increased production of cytokines from macrophages, certain interleukins (IL-2, soluble IL-2R), C-reactive protein, interferon-Y, and tumor necrosis factor-α (24). On the other hand, levels of IL-6 and IL-1b were inconsistent in some studies (24). Depressed patients also show alterations in cellular immunity with leukocytosis and decreased production of NK cells, T and B lymphocytes, along with helper and suppressor T-cells. The function of B cells is also altered in chronic depressive states. There is evidence that behavioral conditioning can modulate immune responses (14).

2.3 Conclusion

Psychodermatologic disorders are multidimensional with complex and, at times, ill-defined etiologies and pathogeneses. Some of the concepts now emerging are fascinating and appear to answer some of the longstanding questions about the mind and skin connection, although there is still much that remains unanswered. This chapter summarizes some of the basic concepts of psychoneuroimmunology and serves as a primer for better understanding discussions on pediatric psychodermatology found in this publication.

References

1. Solarski ST. Living with hidradenitis supprativa. Patient's perspectives. *Dermatol Nurs* 2004; 16(5):447–9.
2. Rodríguez-Cerdeira C, Pera-Grasa JT, Molares A. Psychodermatology: Past, present and future. *Open Dermatol J* 2011;5:21–7.

3. Koblennzer PJ. A brief history of psychosomatic dermatology. Psychodermatology. *Dermatol Clin* 1996;14(3):395–7.
4. Koo J, Lebwohl A. Psychodermatology: The mind and skin connection. *Am Fam Physician* 2001;64:1873–8.
5. Folks DG, Warnock JK. Psychocutaneous disorders. *Curr Psychiatr Rep* 2001;3:219–25.
6. Harth W, Gieler U. *Psychosomatische. Dermatologie.* Heidelberg: Springer, 2006. [German]
7. Locala JA. Current concepts in psychodermatology. *Curr Psychiatr Rep* 2009;11:211–8.
8. Walser A. Bodies in skin: A philosophical and theological approach to genetic skin diseases. *J Relig Health* 2010;49:96–104.
9. Motohashi M, Aoki H, Chiba K. Multipotent cell fate of neural crest-like cells derived from embryonic stem cells. *Stem Cells* 2007,25;2; 402–10.
10. Le Douarin NM, Calloni GW, Dupin E. The stem cells of the neural crest. *Cell Cycle* 2008; 7(8):1013–9.
11. Le Douarin NM. Cell line segregation during peripheral nervous system ontogeny. *Science* 1986;231:1515–22.
12. The Concise Corsini Encyclopedia of Psychology and Behavioral Science. Accessed 2011 Nov 26. URL: http://www.credoreference.com.libproxy.library.wmich.edu/entry/wileypsych/psychoneuro immunology
13. Kyrou I, Tsigos C. Hypothalamic-pituitary-adrenal axis. In: Linos D, Heerden J, eds. *Adrenal glands.* Berlin: Springer, 2005:19–32.
14. Ader R, Cohen N, Felten D. Psychoneuroimmunology: Interactions between the nervous system and the immune system. *Lancet* 1995;345:99–103.
15. Watson SCL, Nance DM, nervous system–immune system interactions. In: Conn PM, ed. *Neuroscience in medicine,* 3rd edn.Totowa, NJ: Humana Press, 2008.
16. Paus R, Theoharides TC, Arck PC. Neuroimmunoendocrine circuitry of the "brain-skin connection." *Trends Immunology* 2008;27(1):32–9.
17. Richards HL, Ray DW, Kirby B. Response of the hypothalamic–pituitary–adrenal axis to psychological stress in patients with psoriasis. *Br J Dermatol* 2005;153:1114–20.
18. Tausk F, Elenkov I, Moynihan J. Psychoneuroimmunology. *Dermatol Ther* 2008;21:22–31.
19. Ginsburg IH, Prystowsky JH, Kornfeld DS, Wolland H. Role of emotional factors in adults with atopic dermatitis. *Int J Dermatol* 1993;32:656–60.
20. Suárez AL, Feramisco JD, Koo J, Steinhoff M. Psychoneuroimmunology if psychological stress and atopic dermatitis: Pathophysiologic and therapeutic updates. *Acta Derm Venereol* 2012;92:7–15.
21. Liverant E. Psychoneurodermatologic disorders. In: Norman RA, ed. *Diagnosis of aging skin diseases.* London: Springer, 2008:213–24.
22. Gober LM, Saini SS. Allergic urticaria. *Clin Basic Immunodermatol* 2008;2:459–77.
23. Yang EV, Glaser R. Stress-induced immunomodulation: impact on immune defenses against infectious disease. *Biomed Pharmacother* 2000;54:245–50.
24. Yang K, Xie G, Zhang Z, Wang C. Levels of serum interleukin (IL)-6, IL-1b, tumour necrosis factor-a and leptin and their correlation in depression. *Aust NZ J Psychiatry* 2007; 41:266–73.

Donald E. Greydanus

3 A clinician's approach to psychocutaneous diseases in adolescents: Untying the Gordian knot

Patients with psychocutaneous disease can be challenging for clinicians. The *sine qua non* of successful management of the adolescent patient with a dermatological condition and potential primary or secondary psychiatric conditions is to acquire a careful medical and psychological evaluation of this patient. Time is necessary for this evaluation and also to develop a clinical rapport with the adolescent to help develop management plans that may change to allow appropriate compliance in this patient. As professionals, physicians need to consider the needs of their patients, and one of the best gifts health care clinicians can provide to their patients is their time. Principles of confidentiality and informed consent must be followed. The therapeutic alliance will be enhanced if both adolescent patient and clinician are engaged in clinical decision-making processes. Patients should be allowed choice of management options where appropriate, while considerable care should be given to adverse effects of medications or other treatment plans. Recalcitrant cases should prompt both a reconsideration of the differential diagnosis but also attention for underlying psychological factors and potential reasons for limited compliance by the often challenging adolescent patient.

"Time is the wisest counselor of all."

Pericles (495–429 BC)

3.1 Introduction

A complete history and physical examination is important to be performed by the competent clinician when evaluating the pediatric patient with clinical concerns including psychocutaneous disorders. A focused history can be utilized as time permits, but sometimes a more comprehensive evaluation is needed to find the correct diagnosis after a succinct differential diagnosis, which leads to selective laboratory testing and the optimal management based on establishing the correct diagnosis.

3.1.1 History taking skills in adolescent patients

The interview process is a key component in evaluation of pediatric patients, particularly the adolescent who presents with dermatological disorders (1). The *medical interview* is typically separated into three core components: information gathering,

Table 3.1: Elements of Physician–Patient Communication (2,3,4)

1. Opening discussion (Kalamazoo Consensus Statement)
2. Process of gathering information
3. Understanding the patient's perspective
4. Sharing information
5. Reaching agreement on problems and plans
6. Providing closure to the encounter

Table 3.2: Patterns of Physician–Patient Communication (4)

1. Narrow Biomedical Interview
2. Expanded Biomedical Interview
3. Biopsychosocial Interview
4. Psychosocial Interview
5. Consumerist Interview

relationship building, and patient education. The six basic aspects of successful clinician–patient communication is identified in Table 3.1 in which the opening discussion is the initial step, followed by the ability to collect key information, in addition to sharing information that the pediatric patient needs to understand for optimal management compliance (2,3,4).

Understanding the patient's perspective is an integral part of this overall process in order to reach a mutual agreement between clinician and patient in regards to identified dermatological problems as well as psychological issues and recommended management plans. This is especially important when dealing with older children and adolescents. The final step in this interaction is properly closing the medical interview to allow the patient (and family for children) to successfully leave the encounter feeling that their questions were answered and that they are willing to return after following the clinician's recommendations.

Table 3.2 lists various clinician–patient communication patterns (4). The least favorite pattern is the "narrow biomedical interview" model since it is very closely clinician-controlled as seen in this mini-scenario:

Clinician: What brings you (the patient) in today?
Patient: I have pimples.
Clinician: Where are the pimples? When did it start? How long has it been bothering you? Are you taking any medications for it?

In this example, the patient is quickly interrupted with a barrage of queries, and the clinician fails to use the "continuer" technique to identify all the issues the patient (and/or family) may have. Also, it fails to appreciate nonverbal patient cues, such as: "You seem upset today – can you tell me about that?"

There is some dialogue on psychosocial and behavioral issues in the "expanded biomedical model"; however, it remains dominated by the interviewer. A much

Table 3.3: Clinical Skills of the Medical Interview (American Academy on Physician and Patient: AAPP): PEARLS (2,3,4)

1. Partnership
2. Empathy
3. Apology
4. Respect
5. Legitimization
6. Support

healthier model is the "biopsychosocial" one in which there is a better balance of control between the adolescent and clinician. Patients control the "psychosocial model" and this is more popular with adult patients. Finally, the model that is often not popular with clinicians is the "consumerist model" since it is fully controlled by the patient who seeks answers to miscellaneous questions.

The American Academy on Physician and Patient (AAPP) has developed the PEARLS mnemonic to review core elements of the medical interview (Table 3.3) (2,3,4). The concept of the link between patient and physician is noted by the term *Partnership*, that is between the patient and clinician. *Empathy* means that the clinician expresses an understanding of the patient (and family) for the newborn, child, or adolescent patient. *Apology* notes that the clinician should apologize for lateness in seeing the patient or lateness in getting laboratory tests. Clinicians should acknowledge the patient's suffering and difficulties as suggested in the term *Respect*, while *Legitimization* means that the clinician acknowledges feelings of the patient or family (i.e. being upset, sad, anxious, others). Finally, *Support* suggests the critical idea that clinicians provide the patient (and family in younger patients) with the concept that s/he will not be abandoned by the clinician in the case of chronic or recalcitrant dermatological disorders (2).

3.2 Interviewing the adolescent patient

It is important to note that the adolescent is in a process of emancipating from parents while becoming more invested in his/her peer group. The clinician's goal with each office visit should be to identify the concerns the patient has with regard to his dermatological condition, seek out other issues related to this concern, provide appropriate clinical recommendations, and deliver an educational experience for the youth as well as his or her family. It is vital to understand the thoughts and feelings of the adolescent patient, especially if there is a link between the dermatological condition and the mental health of this patient, as noted in the many chapters of this publication. It is difficult to develop a beneficial plan for a specific patient if the health care professional has little knowledge of this specific patient.

Key components to improve the office visit are listed in Table 3.4 in a mnemonic format of 6 As (5). Certainly health care providers should be **a**vailable to their patients

Table 3.4: The 6 As of Providing Clinical Care to Youth in the Outpatient Setting (5,6)

1. Availability
2. Accessibility
3. Approachability
4. Acceptability
5. Appropriateness
6. Affordability

in office hours that are convenient or **accessible** to them. Early morning hours may not be good for many adolescents who like to stay up late and get up late if possible. Evening or later afternoon hours may be more acceptable to many of these adolescents. The clinician and office staff should like this age group, and this *approachability* should be evident to the youth and family upon entering the office.

The décor can be "teen-friendly," and the patient should not have to endure a hostile clinician or nurse who may not approve of adolescent dress or behavior. The patient is concerned enough with his/her dermatological condition (and/or other issues) to come to the office and needs a warm and accepting environment from the office setting. For example, the adolescent female taking contraception to prevent pregnancy should not have to encounter an office person who does not approve of teenage sexual behavior.

Acceptability suggests that the clinician understands and accepts the youth's developmental stage and need for increasing autonomy. One should provide *appropriate* health care that deals with the patient's needs and not those of the health care provider. Some time should be spent alone with the adolescent patient to let him or her know he or she is the central figure in this clinician–adolescent patient–family triad. Confidentiality is part of the care of all youth. Certainly, the patient and family need care that is **a**ffordable to them; otherwise recommendations may not be followed, and follow-up appointments may be curtailed.

Though time is money, it is critical that enough time be spent with the adolescent patient to both identify the dermatological issue and begin the process of developing rapport with the adolescent patient (5,6,7). One should be caring and honest with this potentially fragile patient – just being oneself is best while avoiding a false persona that the youth can spot quickly. Once turned off, this patient will not reveal salient (i.e. personal) information and may not follow treatment recommendations. This traveler through adolescence is on a journey, often a trek of turmoil and discovery; s/he needs a comforting health care guide and not a crusty critic! The fundamental clinician who judges the youth and conveys a non-accepting attitude toward the patient's lifestyle does not help this patient on the passage from childhood to adulthood.

Adolescents become very embarrassed when asked to take off clothes and get into a gown. One can spend time alone with the youth who is fully clothed and assess the cognitive and developmental stage of the youth. Is s/he in a Piagetian concrete thinking stage where abstract thoughts and vague questions are not understood well? Failure to answer a question may mean the question was not understood and not a sign of negativity. Non-adherence to a recommended treatment plan may indicate a failure to understand the plan or a conscious (subconscious) effort to sabotage the plan because of conflicts with authorities (i.e. parents) over issues of autonomy. As one gets to know the adolescent patient, it is easier to identify the reasons for such sabotage and ways to overcome it. Education of the youth is important but must be based on knowledge of the patient, which simply takes time. Certainly, time should be spent with the parent (s) or guardian(s) in fact finding and guidance as well.

3.2.1 Confidentiality

Adolescents are not large, still-dependent children, nor are they small, autonomous adults. It is critical for the adolescent patient to understand what is confidential and what is not. Diseases related to sexual or other high-risk, personal behavior require the clinician to establish guidelines with what is and is not shared with parents without the adolescent's permission (8,9,10). This is based on local laws and should be understood by clinicians, adolescents, and parents. Some issues cannot be confidential, such as thoughts of suicide or homicide. Others can be confidential. In such cases, the clinician can ask permission from the youth to share such data with parents. Not respecting the youth's confidentiality can result in the clinician sabotaging management plans.

3.2.2 Parental confidentiality

There are different models of care the clinician can utilize depending on specific circumstances. Parents may request a private meeting if sensitive issues are present. However, meetings without the adolescent present can led to resentment on the part of the youth and failure of this young patient to reveal sensitive data or fully cooperate with treatment plans. One model that can be used is to see parents with the adolescent together, and youth alone, and then, if needed, the parents alone. As the child matures into an adolescent, issues of patient and parental confidentiality must change as well. See Chapter 12.

3.2.3 Health questionnaires

Questionnaires can be very useful to identify family history, past medical history, past surgical history, and other pertinent health information. Indeed, various health care questionnaires have been prepared that youth can complete in private, while parents can complete their own questionnaires (11,12). Considerable clinician and staff time can be saved, and results may provide direction regarding what further details are needed in direct tête-à-tête interviews. If the answers are handled appropriately, confidentiality can be assured and questions can be in a safe, non-threatening tone that may ask for yes/no responses.

3.2.4 Interview techniques

A number of modus operandi can be utilized to aid in the interview process (Table 3.5) (5,6). One well-known one is represented by the *HEADS+ (HEEADSSS)* mnemonic (13). **H** represents *home* (how are things at home?), **E** represents *education* (school) and *eating patterns*, **A** is for *activities*, **D** is for *drugs*, and **S** represents the critical issues of *safety*, *suicidality*, and *sexuality* (5,3,14,15). In a general interview one usually starts with "safe" questions (i.e. general medical issues, school, others) before getting into personal topics as sexuality, drug use, and others. The questions can be directed more specifically if the presenting concern is dermatological; however, sexual behavior or thoughts of suicide should not be missed if the differential diagnosis considers such factors (i.e. gonococcal dermatitis syndrome, dermatitis artefacta, others).

Youth with concrete thinking skills have problems with "time frame" questions such as "How long have you had your rash?" A better approach may be: "Did your rash start before or after. . . .?" One can name an event that would be easily identified by the patient. Some adolescents have difficulty describing severity of symptoms and do better with "On a scale of 1–10 (10 is the worst), what number or range would you use for your pain?"

Sometimes a *mini-Likert* can be useful, such as "How would you compare your school/home performance with your friends?" One could also ask, "Do you feel less

Table 3.5: Useful Tools in the Medical Interview of Adolescents (see the text) (5,6)

1. HEEADSS
2. Time Frame Questions
3. Numerical Rating Scale
4. Mini-Likert Scale
5. Three Wishes Questions
6. Empathic Lead-in Approach
7. Advance Notice of Understanding Approach
8. Indirection and Projection Approach
9. Active Listener Approach
10. Clarifying and Paraphrasing Approach
11. Using Silence Approach

troubled, more troubled, or the same about. . .than your friends?" Some health care professionals use the "*Three Wishes*" approach and ask the adolescent patient to make "three wishes" about their current situation. For example, "If you could change yourself, your friends, your family, and your life, what three things would you change and how?" The answers may vary, but it gives one a sense of the youth's thinking skills and what issues are important.

Another approach that can be useful to identify potentially anxiety-stimulating topics is the "empathic lead-in"; for example, "If I were you, I would feel. . . .Is that true for you?" If the clinician is correct, the discussion from the patient may develop; if one is incorrect, it may prompt the patient to correct the clinician's impression. When told that one is wrong, the clinician can say, "Well, OK, then, can you tell me how it is for you?"

The "advanced notice of understanding" approach may be useful in some situations in which the clinician tells the adolescent patient how s/he will respond to various subjects. For example, the clinician says: "Many adolescents today use drugs or have sex. . .where do you stand on this?" This approach conveys a non-judgmental attitude on the health care professional's part and lets the patient know s/he will not be judged poorly if involved in various high risk behaviors. Also, the "indirection and projection" approach can be useful to reduce patient anxiety about certain subjects. For example, the clinician can say "What do teenagers your age think of sex, pot, (other subjects). . .?" OR "What is going on at your school about. . . .?" The adolescent patient can project his/her own range of experiences in the answers, and the peer group often reflects the specific patient's actions.

3.2.5 Active listening skills

Active listening skills are important to utilize when interviewing patients in which one seeks to hear exactly what the individual is or is not saying in response to questions (5,6). Taking the wrong history by incorrect listening can encourage the wrong diagnosis and wrong management plans. Patients can sort out their issues much better if the clinician is actively listening and interacting with them. One technique is "clarifying" issues in which one repeats the stated problem back to the adolescent; this helps to avoid selective or imaginary listening by repeating what was heard. Repeating allows the adolescent to make corrections or clarifications. If the patient concludes you are not listening, s/he may change answers.

Paraphrasing can be helpful in which clinicians use short paraphrases or summaries about what was said or what one thinks was said. The clinician can say: "If I heard you correctly, you noted. . .Correct?" Or "do you mean you are telling me. . ." Certainly this is done in a gentle manner so the patient does not feel you are questioning the validity or truthfulness of his/her responses. The health care professional can also provide insights into issues; for example, one can note, "You are really worried about this rash," or "You seem very anxious about this condition, is that right?" Also, *silence* can be a very useful technique in some situations. There does not have to be constant chatter or conversation, and if the adolescent stops talking, silence may provide time to gather thoughts or feelings. Silence on the part of the clinician for 10 or 15 seconds may lead the youth to begin further dialogue.

3.3 Concepts of the physical examination

The extent of the physical examination is based on the presenting issues and history of previous examinations. Both the medical history and exam can be used to establish rapport with this patient and provide education in pertinent, important aspects of their health as related to the reason for this health care visit (5,6,14,16,17). Clinicians and staff should seek to avoid unnecessary embarrassment as previously noted. Keep the youth fully clothed while doing the history.

Conduct the physical exam with full respect for the privacy of this patient, and utilize proper draping at all times. Young adolescents may be more developed (i.e. higher sexually maturity rating) than one might think because of age. One breast can be examined while the other is covered. Genitalia and lower extremities can be covered while the abdomen is examined. There are many variations on how to do the specific exam, but seek permission for examination of sensitive areas, and seek to avoid embarrassing this young patient. The issue of chaperonage is done according to local custom as well as the wishes of the patient (5,6,16).

A *mental status examination* affords the opportunity to observe if mental health disorders are complicating the dermatological condition(s) that may be present (18,19,20,21,22,23,24). Is the patient fully oriented (i.e. time, place, person)? Is there a normal or flat affect? Is there good eye contact with the clinician? Is s/he cooperative with the examination? Is s/he dressed appropriately for age and local area? Does s/he appear depressed, angry, upset, and/or express thoughts of suicide? Is there an intact memory, judgment, and intellect? What is the cognitive state (i.e. Piagetian concrete vs formal operational)? Is there evidence of hallucinations or delusions? The rest of the physical exam depends on specific complaints of the patient and need for examination of specific areas of the skin.

3.4 Successful management of the adolescent patient

3.4.1 Informed consent

The rights of patients to consent to various treatments have been defined by the concept of informed consent. This has been a legal as well as medical term in Western medicine that was derived over many centuries out of the Hippocratic tradition.

This practice was based on the concept that clinicians would always act in the best interests of their patients (25). Medicine in the United States gradually focused on rights of patients that included receiving education about their maladies and also included the concept that these patients may agree or not agree to receive recommended treatments. Patients have the right to receive informed consent assuming they are capable of such consent. The atrocities of physicians as examined during the Nuremberg trials (including the Doctors' Trial) of 1945–1947 provided further impetus to rights of patients (25). The term *informed consent* was first used in a medical malpractice trial by Paul G. Gebhard in 1957 in the United States (26).

Those with mental retardation, comatose condition, Alzheimer's disease, childhood age, severe mental illness, and other states or situations provide direct challenges to this concept of informed consent. However, when the clinician is dealing with the adolescent patient, it is vital that this patient understand and agree to management options suggested by the clinician. Subservient to this concept is the principle that the clinician has conducted an appropriate evaluation, knows the patient, and can thus provide the best recommendations to this patient with rights of informed consent.

If the adolescent patient does not understand and agree to the management recommendations, s/he may sabotage the treatment, refuse to follow the suggested plan, and damage any potential therapeutic alliance between patient and clinician. Interwoven in this plan is that principles of confidentiality should be clearly established for this patient that take into consideration rights of the adolescent patient and parents/guardians (8,9). Indeed, confidentiality is never absolute, and the judgment of the knowledgeable clinician who understands the patient is always critical. Laws of the country must be followed, such as HIPAA (Health Insurance Portability and Accountability Act) rules in the United States (27).

3.4.2 Shared decision making

This is a critical concept if the professional clinician seeks successful treatment of the patient with dermatological, psychological, and/or other disorders (28,29). Shared decision making can be complicated when dealing with adolescent patients but must be utilized when dealing with this age and with other patients (30). Youth who do not understand and agree to treatment options may sabotage the management efforts, as noted previously. Even if an adolescent patient cannot legally provide consent in a specific situation, the clinician can still seek an *assent* from the youth that involves soliciting this minor's willingness and choices for management plans (31).

3.4.3 Improving compliance

The dedicated health care professional may find it challenging and even complex to improve management compliance with his/her patients. There is no evidence-based research that recommended plans improve medication compliance (or other treatment compliance) in all cases (32). Clinicians need to spend time to understand the patient and then provide some counseling regarding why the medication or other treatment option is being suggested and work on getting the acceptance from this patient. A rapid response to management failure by quickly changing a dose, changing drugs, or adding more medications without appreciating underlying issues will not improve the clinical outcome for this patient (33). This is particularly critical when complex interplays occur between the potentially thorny triad of developmental needs of adolescents, dermatological diseases, and psychiatric disorders.

Such counseling may change but sometimes must focus on behavioral strategies to improve compliance with proposed treatment options. Based on understanding the specific patient, one can discuss why the medication is important to use. Handouts of the condition(s) can be helpful for some patients (or parents), while others may be helped by additional health care personnel, such as the office nurse or this patient's primary care clinician (34). It does not help to seek any coercion in advocated plans, as this may lead to more refusal to follow the medical plan (35). The key is understanding the patient and underlying issues that may be complicating the patient–clinician alliance. Allowing the patient to choose options may help as well as discussing any side effects of current medications. Changing to medications with minimal side effects can be very beneficial to the patient and increase his/her acceptance of the dermatological and/or psychiatric medication (s). Communication with the teenager via e-mail is often a positive experience for the patient as well (36).

3.5 Conclusion

Patients with dermatological and primary or secondary psychiatric conditions can be challenging as well as time-consuming for clinicians. Indeed, for some clinicians, successful management of this patient may be like untying an intricately interwoven Gordian knot! The *sine qua non* of successful management of the adolescent patient with a dermatological condition is to acquire a careful medical and psychological evaluation of this patient. Time is necessary for this evaluation and also to develop a clinical rapport with the adolescent. Principles of confidentiality and informed consent must be followed. The therapeutic alliance will be enhanced if adolescent patient and clinician are engaged in clinical decision making processes. Recalcitrant cases should prompt both a reconsideration of the differential diagnosis but also a look at underlying psychological factors and potential reasons for limited compliance by the potentially demanding and difficult adolescent patient.

> "Time is the most valuable thing a man can spend."
>
> Theophrastus (371–287 BC)

References

1. Greydanus DE, Feinberg AN, Patel DR, Homnick DN, eds. *The pediatric diagnostic examination.* New York: McGraw-Hill Medial, 2008.
2. Barrier PA, Li JTC, Jensen NM. Two words to improve physician-patient communication: What else? *Mayo Clin Proc* 2003;78:211–4.
3. Makoul G. Communicative skills education in medical school and beyond. *JAMA* 2003;289:93–6.
4. Roter DL, Stewart M, Putnam SM. Communication patterns of primary care physicians. *JAMA* 1997;277:350–6.
5. Greydanus DE, Patel DR, Pratt HD, eds. *Essential adolescent medicine.* New York: McGraw Medical, 2006.
6. Hofmann AD. Communicating with adolescents and their parents. In: Hofmann AD, Greydanus DE, eds. *Adolescent medicine*, 3rd edn. Stamford, CT: Appleton Lange, 1997:40.
7. Mehta R. Approach to an adolescent client. In: Bhave S, ed. *Bhave's textbook of adolescent medicine.* New Delhi, India: Jaypee Brothers Medical Publishers, 2006:16–20.
8. Lyren A, Silber TJ. Consent, confidentiality, and other related issues in the care of adolescents. In: Greydanus DE, Patel DR, Pratt HD, eds. *Essential adolescent medicine.* New York: McGraw-Hill Medical, 2006:29–42.
9. Ford C, English A, Sigman G. Confidential health care for adolescents: Position paper for the Society for Adolescent Medicine. *J Adolesc Health* 2004;35:160–7.
10. McDonnell WM. Adolescent health care. In: Donn SM, McAbee GN, eds. *Medicolegal issues in pediatrics.* Elk Grove Village, IL: American Academy of Pediatrics, 2012:131–9.
11. Elster AB, Kuznets NJ. *AMA Guidelines for Adolescent Preventive Service (GAPS): Recommendations and rationale.* Baltimore, MD: Williams Wilkins, 1992.
12. Chatterjee S, Chatterjee R. Adolescent screening questionnaires. In: Bhave S, ed. *Bhave's textbook of adolescent medicine.* New Delhi, India: Jaypee Brothers Medical Publishers, 2006:21–5.
13. Goldenring JM, Rosen DS. Getting into adolescent heads: An essential update. *Contempor Pediatr* 2004;21:64.
14. Kaul P, Kaplan DW. Caring for adolescents in their office. In: Greydanus DE, Patel DR, Pratt HD, eds. *Essential adolescent medicine.* New York: McGraw-Hill Medical, 2006:17–27.
15. Coupey SM. Interviewing adolescents. *Pediatr Clin North Am* 1997;44:1349.
16. Brown RT. Issues for the male clinician. In: Coupey SM, ed. *Primary care of adolescent girls.* Philadelphia, PA: Hanley Belfus, 2000:81.
17. Greydanus DE, ed. *Caring for your teenager.* New York: Bantam Books and American Academy of Pediatrics, 2003.
18. Harth W, Hillert A, Hermes B, Seikowski K. Niemeier V, Feudenmann RW. Suicidal behavior in dermatology. *Hautartz* 2008;59(4):289–96.
19. Misery L. Consequences of psychological distress in adolescents with acne. *J Invest Dermatol* 2011;131(2):290–2.
20. Chuh A, Wong W, Zawar V. The skin and the mind. *Aust Fam Physician* 2006;35(9):723–5.

21. Sambhi R, Lepping P. Psychiatric treatments in dermatology: an update. *Clin Exp Dermatol* 2010;35(2):120–5.
22. Barankin B, DeKoven J. Psychosocial effect of common skin diseases. *Can Fam Physician* 2002;48:712–6.
23. Gupta MA, Gupta AK, Ellis CN, Koblenzer CS. Psychiatric evaluation of the dermatology patient. *Dermatol Clin* 2005;23(4):591–9.
24. Kieć-Swierczyńska M, Dudek B, Krecisz B, Swierczyńska-Machura D, Dudek W, Garnczarek A, et al. The role of psychological factors and psychiatric disorders in skin diseases. *Med Pr* 2006;57:551–5.
25. Mallardi V. The origin of informed consent. *Acta Otorhinolaryngol Ital* 2005;25(5):312–27.
26. Katz J. *The silent world of doctor and patient.* New York, NY: Free Press, 1984.
27. English A, Ford CA. The HIPAA Privacy Rule and adolescents: Legal questions and clinical challenges. *Perspect Sex Reprod Health* 2004;26(2):80–6.
28. Légaré F, Ratté S, Stacey D, Kryworuchko J, Gravel K, Graham ID, Turcotte S. Interventions for improving the adoption of shared decision making by healthcare professionals. *Cochrane Database Sys Rev* 2010;5:CD006732.
29. Perestelo-Perez L, Gonzalez-Lorenzo M, Perez-Ramos J, Rivero-Santana A, Serrano-Aquilar P. Patient involvement and shared-decision making in mental health care. *Curr Clin Pharmacol* 2011;6(2):83–90.
30. Unguru Y. Making sense of adolescent decision-making: Challenge and reality. *Adolesc Med State Art Rev* 2011;22(2):195–206.
31. Campbell AT, English A. Law, ethics, and clinical discretion: Recurring and emerging issues in adolescent health care. *Adolesc Med State Art Rev* 2011;22(2):321–34.
32. Haynes RB, Yao X, Degani A, Kripalani S, Garg A. McDonald HP. Interventions to enhance medication adherence. *Cochrane Database Syst Rev* 2005;4:CD000011.
33. Lerman I. Adherence to treatment: The key for avoiding long-term complications of diabetes. *Arch Med Res* 2005;36(3):300–6.
34. Eisenmann CM. Revising a medication education program on an inpatient child and adolescent psychiatric unit. *J Psychosoc Nurs Ment Health Serv* 2011;14:1–7.
35. Molodynski A, Rugkåsa J, Burns T. Coercion and compulsion in community mental health care. *Br Med Bull* 2010;95:105–19.
36. Menachemi N, Prickett CT, Brooks RG. The use of physician-patient e-mail: A follow-up examination of adoption and best practice adherence. *J Med Internet Res* 2011;13(1):e23.

Mohammad Khurshid Azam Basra

4 Quality of life issues in children and adolescents with dermatological conditions and their wider impact on the family and society

Skin conditions are very common in children with almost one child in every four having some kind of skin-related problem. Even though the majority of skin conditions are not life threatening, they can have a major impact on the child. This impact may be physical caused by distressing symptoms, psychosocial due to the disfiguring nature of some skin conditions, as well as financial due to direct and indirect costs associated with them. Due to differences in biological and cognitive development, children and adolescents may have some differences in the way their quality of life is affected by skin diseases. This requires age-specific measurement tools for quality of life assessment in children and adolescents. The impact of skin disease has been shown to extend beyond the patients to their immediate caregivers, such as parents and family members, whose own quality of life may be affected due to a child's skin condition. The family impact could be influenced by different factors, such as the nature of the child's skin condition and its severity. For optimal management of children's skin conditions it is important to gauge the impact on parents and family care givers and provide them with appropriate educational, psychological, and social support to enable them to better cope with their child's skin disease, which has been found to result in better medical and social outcomes. Childhood skin conditions such as eczema impose a substantial financial burden on the society that could arise from direct treatment costs to the health care system and indirect costs such as days lost from work by parents. Unfortunately, most of the research to date on the impact of childhood skin diseases on children and families and, in particular, their financial implications has been focused on atopic eczema, and there is a need to study the impact of other skin diseases to have a broader idea of the overall burden of childhood skin diseases.

4.1 Introduction

Changing epidemiology of pediatric diseases, from acute to chronic and from incurable to palliative or curable, has resulted in a growing interest in assessing children's quality of life (QoL). Nowadays, evaluation of QoL is considered a central element of pediatric practice and important for all children i.e. the healthy and the ill (1). In order to understand the QoL issues in children with particular reference to dermatology and the issues surrounding the assessment of QoL in pediatric populations, it important to first understand the concept of QoL. The life time of an individual consists of two fundamental components: quantity of life and quality of life (2). The quantity of life is the number of years from the time of birth to the time of death; the quality of life is the quality of each point in the time between the time of birth and the time of death.

Quality of life is an amorphous term and has different meanings for every individual and culture and differs by context, place, and time (i.e. it may vary within an individual at different points in time). A number of different concepts have been associated with this term, including health-related quality of life, health status, and functional status. Although related and many times used interchangeably, these terms have separate definitions. According to one of the most frequently used definitions, "Quality of life is an individual's perception of their position in life in the context of the cultural and value systems in which they live and in relation to their goals, expectations, and standards and concerns" (3).

In the context of pediatrics, this term refers to "a child's perception and evaluation of performance in relevant life areas and its feelings related to problems in functioning" (4). It has also been described as "A measure of how a child views his/her life in relationship to how they could reasonably expect or desire it to be" (5). Health-related quality of life (HRQoL) could be considered a component of overall QoL that is determined by the individual's health and can be influenced by clinical interventions (6,7). Health status, a related term, indicates a child's level of wellness versus illness (8) and includes the presence of biological dysfunction with or without the level of illness control (9). Finally, functional status could be defined as "a child's ability to perform daily activities that are essential to meet his/her basic needs, fulfil roles and maintain health and well-being" (9).

Since QoL is a purely subjective concept, as expressed by the patient, it is in contrast to other traditional clinical, biological, and radiological measures evaluated by the observers objectively, and it depends on the individual needs as perceived by the patients themselves and not the treating physicians (10). Moreover, being subjective in nature, it can be influenced by a number of factors such as the severity of disease, patient's gender, age, ethnic background, social class, personality type, level of anxiety, education, lifestyle, past experiences, as well as family functioning (11,12,13). Irrespective of contextual differences in their meanings, the terms QoL and HRQoL have frequently been used synonymously in the medical literature and for the sake of simplicity, and because of its wider application, the umbrella term QoL will be used in this chapter to denote HRQoL.

4.2 Pediatric quality of life and its assessment

Children constitute a large proportion of health care consumers, and pediatrics represents a major medical speciality. Assessment of QoL in children is as important as in adults. However, compared to adults, the assessment of QoL in young children is believed to be associated with unique problems and challenges (14). Factors such as age and cognitive and emotional development may compromise children's ability to understand their disease or health in general and the questions asked in a QoL questionnaire in specific. Therefore, there is a concern that children may misinterpret the questions. They may also have time perception problems as well as difficulty in using rating scales and lengthy questionnaires. This conception led to some researchers using proxy data provided by parents to measure children's QoL as their own responses were often considered unreliable or inaccurate (15).

However, the evidence suggests that young children can provide reliable and consistent reports on their QoL using structured questionnaires (16). Moreover, significant areas of discordance exist between children and parents about children's health status, the impact of illness, and QoL (17,18). Based on these observations, it seems important to involve children in management decisions related to their care and equally importantly to rate their own QoL, except in situations where they are either incapacitated or too young to complete the questionnaire themselves. Under these circumstances parents or caregivers may provide valuable information based on their judgment of child's health status and QoL (19). In general, there is better correlation between parental proxy data and child's own response for physical parameters compared with psychological ones (15).

4.3 Skin disease and quality of life

Skin diseases, although not generally life-threatening, frequently have a major impact on patient's psychological and social life as well as everyday activities, which makes QoL and its measurement particularly important in dermatology (20). Herd et al hold the view that QoL seems to be more relevant to dermatology than other diseases due to the reasons that many skin disease patients have chronic and incurable diseases, and the impact of skin disorders on QoL is subjective as well as related to individual circumstances (21). This view is further strengthened by the fact that many skin diseases are more obvious visibly than many chronic systemic diseases. They have the potential to cause direct impact on children's psyche resulting from having negative childhood experiences such as being bullied at school due to their skin appearance. It is, therefore, not surprising to find that some skin diseases in children can have a greater impact on overall QoL than other chronic systemic conditions. For example, using a generic QoL measure, children with generalized eczema were found to have greater QoL impairment than children with cystic fibrosis, asthma, diabetes, epilepsy, and renal disease (22).

4.3.1 Impact of skin diseases on children's quality of life

Childhood is a stage of life characterized by rapid psychosocial development and emotional vulnerability. Any negative experience during this stage may have an impact on an individual's development and QoL impairment in adulthood. Chronic and disfiguring skin conditions in childhood (e.g. eczema, psoriasis, vitiligo, and acne) have the potential to induce negative experiences and problems in social development (23). Although there does not seem to be a great deal of difference in children's QoL based on their gender, younger children seem to have greater impairment of QoL (24).

Most of the research on QoL impact of skin diseases in children has been focused on atopic eczema, possibly due to its high prevalence among children, its chronic and distressing nature, and its economic implications for the family as well as the health care system. Atopic eczema is one of the most common skin conditions affecting young children and has substantial impact on their QoL and the QoL of their parents. The impact on children could be both physiological and psychological. Physical symptoms and psychological problems have been shown to be common issues for children and infants; the physical symptoms include itching and scratching, while the psychological issues include mood changes, feeling sad or upset, embarrassed, and self-conscious, as well sleep disturbance (24,25).

Having eczema can result in lack of self-confidence that could be related to poor self-image and that can ultimately compromise the social development of children (26). In one study, the rate of psychological disturbance was found to be more in children with atopic eczema compared with the control group, and there was a linear relationship with the severity of eczema and the resulting psychological disturbance (27). Moreover, compared with controls, pre-school children with eczema were found to show greater dependency on their parents as well as greater fearfulness (28). An important aspect of childhood is playing games and sports. However, having eczema can adversely impact their leisure activities, such as playing and swimming, which may be either due to the disease exacerbation or related to its psychosocial consequences, such as peer rejection and embarrassment (29).

Pruritus is the predominant physical symptom of eczema and has been shown to result in increased crying, fussiness, and irritability in these children (30). Sleep disturbance is a major issue for children with atopic eczema, which is associated with itching and scratching (27). The abnormalities in sleep pattern not only lead to daytime discipline and behavior problems and impaired performance at school in children, but also result in sleep deprivation and exhaustion in parents as will be discussed later in this chapter (31,32).

Psoriasis is another disfiguring skin condition that can have a devastating impact on the QoL of children and their parents. Physical symptoms of itching and scratching, problems with treatment, and the feeling of embarrassment as well as self-consciousness were found to be the three worst aspects in children suffering from psoriasis (33). The same study showed that the QoL impairment was even greater when psoriasis was accompanied by joint problems.

Another study about the impact of juvenile psoriasis also has shown negative effects of the disease on children's physical, social, and emotional functioning with the majority of children reporting feelings of stigmatization and being bullied (34). Interestingly, in a comparative study from children's perspectives, among various skin diseases, psoriasis followed by atopic eczema caused the greatest QoL impairment, while from parents' perspectives, the highest score was for atopic eczema followed by urticaria and psoriasis (22).

4.3.2 Quality of life assessment in children with dermatological conditions

Quality of life in children can be assessed using generic and disease-specific measures. Generic measures are applicable to any population subgroup with any condition and are thus useful for comparing the QoL impact among different conditions. On the other hand, disease-specific measures are applicable to individuals suffering from a particular disease. These measures are useful for detecting change in the condition over time and are more sensitive to change than generic measures. In between these two types of QoL measures there is a third category that could be labeled as speciality-specific measures, e.g. dermatology-specific measures.

These measures, although less sensitive to change than condition-specific measures, are useful in comparing the QoL impact of different conditions within that speciality, e.g. dermatology. A number of QoL instruments exist to assess the QoL of adults with skin diseases. However, these instruments may not be appropriate for use in children because of the fundamental differences between the conceptualization of children's and adults' QoL. For example, items such as impact of a condition on employment, income, and sexuality will not be applicable to children (19). Therefore, in order to be applied successfully, QoL questionnaires should be developed that have domains specific to different age groups with emphasis on the cognitive, psychological, functional, social, and behavioral characteristics of that age group.

In dermatology, children's quality of life has mostly been assessed using a dermatology-specific QoL measure called the Children's Dermatology Life Quality Index (29); also, for infants suffering from atopic eczema, the Infant's Dermatitis Quality of Life Index has been utilized (25). These two commonly used measures are briefly described in Sections 4.3.3 and 4.3.4. Adolescents have traditionally been categorized with children and their QoL, at least in dermatology, has been assessed either by using the CDLQI (for patients younger than 16 years of age) or the Dermatology Life Quality Index (DLQI, for patients 16 years of age and older) (35). However, as will be discussed later, there are some differences between children and adolescents that warrant separate QoL assessments. It has only been recently that this important difference is acknowledged, and two dermatology-specific measures have been developed specifically for adolescents between the ages of 12 and 19 years, and these will be described later in this chapter.

4.3.3 Children's Dermatology Life Quality Index (CDLQI)

Lewis-Jones and Finlay developed this simple instrument for use in daily clinical practice and clinical trials to assess the impact of skin diseases on the quality of life of school-age (4–16 years) children (29). The CDLQI is usually self-completed, however, and children who are unable to complete themselves may require help from their parents, or it can even be administered as a proxy measure (36). Being a dermatology-specific measure, the CDLQI has the potential to measure the QoL impact of different skin diseases relative to each other and can therefore be used to compare their impact.

The CDLQI has 10 items covering aspects such as symptoms and feelings, school, holidays, leisure, personal relationships, treatment, and sleep. The total scale score ranges from 0–30; a higher score indicates greater QoL impairment. The scores can also be expressed as the percentage of the maximum score. In the original study, the CDLQI scores were highest in scabies patients (mean CDLQI score = 9.5), followed by eczema (mean score = 7.7), and lowest in patients with nevi (mean score = 2.3). The highest scoring individual question was about symptoms and feelings, while the lowest scoring was about friendship.

Test–retest reliability was acceptable and the validity was confirmed by the instrument's ability to differentiate QoL impact between patients and normal controls as well as between inflammatory and non-inflammatory skin diseases. The measure has also shown sensitivity to change following inpatient treatment for atopic eczema and psoriasis and outpatient treatment of acne (37) and following change in clinical severity of the children's eczema (38). The CDLQI has shown strong correlation with both generic QoL measures for children such as the Children's Life Quality Index (CLQI) (22) as well as with disease-specific QoL measures such as Cardiff Acne Disability Index (39).

Recently a set of bands has been proposed to facilitate the clinical interpretation of the CDLQI scores (40). According to this banding system, a CDLQI score of 0–1 = no effect on child's life; 2–6 = small effect; 7–12 = moderate effect; 13–18 = very large effect; and 19–30 = extremely large effect on child's life. A cartoon version of the CDLQI was developed in 2003, which was found to be more easily and more quickly completed (90 seconds vs 120 seconds for text version); thus it was favored by children as well as by their parents (41). This version of the CDLQI has been used in a number of studies, including study of QoL of children with erythropoietic protoporphyria (42).

4.3.4 Infant's Dermatitis Quality of Life Index (IDQoL)

This is a simple proxy-generated disease-specific instrument to measure the impact of atopic eczema on infants (0–4 years old) in the clinical setting and to be used in conjunction with a clinical severity assessment tool (25). The content of the IDQoL was based on parents' views about the QoL impairment of their children caused by atopic eczema. It contains 10 items each with a choice of answers ranging from 0 to 3; 0 = no effect, 3 = very much effect. The questions encompass aspects such as symptoms, sleep, mood, meal times, family activities, treatment, and dressing and bathing the child. All questions pertain to QoL impact over the previous week. There is an additional question that asks for the parent's assessment of the severity of the child's eczema, and it is scored separately on a 0–4 scale, where 0 indicates none and 4 indicates extremely severe. The highest scoring IDQoL items related to the physical symptoms of itching and scratching, mood changes, and sleep disruption (25).

Test–retest reliability and sensitivity to change in a small sample of infants post-treatment was found to be good. In a recent study Beattie and Lewis-Jones have shown the usefulness of the IDQoL in routine clinical practice as well as its sensitivity to change after a consultation with a pediatric dermatologist (43). This study also provided further evidence of the validity of the IDQoL on the basis of a high correlation with the clinical severity of the disease and with the Dermatitis Family Impact (DFI) questionnaire (44).

4.3.5 Impact of skin disease on the quality of life of adolescents

Adolescence may be considered to represent individuals in the age range of 13–18 years of age. Adolescence is a transitional period between childhood and adulthood and has unique physical, psychological, and social characteristics that makes this period of life different from children and adults (45). Some of its differentiating aspects include increasing need for autonomy, intimacy, and sexuality as well as the importance of peers. However, as mentioned earlier, adolescents' QoL has been assessed traditionally together with children or adults, neglecting these specific aspects of this age group.

Thus far, most of the QoL-related research in adolescents has been carried out in the area of chronic illness and the resulting increased incidence of behavioral, psychiatric, academic, and psychosocial difficulties for adolescents (46). As mentioned previously, some of the dominant characteristics of this age include preoccupation with self-image, influence of peers, and the need for intimacy. Consequently, any illness that affects their physical appearance and body image can have a direct impact on social interaction, including relationships with peers and with the opposite sex (47). Furthermore, a negative body image may be associated with a number of psychiatric disorders such as depression and eating disorders among adolescents (48,49,50).

Skin conditions due to their visible nature can have devastating effects on individuals and in particular adolescents who may develop negative body image leading to an adverse impact on QoL. Unfortunately, the QoL research in this important age group in general and specifically in dermatology has been quite disproportionate to the magnitude of general population that this group represents (i.e. 20%). Few studies have empirically investigated the impact that various skin diseases can have on adolescents' QoL (51). Some of the common skin conditions in children and adolescents (such as acne, eczema, and psoriasis) can cause significant QoL impairment (29).

Acne, the commonest skin condition in adolescents, can result in significant morbidity and impairment of QoL in the form of interpersonal difficulties, embarrassment, increased anxiety, shame, and social isolation (20,52). In fact the emotional and social impact of acne has been shown to be comparable with severe disabling conditions like epilepsy and arthritis (53). A skin condition does not have to be physically distressing to affect QoL. Symptomless but highly visible conditions such as vitiligo may induce negative experiences in adolescents in the form of feelings of shame toward peers, avoidance of intimacy, and social as well as sport activities, conflicts with parents, and tendency to do things alone (23).

One of the recent studies with a clear focus on adolescents has identified a number of specific aspects of QoL affecting adolescents with different skin diseases (54). According to the findings of this study, psychological impact of skin disease came up as the most frequently mentioned theme (mentioned by 91% of study subjects) and included different aspects of negative emotions such as feeling of anger, frustration, embarrassment, decreased self-confidence and self-image, being more self-conscious, feeling of being judged, and feeling lonely.

The second most common theme mentioned by study subjects was the physical impact of skin diseases (75%) in the form of itchiness, soreness, pain, etc. that resulted in sleep disturbance in as many as one third of subjects. The other common themes affecting adolescents included impact on socializing, making friends, choice of clothing, avoiding public places, and effect on sporting and other leisure activities, including swimming. Almost one quarter of adolescents felt that their relationships with the opposite sex were affected due to their skin conditions, while 16% felt that their career plans and future aspirations were affected.

4.4 Assessment of adolescents' quality of life in dermatology

The assessment of QoL of teenagers or adolescents using age-specific measures is a recent development in dermatology. There are only two QoL measures so far developed for adolescents: Teenager's QoL (T-QoL) questionnaire (55) and Skindex-Teen (56).

4.4.1 Teenager's QoL questionnaire (T-QoL)

T-QoL is a simple 18-item dermatology-specific QoL measure for adolescents recently developed in Cardiff, United Kingdom (55). The initial 32 items of the measure were based on the content analysis of semi-structured interviews with a cohort of 50 adolescents suffering from various skin diseases. Content validity was established by carrying out a pilot study on another sample of 20 adolescents. The revised 30-item version was subjected to field testing in a new sample of 153 subjects. Further, 12 items, which had suboptimal psychometric properties, were reduced following application of item response and classical test theory models.

Application of Rasch analysis did not support unidimensionality of the measure, and factor analysis identified three domains within the scale. The final 18-item version of T-QoL has 3 response categories: Never = 0; Sometimes = 1; and Always = 3. All questions ask the respondent about the impact of their skin disease on specific QoL aspects at the moment. The score can be presented as an overall summary score (score range = 0–36 with the higher score indicating greater QoL impairment) or as score of individual domains: Domain 1 represents self image (score range = 0–16); Domain 2 represents physical well-being and future aspirations (score range = 0–8); and Domain 3 represents psychosocial impact and relationships (score range = 0–12).

The final validation of T-QoL was carried out in a new cohort of adolescents, and the results have demonstrated promising psychometric properties of the measure in terms of construct validity, internal consistency, and test–retest reliability, as well as sensitivity to change. The authors of the measure see it as a potentially useful measure in routine clinical practice and in research settings.

4.4.2 Skindex-Teen

This is another recently developed "hypothesis-based" 21-item self-administered dermatology-specific QoL measure for teenagers that was developed in the United States (56). The items in the questionnaire inquire about the patients' perception about the impact of their skin condition on various aspects of QoL during the previous four weeks. Each item is scored on a 5 response category: never = 0, rarely = 1; sometimes = 2; often = 3; all the time = 4. The first draft of the questionnaire had 22 items and was formulated based on Skindex, a dermatology-specific measure for adults (57,58). The questionnaire was later revised based on the feedback from 11 dermatology professionals and 20 teenagers.

In the final validation stage, Skindex-Teen was administered to 200 adolescents suffering from various skin conditions. Rasch analysis confirmed the instrument to be multi-dimensional having two factors or domains that were named physical symptoms and psychosocial functioning. The scale can be reported as a total overall score (score range = 0–84; higher score = greater QoL impairment) or by the scores of two individual domains: psychosocial functioning (score range = 0–64) and physical symptoms (score range = 0–20). The final scale has demonstrated good psychometric properties including construct, face, and content validity as well as internal consistency, reliability, and sensitivity to change. The authors of

Skindex-Teen believe that the instrument will prove useful for research and clinical applications (56).

4.4.3 Impact of skin disease on family quality of life: The "greater patient" concept

QoL of individuals is closely related to the QoL of those around them. The relatively new concept of Family Quality of Life (FQoL) originally emerged as an important outcome of services delivery for individuals with disabilities and their families (59,60). FQoL refers to "conditions where the family needs are met and family members enjoy their life together as a family and have the chance to do things which are important to them" (61). Like patients' QoL, family's QoL can be influenced by different factors such as the nature of patient's illness, its severity, as well as personal and socioeconomic and cultural factors.

The studies on care-giving for mentally ill patients have found the impact on family life in the form of disruption of family routine, leisure and social life, financial difficulties, emotional overload, and the stresses on the mental and physical health of other family members (62). Goldstein and Kenet argue that any disease or illness has the potential to disrupt the family life and breaks the family routine, especially when the disease is chronic in nature (63). Therefore, it has been suggested that any attempt to estimate the burden of a disease must also take into account the impact of that disease on the family functioning, and the family's QoL must be analyzed independently and additionally to the patient's QoL (64).

In some specialities, pediatrics for example, the family QoL is regarded as a part of the patient's health (65). However, in dermatology, the awareness of the importance of family QoL is still in its infancy. Due to the chronic nature of many skin diseases, and the way treatment is applied, family members are frequently involved in caregiving, especially in the case of young children. This could result in parents and other close family members being affected by the patient's skin condition (66,67,68). There is evidence to show that parent's QoL is not only related to the severity of the child's skin condition (69) but also to the QoL of children (24). In fact, parent's QoL can actually improve following successful intervention and improvement in children's skin condition (70).

The impact of a patient's skin disease on family members has been studied in only a small number of dermatological conditions (67,71,72,73,74,75) with most attention focused on atopic eczema (72,76). The families of children with eczema have been reported to have lower QoL than families of healthy children (44,77), and taking care of a child with moderate to severe atopic eczema has been found to be more stressful than caring for a child with insulin-dependent diabetes mellitus (78). This is easy to understand when we know that, on an average, parents spend 3 hours per day for treatment of children with moderate to severe eczema (78).

Parents of children with atopic eczema experience a wide range of detrimental effects on their lives (e.g. psychological, social, lifestyle modifications, interpersonal relationships, financial, family activities, sleep, and issues related to the practical care of the patient) (44). According to one study, three of the most common aspects of parents' QoL affected by their children's eczema included helping with the child's treatment, tiredness or exhaustion, and additional expenditure related to treatment and clothes (24). Not surprisingly, the same three aspects were seen as most significant in parents of children suffering from psoriasis (33).

Other common aspects affecting psoriasis patients' families have been reported, including treatment-related issues, psychological pressures, social disruption, and limitations of leisure as well as daily activities (67). In a wider cross section of skin conditions, Basra and Finlay demonstrated that skin diseases can significantly impair the QoL of patients' families in a number of diverse ways, such as emotional distress (98% of the family members), burden of care (54%), effect on housework (42%), social life (48%), holidays (46%), financial difficulties (30%), impact on physical well-being (22%), effect on job/study (40%), restriction of leisure activities (26%), sleep disturbance (20%), effect on sex life (8%), and perceived need for support (12%) (66). In order to highlight the significance of this underestimated and often overlooked aspect of skin diseases (i.e. their impact on a patient's family), the term "Greater Patient" has been proposed that describes the immediate close social group affected by a patient's skin disease (66).

Emotional impact of a child's skin condition on parents is an important issue that can manifest itself in the form of worry, crying, and feelings of guilt, self-blame, anger, sadness, helplessness, and frustration (79). The reaction of people to the patient's skin appearance is a stressful experience for parents and family members and causes a feeling of embarrassment, anger, and frustration (79). Consequently, parents can experience a feeling of social isolation that is mainly due to avoiding people for the fear of having negative and unfriendly interactions with strangers, friends, and family alike (30). The social isolation that family members may experience highlights the need for social and emotional support for these individuals (80). Lewis et al stress that social support for families with a member with chronic illness is of great importance in influencing how the family copes with the situation (81).

Disruption of sleep is another major issue, particularly for the parents of children suffering from eczema, due to frequent scratching and crying of the children in the night. Su et al found that between one and two hours of sleep was lost by parents of children with eczema (78). Sleep was also shown to be a major problem for parents of children with atopic eczema in Lawson's study (44), while Carroll et al have shown that sleep deprivation can affect all family members and that it is a major stress-causing factor for the families (72). The implications for parents can be huge; they may need to miss work or avoid outside work altogether; their social functioning can be damaged; and their relationships with their spouse and other family members can be affected along, with their parenting behavior (77,78).

Financial impact on parents is another consequence of skin conditions in children, and in particular eczema, which has been demonstrated to have a negative effect on the family's financial resources and causes strain on family's budget (44,72). Many parents feel the need to make changes to their lifestyles to adjust with their children's needs, for example, restricting certain diets, making changes in the home, buying special items (i.e. products, clothing, and linens) for the child, and even holiday plans as well as outdoor activities sometimes need additional expenditures (30). The direct financial cost of care of a child having moderate to severe eczema was found to similar to type 1 diabetes but substantially higher than for a child with asthma (78).

In addition to the direct financial impact due to extra expenditure, the household may also be affected indirectly through decreased productivity of family caregivers who require time away from work in pursuit of medical attention for their relative patients. Loss of productivity is an important component of the overall burden of atopic eczema and is directly related to the severity of disease. For example, the cost in the form of loss of productivity to families of patients with moderate and severe eczema has been found to be Australian $894 and $1,290 respectively (78). Moreover, the mean days lost from work per patient are higher for parents of younger children than parents of older children (82). Bickers et al have estimated an annual loss of US$ 986 million due to caregivers' lost workdays (83).

4.5 Assessment of family quality in dermatology

A number of disease-specific instruments to measure the secondary impact on the family have been described for atopic eczema (44,84,85). However, there is only one psoriasis-specific (86) and one "generic" dermatology-specific QoL measure that could be used to measure the "secondary" impact on QoL of families across different skin diseases (87). These tools are briefly described in Sections 4.5.1–4.5.5.

4.5.1 Family Dermatology Life Quality Index (FDLQI)

The FDLQI was developed in Cardiff in 2007 as the first dermatology specific self-administered QoL measure to quantify the impact of patients' skin diseases on their family members (87).The content of the FDLQI was based on family members' reports of how their related patients' skin diseases affected their QoL. It has 10 items covering different aspects of family members' QoL, such as emotional distress, burden of care, effect on relationships, social and leisure activities, and extra house work due to patient's skin disease. Each question asks family member's perception of the impact on their QoL over the last month and is scored on a 4-point scale with a score range of 0–30; higher scores indicate greater QoL impairment.

The measure was shown to be sensitive to change and demonstrated high internal consistency as well as test–retest reliability. The construct validity of the FDLQI was established by its high correlation with patients' DLQI (35) scores and patients' self-assessed disease severity global question scores. Moreover, the measure was able to discriminate between family members based on the nature of patients' skin diseases; family members of patients with inflammatory skin diseases showed significantly higher FDLQI scores compared with family members of patients with non-inflammatory skin diseases. Within-group analysis of FDLQI scores showed that family members of patients with eczema had greatest QoL impairment followed by acne and psoriasis. The measure has further been cross-validated against generic and disease-specific family QoL tools (86,88,89). The brief and simple design of the FDLQI can make it a practical measure for routine clinical use and an additional outcome measure in clinical research.

4.5.2 Dermatitis Family Impact questionnaire (DFI)

The Dermatitis Family Impact (DFI) questionnaire was the first instrument of its kind in dermatology aimed to measure the secondary impact of atopic eczema on the quality of life of parents of children with eczema (44). It was meant to be used as an additional measure in clinical studies and in clinical practice to guide management decisions.

The 10 items of the DFI were derived from intensive qualitative interviews with families of children suffering from atopic eczema and include areas of family life, such as sleep, tiredness, distress, practical difficulties with treatment, and effects on shopping, leisure, housework, family relationships, expenditure, and food. Each question has four possible answers and measures the family impact over the last week only. The total scale score is achieved by summing the scores of individual items; higher score means greater family QoL impairment.

Although the instrument was shown to discriminate between affected families and control families, it was not compared with any other valid QoL instrument for validation purposes; also, neither its reliability nor responsiveness to change was assessed during the initial development process. However, in a recent study, sensitivity of the DFI to change was demonstrated in parents of children with atopic eczema before and after consultation with a pediatric dermatology team (43). The sensitivity of the DFI to change after a dermatology consultation has also been documented by Balkrishnan et al (70), while Ben-Gashir et al showed its sensitivity to change after a change in clinical severity of a child's eczema (69). Further studies have demonstrated good correlation of the measure with other dermatology-specific and disease-specific measures (25,69,90).

4.5.3 Parents' Index of Quality of Life in Atopic Dermatitis (PIQoL-AD)

This is a family/parent oriented QoL measure that was developed simultaneously in several European countries and the United States that adopted a "needs-based" approach (85). This instrument is designed to be completed by parents of children with atopic eczema to assess the impact that their children's eczema and its treatment has on their QoL. The content of the PIQoL-AD was derived from unstructured interviews with parents of children having atopic eczema.

Rasch analysis was applied to reduce the number of items and prove its unidimensionality. The final questionnaire has 28 items in the form of statements and a dichotomous response system. This scoring system was thought to be less burdensome for respondents and also facilitated equivalence of translation. The dichotomous response choices, however, can limit the responsiveness of the instrument. The measure covers a range of affected parents' needs, e.g. need for rest, relaxation, self-respect, independence, personal time and space, control, and also the need for their child to have a safe future.

The test–retest reliability and internal consistency of the PIQoL-AD was demonstrated to be good, and construct validity was established by correlating it with the General Well-Being Index (GWBI) and by the scale's ability to differentiate groups based on parent-perceived eczema severity (85). In a later study of children with atopic eczema treated with pimecrolimus, the PIQoL-AD was shown to be responsive to improvement in children's condition with a 10% reduction in PIQoL-AD scores at baseline and 6 months after using the treatment (91).

A secondary analysis of the data from this and other clinical trials incorporating this measure was used to describe the clinical meaningfulness of the PIQoL-AD scores, which suggests that a change of 2–3 points on the measure should be considered meaningful (92). Although the original measure was intended to be used by parents of children up to the age of 8 years, the authors believe that it could also be used with parents of children up to 12 years.

4.5.4 Childhood Atopic Dermatitis Impact Scale (CADIS)

This is another self-administered "hypothesis-based" instrument to measure the impact of atopic eczema on the QoL of young children and their families (84). The initial 62-item content was derived from published work as well as interviews with affected families and medical professionals. Item reduction was performed by qualitative judgment and psychometric analysis including Rasch analysis. The final 45 items can be explained by a five-scale framework, including three parent-related scales (family and social function, emotions, sleep) and two child-related scales (symptoms and activity limitations and behavior). Each item is scored on a 0–4 scale (0 = never, 4 = all the time) and inquires about the parent's perception of a particular aspect during the last 4 weeks. The internal consistency of all the five scales was acceptable and preliminary evidence of content and construct validity was documented. However, test–retest reliability and responsiveness to change was not assessed at the time of questionnaire development.

4.5.5 Psoriasis Family Index (PFI)

This is a self-administered psoriasis-specific measure to assess the impact of the patient's psoriasis on family members and partners (86). It has 15 items and a 4-point response format from not at all (score = 0) to very much (score = 3); higher scores indicate greater QoL impairment. The items cover different aspects of family members QoL, such as psychological impact, extra house work, social and leisure activities, treatment related burden, effect on daily activities, sleep, choice of clothes, holidays, and family relationships. The preliminary results of psychometric analysis of the measure, including internal consistency, test–retest reliability, and construct validity, are promising. However, further evidence of the scale's performance is required, in particular, its factor structure and sensitivity to change.

4.6 Societal impact of childhood dermatological conditions

Skin diseases are very common in the community. The prevalence in school children and adolescents has been found to be between 26% and 31% (93,94). Two of the commonest skin conditions in this age group are atopic eczema and acne; the former being more common in primary school children and latter in secondary school children and adolescents (93). Both these conditions are known to be chronic in nature and carry substantial morbidity for patients and a significant QoL impact on patients as well as their parents.

Generally, chronic skin conditions and some malignant skin cancers drain considerable health service financial resources in the society. The direct costs of treating skin conditions vary from country to country depending on the local health care systems. So far most of the research on cost estimation of skin diseases has been focused on atopic eczema. It appears that in addition to direct medical costs, atopic eczema may incur indirect costs in the form of days lost from work, purchase of special household products, clothes and linen, over the counter products, special diets, and cleaning agents, as well as additional transport and parking costs to and from hospital and surgery (95).

In the United Kingdom, the annual cost per child was estimated to be £79.59 and included direct and indirect costs such as the cost of prescriptions, NHS consultations, private consultations, purchase of over the counter products, and income loss (96). According to an Australian study, the annual cost of just medical consultations for a child with moderate and severe eczema was estimated at 389 and 642 Australian dollars, respectively, while the annual hospitalization cost for a child with severe eczema was 2,912 Australian dollars (78). The mean direct annual cost of treatment of a child with mild, moderate, and severe eczema was calculated to be 330, 818, and 1,255 Australian dollars and included costs of special diet, medication, dressings, and medical consultations (78). In fact, the same study found that the cost of treating severe eczema in children has been found to be even higher than treating diabetes and asthma (78).

In the United States, the mean annual per patient total costs, including both direct and indirect costs, have been estimated to be approximately $609 (82). Also in the United States, according to a conservative estimate, 364 million dollars are spent annually for the treatment of childhood atopic eczema (97). Finally, in another study comparing the international costs of treatment of eczema the annual per patient treatment costs ranged from $71 in Netherlands to $2,559 in Germany (98).

4.7 Conclusions

Recent advances in medicine have shifted the focus of attention from mortality issues due to acute illnesses such as infectious diseases to long term morbidity issues related to chronic illnesses. The increased survival rates have been accompanied by greater recognition of quality of life of patients as a major outcome. Assessment of quality of life has potential value in evaluating interventions, assessing the outcomes of new therapies, comparing outcomes in clinical trials, and facilitating communication between patients, their family caregivers, and health care professionals. It has also been used as a tool to identify hidden health problems and in monitoring changes in patients' health status and prioritizing health issues for individual patients (99). Equally importantly, it helps in commissioning care programs and in audit work and can also be used as an effective political tool to argue for limited vital resources in a competitive environment in which skin diseases, due to their non-life threatening nature, are not viewed as "important" as other medical conditions.

There is a risk that important information will be missed if clinical measures of disease severity are used alone, neglecting the QoL impact of the disease. Therefore, it is recommended to use simple QoL measures in clinical practice in conjunction with clinical measures when assessing patients with various skin diseases to have an idea of the overall severity. Quality of life assessment is as important in the pediatric population as in the adult population. In situations where it is not possible to cure the disease but to control the symptoms, it is important to determine how the disease and/or its treatment impact on the child's QoL. This can aid in making more appropriate management decisions.

Based on the fact that parents' and children's views differ in their perception of illness and treatment and that parents' views about their children's QoL may be affected by their own emotions and mental health, it is recommended that, wherever possible, children should rate their own QoL (100). Nevertheless, in certain situations it would be quite acceptable to use proxy rating by parents or caregivers, such as when children are too small or incapable to understand and/or respond to questions in the measure.

When measuring the QoL in a pediatric population, it is important to consider the developmental stage of the respondents as particular dimensions may not be equally important in different age groups (e.g. early childhood vs late childhood or adolescence). Adolescents have some specific aspects related to their QoL that are different from adults' and children's QoL; these include physical maturation, autonomy, peer relationship, sexuality, and body image. It is therefore not appropriate to regard this age group as either children or adults, and QoL related research tools should be developed separately for these age groups.

Family members of patients with various skin diseases may be affected in a number of ways by their related patient's conditions, and the assessment of QoL of parents and family members of children is an integral component of comprehensive assessment of the burden of skin disease in the community. It has been suggested that the optimal management of children's skin conditions should also include interventions to reduce the impact on parents and family members if better medical outcomes are to be achieved. Unfortunately, the current health care systems in many countries, including many developed countries, do not provide adequate psychological, social, and financial support to children with various skin conditions and their families.

In order to decrease the burden on this population, there is a need for more structured education programs and specialist care from health care professionals, including dermatologists, general practitioners, pediatricians with special interest in dermatology, psychologists, as well as nurses with special training in dermatology.

In fact, the level of care provided by trained nurse practitioners has been found to be as effective as by dermatologists in improving the severity of eczema as well as QoL outcomes (101).

Having a secure support network with good knowledge of the disease can enable the patients and their families to feel more comfortable and less alone. There is evidence that parent education and psychosocial support can go a long way in reducing illness-related stress among parents, increasing parents' confidence in managing their children's eczema, and, ultimately, in reducing the severity of eczema (102,103). Moreover, patient advocacy groups, wherever available, can be useful in improving patient education and decreasing resource utilization (104).

Finally, most of the research on the impact of childhood skin diseases and especially their impact on family and financial implications has been focused on atopic eczema, and there is a need to study the impact of other skin diseases (such as acne, psoriasis, and genodermatoses) to have a broader idea of the burden of skin disease in this population.

References

1. Harding L. Children's quality of life assessments: A review of generic and health related quality of life measures completed by children and adolescents. *Clin Psychol Psychother* 2001;8:79–96.
2. Torrance GW. Utility approach to measuring health related quality of life. *J Chron Dis* 1987;40: 593–600.
3. World Health Organisation. *Measuring quality of life: The development of the World Health Organisation Quality of Life Instrument (WHOQOL).* Geneva: Author, 1993.
4. Maes S, Bruil J. Assessing the quality of life in children with a chronic illness. In: Rodriguez-Martin J, ed. *Health Psychology and Quality of Life Research.* Alicante, Spain: Health Psychology Department, University of Alicante, 1995:637–52.
5. Collier J, MacKinlay D, Phillips D. Norm values for the generic children's quality of life measure (GCQ). *Qual Life Res* 2000;9:617–23.
6. Juniper EF. How important is quality of life in pediatric asthma? *Paediatr Pulmonol* 1997;15:17–21.
7. Mishoe SC, Baker RR, Poole S, Harrell LM, Arant CB, Rupp NT. Development of an instrument to assess stress levels and quality of life in children with asthma. *J Asthma* 1998;35:553–63.
8. Davis E, Mackinnon A, Reddihough D, Graham HK, Mehmet-Radji O, Boyd R. Paediatric quality of life instruments: A review of the impact of the conceptual framework on outcomes. *Dev Med and Child Neurol* 2006;48:311–8.
9. Drotar D. Validating measures of pediatric health status, functional status, and health-related quality of life: Key methodological challenges and strategies. *Amb Paediatr* 2004;4:358–64.
10. Haliousa B, Beumont MG. Lunel F. Quality of life in dermatology. *Int J Dermatol* 2000;39:801–6.
11. Eiser C, Morse R. A review of measures of quality of life for children with chronic illness. *Arch Dis Child* 2001;84:205–11.
12. Annett RD, Bender BG, Lapidus J, et al. Predicting children's quality of life in an asthma clinical trial: What do children's reports tell us? *J Pediatr* 2001;139:854–61.
13. Sawyer MG, Spurrier N, Kennedy D, Martin J. The relationship between the quality of life of children with asthma and family functioning. *J Asthma* 2001;38:279–84.
14. Mulhurn RK, Horowitz ME, Ochs J, et al. Assessment of quality of life among paediatric patients with cancer. *J Consult Clin Psychol* 1989;1:130–8.
15. Eiser C, Morse R. Can parents rate their child's health-related quality of life? Results of a systematic review. *Qual Life Res* 2001;10:347–57.
16. Juniper EF, Guyatt GH, Feeny DH et al. Minimum skills required by children to complete health-related quality of life instruments for asthma: Comparison of measurement properties. *Eur Respir J* 1997;10:2285–94.
17. Eiser C, Kopel SJ. Children's perception of health and illness. In: Petrie KJ, Weinman JA, eds. *Perceptions of health and illness: Current research and applications.* Singapore: Harwood Academic Publishers, 1997.
18. Simeoni M-C, Sapin C, Antonotti S, Auquier P. Health-related quality of life reported by French adolescents: A predictive approach of health status? *J Adolesc Health* 2001;28:288–94.
19. Connolly MA, Johnson JA. Measuring quality of life in paediatric patients. *Pharmacoeconomics* 1999;16:605–25.
20. Jowett S, Ryan T. Skin disease and handicap: An analysis of the impact of skin conditions. *Soc Sci Med* 1985;20:425–9.
21. Herd RM, Tidman MJ, Ruta DA, Hunter JA. Measurement of quality of life in atopic dermatitis: Correlation and validation of two different methods. *Br J Dermatol* 1997;136:502–7.
22. Beattie PE, Lewis-Jones MS. A comparative study of impairment of quality of life in children with skin disease and children with other chronic childhood diseases. *Br J Dermatol* 2006; 155:145–51.

23. Linthorst Homan MW, de Korte J, Grootenhuis MA, et al. Impact of childhood vitiligo on adult life. *Br J Dermatol* 2008;159:915–20.
24. Ganemo A, Svensson A, Lindberg M, Wahlgren CF. Quality of life in Swedish children with eczema. *Acta Derm Venereol* 2007;87:345–9.
25. Lewis-Jones MS, Finlay AY, Dykes PJ. The infants' dermatitis quality of life index. *Br J Dermatol* 2001;144:104–10.
26. Cotterill J. Psychiatry and the skin. *Br J Hospital Med* 1989;42:401–4.
27. Absolon CM, Cottrell D, Eldridge SM, Glover MT. Psychological disturbance in atopic eczema: The extent of the problem in school-aged children. *Br J Dermatol* 1997;137:241–5.
28. Daud L, Garralda M, David TJ. Psychosocial adjustment in preschool children with atopic eczema. *Arch Dis Child* 1993;69:670–6.
29. Lewis-Jones MS, Finlay AY. The children's dermatology life quality index (CDLQI): Initial validation and practical use. *Br J Dermatol* 1995;132:942–9.
30. Chamlin SL, Frieden IJ, Williams ML, Chren MM. The effects of atopic dermatitis on young American children and their families. *Paediatrics* 2004;114:607–11.
31. Reid P, Lewis-Jones MS. Sleep difficulties and their management in preschoolers with atopic eczema. *Clin Exp Dermatol* 1995;20:38–41.
32. Dahl RE, Bernhisel-Broadbent J, Scanlon-Holdford S, et al. Sleep disturbances in children with atopic dermatitis. *Arch Pediatr Adolesc Med* 1995;149:856–60.
33. Ganemo A, Wahlgren CF, Svensson A. Quality of life and clinical features in Swedish children with psoriasis. *Pediatr Dermatol* 2011;28:375–9.
34. De Jager MEA, de Jong EM, Evers AW, et al. The burden of childhood psoriasis. *Pediatr Dermatol* 2011; early online publication (DOI: 10.1111/j.1525–1470.2011.01489.x).
35. Finlay AY, Khan GK. Dermatology Life Quality Index (DLQI) – A simple practical measure for routine clinical use. *Clin Exp Dermatol* 1994;19:210–6.
36. Lewis-Jones S. Quality of life and childhood atopic dermatitis: The misery of living with childhood eczema. *Int J Clin Pract* 2006;60:984–92.
37. Lewis-Jones MS, Lawson V, Hill G, Finlay AY. Monitoring childhood skin disease handicap. *Br J Dermatol* 1996;135(suppl 45):52.
38. Ben-Gashir MA, Seed PT, Hay RJ. Quality of life and disease severity are correlated in children with atopic dermatitis. *Br J Dermatol* 2004;150:284–90.
39. Walker N, Lewis-Jones MS. Quality of life and acne in Scottish adolescent school children: Use of the Children's Dermatology Life Quality Index (CDLQI) and the Cardiff Acne Disability Index (CADI). *J Eur Acad Dermatol Venereol* 2006;20:45–50.
40. Waters A, Sandhu D, Beattie P, et al. Severity stratification of children's dermatology life quality index scores. *Br J Dermatol* 2010;163(suppl 1):121(abstr PA-8).
41. Holme AS, Man I, Finlay AY, et al. The Children's Dermatology Life Quality Index: Validation of the cartoon version. *Br J Dermatol* 2003;148:285–90.
42. Holme AS, Anstey AV, Finlay AY, et al. Erythropoietic protoporphyria in the UK: Clinical features and effect on quality of life. *Br J Dermatol* 2006;155:574–81.
43. Beattie PE, Lewis-Jones MS. An audit of the impact of a consultation with a paediatric dermatology team on quality of life in infants with atopic eczema and their families: Further validation of the Infants' Dermatitis Quality of Life Index and Dermatitis Family Impact score. *Br J Dermatol* 2006;155:1249–55.
44. Lawson V, Lewis-Jones MS, Finlay AY, et al. The family impact of childhood atopic dermatitis: The Dermatitis Family Impact questionnaire. *Br J Dermatol* 1998;138:107–13.
45. Frisen A. Measuring health-related quality of life in adolescence. *Acta Paediatrica* 2007;96:963–8.
46. Beck AL, Nethercut GE, Crittenden MR, Hewins J. Visibility of handicap, self-concept and social maturity among young adult survivors of end-stage renal cancer. *J Dev Behav Paed* 1986;7:93–6.

47. La Greca AM. Social consequences of pediatric conditions: Fertile area for future investigation and intervention? *J Paediatr Psychol* 1990;15:285–307.
48. Kostanski M, Gullone E. Adolescent body image dissatisfaction: Relationship with self-esteem, anxiety, and depression controlling for body mass. *J Child Psychol Psychiatry* 1998;39:255–62.
49. Halvarsson K, Lunner K, Sjoden P-O. Assessment of eating behaviours and attitudes to eating, dieting and body-image in pre-adolescent Swedish girls: A one-year follow-up. *Acta Paediatrica* 2000;89:996–1000.
50. Stice E, Bearman SK. Body-image and eating disturbances prospectively predict increases depressive symptoms in adolescent girls: A growth curve analysis. *Dev Psychol* 2001;37:597–607.
51. Smith JA. The impact of skin disease on the quality of life of adolescents. *Adolesc Med* 2001;12:343–53.
52. Krowchuk DP, Stancin T, Keskinen R, et al. The psychosocial effects of acne on adolescents. *Pediatr Dermatol* 1991;8:332–8.
53. Mallon E, Newton JN, Klassen A, et al. The quality of life in acne: A comparison with general medical conditions using generic questionnaires. *Br J Dermatol* 1999;140:672–6.
54. Golics CJ, Basra MKA, Finlay AY, Salek MS. Adolescents with skin disease have specific quality of life issues. *Dermatology* 2009;218:357–66.
55. Basra MKA, Salek S, Tanweer Z, et al. Refinement and validation of Teenager's Quality of Life Questionnaire (T-QoL). *J Invest Dermatol* 2011;131:S50(abstr 295).
56. Smidt AC, Lai JS, Cella D, et al. Development and validation of Skindex-Teen, a quality of life instrument for adolescents with skin disease. *Arch Dermatol* 2010;146:865–9.
57. Chren MM, Lasek RJ, Quinn LM, et al. Skindex, a quality-of-life measure for patients with skin disease: Reliability, validity, and responsiveness. *J Invest Dermatol* 1996;107:707–13.
58. Chren MM, lasek RJ, Sahay AP, Sands LP. Measurement properties of Skindex-16: A brief quality-of-life measure for patients with skin diseases. J *Cutan Med Surg* 2001;5:105–10.
59. Park J, Hoffman L, Marquis J, Turnbull AP, Poston D, et al. Towards assessing family outcomes of service delivery; validation of a family quality of life survey. *J Intel Dis Res* 2003;47:367–84.
60. Poston D, Turnbull AP, Park J, et al. Family quality of life: A qualitative inquiry. *Mental Retardation* 2003;41:313–28.
61. Turnbull AP, Turnbull HR, Poston D, et al. Enhancing quality of life of families of children and youth with disabilities in the United States. In: Turnbull AP, Brown I, Turnbull HR, eds. *Families and persons with mental retardation and quality of life: International perspectives.* American Association on Mental Retardation, Washington DC, 2004:51–100.
62. Group for Advancement of Psychiatry. *Family affairs: Helping families cope with mental illness.* New York: Brumer/Mazet, 1986.
63. Goldstein G, Kenet G. The impact of chronic disease on the family. *Haemophilia* 2002;8: 461–70.
64. Verdugo MA, Cordoba L, Gomez J. Spanish adaptation and validation of the Family Quality of Life Survey. *J Intell Dis Res* 2005;49:794–8.
65. Fink R. Issues and problems in measuring children's health status in community health research. *Soc Sci Med* 1989;29:715–9.
66. Basra MKA, Finlay AY. The family impact of skin diseases: The greater patient concept. *Br J Dermatol* 2007;156:929–37.
67. Eghlileb AM, Davies EEG, Finlay AY. Psoriasis has a major secondary impact on the lives of family members and partners. *Br J Dermatol* 2007;156:1245–50.
68. Elliot BE, Luker K. The experiences of mothers caring for a child with severe atopic eczema. J *Clin Nurs* 1997;6:241–7.
69. Ben-Gashir MA, Seed PT, Hay RJ. Is family's quality of life and disease severity related in children with atopic dermatitis? J Eur *Acad Dermatol Venerol* 2002;16:455–62.

70. Balkrishnan R, Manul J, Clarke J, Caroll CL, Housman TS, Fleisher AB Jr. Effects of an episode of specialist care on the impact of childhood atopic dermatitis on the child's family. *J Paediatr Health Care* 2003;17:184–9.
71. Braue A, Ross G, Varigos G, Kelly H. Epidemiology and impact of childhood molluscum contageosum: A case series and critical review of the literature. *Paediatr Dermatol* 2005;22:287–91.
72. Carroll CL, Balkrishnan R, Feldman SR, et al. The burden of atopic dermatitis: Impact on the patient, family, and society. *Pediatr Dermatol* 2005;22:192–9.
73. Fine J-D, Johnson LB, Weiner M, Suchindran C. Impact of inherited epidermolysis bullosa on parental interpersonal relationships, marital status and family size. *Br J Dermatol* 2005;152: 1009–14.
74. Miller AC, Cate IM, Watson HS, Geronemus RG. Stress and family satisfaction in parents of children with facial port-wine stains. *Pediatr Dermatol* 1999;16:190–4.
75. Rakkhit T, Chen S, Lawley L, Freedman S. The impact of Sturge-Weber Syndrome (SWS) on patients and their families. *J Am Acad Dermatol* 2006;54(3):1414(Abstr:121).
76. Warschburger P, Buchholz HT, Petermann F. Psychological adjustment in parents of young children with atopic dermatitis: Which factors predict parental quality of life. *Br J Dermatol* 2004;150:304–11.
77. Lapidus CS, Kerr PE. Social impact of atopic dermatitis. *Med Health R I* 2001;84:294–5.
78. Su JC, Kemp AS, Varigos GA, Nolan TM. Atopic eczema: Its impact on the family and financial cost. *Arch Dis Child* 1997;76:159–62.
79. Chamlin SL. The psychosocial burden of childhood atopic dermatitis. *Dermatol Therapy* 2006;19:104–7.
80. Garwick AW, Kohrman C, Wolman C, Blum RW. Families' recommendations for improving services for children with chronic conditions. *Arch Pediatr Adolesc Med* 1998;152:440–8.
81. Lewis FM, Woods NF, Hough EE, Bensley LS. The family's functioning with chronic illness in the mother: The spouse's perspective. *Soc Sci Med* 1989;29:1261–9.
82. Fivenson D, Arnol RJ, Kaniecki DJ, et al. The effect of atopic dermatitis on total burden of illness and quality of life on adults and children in large managed care organisation. *J Manag Care Pharm* 2002;8:333–42.
83. Bickers DR, Lim HW, Margolis D, et al. The burden of skin diseases: 2004: A joint project of the American Academy of Dermatology Association and the Society for Investigative Dermatology. *J Am Acad Dermatol* 2006;55:490–500.
84. Chamlin SL, Cella D, Frieden IJ, Williams ML, Mancini AJ, Lai J, Chren MM. Development of the childhood atopic dermatitis impact scale: Initial validation of a quality-of-life measure for young children with atopic dermatitis and their families. *J Invest Dermatol* 2005;125:1106–11.
85. McKenna SP, Whalley D, Dewar AL, Erdman RAM, Kohlmann T, et al. International development of the Parents' Index of Quality of Life in Atopic Dermatitis (PIQoL-AD). *Qual Life Res* 2005;14:231–41.
86. Eghlileb AM, Basra MKA, Finlay AY. The Psoriasis Family Index: Preliminary results of validation of a quality of life instrument for family members of patients with psoriasis. *Dermatology* 2009;219:63–70.
87. Basra MKA, Sue-Ho R, Finlay AY. The Family Dermatology Life Quality Index: Measuring the secondary impact of skin disease. *Br J Dermatol* 2007;156:528–38.
88. Basra MKA, Edmunds O, Salek MS, Finlay AY. Measurement of family impact of skin disease: Further validation of the Family Dermatology Life Quality Index. *J Eur Acad Dermatol Venereol* 2008;22:813–21.
89. Tadros A, Vergou T, Stratigos AJ, et al. Psoriasis: Is it the tip of the iceberg for the quality of life of patients and their families? *J Eur Acad Dermatol Venereol* 2011;25:1282–7.

90. Chinn DJ, Poyner T, Sibley G. Randomised controlled trial of a single nurse consultation in primary care on the quality of life of children with atopic eczema. *Br J Dermatol* 2002;146:432–9.
91. Whalley D, Hules J, McKenna SP, et al. The benefit of pimecrolimus (Elidel, SDZ ASM 981) on parents' quality of life in the treatment of paediatric atopic dermatitis. *Pediatr* 2002;110:1133–6.
92. Meads DM, McKenna SP, Kahler K. The quality of life of parents of children with atopic dermatitis: Interpretation of PIQoL-AD scores. *Qual Life Res* 2005;14:2235–45.
93. Fung WK, Lo KK. Prevalence of skin disease among school children and adolescents in a student health service in Hong Kong. *Paediatr Dermatol* 2000;17:440–6.
94. Bechelli LM, Haddad N, Pimenta WP, et al. Epidemiological survey of skin diseases in school children living in the Porus Valley (Acre state, Amazonia, Brazil). *Dermatologica* 1981;163:78–93.
95. Herd RM. In: Williams HC, ed. *Morbidity and cost in atopic dermatitis*. Cambridge: Cambridge University Press, 2000;88–9.
96. Emerson RM, Williams HC, Allen BR. What is the cost of atopic dermatitis in preschool children? *Br J Dermatol* 2001;144:514–22.
97. Lapidus CS, Schwarz DF, Honig PJ. Atopic dermatitis in children. Who cares? Who pays? *J Am Acad Dermatol* 1993;28:699–703.
98. Verboom P, Hakkaart-Van L, Sturkenboom M, et al. The cost of atopic dermatitis in the Netherlands: An international comparison. *Br J Dermatol* 2002;147:716–24.
99. Higginson IJ, Carr AJ. Measuring quality of life: Using quality of life measures in clinical setting. *BMJ* 2001;322:1297–300.
100. Varni JW, Katz ER, Seid M, et al. The Pediatric Cancer Quality of Life Invetory (PCQL). I. Instrument development, descriptive statistics, and cross-informant variance. *J Behav Med* 1998;21: 179–204.
101. Schuttelaar MLA, Vermeulen KM, Drukker N, Coenraads PJ. A randomized controlled trial in children with eczema: Nurse practitioner vs. dermatologist. *Br J Dermatol* 2010;162:162–70.
102. Staab D, von Rueden U, Kehrt R, et al. Evaluation of a parental training program for the management of childhood atopic dermatitis. *Pediatr Allergy Immunol* 2002;13:84–90.
103. Broberg A, Kalimo K, Lindblad B, et al. Parental education in the treatment of childhood atopic eczema. *Acta Derm Venereol* 1990;70:495–9.
104. Kamalpour A, Gammon B, Chen KH, et al. Resource utilization and quality of life associated with congenital ichthyoses. *Pediatr Dermatol* 2011;28:512–8.

Part II: **PSYCHOPHYSIOLOGIC DISORDERS**

Ruqiya Shama Tareen

5 Atopic dermatitis: a psychocutaneous review

Atopic dermatitis (AD) is a very common, multifactorial skin disease affecting about 20% of children. It usually starts in the early formative years, having a relapsing remitting course throughout the childhood, and in about 3% of cases persists throughout their life. Atopic dermatitis provides us with a model of a psychophysiologic disorder with delicate interactions between various factors including genetic predisposition, environmental triggers, acute and chronic psychosocial trauma as well as stress, in addition to its impact on the developing immune system and endocrine system as well as peripheral and central neuromodulators. Atopic dermatitis ultimately results in dermatologic and psychiatric manifestations. This discussion aims to elucidate some of these complex phenomena and how they impact the course and management of atopic dermatitis.

5.1 Introduction

Coca et al first described the term "atopy" in the literature in 1923 while classifying the states of hypersensitiveness (1). Atopy is defined as an inherited preponderance to increased production of IgE immunoglobulin antibodies, which predisposes that person to certain "atopic diseases," including asthma, hay fever, and atopic dermatitis. Atopic dermatitis is a multifaceted disease with an onset before age 5 and with a chronic sometimes lifelong relapsing remitting course. Approximately 50 years ago attention was focused on a possible link between the psychological stress and atopic dermatitis (see Chapter 2); since then our understanding of the intertwining of the emotional state and expression of atopy has improved significantly with increasing evidence pointing toward a psychophysiological origin of atopic dermatitis.

5.1.1 Epidemiology

Atopic diseases in general and atopic dermatitis in particular appear to have rising prevalence in children born after 1980 in European countries. The prevalence rates differ from country to country but generally hover between 10–20% in different parts of Europe. Much higher prevalence rates of up to 35% were found in northern parts of Scandinavia at about 69 N latitude. In the United States, lifetime prevalence was found to be around 17.2% in Oregon in children born during 1987 to 1991 (2). Prevalence rates in countries of Africa were about 11.1%. In Japan prevalence rate was quite different between the two cities studied, ranging from 9.5% to 24% among children of age 5–12 years. In Australia the lifetime prevalence was about 18.7% to

31.9%, depending on the area studied. Atopic disease can occur at any age, but 65% of patients develop atopic dermatitis in the first year of their life (2).

5.2 Pathophysiologic factors in atopic dermatitis

5.2.1 Genetic predisposition

Genetic predisposition is considered the most important risk factor in atopic dermatitis with 77% concordance in monozygotic twins and 15% in dizygotic twins (3). The genetic transmission is quite complex as atopic dermatitis does not have a Mendelian inheritance pattern with an identifiable gene locus. Twin studies have proven the high genetic link, but it appears that genetic susceptibility is the first hit and having a genotype may or may not result in full expression of phenotype unless other risk factors plays a role of second hit. Various candidate genes have been identified, but no definitive associations are found. Maternal transmission is much stronger than paternal, indicating a possibility of genomic transmission, by suppressing the paternal genes (3). Atopic dermatitis is 2.6 times more common in girls than in their age matched counterparts (4).

5.2.2 Socio-economic status

Atopic dermatitis, similar to other atopic diseases, tends to favor the upper socioeconomic strata. A stepwise progression in the prevalence was reported by Freeman in United States and duplicated by many other studies in England, Germany, and Spain (2).

5.2.3 Family size

An inverse relationship has been reported with the number of the siblings and atopic dermatitis. Having three or more siblings was found to be protective against atopic dermatitis (4).

5.2.4 Food allergens

Unlike other atopic diseases, atopic dermatitis is not directly related to food allergens, but a temporal relationship with certain food allergens is reported in up to 15% to 40% of patients with atopic dermatitis, according to different studies. Most common food allergens associated were egg, soy, peanuts, wheat, fish, and cow's milk (4).

5.3 Psychoneuroimmunologic factors

Atopic dermatitis is considered as a neurogenic, cutaneous inflammation resulting from a dysregulated immune system (see Chapter 2). It is hypothesized that exposure to early life stressors (such as neglect, abandonment or inconsistent care giving, or even high family stress) can sensitize the child's immune system. It all starts with over-activation of the hypothalamic-pituitary axis, causing excessive release of cortisol and catecholamine. This in turn leads to over production of the T lymphocyte helper cells (T_H cells), more specifically of T_H2 cells, causing an imbalance of T_H1 and T_H2 cells ratio. T_H2 cells are found in abundance in atopic lesions and are responsible for a cascade of events, including release of several cytokines, increased production of mast cells, and augmentation of eosinophils and B lymphocyte cells production, which in turn produce IgE immunoglobulin.

Newborns who have a genetic predisposition to atopic disease are found to have up to 70% higher levels of IgE in their cord blood. Compared to only 3% of controls, about 10.5% of the genetically predisposed infants developed atopic dermatitis during the first 18 months of life (5). Although IgE seems to be the predominant immunoglobulin in atopic dermatitis, deficiency of IgA in the early few months of infancy allows easy absorption of allergens and primes the subject to produce more IgE in response (6). Various neuropeptides (such as substance P, vasoactive intestinal peptides, neurokinin, leukotriene, neurotensin, and neuropeptide Y) are some of the well known mediators of inflammation released in response to emotional stress causing neurogenic inflammation (7).

5.3.1 Breast feeding

The efficacy of breast-feeding in preventing atopic dermatitis has been proven by several large community based studies. In a study in Belarus of over 1,600 infants, prevalence rate of AD was 3.3% in breast fed infants in comparison to 6.3% in formula fed infants. Some hypoallergenic formulas are also reported to decrease the incidence in infants who had no genetic predisposition to atopic dermatitis (4).

5.3.2 Environmental allergens

Degree of sensitivity to environmental allergens (especially house dust mites) has been shown to have a positive correlation with severity of atopic dermatitis. Conflicting results were reported from different studies about the negative impact of having a furry pet in the household. Having small rodents, rabbits, and guinea pigs in household were found to be associated with increased risk of developing AD in school-aged children. Contradictory to this finding, more recent studies have reported that exposure to animal allergen (especially cat and dog dander) may in fact be protective against developing AD (4). Being raised at a farm has been shown to have a protective effect against atopic respiratory disease, but the correlation was not well established in AD. Several aeroallergens are found to increase the risk of atopic dermatitis, including living near high traffic areas and volatile organic exposure (especially toluene and tobacco exposure); this is particularly increased if the mother smoked during pregnancy and the lactation period (4).

5.4 Psychophysiological aspects of atopic dermatitis

Psychological undercurrents in atopic dermatitis still remain somewhat less clearly defined than some of the other aspect of the disease. For a better understanding of this topic, atopic dermatitis is discussed under four main categories: impact of stress on the immunological system, psychoanalytic hypothesis, biopsychosocial model, and psychological dysregulation due to atopic dermatitis.

5.4.1 Impact of stress on the immunological system

Skin touch is the very first and most important way of communication for the neonate. Most of the neonatal introduction to the world occurs though the tactile communication with others via their skin. A soft touch, a warm cuddle, a comforting lap, and a nestle against the mother's breasts all are some of the earliest experiences that shape an infant's impression of the world outside of mother's womb. Animal studies and behavior studies in premature infants have shown that tactile communication plays an important role in neuronal cell growth and maturation (8).

Histamine, one of the main mediators of the itch and scratch cycle, was released in guinea pigs in response to classical conditioning in response to repeated stress (8). The relationship of stress to atopic dermatitis is bidirectional. Psychological stress, especially early on in infancy, is known to cause an indelible mark on the still evolving neuronal, hormonal, and immunological systems. The first response to any stress is the activation of the sympathetic system with release of catecholamine resulting in increased production of prostaglandins, leukotrienes, and histamine, triggering pruritus and an inflammatory response (9,10). This understanding of neuroimmunological response to stress has been strengthened by the finding that CD8 lymphocyte counts increase in response to psychological stress and stay elevated 1 hour after the initial stressful event in patients with AD, suggesting a heightened autonomic arousal in response to stressful events (10).

Sieffert et al (9) measured this psycho-reactivity in a study of atopic dermatitis patients during acute exacerbations of eczema and then during disease free states; in this study several psychophysiological markers of stress were compared with normal controls. This research failed to confirm that there was a higher psychophysiological response to mental stress in patients with atopic dermatitis; however, it did show that AD patients had higher levels of psychophysiological activation regardless of whether they were in a relapse of atopic dermatitis or were free of their AD. Patients with atopic dermatitis showed higher heart rates and lower rates of heart rate variability, confirming a baseline sympathetic system overstimulation. The atopic dermatitis patients in this study also demonstrated a higher level of anxiety and depression; this is a finding that has been reported by other studies (11,12).

The sensory and autonomic nerves in the epidermis and dermis, when stimulated by exogenous stimuli (such as environmental allergens) or by internal stimulus (such as stress) release a number of neuropeptides (i.e. histamine, tryptase, TNF-α, leukotrienes, and β-endorphins). These mediators exert their inflammatory responses through their specific receptors located on primary afferent neurons (13).

5.4.2 Psychoanalytic hypothesis

The skin is the largest organ in the human body and plays a unique role in our earliest understanding of our world (see Chapter 2). The sense of being touched and caressed promotes a sense of attachment and bonding in the neonate to its primary care giver or object, which in the majority of cases is the mother. The physical contact with the mother is a soothing experience for infants due to the pleasant sensation they derive from tactile, thermal, and pressure senses. A study of mother's behavior toward their atopic children by Rosethental et al (14) showed that mothers of atopic children were less likely to pick up their children when they cried, in comparison to mothers of non-atopic children. Other studies have proposed that mothers of children with atopic dermatitis are conflicted in terms of whether their touch is going to be soothing or will cause more discomfort to the already irritated skin in the case of active disease; also, there could be a sense of repulsion due to the skin condition, however, at a subconscious level.

Psychoanalytic perspective proposes that infants who are not given this soothing physical contact go on to develop a predisposition to atopic dermatitis. Miller et al studied the impact of earliest psychological trauma in the form of a "rejecting mother" and its impact on expression of atopic disease. The rejecting mother was defined as "one whose behavior toward the child is such that she consciously or unconsciously has a desire to be free from the child and considers it a burden." They followed 63 infants with atopic dermatitis with the possibility of being rejected by their mother and found that 98.4% had atopy in comparison to only 24.3% in the control group of children with no atopy (15). A coexisting overprotection by mothers followed by earlier rejection was seen in 57% of infants with atopic dermatitis compared to 10.8% of children with no atopic condition (15).

Object relation theory is a modern take on the Freudian term of *object*. According to this theory the infant arrives in this world in an infantile autistic state where presence of a nurturing, comforting, reliable external object (i.e. a primary caregiver, most likely the mother) is necessary. The infant, when nurtured by this object, proceeds to internalize that primary object to create awareness about self and the surrounding world in context of this object. When object constancy is achieved successfully, it leads to a coherent sense of self. The infant is completely dependent on this object for meeting its needs, and unavailability of this object or even inconsistent fulfillments of the infant's needs may give rise to feelings of abandonment, rejection, anger, and even hostility, which it projects back toward the object. Adequate physical care provision by the mother to the infant along with reassurance and comfort by touch and caressing during this crucial period of development of self enables the infant to regulate its biological function and immunological system. This also allows these systems to not be over burdened in times of stress and, thus, subsequently impact the disease susceptibility in a positive manner (16).

5.4.3 Biopsychosocial model

This contemporary model of mind–body relationship also takes into account various systems surrounding the dyad of mother and baby. This mother–child interaction is impacted by an interactional system that exists between mother and child and that interacts with the immediate surrounding system (such as father, siblings, and other family members), as well as how their interaction with broader systems of structural, financial, spiritual, cultural, and medical systems occurs. The theory proposes that a good relationship with the caregiver is the fundamental determinant of the child's ability to acquire normal physical and emotional health. This theory also takes into account the biological predisposition to disease, such as atopic dermatitis, and other predisposing and perpetuating factors along with the psychological stress in pathogenesis of atopic dermatitis (16).

5.4.4 Psychological dysregulation due to atopic dermatitis

Having a young child with atopic dermatitis creates many complex emotions in the child but also evokes many mixed emotions in parents. An infant with AD needs the physical contact and reassurance by touch of parents more so than infants without AD. On the other hand, the same soft caress can be painful and uncomfortable or perceived in a distorted way by the inflamed and excoriated skin, leading the child to feel as if he or she is being punished or attacked by the mother or caregiver. Since these early sensory perceptions are how the infant perceives his or her sense of self, this unpleasant or bad perception of self could be internalized.

On the other hand, parents perceive infants with atopic dermatitis as somewhat defective as the sense of joy and pride of parenthood is tarnished by the visible skin lesions, constant itching, crying, and discomfort associated with it. The complex interaction between an infant with atopic dermatitis who tends to be more demanding, irritable, and less consolable and the parent who feels resentful, embarrassed, and powerless creates a cycle of negative emotions on both sides. Parents may withdraw from care provision, resulting in an infant with unmet needs who may develop a sense of "bad fit" and resort to self-soothing with self-stimulation of skin by excessive scratching. The parent, when finally identify the unconscious withdrawal from the infant, becomes anxious and guilty and then frantically tries to correct the neglect by showering too much attention; in addition, the parent becomes overprotective toward the child, resulting in another cycle of unhealthy patterns of interaction, where the child becomes excessively demanding, clinging, whining, and taking control of the parent–child relationship (17).

5.5 Clinical features

Atopic dermatitis is characterized by development of an erythematous, papulovesicular rash that initially is weeping and crusting but later becomes lichenified, maculopapular patches due to constant scratching. Atopic dermatitis can involve all of the body, but it typically follows a characteristic distribution according to the age of the pediatric patient. In *infantile* eczema, which occurs in those less than 2 years of age, erythematous, exudative lesions first appear on the face (especially cheeks, forehead, and scalp); lesions then progress to the trunk and extensor surfaces of extremities, sparing the diaper area. In the *childhood* phase, which is from 2 to 11 years of age, lesions are more localized to the flexural surfaces of the limbs and tend to be dry. Perioral region lesions and cheilitis are common, though the rest of the face is usually spared. Hand involvement is common and can be very troublesome for these children. The *adolescent* phase from 12 years onward usually presents with lichenified, macular lesions involving face, neck, upper trunk, and flexures aspects of the extremities. In adolescent girls the first and only manifestation of the AD can be the highly pruritic hand eczema (18).

5.6 Diagnosis

Atopic dermatitis can be difficult to diagnose because of its varied morphologic features and the fact that it lacks a definite laboratory marker. The Hanifin-Rajka Diagnostic Criteria was developed in 1980 to help this difficulty and consists of a set of 4 major and 23 minor criteria for the diagnosis of atopic dermatitis (see Table 5.1). Since its inception, the Hanifin-Rajka Diagnostic Criteria is still the most widely tool used to diagnose atopic dermatitis (19).

Several other studies examined the Hanifin-Rajka Diagnostic Criteria and recommended some modifications in minor criteria based on their findings (19). Several of

Table 5.1: Hanifin-Rajka Diagnostic Criteria

Major Criteria Must meet three or more of the major criteria	• Pruritus • Flexural involvement and lichenification in older children and adolescents and facial and extensor involvement in infants and young children • Chronically relapsing dermatitis • Personal and or family history of atopic dermatitis and other atopic disorders
Minor Criteria Must meet 3 or more of the minor criteria	Typical Skin Manifestations • Xerosis • Cheilitis • Ichthyosis, keratosis pilaris, palmar hyperlinearity • Nipple eczema • Perifollicular accentuation • Facial pallor or erythema • Pityriasis alba • Anterior neck folds • Pruritus with sweating • Dermographism, delayed blanching • Nonspecific hand or foot dermatitis Immune System Related Features • Immediate (type I) skin test reactivity • Elevated serum IgE • Impaired cell immunity (propensity for skin infections esp. Herpes simplex and Staph aureus) • Food intolerance • Wool and lipid intolerance Ophthalmic and Periorbital Features • Keratoconus • Anterior subcapsular cataracts • Recurrent conjunctivitis • Infraorbital fold (Dennie-Morgan) • Orbital darkening Early age of onset Course of disease affected by emotional and environmental factors

Source: Larsen FS, Hanifin JM. Epidemiology of atopic dermatitis. Immunol Allergy Clin North Am 2002;1:1–24

the minor criteria were considered less specific and these include nipple eczema, ichthyosis, cheilitis, anterior subcapsular cataracts, keratoconus, food intolerance, hypopigmented patches (pityriasis alba), and anterior neck folds (19). A simplified diagnostic guideline was introduced by a working group of dermatologists from the United Kingdom in 1990 that included most of the main diagnostic criteria from Hanifin-Rajka Diagnostic Criteria (19). This set of diagnostic criteria was used in epidemiological studies and showed 74% to 84% sensitivity (see Table 5.2) as

Table 5.2: UK Working Party Refinement of Hanifin and Rajka Criteria

Mandatory criteria (must meet)
A self report of itchy skin condition *or*
Parental report of scratching, or rubbing noticed in a child
Plus at least 3 of the following criteria
1. Involvement of flexural folds of elbow, knees, ankles, neck (cheeks in children under 10 years of age)
2. Personal history of another atopic disease like asthma or hay fever *or* Family history of an atopic disease in children under age 4 years
3. History of general dry skin in past year
4. Visible signs of eczema at typical flexural sites *or* Eczema on cheeks, forehead or outer aspects of extremities in children under 4 years of age
5. Age of onset under age of 2 years (not used if child is 4 years of age)
Minor Criteria
Must meet 3 or more of the minor criteria

Source: Larsen FS, Hanifin JM. Epidemiology of atopic dermatitis. Immunol Allergy Clin North Am 2002;1:1–24

well as 97% to 99% specificity in community settings in the United Kingdom (19). Although, when the same criteria were used to study school aged children in Australia, the sensitivity was found to be much lower at 43%, but specificity remained high at 95% (2).

5.6.1 Allergy Testing

5.6.1.1 Skin prick test (SPT)

Mast cell-bound IgE medicated food allergy can be diagnosed by introduction of food allergens via skin prick testing; the resulting atopic reaction is found to be 100% predictive of a particular food allergy. A positive reaction is identified in children over 2 years of age when exposed to cow's milk if they develop a SPT weal diameter >8 mm and under 2 years of age with an SPT weal of >6 mm in diameter. However, SPT is found to be unreliable when used in infants (20).

5.6.1.2 Atopy patch test (APT)

The atopic patch test (APT) is useful in the diagnosis of aeroallergens and food allergies that involve T cell and dendritic cell mediated inflammatory processes. APT can increase the accuracy of the diagnosis substantially when used in combination with SPT. APT is especially useful in identifying late phase clinical reactions with a specificity of 95%. APT has higher specificity, up to 92%, compared to SPT with a 53% and IgE level with 64%. The European Task Force on Atopic Dermatitis (ETFAD) has developed a protocol to standardized APT administration, using 5,000

Table 5.3: Differential diagnosis of atopic dermatitis

Condition	Clinical Features	Pruritus	Common Sites
Atopic Dermatitis	May be associated with asthma and allergic rhinitis.	+++	Flexor aspects of limbs. Face, scalp and trunk in children under 2 years.
Contact Dermatitis	History of contact with irritant, exposed surfaces	+++	
Seborrheic Dermatitis	Reddish pink, greasy, punctate lesions coalesces to form diffuse lesions	+/−	Scalp, scalp, skin folds, behind ears
Psoriasis	Discrete, raised reddish pink lesions with fine silver scales	+	Extensor surfaces of extremities
Icthyosis vulgaris	Generalized dry skin, positive family history	++	Extensor surfaces of limbs
Scabies	Crowded conditions, burrows	+++	Interdigital spaces

to 7,000 PNU/g in adults and proposes its use with half of this concentration in children. ETFAD supports using 12 mm diameter chambers and does not advocate use of any pretreatment. Some reaction may be observed in 48 hours, but maximal response may not be observed until 72 hours (20).

5.6.1.3 Double blind placebo controlled food challenge (DBPCFC)

Regarded as a gold standard in early studies, the Double Blind Placebo Controlled Food Challenge (DBPCFC) still remains the most definitive test for food allergy. Reasons for limited use of DBPCFC include the inherent risk involved in exposure to potentially life threatening allergic reactions, the amount of resources needed to undertake this test, and the development of SPT testing (20).

5.6.2 Differential Diagnosis

The differential diagnosis of atopic dermatitis is outlined in Table 5.3.

5.7 Management

5.7.1 Prevention of relapse

Avoidance of the offending irritants and allergens is the first step in the management of atopic dermatitis. Taking a thorough history and identifying the offending agents are the most important components of a successful treatment plan (21).

5.7.2 Food allergens

About 30% to 50% of children with AD have defined food allergies, which perpetuates the atopy (20). Some of the most common food allergens are cow milk, peanuts, eggs, fish, soy, wheat, and nuts (21). Exhaustive protection from food allergens has not been proven to be very effective, and overzealous attempts to avoid food allergens may lead to nutritional deficiencies, complicating the clinical presentation (20). It is not prudent to attempt challenging exposure to allergens to establish food allergy as in the case of severe allergies, which may lead to severe reactions, such as anaphylaxis. In high risk infants, recommendations to delay or even prevent the onset of atopic dermatitis include postponing the introduction of solid food until 6 months of age, feeding completely on breast milk, and, when breast feeding is not possible, using hydrolyzed hypoallergenic formula (20).

5.7.3 Aeroallergens

House dust with 13 species of identified dust mites is known to be the most common aeroallergen implicated in atopic disease. High levels of Der p1 specific antibodies were detected in 95% of AD patients and correlated well with the severity of the disease (22). Bedding, overstuffed furniture, carpets, and other items provide the perfect breeding ground for these fomites (22). Covering of mattresses, diligent vacuuming, and removal of carpets can significantly improve the prognosis of the atopic dermatitis.

5.7.4 Optimizing the epidermal barrier (EB)

The epidermis is the first line of defense against any percutaneous invasion of allergens, infective agents, irritants, chemicals, and other substances. The epidermal skin barrier is a protective shield that is located in the deeper part of the stratum corneum. The efficacy of this barrier in resisting the penetration of these molecules depends on the thickness of stratum corneum. There are wide inter-individual variations in the efficacy of the EB according to different areas of the body as well as intra-individual variations. Many enzymes are needed to maintain the integrity of the EB, and these enzymes are pH dependent (23). Any disruption of the normal skin pH of 7.0 can cause increase in the activity of enzymes (such as proteases), which can lead to thinning of the stratum corneum and impairment of the EB (23). Commonly used soaps and other agents to cleanse skin can disrupt this pH, and repeated use can cause significant thinning of the EB. Avoidance of soap and detergents as well as use of emollient wash products (such as hyroxyurea, soft paraffin, mixture of soft and liquid paraffin, and mineral oils with or without any active ingredients) can be key factors in successful treatment of atopic dermatitis. See Box 5.1.

Box 5.1 Commonly used emollients for maintaining the epidermal barrier

Cream ®
Hydromol products ®
Lipobase ®
Oilatum Plus ®
Balneum Plus ®
Aquaphor®
Eucerine ®
Petroleum Jelly®

5.7.5 Hydration therapy

Due to the damaged epidermal barrier and decreased levels of ceramide in their skin, children with atopic dermatitis have a tendency to have low skin water content, leading to excessive dryness of skin or xerosis, leading to a relapse of the atopic dermatitis (24). Keeping the skin hydrated to prevent a relapse or to improve healing during an acute episode of atopic dermatitis is very important. Soaking baths are beneficial, although showers can be used in milder cases. Soaking baths in lukewarm water followed by gentle pat drying and applying an occlusive sealer (such as petroleum jelly or a urea containing moisturizer) to seal the water in the epidermis is the best way to optimize hydration of skin. In cases of localized atopic dermatitis, the affected body area, such as an arm or leg, can be soaked in a water basin (24).

5.7.6 Management of pruritus

Pruritus or itch is almost synonymous with atopic dermatitis, affecting almost 100% of the patients with atopic dermatitis. The unrelenting itch and scratching further damages the skin, exacerbating dermatitis as well as perpetuating an unending "itch–scratch" cycle. Pruritus is particularly troublesome at night. Several mechanisms are at interplay behind this cycle of itch and scratch, including peripheral mediators of itch, such as histamine, various neuropeptides, acetylcholine, tryptase, cytokines, neurotphin-4, eosinophils, platelet aggravating factor, cannabinoids, opioids peptides, interferon gamma vanilloids, and calcineurin inhibitors (25).

Since the mechanism of the pruritus is so complex, it is of no surprise that traditional remedies such as antihistamines are often not effective. The current approach is to focus on the reduction of inflammation in the skin and thus decrease the intensity of the pruritus. The most commonly used and effective anti-inflammatory agents are topical corticosteroids. Recently immunomodulatory agents inhibiting calcineurin (such as tarcolimus and pimecrolimus) have been shown to abort the acute attacks of atopic dermatitis by decreasing pruritus and stopping the itch–scratch cycle (25).

Other inhibitors of mediators of pruritus (such as interferon gamma, capsaicin, opiate receptors antagonists, and leukotriene antagonists) have also been shown to decrease the pruritus and favorably impact the atopic dermatitis. Systemic treatment with immunomodulators (such as cyclosporine, glucocorticoids, tarcolimus, and pimecrolimus) has been used in treatment for refractory atopic dermatitis; however, topical therapy is the mainstay of treatment (25).

5.7.7 Topical corticosteroids

Since the discovery of hydrocortisone in the 1950s, the glucocorticoids are the most important medical discovery in the history of dermatologic therapies. Later, the development of halogenated corticosteroids opened the door for even more potent agents. When used inappropriately corticosteroids can induce various systemic side effects, and this has led to a serious debate about which corticosteroids are for which part of the body and for how long should they be used without causing any deleterious lifelong adverse effects.

Corticosteroids are lipophilic and are easily absorbed from the epidermis; after entering the cells they bind to the DNA binding glucocorticoid receptors, causing down or up-regulation of gene expression. The genes that are expressed encode various enzymes leading to four main mechanisms of actions of corticosteroids: immunomodulation, vasoconstriction, anti-inflammation, and anti-proliferation (26). Any decision in regards to initiation of treatment with corticosteroids and which ones to use depend on various factors, discussed in Sections 5.7.7.1–5.7.7.6.

5.7.7.1 Age

The younger the child, the greater is the absorption of the corticosteroids from the epidermis. This, along with the relatively larger body surface area that young children have, readily predisposes them for serious local and systemic side effects. Thus, in infants and younger children, first all the alternative treatment options should be employed; only when all other measures fail, should use of corticosteroids (steroids) be considered.

When indicated, the lowest potency corticosteroid should be used, although moderate potency agents (such as methylprednisolone acetate or prednicarbate) can be used as they have a better side effect profile if used for a limited time. The relapsing, remitting nature of atopic dermatitis requires the treating physician to be mindful that the need for a course of corticosteroids (steroids) may arise multiple times during the course of disease; however, great care should be taken that individual courses of corticosteroid treatment should not be longer than 3 weeks at a time (27,28).

5.7.7.2 Potency of corticosteroids

Corticosteroids are divided into seven classes based on their potency on vasoconstrictor assay, class 1 being the most potent. As a general rule, the use of potent corticosteroids in children is reserved only for very severe, recalcitrant disease that has not responded to other forms of treatment. When a decision is made to use a potent corticosteroid, the effort should be made to use it for the minimal effective period to avoid topical and systemic side effects. Children have a low body volume to skin surface area ratio, which can predispose them to higher rates of steroid absorption; this effect, when combined with a higher potency steroid application, can produce deleterious side effects even in short term therapy (27,28). See Table 5.4.

5.7.7.3 Site of topical application

Penetration and absorption of steroids is much more rapid and complete from the sites where the skin is thinner – such as the face, eyelids, forehead, axillae, and genital area. Use of high to medium high potency corticosteroids (class 1–5) should be avoided in such areas. Lowest potency of steroids and shorter treatment time can reduce the risk of topical side effects, such as skin thinning and atrophy (27,28).

5.7.7.4 Frequency of application

The stratum corneum serves as a reservoir that can release the active ingredient over time; thus, once daily application may be sufficient in most cases, while highly active disease may require twice daily application. Frequency of application should be tapered gradually until stopping the medication in order to prevent any rebound of the atopic dermatitis (27,28).

5.7.7.5 Type of application

It is important to select the right medium of delivery for the steroid being prescribed to optimize the therapeutic effects. Ointments are most viscous as they are oil based and are the best choice to provide occlusion of the dry xerotic type of lesions. Creams, being less viscous, have more acceptance from patients and caregivers. Creams are well suited for the lesions that are wet and oozy. Lotions and gels are water based and are generally not suited for dry lesions or xerotic skin but can be of use in areas where creams and ointments cannot be used, such as the scalp or other hairy areas (27,28).

5.7.7.6 Amount of application

Generally used, a "fingertip unit" (FTU) is a reliable and effective way of gauging the amount to be applied. One FTU is considered enough to treat an area of skin twice the size of an adult's hand. It is estimated that 2 FTU are approximately equal to

Table 5.4: Classification of topical corticosteroids by potency

Class	Potency	Corticosteroid	Strength
I	Very High	Betamethasone dipropionate	0.05%
		Clobestol propionate	0.05%
		Diflorasone diacetate	0.05%
		Halobetasol propionate	0.05%
II	High	Amcinonide	0.1%
		Betamethasone dipropionate	0.05%
		Desoximetasone	0.05%
		Desoximetasone	0.25%
		Fluocinonide	0.05%
		Halcinonide	0.1%
		Mometasone furoate	0.1%
		Triamcinolone acetonide	0.5%
III	High-Medium	Amcinonide	0.1%
		Betamethasone valerate	0.1%
		Diflorasone diacetate	0.05%
		Fluticasone propionate	0.005%
		Clocortolone pivalate	0.1%
		Triamcinolone acetonide	0.1%
IV	Medium	Betamethasone valerate	0.12%
		Flucinolone acetonide	0.025%
		Flurandrenolide	0.05%
		Hydrocortisone valerate	0.2%
		Mometasone furoate	0.1%
V	Low-Medium	Hydrocortisone butyrate	0.1%
		Hydrocortisone probutate	0.1%
		Prednicarbate	0.1%
VI	Low	Alcometasone dipropionate	0.05%
		Desonide	0.05%
		Flucinolone acetonide	0.01%
VII	Lowest	Dexamethasone	0.1%
		Hydrocortisone	0.25%
		Hydrocortisone	0.5%
		Hydrocortisone	1%
		Hydrocortisone acetate	0.5%
		Hydrocortisone acetate	1%

1 gram of corticosteroid. Recommended maximal dose in grams depends on patient age, the amount of the body surface area covered with atopic dermatitis, the site of lesions, disease severity, and steroid potency. As a general rule a corticosteroid prescription should not exceed 50 grams at one time. Close monitoring and frequent visits are keys in avoiding the long term local and systemic side effects in children requiring frequent corticosteroid prescriptions (26,27,28).

5.7.8 Topical immunomodulators

Calcineurin inhibitors (such as tarcolimus and pimecrolimus) act by binding to cytosolic immunophilin receptors and inhibiting calcineurin; this action results in decreasing inflammation by down regulation of inflammatory mediators such as interleukins (IL-2, IL-4, & IL-8), along with tumor necrosis factor alpha (TNFα), interferon gamma (INFγ), lymphocytes (TH1, T_H1 and T_H2), and granulocyte–macrophage colony stimulating factor.

5.7.8.1 Tarcolimus

The efficacy of tarcolimus alone or in combination with steroids has been shown by multiple studies. Tarcolimus ointment (0.03% and 0.1%), when used twice daily in pediatric patients 2–15 years of age, was shown to be more effective than 1% hydrocortisone (29). Tarcolimus has also shown superiority when compared to 0.005% fluticasone pivalate ointment in the pediatric population (29). Tarcolimus (0.1% ointment) has been shown to be effective and safe for up to 12 months to 3 years of treatment in those aged 2–15 years (27). The most common side effect, reported in 29.9% of children, was a burning sensation at the site of application followed by transient pruritus in 23%, which improved in a few days (29).

5.7.8.2 Pimecrolimus

When pediatric patients 2–17 years old with mild to moderate atopic dermatitis were treated with pimecrolimus 1% cream twice daily for 6 weeks, 34.8% became clear or almost clear of atopic dermatitis (27). Pimecrolimus was effective when used in those 3–23 months of age and others 2–17 years of age. Infants with atopic dermatitis showed 61% improvement at week 6 and >80% improvement at 12 months when pimecrolimus was applied twice daily along with a moderately potent corticosteroid. After the active treatment period ended, fewer infants had a relapse when compared to the control group. It was also reported that pimecrolimus seems to be more effective in treating lesions on the face. About 2.5% of infants and 10.5% children reported burning sensation at the site of application that improved in 1–3 days (27,29).

5.8 Systematic treatment of atopic dermatits

5.8.1 Antihistamines

Histamine is the most well known mediator of cutaneous inflammation. It is released from mast cells in response to an atopic challenge causing pruritus, vasodilation, and edema. Most atopic effects are mediated by H_1 receptors, and all antihistamine used in atopic conditions works at H_1 receptors. The first generation antihistamine readily crosses the blood brain barrier, thus causing side effects such as sedation, daytime drowsiness, motor incoordination, and others. The main concern when using histamine in pediatric populations is the paradoxical irritability and hyperactivity that can occur after the immediate sedative effects wear off. Diphenhydramine is the first antihistamine introduced in 1947 followed by chlorpheniramine, promethazine, cyproheptadine, and hydroxyzine. The second generation of antihistamine became popular after they came on market in the 1980s due to their low penetration of the blood brain barrier, making them comparatively non-sedative. Loratadine, desloratadine, cetirizine, and fexofenadine are beneficial especially when there are other comorbid atopic conditions. Fexofenadine has shown an edge in this group of antihistamines in terms of reduction in pruritus due to atopic dermatitis (30).

5.8.2 Phototherapy

Ultraviolet B (UVB) therapy with a wavelength of 290–320 nm has been used effectively in the treatment of atopic dermatitis for many years. Phototherapy doses are defined as minimal erythema doses (MED) and 0.5–1 MED is considered effective (31). UVB works by causing apoptosis of T lymphocytes, immunosuppression by its effect on cytokines and interleukin and by its antimicrobial action, as well as possible thickening of epidermis enhancing the EDB. Clayton et al, in a 6 years retrospective review of children with AD treated with narrow band UVB (NB-UVB), showed a response rate of 40% with improvement sustaining at 3 months follow up. However, the children were also using emollients and topical steroids during active treatment (32).

Combination UVA and UVB (UVA/B) has shown effectiveness against atopic dermatitis; however, when NB-UVB was used in combination with UVA, it resulted in more than 90% reduction in atopic dermatitis symptoms. When NB-UVB/A was used in combination with topical corticosteroids, the need for UVB dose decreased without affecting the overall response and remission rates (33). There is a risk of developing cataracts in children with severe atopic dermatitis that peaks between 15–25 years of age; thus, a slit lamp examination is necessary to rule out any cataracts before the initiation of phototherapy, and optimal use of eye protection gear during treatment is necessary (34). Concomitant use of any topical immunosuppressants is contraindicated due to the increased risk of skin malignancies (34).

5.8.3 Antibiotics

Atopic dermatitis skin is highly susceptible to colonization with *Staphylococcus aureus* resulting in frequent secondary infections. Widespread infection will require systemic antibiotics; a 7–10 day course of cephalosporin and synthetic penicillin is usually effective. For penicillin allergic patients, fusidic acid and clindamycin are effective alternatives (35).

5.8.4 Systemic corticosteroids

The literature is quite sparse in terms of use of systemic steroids in children. Two randomized clinical trials of short term use of high potency systemic steroids showed modest improvement. No clinical studies are available for use of prednisone in children. Due to the concerns about the systemic side effects (especially the suppression of the hypothalamic-pituitary-adrenal axis), systemic corticosteroids should only be used to control severe flare ups at the smallest effective dose and for the shortest duration possible in order to optimize positive results (35).

5.8.5 Immunomodulators

The majority of pediatric patients respond well to topical treatments; however, a very small percentage of children with severe recalcitrant atopic dermatitis may require systemic treatment with such agents as immunomodulators. As systemic treatment carries the risk of some very serious long term side effects, the decision to embark on such therapy has to be weighed very carefully in terms of benefits of symptom improvement and gain in quality of life versus risks of immunosuppression,

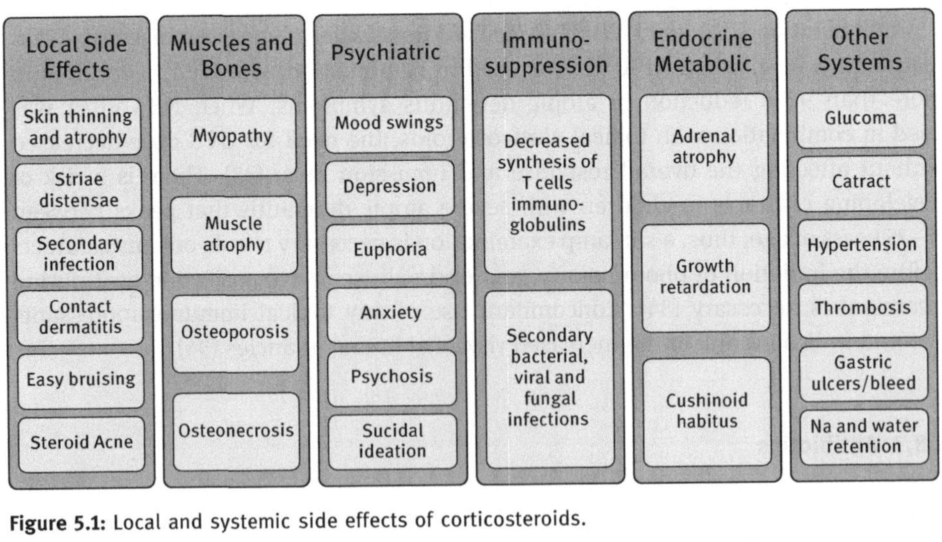

Figure 5.1: Local and systemic side effects of corticosteroids.

renal insufficiency, and malignancy. Sexually active female adolescents should be screened for pregnancy. In general, such treatment should only be used in difficult-to-treat or recalcitrant cases and only with the lowest effective dose for the shortest possible time frame, in addition to close monitoring by appropriate specialists (35,36).

5.8.6 Cyclosporine

The very first calcineurin inhibitor, cyclosporine, is a non-cytotoxic immunosuppressant, which acts by inhibiting lymphocyte activation. Careful selection of patients is necessary to exclude ones with any contraindication to cyclosporine, including any renal insufficiency, uncontrolled hypertension, history of hepatitis B or C, or any malignancy. Patients 2–16 years of ages have been treated with doses of up to 5 mg/kg/day; this was well tolerated and was efficacious in studies both in short term cases of 12 weeks and in long term continuous treatment of up to 12 months (35,36). Quality of life improvement was seen in both short term and long term treatment at 12 weeks (35,36). Cyclosporine is the only systemic treatment with convincing evidence to support its use in children with severe treatment refractory atopic dermatitis (35,36).

5.8.7 Azathioprine

An inhibitor of purine synthesis and subsequently of cellular DNA and RNA, azathioprine is shown to be effective in severe atopic dermatitis. Before using this medication, it is necessary to get such screening tests as a complete blood count, liver function tests, and assay of thiopurine methyltransferase (TPMT) to assess for bone marrow function at base line; this is followed by continued monitoring weekly for the first 6 weeks and then at 3 month intervals (37). When used in doses of 2–3.5 mg/kg/day in patients 6–16 years old, good response was seen in 41 out of 48 children in 2–6 weeks (37). Adverse events include gastrointestinal upset, transient elevation of liver function, anemia, thrombocytopenia, hypersensitivity phenomenon, and increased risk of lymphoreticular malignancy (37).

5.8.8 Infliximab

Infliximab is a monoclonal antibody that neutralizes the tumor necrosis factor α (TNF α) and is found to be effective in other atopic disorder such as asthma; however, its use in atopic dermatitis is relatively new and appears to be promising (35).

5.8.9 Interferon-γ

Interferon γ (INF γ) causes inhibition of IgE production that theoretically should restore immune balance in patients with atopic dermatitis who show a deficiency of INF γ. There is lack of good controlled trials to support the use of INF γ at this time unless the patients are not eligible for other proven systemic therapies (35).

5.8.10 Leukotriene inhibitors

Since patients with atopic dermatitis produce leukotrienes in abundance, which are strong inflammatory mediators, the idea of using a leukotriene antagonist to counter this pro-inflammatory response and potentially diminish atopy is appealing. One study of pediatric patients 6–16 years of age with moderate to severe atopic dermatitis who were treated with montelukast for 4 weeks at a dose of 5 mg daily showed a significant reduction in severity of atopic dermatitis; however, another study failed to replicate these positive results (35).

5.9 Psychiatric comorbidities

Atopic dermatitis, due to its early manifestation in life in addition to severity and course of illness, tends to cause everlasting temperamental and psychological changes in both younger and older children. The dilemma of a child with atopic dermatitis is not that he or she is not getting enough attention by parents but that at times too much attention is received, which can be misguided or even negative in some situations. Most of the attention is focused on the skin and its care at the cost of neglecting the emotional and developmental needs of the child (16). Also, providers may be mainly focused on treating the skin disorder based on the severity of its lesions and never attempt to go deeper than the skin to take care of the emotional and psychosocial wounds contributing to the atopic dermatitis.

Several psychiatric disorders are found to have higher prevalence in children with atopic diseases. Children with atopic dermatitis are more prone to develop depression as well as various nonspecific psychosomatic symptoms when compared to age matched controls (38). Behavioral problems are also an issue in these children. A study of school aged children in the United Kingdom found a twofold risk of having psychological problems in children with atopic dermatitis in comparison to the children without this dermatological condition (39).

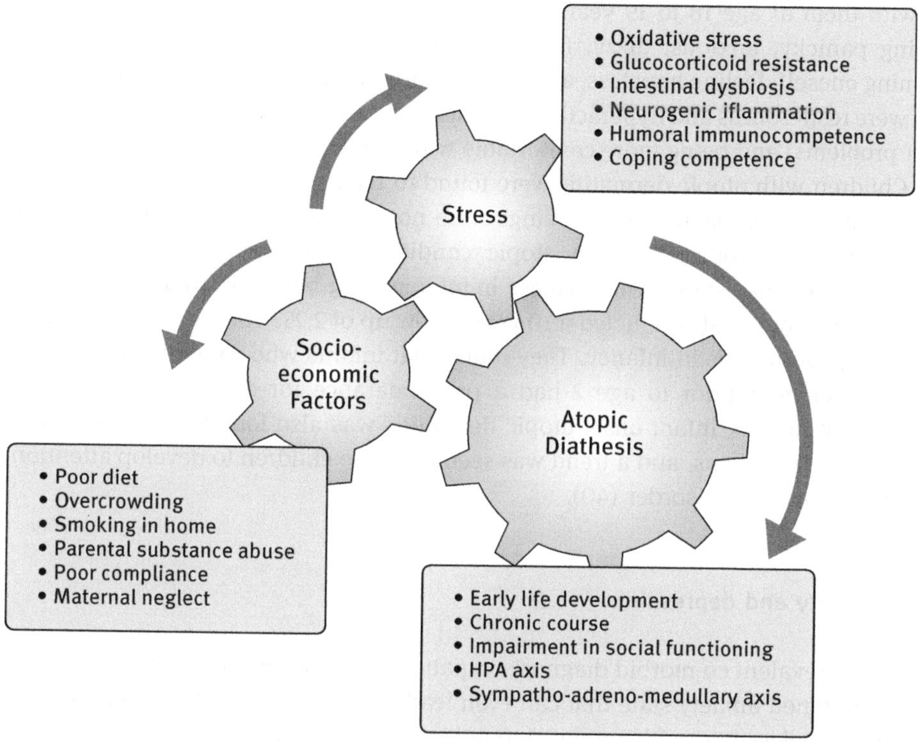

Figure 5.2: Bidirectional interaction of different factors contributing to psychological issues.

5.9.1 Family dynamics

The strain on any family unit dealing with a child with atopic dermatitis is challenging, and when you add other psychosocial stressors (i.e. associated economic burdens) it can become overwhelming. Families with low socioeconomic levels can be overburdened with the caregiving more quickly, leading to unhealthy coping styles and negative parenting; these results can have damaging long term psychological impact on the child during the most important formative years of his or her life when the foundations for personality, temperament, and coping mechanisms are being established (39).

5.9.2 Internalizing and externalizing behaviors

All atopic conditions are known to be associated with internalizing behaviors and to a lesser degree with externalizing behaviors. Lien et al conducted a base line survey of 3,674 high school Norwegian students who were 15 to 16 years of age and followed up with them at age 18 to 19 years (39). Internalizing behaviors were identified as feeling panicky, anxious, dizzy, feeling tense, sadness, sleeplessness, worthless, blaming oneself, feeling hopeless, and finding everything a burden. Externalizing factors were restlessness and hyperactivity, inattention, peer relationship problems, conduct problems, and being more comfortable with adults than age appropriate peers.

Children with atopic dermatitis were found to have more likelihood of developing internalizing behaviors, but findings were not as robust as in asthma. No clear relationship was found between atopic conditions and externalizing behaviors (39). The study also showed an increase in internalizing behaviors at a 3 year follow up study. Schmitt et al conducted a 10 year follow up of 2,252 children first identified with atopic dermatitis in infancy. They found that infants who were diagnosed with this skin disorder prior to age 2 had a preponderance for developing emotional problems at age 10. Infant-onset atopic dermatitis was also found to be associated with conduct problems, and a trend was seen for these children to develop attention deficit hyperactivity disorder (40).

5.9.3 Anxiety and depression

The most prevalent co-morbid diagnosis in patients with atopic dermatitis appears to be a heightened anxiety state that can even lead to development of an overt anxiety disorder. Adolescents with atopic dermatitis have lifetime rates of anxiety and depression that are increased over controls. Studies have reported 46% of adolescents with atopic dermatitis have anxiety and 17% suffer from depression (41). Anxiety levels tend to decrease with the improvement in skin condition only to revert back to the high levels after the relapse. Linnet et al reported higher levels of state and trait anxiety in children with atopic dermatitis that correlated well with severity of illness (42). Association of atopic dermatitis with depression has not been as robust as it has been seen in other chronic dermatologic conditions, such as psoriasis and acne. When depression is seen in children with atopic dermatitis, it is more likely comorbid with heightened anxiety, especially related to social situations (43).

5.9.4 Personality traits

An atopy-specific personality has been proposed for children suffering from atopic disorders. It has been postulated that an infant with atopic dermatitis who is irritable due to skin lesions needs physical contact from a parent for reassurance and comfort; also, a parent's feelings of disappointment and failure along with reluctance to touch in fear of aggravating the illness leads to a sense by the infant of being rejected by the mother. This leads to elevated anxiety and hostility in the infant or child giving rise to the foundation of some specific personality traits. The atopic personality is said to have traits of hypersensitivity, aggressiveness, sense of inferiority, insecurity, mood labiality, and cognitive rigidity. These individuals have difficulty dealing with anger and hostility in interpersonal relationships. Further studies have failed to agree on such specific personality disorders, and there is concern that these personality traits are not specific to atopic dermatitis or atopic disease but are more of a representation of chronic illnesses, such as autoimmune disorders or cancers.

5.10 Management of psychiatric comorbidities

5.10.1 Multidisciplinary approach

Chronic dermatologic diseases, such as atopic dermatitis, are best served with a multidisciplinary approach. Including professionals from different areas of health care and providing a comprehensive interdisciplinary approach to management can reduce the frequency and severity of relapses as well as avoid complications from this skin disorder. A typical team should include a clinical social worker, psychologist, and psychiatrist to address psychosocial and psychiatric issues. The dermatologist or the primary care physician leads the team with an ability to convene the team or consult with individual professionals as needed. Some major concerns in maintaining a multidisciplinary team are turf as well as territory issues, conflict communication, and organizational constraints (44).

5.10.2 Psychoeducation

Psychoeducation of the child, adolescent, and the family should be the integral part of a multidisciplinary treatment plan of a child or adolescent with atopic dermatitis. Psychoeducation can play a major role in situations with more frequent and severe relapses, which are difficult to manage, not only by particularly focusing on a good understanding of the physiologic and pathologic factors at play in their illness in terms understood by family members, but also by improving some understanding of the role of stress and its negative interactions. Education on specific techniques (such as relaxation, assertive communication, self-control of itching and scratching, and stress management) can lead to improved disease outcome (45).

5.10.3 Psychosocial assessment

A thorough psychosocial assessment is necessary to understand the family interaction and dynamics. Gustaffson et al proposed a family interaction evaluation using standardized family testing comprising tasks related to skills of decision making, conflict resolution, cooperation, and differences of opinion about likes and dislikes among family members. Social network and support system assessment was also conducted, asking parents to list individuals outside of the immediate family, their availability, geographic proximity, and the importance of their relationship with that particular individual; this was done to outline a weak versus healthy social support network (46). Evaluation of socioeconomic status is also important as low income levels along with other associated factors (i.e. overcrowded living conditions, poor nutrition, negative family interactions, substance abuse, smoking by parents, and non adherence to the treatment plan) can adversely impact the prognosis (46).

5.10.4 Psychiatric symptoms review

It is imperative to assess children and adolescents with atopic dermatitis for any comorbid psychiatric conditions because of the high incidence of associated general anxiety, social anxiety, depression, and personality traits. Many psychometric scales are available that can be readily used in different clinical settings with high reliability in identifying comorbid illnesses.

5.10.5 Quality of life assessment

Children with atopic dermatitis are shown to have a significant reduction in quality of life (QoL) when compared to their age matched counterparts (see Chapter 4). Assessment of QoL encompasses all domains of their life, including family interaction, school performance, ability to engage in extracurricular activities, participation in physical contact sports, as well as interpersonal and social relationships. QoL research has shown that children with atopic dermatitis have much higher impairment in this regard not only when compared to patients suffering from other chronic dermatologic conditions but also when compared with those suffering from other chronic illnesses, such as malignancies (11).

5.10.6 Psychodynamic therapy

It is important to help patients with atopic dermatitis understand the unrecognized and unconscious meaning of their illness and its impact on their understanding about themselves and their interaction with others (see Chapter 23). Children, based on their level of development, may not be able to engage in any in-depth psychodynamic therapy; however, such therapy may be beneficial to adolescents with atopic dermatitis. Psychodynamic-based group therapy is more beneficial when working on neuroticizing and pathological relationships, issues of transference, and counter transference that can be worked out in a group setting (11).

5.10.7 Cognitive behavioral therapy

Exploring the negative schema the patients have developed over many years about self, caregivers, and the world itself as well as attempting to change these issues in a positive direction will help develop a better understanding of their illness, compliance with treatment, and ultimate disease outcomes. The aim of therapy is to help children and adolescents with atopic dermatitis recognize automatic negative thoughts, dysfunctional assumptions about self-image, and self-depreciatory as well as blaming attitudes; therapy then replaces them with more positive attitudes. This approach will give rise to a more balanced understanding of self and illness, which will help the patient develop improved coping skills and decrease the social phobia, depression, and anxiety along with other avoidance behaviors.

5.10.8 Behavioral modifications

Relaxation techniques are shown to have some effectiveness in decreasing the itch and scratch cycle; these techniques include progressive muscle relaxation, autogenic training, electromyographic (EMG) biofeedback training, and cue controlled relaxation (11) (see Chapter 23). Strategies to teach more self control and scratch avoidance led to these children being symptom free for prolonged periods; these strategies include rewarding children for not scratching and ignoring the scratching behavior (11).

5.10.9 Psychotropic medications

Use of psychotropic medication will be necessary in a small number of pediatric patients with severe anxiety spectrum or depressive disorders who have failed to respond to psychotherapeutic approaches. *Selective serotonin reuptake inhibitors* (SSRIs) are now considered the first line medications for the management of anxiety and depression in these patients. In terms of efficacy, all of the available SSRIs are considered equal, but only a few are officially approved for use in the pediatric population. At present fluoxetine is approved for use in those ≥8 years for depression and in those ≥7 years for obsessive compulsive disorder (OCD). Fluvoxamine is approved in patients ≥8 years, sertraline in patients ≥6 years, and escitalopram for adolescents ≥12 years for OCD.

Tricyclic antidepressants (TCAs) are older antidepressants and are less commonly used in this early part of the twenty-first century, mostly because of their unfavorable side effects profile but also because SSRI antidepressants are better tolerated and have fewer drug–drug interactions. In fact, TCAs are very effective antidepressants; doxepin and imipramine are approved for OCD and depression in those ≥12 years of age, and clomipramine is approved for OCD in patients ≥10 years of age (47).

How one decides to choose an SSRI depends on various factors, such as the specific side effect profile, whether this medication has been used with good results in this patient before or has shown a good response in a family member, any contraindications, availability as an acceptable formulation (i.e. solution or suspension), and medication costs. In order to improve patient compliance, prescribing a medication with daily dosing is usually preferable to two or three times a day dosing (47). The United States Food and Drug Administration (FDA) has issued an advisory and black box warning about emergence of suicidal ideation during the initial phase of SSRIs treatment; this development has changed the prescribing behaviors of many primary care physicians and pediatricians in recent years leading to a reluctance in some to prescribe SSRIs. It is, however, recommended that the use of SSRIs in children and adolescents should be taken in consideration in situations where it is really indicated, and these pediatric patients should be followed closely, especially in the earlier phase of treatment, to monitor for any suicide risk.

5.11 Conclusion

Atopic dermatitis is a chronic, relapsing, remitting disease starting in very early childhood, and 20–40% of those afflicted continue to suffer throughout their life. It affects every aspect of these patients' lives with resultant decrease in their quality of life. The impact of illness extends beyond the skin management alone and can lead to neglecting other aspects of disease, especially the known psychophysiologic and psychoneuroimmunologic links with psychiatric disorders. A comprehensive multidisciplinary approach is necessary, including a psychiatric perspective, to enhance the success of any treatment plans for atopic dermatitis.

References

1. Coca AF, Cooke RA. On the classification of phenomena of hypersensitiveness. *J Immul* 1923;8:163–82.
2. Larsen FS, Hanifin JM. Epidemiology of atopic dermatitis. *Immunol Allergy Clin North Am* 2002;1:1–24.
3. Larsen FS. Clinical genetics of atopic eczema. In: Ring J, Przybilla B, Ruzicka T, eds. *Handbook of atopic eczema*, 2nd edn. Berlin, Heidelberg: Springer, 2006:235–43.

4. Schäfer T, Ring J. Epidemiology of atopic eczema. In: Ring J, Przybilla B, Ruzicka T, eds. *Handbook of atopic eczema,* 2nd edn. Berlin, Heidelberg: Springer, 2006:21–30.
5. Croner S, Kjellman NIM, Erikkson B, Roth A. IgE screening in 1701 newborn infants and the development of atopic disease during infancy. *Arch Dis Child* 1982;57:364–8.
6. Chapman RH, Parish WE. Atopic dermatitis. In: Chapman RH, Burton JL, Ebling FJ, eds. *Textbook of dermatology.* London: Blackwell, 1992;5:589–610.
7. Novak N, Bieber T. The pathogenesis of atopic dermatitis. In: Reitamo S, Lugar TA, Steinhoff M, eds. *Textbook of atopic dermatitis.* London: Informa Healthcare, 2008:210–20.
8. Schneider G. Psychosomatic aspects and psychiatric conditions. In: Misery L, Ständer S, eds. *Pruritus.* Berlin: Springer, 2010:211–5.
9. Arndt J, Smith N, Tausk F. Stress and atopic dermatitis. *Curr Allergy Asthma Rev* 2008,8:312–7.
10. Seiffert K, Hilbert E, Schaechinger H. Psychophysiological reactivity under mental stress in atopic dermatitis. *Dermatology* 2005;210:286–93.
11. Gieler U, Ehlers A, Hohler T, Burkard G. The psychosocial status of patients with endogenous eczema: A study using cluster analysis for the correlation of psychological factors with somatic findings. *Hautarzt* 1990;41:416–23.
12. Faulstich ME, Williamson DA, Duchmann EG, Conerly SL, Brantley PJ. Psychophysiological analysis of atopic dermatitis. *J Psycho-Som Res* 1985;29:415–7.
13. Steinhoff A, Steinhoff M. Neuroimminuology of atopic dermatitis. In: Granstein RD, Luger TA, eds. *Neuroimmunology of skin: Basic sciences to clinical practice.* Berlin: Springer, 2008:197–207.
14. Rosenthal MJ. Psychosomatic study of infantile eczema: I. Mother child relationship. *Pediatrics* 1952;10:581–91.
15. Miller H, Baruch DW. Psychosomatic studies of children with allergic manifestations: I Maternal rejection; a study of 63 cases. *Psychosom Med* 1948;10:275–88.
16. Howlett S. Emotional dysfunction, child–family relationships and childhood atopic dermatitis. *Br J Dermatol* 1999;140:381–4.
17. Marmor J, Ashley M, Tabachnik N, et al. The mother-child relationship in the genesis of neurodermatitis. *Arch Dermatol* 1956;74:599–605.
18. Jones SM, Buchanan A, Burke AW. Atopic dermatitis. In: Lieberman P, Anderson JA, eds. *Current clinical practice: Allergic diseases: Diagnosis and treatment,* 3rd edn. Totowa, NJ: Humana Press, 2007:217–47.
19. Rothe MJ, Grant-Kels JM. Diagnostic criteria for atopic dermatitis. *Lancet* 1996;348:769–70.
20. Heine RG, Hill DJ, Hosking CL. Role of food allergens in atopic dermatitis. In: Reitamo S, Lugar TA, Steinhoff M, eds. *Textbook of atopic dermatitis.* London: Informa Healthcare, 2008:85–99.
21. Peterson JD, Chan LS. A comprehensive management guide for atopic dermatitis. *Dermatol Nurs* 2006;18(6):531–42.
22. Mrabet-Dahbi S, Renz H. Role of inhalant allergens in atopic dermatitis. In: Reitamo S, Lugar TA, Steinhoff M, eds. *Textbook of atopic dermatitis.* London: Informa Healthcare, 2008:101–15.
23. Cork MJ, Danby S, Vasilopoulos Y. Epidermal barrier dysfunction in atopic dermatitis. In: Reitamo S, Lugar TA, Steinhoff M, eds. *Textbook of atopic dermatitis.* London: Informa Healthcare, 2008:35–58.
24. Boguniewicz M, Nicol N. General management of patients with atopic dermatitis. In: Reitamo S, Lugar TA, Steinhoff M, eds. *Textbook of atopic dermatitis.* London: Informa Healthcare, 2008: 147–64.
25. Ständer S, Lugar TA, Steinhoff M. Itch–pathophysiology and treatment. In: Reitamo S, Lugar TA, Steinhoff M, eds. *Textbook of atopic dermatitis.* London: Informa Healthcare, 2008:117–29.
26. May E, Zollner T, Schäcke H. Mode of action of glucocorticoids. In: Reitamo S, Lugar TA, Steinhoff M, eds. *Textbook of atopic dermatitis.* London: Informa Healthcare, 2008:165–79.

27. Paller, AS. *The 2004 process of care: Treatment options for the management of atopic dermatitis.* New York: Millennium CME Institute, 2004.
28. Peterson JD, Chan LS. A comprehensive management guide for atopic dermatitis. *Dermatol Nurs* 2006;18(6):531–42.
29. Reitamo S, Van Leent EJ, Ho V, et al. Efficacy and safety of tacrolimus ointment compared with that of hydrocortisone acetate ointment in children with atopic dermatitis. *J Allergy Clin Immunol* 2002;109:539–46.
30. Maurer M, Worm M, Zuberbie T. Antihistamines in atopic dermatitis. In: Reitamo S, Lugar TA, Steinhoff M, eds. *Textbook of atopic dermatitis.* London: Informa Healthcare, 2008:210–20.
31. Grundmann SA, Beissert S. Phototherapy of atopic dermatitis. In: Reitamo S, Lugar TA, Steinhoff M, eds. *Textbook of atopic dermatitis.* London: Informa Healthcare, 2008:187–95.
32. Clayton TH, Clark SM, Turner D, Goulden V. The treatment of severe atopic dermatitis in childhood with narrowband ultraviolet B phototherapy. *Clin Exp Dermatol* 2007;32:28–33.
33. Valkova S, Velkova A. UVA/UVB phototherapy for atopic dermatitis revisited. *J Dermatol Treat* 2004;15:239–44.
34. Holmes SA, Anste AV. Phototherapy and PUVA photochemotherapy in children. *Photodermatol Photoimmunol Photomed* 2004;20:69–75.
35. Ricci G, Dondi A, Patrizi A. Systemic therapy of atopic dermatitis in children. *Drugs* 2009; 69(3):297–306.
36. Harper JI, Ahmed I, Barclay G. Cyclosporin for severe childhood atopic dermatitis: Short course versus continuous therapy. *Br J Dermatol* 2000;142(1):52–8.
37. Murphy LA, Atherton D. A retrospective evaluation of azathioprine in severe childhood atopic eczema, using thiopurine methyltransferase levels to exclude patients at high risk of myelosuppression. *Br J Dermatol* 2002;147:308–15.
38. Hashiro M, Okumura M. Anxiety, depression and psychosomatic symptoms in patients with atopic dermatitis: Comparison with normal controls and among groups of different degrees of severity. *J Dermatol Sci* 1997;14:63–7.
39. Lien L, Green K, Thoresen M. Atopic conditions and mental health problems: A 3-year follow-up study. *Eur Child Adolesc Psychiatry* 2010;19:705–13.
40. Schmitt J, Apfelbacher C, Chen CM. Infant-onset eczema in relation to mental health problems at age 10 years: Results from a prospective birth cohort study (German Infant Nutrition Intervention plus). *J Allergy Clin Immunol* 2010;125(2):404–10.
41. Slatter MJ, Hetzel S, Essex MJ. Anxiety and depression in adolescents with atopic dermatitis. *Brain Behav Immunity* 2009;23:25–6.
42. Linnet J, Jemec A. An assessment of anxiety and dermatology life quality in patients with atopic dermatitis. *Br J Dermatol* 1999;140:268–72.
43. Gupta MA, Gupta AK. Depression and suicidal ideation in dermatology patients with acne, alopecia areata, atopic dermatitis and psoriasis. *Br J Dermatol* 1998;139:846–50.
44. Lewallen JP, Tuturro CT, Turturro A. Working with other healthcare providers. In: Norman RA, ed. *Preventive dermatology.* London: Springer, 2010:47–56.
45. Habib S, Morrissey S. Stress management for atopic dermatitis. *Behav Change* 1999;16(4):226–36.
46. Gustafsson PA, Kjellman N-IM, Bjorksten B. Family interaction and a supportive social network as salutogenic factors in childhood atopic illness. *Pediatr Allergy Immunol* 2002;13:51–7.
47. Kamboj MK, Tareen RS. Management of nonpsychiatric medical conditions presenting with psychiatric manifestations. *Pediatr Clin North Am* 2011;58:219–41.

Sandra Ros and Eulalia Baselga

6 Psoriasis and children: A psychological approach

Psoriasis is one of the most important dermatological inflammatory diseases in children and adolescents. Its appearance in this pediatric age group has considerable psychological effects on the patient as well as the family. This chapter reviews these issues and provides recommendations for management. Basic areas of intervention involve focusing on facilitating and managing stress, developing self-control skills, improving self-esteem, strengthening adaptive features of each child or adolescent, stabilizing the psycho-emotional condition of the child, and providing or facilitating problem solving and social skills.

6.1 Introduction

Psoriasis is one of the most important dermatological inflammatory diseases in children and adolescents. Psoriasis is an inflammatory inherited dermatosis, characterized by erythematous scaly papules and plaques that usually follow a chronic fluctuating course with flares of variable duration and severity. Psoriasis is a multifactorial genetic disorder triggered by several environmental factors such as trauma, infections, or stress (1,2,3). Childhood psoriasis is a well-recognized entity, but its true prevalence is not known, and the studies carried out yield various percentages.

There is not much literature on the impact of psoriasis in children and adolescents compared with that found in adults; in spite of this, our experience shows that considerable emotional vulnerability exists in the pediatric population, which has been extensively studied in other diseases such as oncological processes (4).

In order to understand the scope that psoriasis has on the child or adolescent, we must not only measure and treat the physical damage of psoriasis, but we must also assess how this disease affects the child's emotional development and his vital areas such as social development, family health, and education (5,6). Psoriasis can affect physical appearance and growth, resulting in reduced activity, pain, itching, the need for regular therapy, and sometimes, unpleasant procedures as well as possible loss of school attendance.

For this purpose, in this chapter we emphasize the relationship between psoriasis and stress, the aspects derived from the visibility of lesions, the child's psycho-emotional aspects (e.g. body image and self-esteem) and, finally, the relationship with his family environment. The latter will partly determine how the child lives and faces this disease and its treatment. It is important to remember that because of the chronicity of this disorder, health education, family support, and coping strategies will help these children to a better acceptance of a disease that they have not chosen. For this reason, patients with childhood psoriasis as well as their families require special attention.

6.1.1 Epidemiology

Psoriasis in childhood is not uncommon (7,8,9,10,11,12). The prevalence in the general adult population ranges from 1–3% (13), but the exact prevalence of psoriasis in childhood is unknown, largely because diverse age definitions have been used in different studies (14,15,16,17,18). Furthermore, psoriasis may be underdiagnosed in childhood. Psoriatic diaper rash may be diagnosed as diaper dermatitis, and inverse, scalp psoriasis may be confused with infantile seborrheic dermatitis.

In the prevalence study carried out by Gelfand et al in the United Kingdom, the data show an estimate of psoriasis of 0.6% in children from 0–9 years old and 1.4% in those between 10–19 years old (18). Other results are those obtained by the group of Augustin in Germany, who found a prevalence of 0.71% in pediatric patients under 18 years old (3). Farber and Nall reported that in the United States, 35% of patients with psoriasis had the disease onset before the age of 20 (2% in infants, 8% in childhood, and 25% in adolescence) (15). Overall, it may be said that at least one third of psoriatic patients develop the disease during childhood (10,15). Congenital psoriasis has been reported, but it is rare (19,20,21). It has been postulated that based upon age of onset, psoriasis vulgaris can be divided in two groups: early onset psoriasis, presenting before the age of 40; and late onset psoriasis, presenting after the age of 40 (10,22). Clinical features seem also to support this classification (7,10).

Childhood psoriasis seems to be more prevalent in girls than in boys, approaching a 2:1 ratio (14,17). This female preponderance has not been confirmed by others (11,16). Among the infant population (0–18 years old), the mean age of psoriasis onset ranges between 7 and 10 years old (23,24,25).

Swanbeck et al found that the lifetime risk of inheriting psoriasis, if no parent, one parent, or both parents have psoriasis, is 4%, 28%, and 65%, respectively (26). If there is already one affected child in the family, the corresponding risks are 24%, 51%, and 83%, respectively. Family history of psoriasis also predicts an early disease onset (27,28). Spontaneous remissions are more frequent in children (17).

6.2 Dermatological clinical features

The lesions of psoriasis consist in well-demarcated erythematous, scaly papules and plaques. The scales have a characteristic silvery aspect and the so-called Auspitz's sign is seen after removing them by scratching punctate hemorrhages. This phenomenon is useful for diagnosis. Another useful clinical sign is the presence of erythema and/or fissuring at the intergluteal fold (Brunsting's sign).

The distribution is frequently symmetric. The areas of predilection are the scalp and extensor surfaces of the extremities. Psoriasis tends to develop in areas of previous trauma (Koebner phenomenon). Psoriatic plaques, although usually asymptomatic in adults, may be pruritic in a high percentage of children (16,17). Several clinical sub-types of psoriasis have been described both in adults and children: plaque-type, guttate, erythrodermic, pustular, inverse psoriasis, and arthropatic psoriasis. The clinical aspects depend also on the location. Therefore, further topographic variants may also be defined: scalp, facial, napkin, palmo-plantar, nail, fingertip, and folicular psoriasis.

6.2.1 Plaque psoriasis

Plaque psoriasis is the most common variant in children (11,16). Plaques of psoriasis in children tend to be thinner, with finer scales than in adults, and may be confused with eczematoid lesions. Erythematous, squamous plaques of different sizes appear most commonly on extensor aspects of the extremities, knees, elbows, and scalp. The face is very often affected in children.

6.2.2 Guttate psoriasis

Guttate psoriasis is characterized by the sudden appearance of small, teardrop, erythematous, scaly papules and plaques on the trunk and proximal extremities. The face may also be affected. It may be the only and initial manifestation of psoriasis, or may develop on pre-existing plaque-type psoriasis. Guttate psoriasis commonly occurs 1 or 2 weeks after an upper respiratory tract infection, usually streptococcal pharyngitis. Triggering by streptococcal perianal dermatitis has been also described (29,30).

Guttate psoriasis responds rapidly to treatment with either antistreptoccocal antibiotics or phototherapy. Even without treatment it resolves spontaneously in several months, after which the child may remain in remission for several years. In children in whom there is a streptococcal infection triggering the disease, it is common to see a bout of guttate psoriasis every time the child has pharyngitis (16).

6.2.3 Erythrodermic psoriasis

Psoriasis can progress to involve the entire skin with erythema and exfoliation. This form of psoriasis is exceedingly rare in children (7,31). Precipitating factors in children with pre-existing psoriasis include certain drugs (such as antimalarials, gold therapy, and lithium), stress, phototoxicity, and sudden withdrawal of corticosteroid treatment. A few congenital cases have been reported; these congenital forms are usually very severe, respond poorly to treatment, and commonly develop arthropathy at a later age (11,32).

6.2.4 Pustular psoriasis

Pustular psoriasis is an uncommon form of psoriasis that represents about 1% of childhood psoriasis (7,11,32). It can be divided into generalized and localized forms (33,34,35). Generalized pustular psoriasis is further subdivided in generalized pustular psoriasis (Von Zumbush type), circinate, or annular pustular psoriasis (Bloch-Lapiére type), and localized forms of generalized pustular psoriasis (not acral or palmoplantar). Mixed forms may also occur. Localized pustular psoriasis can be subdivided in palmoplantar pustulosis of Barber and acrodermatitis continua of Hallopeau, affecting the distal aspect of one or two fingers.

In generalized pustular psoriasis Von Zumbush type, there are widespread, 1 to 2 mm sterile pustules of abrupt onset. Individual pustules may coalesce to form lakes of pus. Mucous membrane lesions are common, and geographic tongue has been described (33,36,37). During the acute flares, the patients are often ill, with high fever, malaise, and pain, secondary to their exfoliating skin. Individual lesions resolve within 3 to 4 days, with recurrent flares of inflammation. The conversion to psoriatic erythroderma is possible (37). This form of pustular psoriasis tends to occur more commonly in infants and toddlers. Some of them go on to develop psoriasis vulgaris at a later age (7,32,35).

Generalized pustular psoriasis has been described in children with non bullous congenital erythroderma (7,32,38), and rare congenital cases have been reported (7,12). Several provocative factors have been recognized in children with generalized pustular psoriasis. Infection, not only streptococcal, seems to be the most common trigger (32,33). Other factors include irritating local treatment with coal tar or anthralin, sun exposure, or drugs.

Annular pustular psoriasis (Bloch-Lapiére) is a milder generalized variant characterized by gyrate, annular lesions with a pustular border. Onset and clinical course is often subacute and affects children of older age (32,34). Systemic symptoms may be present, although they are usually less severe than in the Von Zumbush form. Annular pustular psoriasis may follow acute von Zumbush forms. Localized forms of generalized pustular psoriasis include those plaques of psoriasis not acrally located that develop pustules on top (psoriasis with pustules). This may be seen after local treatment with anthralin or coal tar. Diaper psoriasis may also develop pustules in instances of secondary candida infection.

Localized acral pustular psoriasis, both Barber type or acrodermatitis continua of Hallopeau, have been considered exceptional in children. However, in a recent pediatric series, acral pustular psoriasis was seen in 5% of patients (11). In palmoplantar pustular psoriasis of Barber there are recurrent crops of pustules, 2–4 mm in diameter, on normal appearing skin of the palms and soles. Older pustules become dark brown in color and are finally shed. The eruption is usually symmetric, and the preferred sites of occurrence are the thenar and hypothenar eminences on the palms and the insteps on the soles. Palmoplantar pustulosis may coexist with sternocostoclavicular arthritis and chronic recurrent multifocal osteomyelitis (39).

Achrodermatitis continua of Hallopeau may be slightly more common than palmoplantar pustulosis. In this form, pustules develop on the tips of one or two fingers or toes. Pustulation of the nail bed and nail folds leads to progressive nail destruction. Psoriatic-form scaling develops upon desiccation of pustules. Bony changes may occur with progressive tapering of the finger tips. The disease remains localized to the same finger for months or years.

6.2.5 Psoriatic arthritis

Psoriatic arthritis is one of the well-known complications of psoriasis (40,41,42). Arthritis and psoriasis appear in about 2% to 4% of children with chronic arthritis (43). Skin manifestations, usually mild, most commonly precede or occur simultaneously with articular symptoms, which are diagnostically useful. Nail changes are more common in children with arthritis than in those without it.

Five different clinical subsets have been recognized in psoriatic arthropathy: (a) predominant distal interphalangeal (DIP) joint involvement, (b) arthritis mutilans, (c) symmetric polyarthritis similar to rheumatoid arthritis (but seronegative), (d) asymmetric oligoarthritis, and (e) ankylosing spondylitis. Mixed forms may also occur (44). A joint pattern with asymmetric arthritis of large and small joints and a high rate of dactylitis (sausage finger) is prototypical for the disease (43). Children with psoriatic nail disease have higher incidence of DIP joint involvement. Fortunately, in juvenile psoriatic arthritis, systemic manifestations are extremely rare.

6.2.6 Inverse psoriasis

In some patients psoriasis may almost exclusively affect skin folds such as the inguinal, axillary, suprapubic, and intergluteal folds. Psoriatic diaper dermatitis is a particular form of inverse psoriasis that is very common in infants. Small folds such as the retroauricular folds, interdigital folds, the external canthi, lip comissure, and the periumbilical area may also be affected. Due to the natural maceration of the skin in those areas, inverse psoriasis lacks scaling and is thinner and of a brighter red than in other areas.

6.3 Psychological clinical features

The relationship between psycho-emotional factors, psycho-social impact, and psoriasis in adults has been extensively described by different authors (45,46,47,48,49). However there is little scientific literature regarding its involvement in childhood and adolescence (4,5,50,51). Although certain factors can be extrapolated to children and adolescents, there are some differentiated features due to disease impact on an emotional level in leisure time activities being reduced as well as less time spent in other areas (i.e. at school, in social relationships, in sleeping); also, there are other inconveniences caused by the symptoms and treatments in this population. We will highlight some of the most representative and relevant aspects such as the role of the family, the role of stress, and the visibility of the lesions. Our experience shows that the diagnosis of a chronic disease such as psoriasis in children and adolescents can cause a strong emotional impact on the child and his familial environment. This is why special attention to features of the child's familial environment has to be drawn.

The family plays a vital role in the course of the disease, whether or not there are family members affected with psoriasis. In the first stage it will be important to understand how the family experiences the diagnosis because it can help to mitigate the emotional impact of the disease on the child or adolescent, or on the contrary, create a situation of overprotection, anxiety, and stress. Later, the family involvement will influence how the parents and/or caregivers live the child's disease. We must take into account that the deterioration of health that involves a chronic disease and the visibility of lesions typical of psoriasis in children can create clinical conditions of anxiety and depression in parents that will probably require psychological treatment. The family also will have a crucial role in the child's treatment, which may be complex due to the time spent on treatment, the disease perseverance, the financial difficulties in paying the medical services as well as treatments, and the changes in certain routines and family habits (5).

Stress is another factor to consider when we talk about childhood psoriasis. In the same line of what happens in adults, stress plays an important role in the adaptive system overload of the body, accelerating the onset of psoriasis and exacerbating the symptoms. However, we must also highlight that the disease itself is creating a stressful situation in the child or adolescent.

Due to nervous-psychic genesis of psoriasis stress situation, it initiates the cascade of biochemical and immunological reactions leading to a psoriasis focus. The stress situations in children can be generated by family situations, school problems, and difficulties in the relationship with the parents or siblings. The beginning and exacerbations of these dermatoses depend on many psycho-social risk factors in children (6). The psychotherapeutic treatment of stress in children and adolescents will facilitate a better management of stressful situations, whether they are derived from psoriasis or exogenous situations.

The body image disturbance suffered by children and adolescents with psoriasis due to the visibility of their lesions is one of the characteristic aspects of the psoriasis that makes it different from other chronic diseases. Thus, we find studies that demonstrate that children with psoriasis have a worse quality of life than children with diabetes or epilepsy (see Chapter 23). Visibility of the lesions may result in a child's sense of differentiation from his close environment, feeling that his skin is different; also, in some cases, psoriasis limits his or her participation in games, sports, and even in school activities. This sense of differentiation and the limitations can affect the child's self-esteem and his emotional development. The role of the family is fundamental to mitigate and face these situations, which are not only confronted by the child, but the parents, who have to accept the visible disease of their child. However, we must consider that young children do not feel ashamed about their image, although eventually and as they grow, such negative feelings will appear (52).

Adolescence is more vulnerable (53). It is a life stage in which the body image is really important. The adolescent begins to go outside, leaving aside the family protection, and a visible disease such as psoriasis seriously affects the development of the self-concept, self-image, and self-esteem. It is a life stage in which social relationships play a leading role. The adolescent with psoriasis may show fear of rejection, social isolation and inhibition, and shame due to the psoriasis. All of this may have its psychopathological correlate: some teens may present symptoms of anxiety and depression reactive to psoriasis and even medical conditions that can be diagnosed by criteria from the American Psychiatric Association's (APA) Diagnostic and Statistical Manual of Mental Disorders (DSM IV-R). The presence of this emotional distress can affect the academic performance (i.e. concentration problems due to anxiety). Difficulties in the sleep area due to psychopathology or also due to certain disease symptoms such as itching are also common (5,54). The presence of this psychopathology can also affect family unity in a time of life where the parent–child relationship is highly sensitive.

It would be interesting to perform a psychological profile of pediatric patients with psoriasis, yet it is not possible because we cannot forget that every patient, every child, and every adolescent is different, as are familial, social, and educational environments. The premorbid psychopathological characteristics and personality traits of children or adolescents will also be protective, and risk factors may exert a modulatory role in this network. Therefore, to generalize attitudes, feelings about the disease, fears, frights, and concerns seems an unattainable task. There will be so many profiles of children and adolescents with psoriasis equivalent to existing children and adolescents.

The psycho-emotional support to face this situation is vital for the adaptation to the disease situation. However, an assessment focused on two aspects is necessary: the first one is unmistakably focused on the child or adolescent to determine potential emotional damage, levels of anxiety, depression, and stress; also important is the detection of internalizing behavior problems (i.e. anxious, depressive, and overcontrolled) or externalizing (i.e. aggressive, hyperactive, noncompliant, and undercontrolled) and self-esteem. The second aspect will be the family. An extensive analysis of familial relationships, how parents and siblings are living the disease, and what changes occurred at the familial level since the diagnosis is very helpful to establish an effective psychological intervention.

6.3.1 Differential diagnosis

The diagnosis of psoriasis is usually made by clinical appearance. In children, some other diseases may be considered, and in case of doubt, a skin biopsy would be necessary. Guttate psoriasis may be confused with pityriasis rosea and chronic pityriasis lichenoides. In pityriasis rosea there is a herald patch, the lesions are oval as well as distributed along skin lines, and they usually have a shorter duration. In chronic pityriasis lichenoides, papules are brownish with a central crust or scale.

Follicular psoriasis on the elbows and knees as well as scalp psoriasis may be confused with pityriasis rubra pilaris, frictional dermatitis, or lichen spinulosus. The constant involvement of the palms and soles and the typical salmon hue of the lesions may differentiate pityriasis rubra pilaris. Napkin psoriasis may be very difficult to differentiate from seborrheic dermatitis. Psoriatic diaper rash is usually brighter red, better demarcated, and shinier than seborrheic dermatitis and lacks the yellow scale. Candidiasis should also be ruled out; satellite pustules and peripheral scaling are highly suggestive of Candida infection.

Eczema of the palms and soles may be impossible to differentiate from psoriasis. In many cases there is a true overlap of both diseases. If vesicles are present, it is highly suggestive of eczema as vesicles are not a feature of psoriasis. Palmoplantar psoriasis in children may manifest with glazed erythema of the palms and soles as in juvenile plantar dermatitis. Hyperkeratotic eczema is very difficult to differentiate. Nummular eczema may be considered in the differential diagnosis of plaque type psoriasis.

Acral pustular psoriasis has to be differentiated from acropustulosis of infancy, scabies, and tinea pedis. In acropustulosis, each crop of lesions resolves spontaneously in a few days, while pustular psoriasis is more persistent. Tinea pedis is usually asymmetric and a direct potassium hydroxide examination allows a rapid differentiation in case of doubt. Scabies usually shows lesions elsewhere, and scraping helps to establish the diagnosis. Erythrodermic psoriasis, especially if congenital, is very difficult to differentiate from other forms of erythroderma, such as icthyosis, metabolic disorders, or immunodeficiencies. Skin biopsy may not be useful in these situations, and only observation over time will confirm the correct diagnosis.

6.3.2 Psychotherapeutic intervention

It is clinically challenging to provide psychological care to children and adolescents with psoriasis who present with various psycho-emotional difficulties. These difficulties are mainly due to two barriers: the lack of specialized professionals connected to dermatology departments, and the resistance shown by the families of children and adolescents because of the stigma associated with the psychological treatment. It is important to note that contributing to the family resistance barrier is that many parents feel that they are being blamed for not managing the child's condition well enough. The last aspect can be redirected by giving the family support and information about the difficulties and the potential stress at the family level in the care of a child with a chronic, visible disease such as psoriasis.

In order to improve the knowledge on psoriasis, treatments and expectations will be of vital importance in this first stage. It is important to explain to the family, especially the parents, that the multidisciplinary approach utilized by the dermatologist and psychologist can help the child achieve a better coping mechanism with resultant adaptation to the disease and to situations generated by childhood psoriasis, and a reduction of the associated psychopathology (i.e. anxiety and sadness). This makes it easier for the parents to understand and appreciate the necessity for this type of treatment without the feeling of being judged in any way.

We must not forget to explore the relationships established at the familial level of the onset and course of psoriasis, which will be very helpful for future psychotherapeutic interventions. The attitude of the family regarding the child may be permissive, inducing a dependent behavior, or overprotective, inducing infantile behaviors that can prevent social autonomy and hinder the adherence to self-care (i.e. skin hydration). Difficulties in mother–child relationships could emerge as, for example, negative attitudes from the parents focused on the disease and the symptoms, distancing from other family members, and psychopathology in the closest family environment.

Another point of vital interest in our psychotherapeutic intervention should be focused on how parental stress and anxiety directly affect the child. For this reason, the programs with pediatric patients should also be oriented to the parents to achieve two main objectives:

(a) to reduce stress, depressive and anxiety symptoms, or the medical condition (anxiety and mood disorders). The presence and intensity of psychopathological factors will determine the father–child relationship and may even facilitate the appearance of these symptoms in the pediatric patient.

(b) to teach the parents procedures to help their children and themselves cope with the disease. We know that the diagnosis of psoriasis creates a start up of coping mechanisms and important adjustments in family dynamics. Psoriasis is a disease that even if not disabling, involves a chronicity, visibility, as well as social stigma that can severely affect ones self-esteem. Therefore, an inadequate coping of the psoriasis by the parents can lead the family to become a risk factor and not a protector factor against the potential psycho-emotional involvement of the child. The psychotherapeutic treatment needs to reduce anxiety and stress of parents. Therapy in a group or individual format will correct some of the maladaptive behaviors of parents toward the child, improving the quality of life of parents and ensuring the emotional bonding with the child.

When performing a psychotherapeutic intervention in children with psoriasis, we must have the child's age in mind. In the younger pediatric population, the intervention is focused on the family and the child. In the older pediatric population, the intervention will be focused on the adolescent, clearly separating the psychotherapeutic space of the patient from the psychotherapeutic space of the family (55,56). In our clinical practice the psychotherapeutic intervention in the pediatric patient is focused on two constructs: progressive relaxation techniques and psychotherapy.

In progressive relaxation techniques (i.e. autogenic and progressive muscle relaxation), the objective is to train children in different relaxation techniques to learn how to manage and/or reduce the tension produced by daily events of life, associated with psoriasis as well as stressful situations that may arise in their environments. Through them, we teach the child or adolescent to control his body physically through progressive relaxation and to identify the stressful situations. We know, as we mentioned previously, the important role of stress as it can precipitate or exacerbate outbreaks. Through the progressive relaxation technique adapted to children, we can provide our patients with a useful and necessary tool to feel able to regulate their levels of anxiety.

6.3.3 Psychotherapy

Pediatric patient-oriented psychotherapy starts with the psychological interview in which the clinician assesses, in addition to an existing psychopathology, the cognitive abilities, personal resources, and protective factors, such as family support and, in the case of adolescents, social support (see Chapter 23). Children with emotional and behavioral problems prior to psoriasis, with pediatric psychiatric disorders and history of psycho-social maladjustment as well as a tendency to anticipatory fears, can show the clinician or clinician team certain vulnerability to maladjustment when facing new situations. An early intervention when detecting these potential risk factors can help to minimize the impact of psoriasis later in life, even when we do not detect psycho-emotional alterations due to a skin disease.

The objective of psychotherapy is to identify the stressful situations related to the psoriasis perceived by the adolescent, such as avoidance behavior, social isolation, and even the anticipation to social rejection. At such a vital stage of personal development in which the adolescent walks toward socialization and emotional autonomy, adolescents with psoriasis face a situation of vulnerability linked to the visibility of psoriasis, different treatments, and distressing physical symptoms. These three variables will affect most of our patients as stress generators.

In psychotherapy, it is a priority to analyze each of these factors through a comprehensive dialogue with the adolescent, creating a safety climate that promotes the active involvement of the patient; there is a space in which the adolescent may freely express all those situations that generate anxiety and fear. Although every patient is unique in his or her innermost core, it is true that certain similar stressful situations are commonly perceived in this population. Stressful situations comprise social avoidance behaviors due to fear of rejection together with a cognitive anticipation of social rejection. Hiding the lesions by using specific clothes also causes a stressful situation in the adolescent with psoriasis. In the case of lesions not affecting exposed areas, we can identify this constant anticipatory anxiety, focused on the thought that it may affect those exposed areas or the fear of being discovered.

The physical limitations generated by the symptoms of psoriasis (i.e. skin tension, bleeding lesions, itching, and pain) will necessarily modify some daily activities as sport or leisure of our patients, generating for them more tension, stress, and rejection because of the disease. Physical symptoms may alter the sleep area: frequent awakenings occur during the night, and these symptoms hinder the normal resting cycle of adolescents or children, thus facilitating more emotional distress and irritability.

All these factors may facilitate social isolation or withdrawal of adolescents because of the fear of being discovered and thus being isolated from their environment. Expressing all these situations in a therapeutic environment, as a catharsis, helps the adolescent to be aware of his or her emotional state. Often on the first visit the adolescent unconsciously denies having any suffering. The goal of psychotherapy is to be able to work on these situations at both cognitive and behavioral levels so that the adolescent can generate coping tools that help him or her deal with the stressful situation.

At the cognitive level, the therapist works on the identification, expression, and confrontation of the feelings generated by psoriasis in adolescents. Fear of worsening of the disease, physical imperfection feelings induced by not following the current aesthetic canons, rejection of one's own body image, and maladaptive thoughts that accompany these feelings directly influence the presence of symptoms of anxiety and depression. These symptoms can emerge as a result of personal insecurity; these involve feelings of stigmatization mentioned previously and alteration of the socialization process and are the key to the psychotherapeutic approach and to the prevention of authentic clinical diagnosis according to classification by the APA's DSM-IV-R.

The last aspect on which we have to focus the psychological intervention is to differentiate the identity of the patient from the disease. Adolescent patients often do not feel like teenagers with a chronic disease – they feel "psoriatic." This establishes limits because everything in their life revolves around the disease. This is certainly the most intimate and committed process in psychotherapy. The therapeutic relationship with adolescents having psoriasis should indeed be intense in order to be able to work out this differentiation aspect between "I" and "psoriasis."

The establishment of the positive and valuable aspects of every adolescent and his strengths at the personal and social level are important to establish. Also, it is helpful to strengthen those personality characteristics that are favorable at the relational level; this will allow him to see by himself the negative aspects (of his own and of the disease) in which until now he has based his reality, but also his own positive and adaptative aspects, which until this moment have been ignored.

In order to understand and respect the difficulty and hostility that the acceptance of a chronic disease as psoriasis represents for the adolescent, it will help us as professionals to understand the nature of the disease and to facilitate the adolescent's assumption of psoriasis as part of his or her life and person instead of an acceptance of a disease that has been imposed. Therefore, it is necessary to encourage the positive and negative feelings that these patients experience.

Helping the adolescent to develop coping strategies with the disease and the typical situations that every adolescent (with or without a chronic disease) faces in this stage of life probably is the last step of psychotherapy. At this point the therapist works on the autonomy of the adolescent and the active involvement in the treatment of psoriasis. This facilitates the adolescent to express to the dermatologist the difficulties that the treatment involves and that can reduce the treatment adherence.

In summary, psychotherapy focuses on generating an adequate space without prejudice where the therapist and the adolescent can work together, facilitating the expression of the feelings caused by psoriasis, either internalizing (fears, anxious-depressive symptoms, withdrawal, low self-concept) or externalizing disorders (failure, challenges, irritability, self-harm), as well as facilitating the adaption to the disease and the management of emotions generated by psoriasis in this population of patients who are so vulnerable at this moment of their lives.

In patients in whom psoriasis appears at a younger age, the intervention focuses on these issues: facilitating the adoption of active coping mechanisms to psoriasis, the adjustment to a new family situation due to the appearance or the course of psoriasis in the pediatric patient, the prevention and/or treatment of the potential psychopathological symptoms that could appear in parents or caregivers of the child because of the emotional overload that represents the appearance of the chronic disease as well as the treatments and the loss of the child's health, and the strategies to promote necessary self-care in psoriasis tailored to each pediatric patient age.

6.4 Conclusions

We know that the diagnosis of psoriasis can cause a strong psychological impact on any stage of life and involves a large variety of psychological adjustments in the individual who suffers from it. When this chronic and visible skin disease appears in childhood and adolescence, it involves both the family and the child or adolescent. Finally, it can be said that the complete therapeutic approach aims to facilitate a process of normalization of the different members of the family throughout the course of the disease. However, we know that each situation is different, that psoriasis can enhance or worsen certain pre-existing aspects, and that each family will find a variety of strategies to accept the situation of the disease in the most optimal manner.

The basic areas of intervention in pediatric patients primarily focus on facilitating and managing stress as well as self-control skills, improving self-esteem, strengthening adaptive features of each child or adolescent, stabilizing the psycho-emotional condition of the child, and providing or facilitating problem-solving as well as social skills. Finally, it is important not to forget that each of our pediatric patients is unique and that it is important to understand as well as respect each of their situations.

Acknowledgments

I would like to thank the editors, especially Dr. Jafferany, for giving me the opportunity to collaborate in this project. I also would to thank Dr. Malouf and Dr. Puig for his continued support, encouragement, and feedback throughout the development of this chapter. And finally I would like to thank Dr. Wulff, my mentor, for his support, assistance, and training in the field of psychosomatics.

References

1. Baselga E, Mascaro JM. Dermatosi infiammatorie: La psoriasis nell'età pediatrica. In: Abrizi G, ed. *Dermatologia pediatrica*. Milano: Masson, 2003:367–80. [Spanish]
2. Gudjonsson JE, Elder JT. Psoriasis: Epidemiology. *Clin Dermatol* 2007;25:535–46.
3. Augustin M, Krüeger K, Radtke MA, et al. Disease severity, quality of life in health care in plaque psoriasis: A multicenter prospective cross-sectional study in Germany. *Dermatology* 2008;216: 366–72.
4. Beattie PE, Lewis-Jones MS. A comparative study of impairment of quality of life in children with skin disease and children with other chronic childhood disease. *Br J Dermatol* 2006;155:145–51.
5. Ganemo A, Wahlgren CF, Svensson A. Quality of life and clinical features in Swedish children with psoriasis. *Pediatric Dermatol* 2011;28:375–9.

6. Nyfors A, Lomholt K. Psoriasis in children. A short review of 245 cases. *Br J Dermatol* 1975;72: 437–42.
7. Beylot C, Puissant A, Bioulac P, Saurat JH, Pringuet R, Doutre MS. Particular clinical features of psoriasis in infants and children. *Acta Derm Venerol* 1979:Suppl 87:95–7.
8. Farber EM, Mullen RH, Jacobs AH, Nall L. Infantile psoriasis: A follow-up study. *Pediatr Dermatol* 1986;3:237–43.
9. Farber EM, Nall L. Childhood psoriasis. *Cutis* 1999;64:309–14.
10. Swanbeck G, Inerot A, Martinsson T, Wahlstrom J, Enerback C, Enlund F, et al. Age at onset and different types of psoriasis. *Br J Dermatol* 1995;133:768–73.
11. Morris A, Rogers M, Fischer G, Williams K. Childhood psoriasis: A clinical review of 1262 cases. *Pediatr Dermatol* 2001;18:188–98.
12. Verbov J. Psoriasis in childhood. *Arch Dis Child* 1992;67:75–6.
13. Farber EM, Nall L. Epidemiology: Natural history and genetics. In: Roenigk HH, Maibach HI, eds. *Psoriasis*. New York: Marcel Dekker, 1998:107–57.
14. Al Fouzan AS, Nanda A. A survey of childhood psoriasis in Kuwait. *Pediatr Dermatol* 1994;11: 116–9.
15. Farber EM, Nall ML. The natural history of psoriasis in 5600 patients. *Dermatologica* 1974;148: 1–18.
16. Nanda A, Kaur S, Kaur I, Kumar B. Childhood psoriasis: An epidemiologic survey of 112 patients. *Pediatr Dermatol* 1990;7:19–21.
17. Raychaudhuri SP, Gross J. A comparative study of pediatric onset psoriasis with adult onset psoriasis. *Pediatr Dermatol* 2000;17:174–8.
18. Gelfand JM, Weinstein R, Porter SB, et al. Prevalence and treatment of psoriasis in the United Kingdom: A population-based study. *Arch Dermatol* 2005;141:1537–41.
19. Lehners-Weber C, de la Brassine BM, Dezfoulian B, Richert B, Bonardeaux C, Willemaers V. Congenital psoriasis following the lines of Blaschko. *Pediatr Dermatol* 1996;13:219–21.
20. Lerner MR, Lernr AB. Congenital psoriasis: Report of three cases. *Arch Dermatol* 1972;105: 598–601.
21. Chang SE, Choi JH, Koh JK. Congenital erythrodermic psoriasis. *Br J Dermatol* 1999;140:538–9.
22. Henseler T, Christophers E. Psoriasis of early and late onset: Characterization of two types of psoriasis vulgaris. *J Am Acad Dermatol* 1985;13:450–6.
23. Fan X, Xiao FL, Yang S, et al. Childhood psoriasis: A study of 277 patients from China. *J Eur Acad Dermatol Venereol* 2007;21:762–5.
24. Seyan M, Coskum BK, Saglam M, et al. Psoriasis in childhood and adolescence: Evaluation of demographic and clinical features. *Pediatr Int* 2006;48:525–30.
25. Kumar B, Jain R, Sandhu K, et al. Epidemiology of childhood psoriasis: A study of 419 patients from northern India. *Int J Dermatol* 2004;43:654–8.
26. Swanbeck G, Inerot A, Martinsson T, Enerback C, Enlund F, Samuelsson L, et al. Genetic counselling in psoriasis: Empirical data on psoriasis among first-degree relatives of 3095 psoriatic probands. *Br J Dermatol* 1997;137:939–42.
27. Altobelli E, Petrocelli R, Marziliano C, et al. Family history of psoriasis and age at disease onset in Italian patients with psoriasis. *Br J Dermatol* 2007;156:1400–1.
28. Henseler T, Christophers E. Disease concomitance in psoriasis. *J Am Acad Dermatol* 1995;32: 982–6.
29. Herbst RA, Hoch O, Kapp A, Weiss J. Guttate psoriasis triggered by perianal streptococcal dermatitis in a four-year-old boy. *J Am Acad Dermatol* 2000;42:885–7.
30. Patrizi A, Costa AM, Fiorillo L, Neri I. Perianal streptococcal dermatitis associated with guttate psoriasis and/or balanoposthitis: A study of five cases. *Pediatr Dermatol* 1994;11:168–71.
31. Prystowsky JH, Cohen PR. Pustular and erythrodermic psoriasis. *Dermatol Clin* 1995;13:57–770.
32. Zelickson BD, Muller SA. Generalized pustular psoriasis. A review of 63 cases. *Arch Dermatol* 1991;127:1339–45.

33. Tay YK, Tham SN. The profile and outcome of pustular psoriasis in Singapore: A report of 28 cases. *Int J Dermatol* 1997;36:266–71.
34. Baker H, Ryan TJ. Generalized pustular psoriasis: A clinical and epidemiological study of 104 cases. *Br J Dermatol* 1968;80:771–93.
35. Judge MR, McDonald AM, Black MM. Pustular psoriasis in childhood. *Clin Exp Dermatol* 1993;18:97–9.
36. Langtry JA, Carr MM, Ive FA, Gordon P, Hunter JA, Harper JI. Ichthyosiform erythroderma associated with generalized pustulosis. *Br J Dermatol* 1998;138:502–5.
37. Juanqin G, Zhiqiang C, Zijia H. Evaluation of the effectiveness of childhood generalized pustular psoriasis treatment in 30 cases. *Pediatr Dermatol* 1998;15:144–6.
38. Langtry JA, Carr MM, Ive FA, Gordon P, Hunter JA, Harper JI. Ichthyosiform erythroderma associated with generalized pustulosis. *Br J Dermatol* 1998;138:502–5.
39. Job-Deslandre C, Krebs S, Kahan A. Chronic recurrent multifocal osteomyelitis: Five-year outcomes in 14 pediatric cases. *Joint, Bone, Spine* 2001;68:245–51.
40. Scarpa R, Mathieu A. Psoriatic arthritis: Envolving concepts. *Curr Opin Rheumatol* 2000;12: 274–80.
41. Southwood TR, Petty RE, Malleson PN, Delgado EA, Hunt DW, Wood B, et al. Psoriatic arthritis in children. *Arthritis Rheum* 1989;32:1007–13.
42. Shore A, Ansell BM. Juvenile psoriatic arthritis – an analysis of 60 cases. *J Pediatr* 1982;100: 529–35.
43. Hafner R, Michels H. Psoriatic arthritis in children. *Curr Opin Rheumatol* 1996;8:467–72.
44. Scarpa R, Lubrano E, Cozzi R, Ames PR, Oriente CB, Oriente P. Subcorneal pustular dermatosis (Sneddon-Wilkinson syndrome): Another cutaneous manifestation of SAPHO syndrome? *Br J Rheumatol* 1997;36:602–3.
45. Gupta MA, Gupta AK. Depression and suicidal ideation in dermatology patients with acne, alopecia areata, atopic dermatitis and psoriasis. *Br J Dermatol* 1998;139:846–50.
46. Kimball A, Jacobson C, Weiss S, Vreeland MG, Wu Y. The psychosocial burden of psoriasis. *Am J Clin Derm* 2005;6:383–92.
47. Ginsburg IH, Link BG. Psychosocial consequences of rejection and stigma feelings in psoriasis patients. *Int J Dermatol* 1993;32:587–91.
48. Gupta MA, Gupta AK, Watteel GN. Perceived deprivation of social touch in psoriasis is associated with a greater psychologic morbidity: An index of the stigma experience in dermatologic disorders. *Cutis* 1998;61:339–42.
49. Vardy D, Besser A, Amir M, et al. Experiences of stigmatization play role in mediating impact of disease severity on quality of life in psoriasis patients. *Br J Dermatol* 2002;147:736–42.
50. de Jager ME, van der Kerkhof PCM, de Jong EMGJ, Seyger MMB. Psoriatic arthritis: evolving concepts. *Br J Dermatol* 2010;163:1099–1101.
51. Bilgic A, Bilgic Ö, Akış HK, Eskioğlu F, Kılıç EZ. Psychiatric symptoms and health-related quality of life in children and adolescents with psoriasis. *Pediatr Dermatol.* 2010;27:614–7.
52. Walters E. Problems faced by children and families living with visible difference. In: Lansdown R, Rumsey N, Bradbury E, Carr T, Oartrudge J, eds. *Visibly different: Coping with disfigurement.* Oxford: Butterworth-Heinmann, 1997.
53. Smith JA. The ipact of skin disease on the quality of life of adolescents. *Adol Med* 2001;12: 343–353.
54. Weisshaar E, Seeliger S, Diepgen TL, et al. Pruritus in childhood. A diagnostic and therapeutic challenge. *Haurtarzt* 2004;55:855–68.
55. Rauch PK, Jellinek MS. Pediatric dermatology: Developmental and psychological issues. *Adv Dermatol* 1989;4:143–56.
56. Czyzewski DJ, Lopez M. Clinical psychology in the management of pediatric skin disease. *Pediatric Dermatol* 1998;3:619–29.

Donald E. Greydanus

7 The acnes: Acne vulgaris, acne rosacea, and acne excoriée

Acne vulgaris is a chronic inflammatory disorder of sebaceous units and hair follicles (obstruction of pilosebaceous units) found in the majority of adolescents and many adults. Acne vulgaris involves abnormal keratinization, androgen stimulated sebum production, *Propionibacterium acnes* colonization, and abnormal host immune response to inflammation. Management involves use of various topical and systemic medications. Topical medications include benzoyl peroxide, various retinoids (tretinoin, tazarotene, adapalene), azelaic acid, and topical antibiotics (erythromycin and clindamycin among others). Systemic agents include various antibiotics, oral contraceptives, and isotretinoin. Management of comorbid conditions that worsen acne should be carefully managed, such as causes of hyperandrogenemia. Drugs that worsen acne should be stopped and substituted for if at all possible. Psychological impact can be considerable and should be an important part of the overall management for this disorder. Development of scars is very upsetting to patients, and management should be directed to scar prevention early in the course of acne management. Acne rosacea, acne excoriée, and other acne variants are also considered.

> It is far more important to know what person the disease has than what disease the person has.
>
> Hippocrates (460–370 BC)

7.1 Acne Vulgaris

7.1.1 Introduction

Acne vulgaris is a chronic, multifactorial, inflammatory disorder of the sebaceous glands as well as ducts and the hair follicles with a strong genetic predisposition (1,2,3,4,5). It is found in areas of increased sebaceous density, i.e. the face, chest, upper arms, and back. Though acne can be seen at any age, it typically begins at puberty and its onset, and severity is influenced by genetic factors as well as the host immune response to inflammation.

7.1.2 Epidemiology

Acne can be found in all ages of childhood (neonatal, infantile, childhood) and adulthood (6,7,8). Acne vulgaris is found in as many as 40% in those between

8 and 10 years of age, 90% of mid-adolescent males (i.e. ages 13 to 17), and 80% of similar aged females; severe acne is noted in 10% of adolescents and young adults. Severe acne may occur in young adults even if they only had mild acne as adolescents. Concern with acne accounts for 14% of visits to primary care clinicians and 27% of visits to dermatologists. Table 7.1 provides a classification of acne and its many variants. The direct cost of acne management is over $2.2 billion per year in the United States (9). Acne rosacea is reviewed in the next section (10).

Table 7.1: Classification of acne and variants*

Type	Comment
• ACNE VULGARIS (GROUP I)	
Comedonal acne vulgaris	Disorder of sebaceous follicles with horny impactions. Graded according to percent of face involved: I=10%; II=10%-25%; III=25%-50%; IV=more than 50%.
Papulopustular acne	Rupture of the distended sebaceous gland (inflammatory acne) with varying degrees of inflammation.
Graded V-VIII.	
Acne conglobata	Severe nodulocystic acne vulgaris. Described in 3% of white adolescent males, with severe scarring. Extremities and buttocks often involved, as well as groin, scalp and axilla. Persistence into adulthood can occur.
SAPHO	syndrome of acne, pustulosis, hyperostosis, and osteitis; this is classified as a seronegative spondylarthritis.
Acne tropicalis (tropical acne)	Severe inflammatory acne vulgaris seen in those exposed to tropical conditions.
Acne fulminans (acute, febrile, ulcerative conglobate acne)	Rare variant described in males, ulcerative conglobate acne characterized by large nodules with scarring on trunk and sometimes face; also fever, ulcers, polyarthritis or arthralgia and leukocytosis. Sacroilitis often noted. Osteolysis and periosteal reaction can occur.
• ACNE VULGARIS VARIANTS (GROUP II)	
Infantile acne (acne neonatroum)	Comedonal acne on malar region of males during first few weeks to year of life. Occasionally noted in either sex from 1–2 years of age. Acne neonatorum refers to acne limited to the first month of life.
Premenstrual acne	Cyclical microcomedonal acne developing before the menstrual period.
Gram-negative folliculitis	Associated with long-term broad-spectrum antibiotic use. Variable patterns of facial nodules due to *Proteus, Pseudomonas, Klebsiella,* or *Enterobacter* organisms. Treat with isotretinoin or high-dose ampicillin or amoxicillin or other antibiotics.
Excessive androgen acne	Severe acne related to high androgen levels (eg, polycystic ovary syndrome). Treatment with antiandrogens such as cyproterone

(*Continued*)

Table 7.1: Classification of acne and variants* (*Continued*)

Type	Comment
	acetate; see text; close medical supervision is necessary due to adverse drug effects.
Folliculitis keloidalis	Chronic, recurrent low-grade pustular dermatitis of the occipital and posterior neck regions. May result in scarring, keloid formation, and alopecia. Most commonly noted in black males with closely shaved areas and ingrown hairs. Avoid certain shaved hairstyles and occlusive hair oils; topical or systemic antibiotics may be necessary. Intralesional corticosteroids or surgical excision of scar or keloids may be necessary.
Acne mechanica	Exacerbation of acne vulgaris by excessive rubbing to cause friction, as with overzealous face washing or even tight helmets or clothing (leotards); use of absorbent material under the occlusion can help, such as a cotton T-shirt under a leotard.
Chemical acne	Exacerbation of acne vulgaris by cosmetics, detergents, hair creams or oils, chlorinated hydrocarbons, tars, emollient skin or bath oils. Pomade acne refers to hair oil or grease inducing comedonal acne at the hair line and forehead. High-potency steroid cream should *never* be used on the face.
Acne due to physical agents	Exacerbation of acne vulgaris by sunlight, ionizing radiation; Mallorca acne (acne aestivalis) is a sunlight-induced, winter variant with papular folliculitis of arms, shoulders, and trunk; no comedones, nodules or scarring.
Drug-induced acneform rashes	Iodides, bromides, barbiturates, rifampin, phenytoin, lithium; others may be associated. Steroid acne can occur secondary to steroid (systemic, oral) use and responds poorly to antibiotics. Fluorinated steroids are particularly implicated, but fluorinated creams should *never* be used on the face! Patients with acne should be screened for medications and foods that might contain high levels of "acnegenic" substances. Athletes should be advised to avoid anabolic steroid use, which has many side effects, including a drug-induced acneform disorder.
• NONACNE ACNEFORM RASHES (DIFFERENTIAL DIAGNOSIS)	
Pyoderma faciale	Progressive facial inflammatory lesions (nodules, hypertrophic scars, and absence of comedones) occurring in adult females 20–40 years of age.
Acne rosacea	Facial papules and pustules associated with dilated blood vessels in the nasolabial areas in adults age 30–50. See text.
Folliculitis-associated Immunological defects	*Example*: Chronic granulomatous disease.
Periofolliculitis capitis abscedens suffodiens	Diffuse, explosive scalp cellulitis associated with severe acne and hidradenitis suppurativa. Treat with antibiotics and retinoic acid.

(*Continued*)

Table 7.1: Classification of acne and variants* (*Continued*)

Type	Comment
Hidradenitis suppurativa	Keratin obstruction of aprocrine ducts with secondary infection of apocrine glands in axillae, areolae, labiae, scrotum, or perineum. Fluctuant nodules with purulent drainage and sinus tract formation. Associated with obesity, severe acne vulgaris, tropical climates, poor hygiene. Unusual cases can be associated with fever, anemia, and arthralgia. Treatment is as for abscesses in general; intralesional steroid injection, exteriorization of sinus tracts, or excision of involved tissue may be required. Acne surgery is the ultimate choice for most, though oral isotretinion (40 mg, bid) is helpful to some. Oral antibiotics (tetracycline 1-2 g/day) can also help some. Avoid tight clothes over affected areas. Antibacterial soaps may help. Hygiene and aluminum chloride (6.25% in anhydrous alcohol) may help to reduce perspiration. Benzoyl peroxide and topical antibiotics may be helpful for a few patients, but not the majority. Response to all treatment measures is variable, see Chapter 16.
Pseudofolliculitis barbae	Chronic folliculitis in beard area (especially black males) aggravated by shaving. Treat by growing a beard, avoiding a close shave, clipping hairs, and systemic antibiotics if pronounced. Electric razor use is essential for most, though some may find frequent straight-edge razor changes acceptable. Multiple small keloids may form in persons predisposed to keloid formation.
Trichostasis spinulosa	Facial eruption resembling blackheads but made up of follicular papules containing vellus hairs, keratin, and melanin; distributed over the nose and malar regions. Treat with isotretinoin.
Adenoma sebaceum	Pinkish yellow sebaceous papules on face; commonly clustered in groups around the nose. One of the classic stigmata of tuberous sclerosis.
Keratosis pilaris	Hereditary, self-limiting, hair follicle keratinization disorder which peaks in adolescence. Can be associated with atopic dermatitis or ichthyosis vulgaris. Flesh-colored 1–2 mm papules are noted on lateral upper arms, anterior thighs, or the face. The lesions can be red or white. Moisturizers (with lactic acid), topical keratolytics (with propylene glycol) and tretinoin may be helpful.
Neurotic exorciations	Superficial excoriation or deeper ulcer in acne areas and other generalized areas. Found in individuals with severe mental illness. Some distributed individuals use cigarettes, knives, acids, or alkalis to produce facial injury often called factitial dermatitis. Treatment is attention to the injured skin with psychiatric treatment. See text.

Also see molluscum contagiosum and verrucae (Chapter 1).

* Used with permission from: Greydanus DE: Disorders of the skin. In: AD Hofmann, DE Greydanus (eds). Adolescent Medicine, 3rd Edition. Stanform, CT: Appleton & Lange, 1997; ch. 18:377.

7.1.3 Pathogenesis

The pathogenesis of acne vulgaris involves three main components: sebum, keratin plug, and the microbial skin flora (11). Sebum is made by the sebaceous glands and is composed of approximately two thirds triglycerides and one third wax esters along with steroid esters and squalene. The protein secreted by keratinocytes is called keratin, while sebum is secreted into hair follicles through the sebaceous duct. Sebum production is influenced in adolescence by the adrenal and gonadal androgens. Acne is an inflammatory condition and starts with follicular keratinocytes becoming so sticky that a keratin plug forms, which then occludes the follicle with trapping of sebum. Trapped sebum leads to perifollicular inflammatory and secondary impaction. Seborrhea may be mild to severe and is not specifically linked to acne vulgaris.

Local bacteria contribute to the acne process, and this flora includes *Propionibacterium acnes* (formerly known as *Corynebacterium acnes*), which has been implicated in acne pathogenesis since 1896. This bacterium is an anaerobic Gram-positive diphtheroid that increases during adolescence and colonizes at pilosebaceous follicles. This important microbe converts triglycerides to free fatty acids and produces mediators as well as chemotactic factors that leads to the inflammatory nature of acne (*vide infra*). Other flora implicated in acne include coagulase-negative *Staphylococcus epidermidis* and the yeast *Pityrosporum ovale*.

An important etiologic component in adolescent acne development is the increasing level of plasma testosterone in which testosterone is converted in the skin to dihydrotestosterone by 5-α-reductase. This conversion leads to direct stimulation of sebaceous gland enlargement via a cyclic cAMP (adenosine monophosphate) mechanism. Estrogen can inhibit gland stimulation, and acne exacerbations in females may occur during periods of reduced estrogen stimulation, such as before menstruation. Youth can have normal hormonal levels but still have severe acne, partially due to increased free testosterone levels and DHEAS along with lowered levels of SHBG (sex hormone-binding globulin).

Acne vulgaris typically initiates with the development of microcomedones, the primary, noninflammed acne lesions, which are due to occluded hair follicles. The microcomedone is due to excessive sebum from desquamated epithelial cells in the follicular wall, as noted previously; microcomedones become overt comedones. Closed comedones are called whiteheads, while open comedones or blackheads have pigmented epithelial cells and are due to retained melanin. The open or closed comedo obstructs the follicle duct and sebum outflow leading to follicle distention and potential rupture.

7.1.3.1 Inflammatory Pathogenesis

Ongoing distention results in local tissue injury that is worsened by conversion of sebum triglycerides to irritant free fatty acids. The follicle ruptures, which allows bacterial infection or invasion of the follicle and surrounding tissues; this is complicated by *Propionibacterium acnes*, which stimulates chemtactic substances that enhance polymorphonuclear neutrophils (PMNs). *P. acnes* interacts with Toll-like receptors (TLRs) in this process (9,12). TLRs are a class of proteins playing a significant role in the immune system and recognize molecules from microbes.

The pathogenesis of acne vulgaris involves inflammation with genetic overlay. Proinflammatory lipids, chemokines, and cytokines assume the role of mediators in this process that develop acne lesions with the stimulation of bacterial antigens (13). Current research invokes the influence of neuropeptides and peroxisome proliferator-activated receptor (PPAR) ligands. Those with acne have peripheral blood mononuclear cells (PBMCs) with increased interferon-gamma, and interleukins (IL-12p40 and IL-8). Antimicrobial and proinflammatory cathelicidins are involved in acne pathogenesis, and these are a family of polypeptides found in lysosomes of macrophages and polymorphonuclear leukocytes; they are important parts of the immune system, protecting against bacterial invasion (14).

The result of this complex inflammatory process that is initiated by rising androgens of adolescence and influenced by environmental and genetic factors is varying degrees of erythematous papules, pustules, nodules, cysts, scarring, and depigmentation that characterize inflammatory acne vulgaris. The severity is influenced by genetic factors, sexual maturity rating of the individual, and sebum production rate. Both dermatological and emotional scaring may also result. Scars can hypertropic (keloid) or atrophic (i.e. rolling, boxcar, or icepick-types) (15).

7.1.4 Classification

Noninflammatory acne (Grade I) involves acne with both closed and open comedones. Further grades of inflammatory acne can result from the closed comedone (whitehead). Grade II (early inflammatory acne) reflects comedones and papules; papules are raised, red lesions that are obstructed follicles. Moderate, localized inflammatory acne with pustules defines Grade III, while Grade IV refers to severe, generalized acne vulgaris with cysts that are typically painful and warm. A wide variety of scoring systems have been used by clinicians over the years, such as the Investigator's Static Global Assessment Scale (16).

7.1.5 Management

7.1.5.1 Overview

The course of a patient's acne vulgaris and its management runs a highly individualized pathway. Clinicians should be sure of the diagnosis and of the differential diagnosis of acne vulgaris that includes drug-induced acneiform eruptions, acne rosacea, bacterial folliculitis, perioral dermatitis, angiofibromas, trichostasis spinulosa, adenoma sebaceum, keratosis pilaris, and various acne variants (17) (Table 7.1). One clue to acne vulgaris is to find the presence of both open and closed comedones. Some individuals have a mild course with comedonal lesions lasting only 1 or 2 years. Those at the other end of this spectrum have extensive, persistent disease with pustules and cysts lasting many years as well as emotional scars lasting a lifetime. Acne vulgaris may continue or even begin in adulthood.

Management seeks to control and not cure the acne in which primary goals involve improvement in appearance as soon as possible as well as prevention of scarring (18). Various recommendations are given that include gentle face washing and use of topical agents (bacteriostatic and/or peeling). Careful attention to skin color is important as skin of color is at risk for hyperpigmentation due to acne lesions and irritating topicals (19).

Improvement of simple Grade I acne vulgaris may be seen with gentle washing of the face or other involved areas two to three times a day with mild soap (i.e. Neutrogena, Basis, Purpose, Aveeno Emulave). Instruct the patient to avoid excessive or harsh washing as this may irritate the skin and lead to *acne mechanica* (Table 7.1). Also, the patient should avoid irritating the skin by rubbing alcohol, mechanical abrasives, or astringents. Teach the teenager to avoid squeezing or otherwise injuring the comedones since this increases damage to skin tissue and introduces more infection; a comedonal extractor can be helpful to safely remove unsightly comedones. Teach the patient that acne is not due to poor hygiene or dirty skin. Teach that acne is not a disease of shame but, in fact, a complex disorder of the skin that affects billions of humans.

Diet per se is not usually causative in acne, though some patients anecdotally noted that certain foods do exacerbate their acne, such as soft drinks, chocolate, French fries, nuts, or others (17). Research is evaluating such issues as the role of lipid-soluble antioxidants (vitamin A and E), omega-3 fatty acids, low fat/low glycemic foods, and other potential dietary factors (17). Cosmetics should be cautiously used, and only apply oil-free or water-based types; avoid oily creams and any topical that consistently irritates the skin. For example, pomade acne (Table 7.1) can be improved by instructing the patient to use a less oily gel or lotion on hair ends. Also, less grease or oil exposure in restaurants or automobile shops can be beneficial to some persons with acne.

A wide variety of regimens are utilized by different clinicians in the care of patients with acne vulgaris. Management of inflammatory acne typically involves topical and systemic antibiotics along with retinoic acid and/or benzoyl peroxide. Retinoic acid is the acid form of vitamin A and is also called all-trans retinoic acid (ATRA) (20,21). There are a variety of over-the-counter topicals that can be used, such as combinations of resorcinol and sulfur. Application of topicals is usually with a pea sized amount on a finger split into four parts of the face and a thin application gently applied over the face. Some patients (such as some males) are reluctant to consistently apply topical medication to their face because this is equated with a feminine task. They can be taught that this is simply applying medication and has nothing to do with masculine or feminine tasks. Clinicians should never underestimate the fact that acne scars (or scars from any cause) are very upsetting to patients, and aggressive management is necessary to enhance scar prevention early and throughout the treatment course (22).

Table 7.2 outlines basic acne vulgaris medical management. Combination products include clindamycin or erythromycin with benzoyl peroxide. These antibiotics are generally not used alone for a long time since this may increase risk for antibiotic resistance. Typical dose of tetracycline or erythromycin is 250 to 500 mg daily (vida infra). The combination of benzoyl peroxide and oral antibiotics may reduce the risk for emergence of antibiotic resistant *P acne*. Various anti-acne vulgaris medications are now reviewed.

Table 7.2: Outline of acne vulgaris management

1. **Grade I or Mild comedonal Acne**
   a. Benzoyl peroxide (5% – 10%) once or twice a day OR
   b. Tretinoin (Retin-A): once or twice a day
   c. Caution using benzoyl peroxide and tretinoin together as this will increase skin irritation and erythema
   d. Azelaic acid as monotherapy
2. **Grade II**
   a. Benzoyl peroxide (5% –10%) with topical antibiotics (twice a day)
   b. Tretinoin with topical antibiotics twice a day; antibiotics are used for the inflammatory component of acne; increase tretinoin strength if necessary and tretinoin can be helpful for inflammatory component as well
   c. Can use product that combines benzoyl peroxide and topical antibiotic
   d. Azelaic acid with topical antibiotics
3. **Grade III**
   a. Antibiotics (oral) with 10% Benzoyl peroxide (twice a day)
   b. OR oral antibiotics with tretinoin (once or twice a day); increase Tretinoin strength as needed.
4. **Grade IV**
   a. Use Grade III scheme.
   b. Use isotretinoin (Accutane)
   c. Dermatology consultation

7.1.5.2 Benzoyl Peroxide

Benzoyl peroxide is a commonly used organic compound of the peroxide family consisting of two benzoyl groups connected via a peroxide link. It is listed in the World Health Organization Model Lists of Essential Medicines. Benzoyl peroxide is useful for comedonal acne because it leads to keratin dehiscence with resultant desquamation; benzoyl peroxide is also bacteriostatic (antimicrobial), anti-inflammatory, and leads to local reduction of free acid levels in the skin (23,24). Its work as a peeling agent leading to heightened skin turnover, pore clearing, and reduction in amounts of local bacteria.

Benzoyl peroxide is available in different formulations (cream, gel, foam, and wash) and topical concentrations: 2.5%, 5%, or 10%. Water-based gels are less irritating than acetone or alcohol-based gels. It is also found as soap or a 5% and 10% wash that is very useful for back acne or application to other large areas. It is also available in different combinations with other chemicals, such as sulfur, salicylic acid, adapalene, vitamin A, and antibiotics (erythromycin or clindamycin) (23).

Side effects of this chemical include dryness and erythema particularly in atopic, black, and/or fair-skinned individuals. Liquid and cream forms are less irritating than gel forms, though gel forms seem to be more efficacious. Other side effects include excessive peeling, pigmentary changes, transient acne worsening by stimulation of existing comedons, and increased photosensitivity. Benzoyl peroxide can lead to bleaching of colored articles (i.e. towels, clothes, bed coverings).

One regimen is to advise the patient to start with a thin layer of 5% benzoyl peroxide and use it for a few hours a day or every other day; then, use a gradual build-up plan as tolerated to an overnight application and eventually to a twice a day regimen that allows comfortable dryness and peeling but avoids excessive redness, chapping, cracking, or discomfort. Eventually seek to use a 10% gel formulation. Combination products as noted may be helpful in recalcitrant situations.

7.1.5.3 Tretinoin

Tretinoin is also called all-trans retinoic acid (ATRA) and is the acid form of vitamin A. It is very commonly used in the treatment of acne as a cream or gel and is also used for other dermatological conditions such as alopecia, stretch marks, and wrinkling associated with aging. It is also used in capsule form to treat acute promyelocytic leukemia. A number of brands are available in its topical form such as Retin-A, Renova, Atinac, Avita, and others. Tretinoin is available in increasing potency: cream (0.025%, 0.05%, 0.1%), gel (0.01%, 0.025%), micro-gel (0.04%, 0.1%), and liquid (0.05%).

Tretinoin targets the main factors of pathogenesis for acne: it heightens the rate of cell turnover in the follicular epithelium, reduces the cohesiveness of the epithelial cell, thins the skin horny layer, heightens antibiotic activity, and leads to less formation of comedones. Many clinicians use tretinoin or other topical retinoids as the first line of management for acne since topical retinoids target the microcomedo, which is the precursor to other acne lesions; other advantages to topical retinoids include their anti-inflammatory and comedolytic effects. Topical retinoids are combined with oral antibiotics for moderate to severe acne with discontinuation of the antibiotic within 8 to 12 weeks; the retinoid can then be continued as maintenance management (18).

Tretinoin topical application may lead to skin erythema, itching, scaling, burning, and even a severe sunburn. Thus, a gradual increase in its use (as noted with benzoyl peroxide) is recommended, and appropriate sunscreen is needed with sun exposure. Avoid para-aminobenzoic acid (PABA) sunscreens due to increased hypersensitivity risks. A post-inflammatory increase or decrease in pigmentation may be seen in darker-skinned patients. Side effects may be reduced with lower strength formulations. Evidence of teratogenicity is unclear at this time, and it is listed with a category C classification.

Patients using tretinoin should avoid hair removal waxing since removal of the wax leads to removal of the epithelium leading to more erythema and pain. Cautiously use tretinoin with benzoyl peroxide; for example, benzoyl peroxide is used in the morning and then tretinoin at night; however, use of both products increases the risk of severe skin sensitivity.

Use a mild soap (as previously noted) and also use a 30 to 45 minute delay between face washing and tretinoin application to reduce skin irritation risks. Liquid or solution forms are most irritating to the skin. Start with a less concentrated form with gradual build-up from once every second or third day to every day as tolerated. Educate the patient that initial use can lead to transient irritation of formed comedones with a temporary pustular rash within 2 to 3 weeks of use. This can occur in half of those using tretinoin and may lead to discontinuation because of complaints that the medication made their acne worse. The skin should be dry before coming into contact with bed sheets or clothes due to potential bleaching action of tretinoin.

7.1.5.4 Adapalene

Adapalene (Differin, Teva) is a third-generation topical, antiinflammatory retinoid used to treat mild to moderate acne vulgaris because of its ability to reduce microcomedone development. It is available as a 0.1% cream, 0.1% gel, and 0.3% gel. In contrast to tretinoin, adapalene can remain effective even when applied at the same time as benzoyl peroxide. It can heighten the effectiveness of topical clindamycin, though increased side effects may result. It can be used with antibiotics (topical or oral) for mild to moderate acne and combined with oral antibiotics for moderate to severe acne (25). Adapalene was FDA-approved for acne in 1996 and is also used to treat keratosis pilaris.

7.1.5.5 Tazarotene

Tazarotene (Avage, Tazorac, Zorac) is another topical, anti-inflammatory retinoid used to treat mild to moderate acne vulgaris; it is also FDA-approved to treat psoriasis and skin damaged from sun exposure. It is available as a gel or cream and has side effects similar to other topical retinoids; for example, severe skin dryness and cracking may be seen. It is available in two concentrations, 0.05% and 0.1%, and it is usually applied once at night after using a mild face cleanser. As with other retinoids and benzoyl peroxide, it may take some weeks for clear evidence of improvement to be seen, often leading to patients becoming discouraged and prematurely stopping the medication. Education by the clinician about this possibility may reduce such compliance issues.

7.1.5.6 Azelaic acid

Azelaic acid is part of the dicarboxylic acid group and is used for mild to moderate acne vulgaris. It is developed from the yeast *Pityrosporum ovale* (*Malassezia furfur*), which lives on normal skin and is industrially made by oleic acid ozonolysis. It is also found in barley, rye, and wheat. Azelaic acid prevents skin pore occlusion (i.e. anti-comedonal) and reduces local bacterial growth (i.e. anti-bacterial). It is available in a 20% cream or 15% gel form and can be used twice a day as tolerated. Its use may cause tingling, burning, stinging, or itching of the skin, which is usually temporary. Hypopigmentation is also reported especially in those with dark skin. However, it is also used to treat skin pigmentation disorders since it is a tyrosinase inhibitor that decreases melanin production. Thus, a major benefit of this product is to improve hyperpigmented lesions.

7.1.5.7 Antibiotics: Overview

Antibiotics are not utilized for mild comedonal acne but are indicated in mild to moderate acne with inflammatory and/or cystic lesions often with other medications (i.e. benzoyl peroxide or retinoids) (Table 7.2) (26,27). Oral formulations are used for moderate to severe acne and may take 1 to 2 months to see improvement and can be used for many months.

Improvement occurs because of *P. acnes* suppression, bacterial lipase inhibition, and interference with neutrophil migration by local chemotaxis improvement. Topical formulations should be used for short term use (as under 3 months) and not combined with the same antibiotic in oral form to reduce the risk of antibiotic resistance, which is especially noted with topical erythromycin and clindamycin. Such resistance may also be lowered with the combination of antibiotics with topical benzoyl peroxide or topical retinoid. The development of such resistance leads to poor response to anti-acne treatments.

Topical forms of erythromycin (Emgel, Erycette, A/T/S, Eryderm, others: 1.5%–3.0%), or clindamycin (Cleocin T, 1%) are used as well as oral forms of tetracycline, erythromycin, doxycycline, and minocycline. Irritation and dryness may occur with topical formulations. Pseudomembraneous enterocolitis is an unusual side effect to use of topical clindamycin. A gel form may be more efficacious for those with oily skin. Combination with benzoyl peroxide is available as seen with erythromycin (Benzamycin) or clindamycin (Benzaclin).

7.1.5.8 Oral tetracycline

Tetracycline hydrochloride has been a commonly used oral antibiotic for acne vulgaris with a dose usually between 250 to 1,000 mg per day. Dosages over 1 gram per day are seldom used. One regimen is to use 250 mg four times a day (500 mg twice a day) with gradual reduction to 250 mg once a day as efficacy is seen. Occasional patients require 2 to 3 grams per day for significant improvement. Inhibition of MMP (matrix metalloproteinase) enzymes are part of the effectiveness of tetracyclines in acne treatment (28).

Optimal absorption is seen when taken on an empty stomach (i.e. 2 hours after a meal or 1 hour before a meal). It may take 2 to 4 weeks for improvement to be appreciated. Failure of efficacy may arise because of issues with compliance, antibiotic resistance, absorption problems, and/or persistence of deep nodular lesion.

Tetracycline has proved to be a safe antibiotic that can be used for many years. Periodic screening should be done that includes a complete blood count (CBC), blood urea nitrogen, creatinine, and liver enzymes. Side effects tend to be dose-related, particularly if daily doses are over 500 mg (Table 7.3). Carefully monitor for gastrointestinal (esophageal) irritation, photosensitivity, and, with chronic use, renal complications as well as microbial resistance. It should be taken on an empty stomach with a large glass of water; avoid taking it with an antacid or with dairy products. Gram-negative folliculitis (especially around the nose) may occur in some with severe acne taking tetracycline chronically. Using with ibuprofen may heighten the efficacy of tetracycline.

Monilial vaginitis responds to anti-fungal treatment, and tetracycline discontinuation is usually not necessary. Tetracycline is not used in those under age 9 years since it may cause enamel defects in unerupted teeth and can be deposited in teeth as well as bones of a fetus of a pregnant individual. Tetracycline is contraindicated in pregnancy. Anecdotal cases of pregnancy are reported in females on both oral contraception and tetracycline and has been attributed to tetracycline-altered gastrointestinal flora with potential of lowered efficacy of oral contraceptives; however, there is no clear evidence-based research that antibiotics, such as tetracycline, actually reduce efficacy of oral contraceptives.

Table 7.3: Potential side effects of tetracycline

Allergic reactions
Bacterial resistance
Esophagitis
Gastrointestinal irritation
Gram-negative folliculitis
Headache
Hemolytic anemia
Inhibition of leukocytosis during acute infections
Monilial vaginitis
Photo-onycholysis – separation of the nail from its plate after sun exposure (rare)
Photosensitivity
Pseudotumor cerebri
Teeth discoloration (do *not* use in those younger than 9–12!)
Transient blood urea nitrogen elevation
Transient leucopenia
Transient liver enzyme elevation

7.1.5.9 Other oral antibiotics

Erythromycin is also widely used for acne vulgaris and is used in doses of 500 to 2,000 mg per day. Erythromycin may also lead to gastric irritation, including when taken on an empty stomach. Side effects also include nausea and diarrhea, which can be reduced by taking enteric-coated erythromycin. It can be given at any age.

Doxycycline (50 mg twice daily), trimethoprim-sulfamethoxazole, and minocycline (50–300 mg per day) have also been used. *Doxycycline* has similar side effects to tetracycline, though with less dental staining. Gastrointestinal upset, photosensitivity, and photo-onycholysis are well known as adverse effects. Do not give to those under 9 years of age. Oral *clindamycin* (150–600 mg per day) is not used for acne since it can lead to colitis. Bacterial resistance is a growing phenomenon, and it is recommended to avoid using oral or systemic antibiotics over 3 months in attempts to control this problem.

Minocycline can lead to dizziness, headaches, photosensitivity, vertigo (vestibular disturbance), tooth discoloration, and, with chronic use, increased skin pigmentation as well as localized facial marks that are dark bluish; also rarely seen are autoimmune syndromes with hepatitis, serum sickness-like reaction, lupus-like syndrome, and a hypersensitivity syndrome. It should be given on an empty stomach, and avoid taking it with dairy products. It should not be given to those under 9 years of age. Dosage is 50 to 100 mg twice a day. Its high price and significant potential adverse effects both suggest it is a second-line oral antibiotic for acne vulgaris treatment (29).

Trimethoprim-sulfamethoxazole can be given at any age but should only be used as a second-line drug for acne vulgaris. It can lead to drug hypersensitivity reaction, bone marrow suppression, GI upset, hepatitis, and renal toxicity; Avoid in glucose-6-phosphate dehydrogenase (G6PD) deficiency and use only as a second-line antibiotic. Dosage is once or twice daily of the 80/400 or 160/800 mg formulations. Some clinicians prescribe *cephalexin* at 250–500 mg twice a day; it can be used at any age but can lead to GI upset, and it is considered as a second-line drug.

7.1.5.10 Dapsone

Dapsone (diamino-diphenyl sulfone) is a white to creamy white, odorless crystalline powder used to treat a number of disorders, including mild to moderate acne vulgaris as a 5% gel (Aczone). Oral dapsone is also used for acne fulminans and acne conglobata if other treatments do not work; it is used for its anti-inflammatory and immunomodulatory effects.

7.1.5.11 Miscellaneous acne treatments

Oral zinc sulfate has been used with mixed results by clinicians and has been limited by gastrointestinal side effects (17). The role of topical sulfur, salicylic acid, and resorcinol remains unclear, though they have been used for many years (17). Patients with severe cystic acne and thick walls can be improved with intralesional steroid injection (triamcinolone acetonide) or incision and drainage. Use of antiandrogens may be helpful in some, such as spironolactone (50–200 mg per day) or cyproterone, which can reduce sebum production (*vida infra*).

Oral contraceptives can improve acne vulgaris by lowering gonadotropin secretion with reduced ovarian-induced androgens and also by increasing SHBG (sex hormone-binding globulin) levels that lower free testosterone levels. Oral contraceptives can serve as an adjuvant treatment for acne, particular in a female who is sexually active. Pills with low androgenic progestin are recommended, such as norgestimate (Ortho Tri-Cyclen) which is FDA approved for the treatment of acne vulgaris (3,30,31). Other contraceptives are efficacious, such as ethinyl estradiol combined with chlormadinone acetate, which is available in Europe (32). Sexually active females with acne may notice worsening of this condition if placed on long-acting progestin implants or depo-medroxy-progesterone acetate (Depo-Provera).

Ultraviolet light therapy does not significantly improve acne vulgaris and may lead to skin aging and possibly melanoma. Research is focusing on newer research treatments such as use of low-dose isotretinoin plans, chemical peels, photodynamic therapy (PDT), light and laser treatments, anti-inflammatory agents as lipooxygenase inhibitors, insulin sensitizing drugs, 5-alpha-reductase type I inhibitors, oral probiotics, and others (33,34,35). PDT uses a photosensitizer, light source, and molecular oxygen to kill specific cells in the pilosebaceous units and is being used by dermatologists to treat inflammatory acne vulgaris (36). Scars can be treated with a chemical peel, dermabrasion, collagen injection, or intralesional steroids for keloids.

7.1.5.12 Isotretinoin (13-cis-retinoic acid)

Isotretinoin (Accutane; Claravis; Amnesteem; Sotret) is a powerful anti-acne medication identified since the 1980s to be effective in many cases of severe, recalcitrant, nodulocystic acne; milder acne resistant to other more traditional treatments; and various forms of acne with scarring and psychological distress (37,38,39). It is a derivative of vitamin A and is used in other conditions, including hidradenitis suppurativa, acne rosacea, acne fulminans, acne conglobata, some forms of ichthyosis, and others. Its precise mechanism of action is unclear but may be related to its effect on NGAL (neutrophil-gelatinase associated lipocalin) in skin, which lowers sebum production and exerts an antimicrobial effect on *P. acne*. It decreases sebum production and shrinks sebaceous glands in addition to having anti-inflammatory effects; it also improves abnormal keratinazation. Though its effect on sebum production is temporary, the remission on acne can be permanent.

Dosage includes 0.5 to 1.0 mg (up to 2.0 mg) per kg per day over a twice a day course for 15 to 24 weeks (up to 9 months); improvement is typically seen with an accumulative dose of 100 to 150 mg per kilogram. A second course is occasionally needed after 2 months or more off the medication. Most patients receive significant improvement, including 40% or more with complete acne resolution. Lower doses (i.e. half the usual dose) may be effective in some with lower side effects but a higher relapse rate. Prior to isotretinoin prescription the clinician should order a complete blood count (CBC), chemistry profile (including liver function tests), and fasting lipids (triglycerides and cholesterol). The CBC and chemistry profile are typically obtained again at 4 to 6 weeks into treatment with isotretinoin. This medication has a short half life and is cleared from the body in a few days.

A large number of side effects are possible with isotretinoin (Table 7.4). Triglycerides are particularly increased in those with diabetes mellitus, alcohol abuse, obesity, and/or positive family history for hyperlipidemia. Patients with a history of intestinal disorders may develop severe diarrhea or rectal bleeding; some research notes a possible link to inflammatory bowel disease in some patients that includes both ulcerative colitis and Crohn's disease. Diffuse skeletal hyperostosis may develop with prolonged use of isotretinoin. There is an association between pseudotumor cerebri with tetracyclines and isotretinoin; vitamin A supplements may increase this toxic risk as well. Final closure of epiphyses may not occur in youth until the late teens or even early 20s, and thus, use of isotretinoin in this age group may result in decreased potential growth by reducing long bone growth.

Table 7.4: Potential side effects of isotretinoin

TERATOGENICITY (see text)
Cheilitis (90%)*
Severe dry skin and pruritus (80%)*
Dry nose and mouth along with epistaxis (80%)
Conjunctivitis (40%)
Dry eyes*
Decreased night vision*
Difficulty with contact lenses (40%)
Increased cholesterol and triglycerides (25%)*
Musculoskeletal aches (16%)
Alopecia and hair thinning (10%)*
Photosensitivity
Arthralgia*
Corneal opacities (5%)
Headache (5%)
Fatigue (5%)
Depression (<5%)*
? Suicide risk?
Elevated liver enzyme and blood sugar levels
Severe rectal bleeding and diarrhea
Acne rosacea* (with high doses of isotretinoin)
Inflammatory bowel disease* (including exacerbation of previous disease)
Low back pain
Keloids*
Degenerative disc disease*
Increased susceptibility to sunburn
Osteopenia*
Peeling of palms and soles
Pseudotumor cerebri (especially when combined with oral antibiotics)
Premature epiphyseal closure
Cervical spine hyperostosis
Erectile dysfunction*
Others

*May be permanent side effects

High doses of isotretinoin can result in toxicity that looks like vitamin A toxicity. It is not used with a history of allergy to paraben because paraben is used as a preservative in the isotretinoin gelatin capsule.

Frequent (even hourly) application of white petrolatum to the lips is helpful in dealing with the often present cheilitis due to isotretinoin; steroid ointment may be helpful such as 1% hydrocortisone or stronger formulations. Xerosis may improve with application of lipid free moisturizers or lotions (i.e. Cetaphil, Aquanil) without worsening the acne. Ocular dryness may improve or stabilize with artificial tears. The risk of photosensitivity is lowered with use of sunscreens in an oil free, non-acnegenic base. A lower dose of the isotretinoin may be necessary to deal with such irritating adverse effects. Use of isotretinoin can lead to the appearance of lesions that look like pyogenic granulomas and may require discontinuing the isotretinoin if steroids do not ameliorate this development. Apply antibiotic ointment (i.e. mupirocin) to the nose two times a day to reduce *Staphylococcus aureus* infections, which, if this develops, requires appropriate antibiotics. The clinician should be vigilant in observing and managing these potentially serious infections.

7.1.6 Teratogenicity and isotretinoin

Isotretinoin is a major teratogenic agent, and Table 7.5 outlines some of these defects; it is contraindicated in pregnancy and is classified as an FDA Pregnancy Category X and ADEC Category X. The use of this drug during pregnancy leads to a 25-fold increase in teratogencity that includes mental subnormality in 50% even with no external evidence of other defects. Isotretinoin does affect the fetal dividing cells but not the spermatozoa or ova.

Table 7.5: Teratogenic effects of Isotretinoin?

Affected Area of the Body	Teratogenic Effects
Head	Microcephaly, abnormal cranium, anencephaly, seizures, psychomotor retardation.
Eyes	Microphthalmia, blindness, down-slant of palpebral fissures.
Ears	Atretic ears, hypoplastic auditory meatus, absent eighth nerve, deafness, rudimentary, or malformed pinnae.
Mouth	Cleft palate, lip micrognathia.
Heart	Patent ductus arteriosus, atrial septal defects, ventricular septal defects, truncus arteriosus, others.

Used with permission from: Greydanus DE: Disorders of the skin. In: AD Hofmann, DE Greydanus (eds). Adolescent Medicine, 3rd Edition. Stanform, CT: Appleton & Lange, 1997; ch. 18:380.

The FDA announced the *iPLEDGE* program in 2005 to emphasize the need for pregnant females to avoid taking isotretinoin. Since 2006 only clinicians officially listed in this program can prescribe this drug, and only patients who are officially registered can receive this drug. This also includes males, though there is no evidence that their sperm is affected. Females taking isotretinoin should have negative pregnancy test(s) at least 2 weeks prior to its initiation and should take two types of contraception at the same time for at least 30 days prior to starting it and for at least 30 days following use of this drug. If one is taking isotretinoin, s/he is not allowed to donate blood during the time on this drug and also for at least 30 days after stopping it. The program for isotretinoin management recommended by the manufacturer is called *S.M.A.R.T.* (System to Manage Accutane Related Teratogenity) (20,40).

7.1.7 Depression, suicidality, and isotretinoin

Isotretinoin has been linked by anecdotal data to depression, psychosis, and even suicide in some patients. However, research in general has failed to establish a clear link between use of this drug and overt depression as well as suicide (41,42,43). Anecdotal cases of suicide in patients taking isotretinoin fuel the ongoing debate. It is clear that patients with acne have increased risk for depression because of the distress that this condition can induce. It is also clear that depression and suicide are real phenomena among adolescents and young adults around the world. Separating out the role of isotretinoin as a cause of depression and/or suicide in those with severe, cystic, disfiguring acne from other factors is very difficult. Even those with so-called mild acne can have major distress because of negative reactions to this disorder. Clinicians should be aware of the real presence of depression and suicide in this age group and should be aware of the potentially negative effects of severe acne itself. Thus, those taking this drug and all patients with acne should receive careful and ongoing screening for depression and suicidality.

7.1.7.1 Management of acne vulgaris comorbid conditions

Another part of the overall management plan for acne is to treat underlying or comorbid conditions. For example, acne can be very severe in disorders with increased androgens, such as congenital adrenal hyperplasia, polycystic ovary syndrome (PCOS), Cushing's disease, Syndrome X (hyperlipidemia, obesity, hypertension, and insulin resistance), and other states of hyperandrogenemia (Table 7.6) (1,2,20).

Acne may be the first significant sign of PCOS or adrenal hyperandrogenism. Underlying endocrine disorders should be carefully managed, and appropriate medications can be very helpful in acne treatment as well; these medications include low dose prednisone, oral contraceptives, anti-androgens (i.e., cimetidine, spironolactone, or cyproterone acetate), or even GnRH (gonadotropin-releasing hormone)

Table 7.6: Causes of hyperandrogenemia in females with potential of severe acne*

Genetic and familial increased androgen sensitivity
Adrenal androgens
Congenital adrenal hyperplasias
21-hydroxylase deficiency
Classic
Late-onset
3-β hydroxysteroid dehydrogenase deficiency
Classic
Late-onset
11β-hydroxylase deficiency
Classic
Late-onset
Adrenal tumors
Adrenocortical carcinoma
Testosterone-secreting adenoma
Adrenal rest adenoma and carcinoma
Cushing's disease
Ovarian androgens
Polycystic ovary syndrome (PCOS)
Conditions associated with PCOS
PCOS with ovarian tumor
Pineal gland hyperplasia and diabetes
Congenital lipoatrophic diabetes
Hyperprolactinemia
Hyperthyroidism
Hypothyroidism
Androgen-secreting cysts and hyperplasias
Stromal hyperplasia and hyperthecosis
Solitary follicle cyst
Hyperreaction luteinalis of pregnancy
Androgen-secreting ovarian tumors
Arrhenoblastoma (androblastoma)
Thecoma-fibroma group tumors
Granulosa cell tumors
Lipoid cell tumors
Gynandroblastoma
Epithelial tumor

(*Continued*)

Table 7.6: Causes of hyperandrogenemia in females with potential of severe acne *(Continued)*

Luteoma of pregnancy
Testicular androgens in XY females
5-α reductase deficiency
Mixed gonadal dysgenesis
True hermaphroditism
17-β hydroxysteroid dehydrogenase deficiency
Other rare intersex conditions
Exogenous androgens
Medical
Hypoplastic anemias
Growth stimulation
Adrenal replacement
Danazol
Synthetic progestins in oral contraceptives
Adrenocorticotropic hormone (ACTH) therapy
Nonmedical
Bodybuilding and athletic anabolic steroids

Source: Used with permission: Greydanus DE, Patel DR. Acne vulgaris and chronically ill Adolescents. Internat J Disabil & Hum Devel 2008; 7(3): 322.

agonists. Side effects of these various medications must be kept in mind; for example, adverse effects of spironolactone include menstrual irregularity, fatigue, hyperkalemia, and breast tenderness. Also, some medications can worsen acne (Table 7.7), and these should be discontinued if possible and alternative drugs used that do not worsen the dermatological condition.

7.1.7.2 Management of Well-Being in Acne Patients

Depression is a common aspect in human beings and also those with acne (44). Acne develops intense feelings of sadness, guilt, shame, and anger in adolescence at a time when the youth's sense of self is emerging (45,46,47,48,49,50). Approximately 25% of adolescents with acne have some scarring by late adolescence, adding to their sense of distress over this disease (51,52). The development of acne is a major problem for both the adolescent and the adult and can have an immensely negative impact on their psychosocial development that can last a lifetime. The art and science of managing acne patients demands that the clinician address this feature in addition to the formal and classic medical task of prescribing anti-acne drugs.

Table 7.7: Medications/chemicals that worsen acne*

Androgenic steroids
Barbiturates
Bromides
Diphenylhydantoin
Glucocorticoids
Iodides
Isoniazid
Kelp and other seaweed
Lithium
Rifampin
Synthetic progestins
Vitamin B12
Others

*Used with permission: Greydanus DE, Patel DR. Acne vulgaris and chronically ill Adolescents. Internat J Disabil & Hum Devel 2008; 7(3): 323.

Effective management of all with acne is important, and its value should never be underestimated. Youth should be asked and taught about acne treatment even if the patient does not ask about management options. As noted, it is difficult to separate out depression that may occur in any person from depression worsened by the skin condition itself. It is also difficult to separate out suicidality that occurs in many youth and adults from that stimulated by acne itself. Those with acne should be evaluated for depression, suicidality, anxiety, body dysmorphic disorder, self-injury (acne excoriée – vida infra), and other mental health issues (53,54,55,56).

Successful treatment of acne includes the *sine qua non* principle that acne management is not only prescription of dermatological agents but careful and persistent attention to the psychosocial and mental health status of this patient whose feelings can be more sensitive than the acne skin (57). The emotional health of these patients should be evaluated and monitored as the acne management is developed. For example, stress can trigger and worsen acne by androgen hormone activation. Some patients may need overt mental health treatment with therapy and/or psychopharmacologic management (58,59,60).

7.1.7.3 Acne excoriée

Acne excoriée refers to acneform lesions on the face and other parts of the body due to deliberate self-injury on normal and/or abnormal skin (see Chapter 11). It is part of a wide range of self-induced skin diseases that includes dermatitis artefacta, neurotic self-mutilation (neurotic excoriation), self-mutilation associated with psychotic features (i.e. hallucinations or delusions), nail biting (onychophagia), Munchausen syndrome, and acne excoriée (61). The patient may present with multiple excoriated or acne-form lesions over the face (as well as upper arms, forearms, other areas) with or without a history of previous lesions. There may be a history of mental illness such as obsessive compulsive disorder, depression, psychosis, or other disorders. A careful medical history reveals that the patient may have an uncontrollable urge for self-mutilation and underlies the need for the clinician to know the patient carefully and not just injudiciously provide medical prescriptions (62).

The patient typically does not complain of these lesions even if they appear to be painful or unsightly (63). There may be lesions that do not heal despite appropriate treatment such as antibiotics, and the clinician should be highly suspicious of dermatological features (including ulcers and scars) that do not conform to known patterns of physiologic illness (64). The mentally disturbed patient may develop habits that directly lead to skin trauma of various degrees that can lead to linear and stellate facial ulcers, hypertrophic scars, and other lesions (65). If treatment does not occur, the condition may continue for many years. The patient may admit to the self-injury if carefully asked and may note squeezing, rubbing, or picking at lesions. Self-destructive behavior is common in mentally retarded patients (66).

Management begins with suspicion on the part of the clinician because of lesions that do not fit known disorders and/or do not heal properly with treatment. A mental status, medical history, and careful examination are needed for all these patients. Treatment is needed for the underlying behavioral/psychiatric disorder(s) and may include psychotherapy and/or psychopharmacology (61,62,63,64). As the underlying psychopathology is improved, the scars can be treated with dermatological treatments such as resurfacing (chemical peels, lasers, light therapy, cryotherapy), dermal fillers, and surgery (i.e. dermabrasion, subcision or punch excision) (14,67,68,69).

7.2 Acne Rosacea

Acne rosacea, a condition known for centuries, is a chronic, inflammatory dermatological condition mainly observed in adults that is distinct from acne vulgaris and is characterized by flushing, central facial erythema (transient or persistent), dilated (visible) blood vessels (telangiectasias; couperosis), burning pain, comedones, papules, pustules, and/or facial skin fibrosis (10,70). There can also be ocular involvement (30% to 50%) with thickened skin and the enlargement (phymas) of the nose called rhinophyma (bulbous nose, phymatous rosacea). The cause of the bulbous nose (i.e. enlarged, bulb-shaped, erythematous) is unclear, was erroneously linked for centuries with excess alcohol, and is now linked with being a rare part of severe rosacea. *Phyma* comes from the Greek and means “mass” (swelling or bulb). The nose can contain many oil glands that present a yellow or waxy appearance. The development of malignancy within a rhinophyma has been reported (71,72).

The term “rosacea” denotes the facial telangiectasias with or without facial erythema, and acne rosacea was separated from acne vulgaris in the twentieth century as more understanding of these conditions emerged (73). The red face has historically been used by novelists and others to denote negative traits of persons, adding to the stigmata of rosacea that continues to the present (73).

Current studies present a range of epidemiologic data based on criteria used for the diagnosis. Acne rosacea classically is first noted around 30 years of age and affects 1% to 20% of the adult population to some extent (74). Though less common, acne rosacea, including ocular rosacea, can occur in children as young as 1 year of age (75). A positive family history and having very light skin (“Celtic” skin type) increase the risk for this disorder, while the often indicted coffee and alcohol are not risk factors (74).

Four types of acne rosacea have been established based on the National Rosacea Society’s Expert Committee on the Classification and Staging of Rosacea: erythemato-telangiectatic, papulopustular, phymatous, and ocular (76,77,78,79,80). Other variants are noted, such as lupoid or granulomatous types, which may represent different rosacea stages or overlapping syndromes (80).

7.2.1 Pathophysiology

The cause of acne rosacea is unclear at this time but is currently linked to various factors such as inflammatory, genetic, environmental, vascular, and microbial (i.e. *Helicobacter pylori* and *Demodex folliculorum*) (76). Some with rosacea have a light phototype, which is sensitive to various climate changes, while others have genetic proclivity for primary vascular anomalies, which are then influenced by a variety of factors such as ultraviolet ray exposure, skin flora, and/or climate changes (81). A precipitating factor in some may be reactive oxygen species that includes superoxide and hydroxyl radicals, hydrogen peroxide, and singlet oxygen (82).

Rosacea swelling or edema allows colonization and growth of microbes (as *Demodex folliculorum*), which can lead to inflammation that contributes to rosacea papules, pustules, and granulomas (81,83). *Demodex folliculorum* is a species of face mite that increases in amount during early adolescence due to the increase in sebaceous glands; they are found in increased concentration in the central part of the face, and their food is sebaceous secretions and dead cells.

Recent research in molecular biology provides etiologic links with inflammatory and vascular factors because of immune dysfunction (77). Research also notes dysregulation of mediators and receptors involved in neurovascular as well as neuro-immune communication in early stages of rosacea; it may be a neurogenic inflammatory disorder due to sensory nerve disease because of abnormal release of key neuromediators (84). Other researchers describe acne rosacea as a disorder of cathelicidins and skin innate immunity (85). Those with rosacea have increased levels of these polypeptides called cathelicidins (vida supra) and also increased levels of stratum corneum tryptic enzymes (SCTEs). SCTEs are an important part of the desquamation process in human skin, which involves production of corneocytes and their shedding from skin.

Further understanding of the pathophysiology of acne rosacea will enhance our understanding of connections between the human immune, nervous, and cutaneous vascular systems (86). For example, the development of skin fibrosis in some rosacea patients indicates a powerful link between chronic *inflammatory* mechanisms and the development of fibrosis in the skin. The vascular defects in rhinophyma can lead to local development of TGF-β1 (transforming growth factor β1) that induces skin fibrosis and skin thickening (82). TGF-β1 is a protein controlling cellular differentiation, proliferation, and other functions in most cells.

Steroid-induced rosacea (iatrosacea) is described in patients using chronic facial steroids, particularly potent topical steroids, which can lead to facial erythema, telangiectasias, photosensitivity, hyperpigmentation, and xerosis (87). The underlying etiology with iatrosacea is linked to steroid-induced rebound vasodilatation and proinflamatory cytokine release (87).

7.2.2 Management of acne rosacea

The purpose of therapy is to improve the patient's quality of life by improving this disease in which there is noticeable reduction in erythema, papules, pustules, and overt physical discomfort (77). The skin should be protected from harmful effects of sunlight, and the patient should avoid known triggers for disease exacerbation (78). Triggers in some patients include ultraviolet radiation, stress, microbes, heat, cold, and/or spicy foods that can precipitate rosacea pathophysiologic mechanisms noted earlier and involve the cytokine as well as chemokine network (88). Management of steroid-induced rosacea is stopping the topical steroid and use of topical tacrolimus and oral antibiotics (87).

Evidence-based research suggests effective results for acne rosacea can be seen with the use of acne medications such as doxycycline (40 mg) and azelaic acid (15% gel) as well as topical metronidazole. Ocular rosacea may improve with cyclosporine (0.5% ophthalmic emulsion) and 40 mg doxycycline (slow release form) (71,72,75,89). Sodium sulfacetamide 10%-sulfur 5% (emollient foam) is also used by clinicians for acne rosacea, while second-line management drugs include clindamycin, benzoyl peroxide, permethrin, and calcineurin inhibitors (77). A synergistic effect has been reported with the combination of azelaic acid as well as topical metronidazole with doxycycline (78,90). Improvement with both azelaic acid and doxycycline has been linked to the ability of these drugs to downregulate antimicrobial and proinflammatory cathelicidins (14).

Pimecrolimus (Elidel) is an immunomodulating topical agent (1% cream) used to treat atopic dermatitis with recent research noting some efficacy in rosacea (91). New products continue to be evaluated, such as brimonidine tartrate gel (0.5%); this α-2-adrenergic agonist has vasoconstrictive activity and has been shown to be efficacious in the management of rosacea (92).

Choosing the right soothing vehicle or formulation that includes cleansers, moisturizers, and facial foundation products is important to the overall management success in providing efficacy with minimal skin irritation that will increase patient compliance (93,94). It is also important to provide decongestant active ingredients and appropriate medical makeup to improve the red face appearance (95).

Oral isotretinoin is also used for phymatous rosacea and other types of acne rosacea recalcitrant to other treatments (76,78,96). Erythematous skin and telangiectasias are also managed with light-based therapies (i.e. pulsed dye laser and intense pulsed light) (78,97). Treatment of rhinophyma is with surgery to correct the nasal appearance using laser surgery or dermabrasion (rotating brush) as well with anti-acne medications. Surgery may be requested by the patient because of cosmetic concerns, issues with airway obstruction, or eating difficulty (98).

7.3 Acne Variants

Table 7.1 lists a variety of acne variants. For example, *acne conglobata* may improve with sulfone, oral steroids, and/or oral isotretinoin. *Acne fulminans* is also called acute febrile, ulcerative, conglobate acne in which there can be an acute onset of hemorrhagic and ulcerative acne that involves the face, chest, back, and other areas. It can be the skin manifestation of SAPHO (acute fulminans with synovitis-acne-pustulosis-hyperostosis-osteitis) (99). Acne fulminans may be improved with acne measures already reviewed along with salicylates (for fever and/or muscle–joint symptomatology), oral corticosteroids (topical and systemic), dapsone (diaminodiphenyl sulfone), nonsteroidal anti-inflammatory drugs (NSAIDs), infliximab, methotrexate, and/or isotretinoin (see further on) (99,100,101). Table 7.1 outlines other acne variants and acneform disorders and outlines management concepts.

7.4 Conclusion

Acne vulgaris relates to abnormal keratinization, androgen-stimulated hormone sebum production, follicular plug development (pilosebaceous unit obstruction), colonization with *P. acnes*, host response to inflammation, and genetic factors. Management is individualized based on disease severity, motivation of the patient for treatment, and comorbid conditions. Recommended treatment options are likely to be continued if the patient is bothered by this dermatological condition and perceives that management leads to significant improvement. Patients must be taught that treatment may take some weeks before positive results can be appreciated. Time must be spent by clinicians in explaining the cause of acne and dealing with challenging compliance issues in some patients. The time is worthwhile for the clinician and patient since acne can have lifelong negative consequences for the youth and his or her overall well-being in adulthood.

Fortunately, most persons can be effectively treated with a combination of topical agents (i.e. benzoyl peroxide, topical retinoids, azelaic acid, antibiotics) and oral agents (i.e. oral contraceptives, oral antibiotics). Oral isotretinoin is a powerful drug for severe and/or resistant acne that is both beneficial for most but also fraught with many potential side effects including teratogenicity. Consultation with dermatology is necessary for dealing with situations not responsive to basic acne measures and for dealing with isotretinoin. Fortunately, most patients with acne will see improvement with currently available options. However, successful management of acne is not just prescribing dermatological agents but includes judicious attention to the psychosocial well-being of this patient who can be physically but even more seriously emotionally scarred for life by this most common of skin disorders. The website for treatment of acne from the American Academy of Dermatology is available at www.skincarephysicians.com/acnenet.

References

1. Greydanus DE. Disorders of the skin. In: Hofmann AD, Greydanus DE, eds. *Adolescent Medicine*, 3rd edn. Stanford, CT: Appleton Lange, 1997:375–407.
2. Greydanus DE, Patel DR. Acne vulgaris and chronically ill adolescents. *Int J Disabil Hum Devel* 2008;7(3):319–27.
3. Williams HC, Dellavalle RP, Garner S. Acne vulgaris. *Lancet* 2012;379:361–72.
4. James WD. Acne. *N Engl J Med* 2005;352:1463–72.
5. Krowchuk DP, Gelmetti C, Lucky AW. Acne. In: Schachner LA, Hansen RC, eds. *Pediatric Dermatology*, 4th edn. Philadelphia, PA: Mosby, 2011:827–50.
6. Ascenso A, Marques HC. Acne in the adult. *Mini Rev Med Chem* 2009;9:1–10.
7. Friedlander SF, Baldwin HE, Mancini AJ, Yan AC, Eichenfeld LF. The acne continuum: An age-based approach to therapy. *Semin Cutan Med Surg* 2011;30(3 Suppl):S6–11.
8. Schnopp C, Mempel M. Acne vulgaris in children and adolescents. *Minerva Pediatr* 2011;63: 293–304.
9. Bhambri S, Del Rosso JQ, Bhambri A. Pathogenesis of acne vulgaris: Recent advances. *J Drugs Dermatol* 2009;8:615–8.
10. Powell FC. Rosacea. *N Engl J Med* 2005;252:793–803.
11. Feinberg AN. The integument system: Skin, hair, nails. In: Greydanus DE, Feinberg AN, Patel DR, Homnick DN, eds. *The pediatric examination*. New York: McGraw-Hill, 2008:570.
12. Bellew S, Thiboutot D, Del Rosso JQ. Pathogenesis of acne vulgaris: What's new, what's interesting, and what may be clinically relevant. *J Drugs Dermatol* 2011;10:582–5.
13. Zouboulis CC. Modern aspects of acne pathogenesis. *J Dutsch Dermatol Ges* 2010;8(Suppl 1): S7–14.

14. Fleischer AB Jr. Inflammation in rosacea and acne: Implications for patient care. *J Drugs Dermatol* 2011;10:614–20.
15. Basta-Juzbašić A. Current therapeutic approach to acne scars. *Acta Dermatovenerol Croat* 2010;18:171–5.
16. Newman MD, Bowe WP, Heughebaert C, Shalita AR. Therapeutic considerations for severe nodular acne. *Am J Clin Dermatol* 2011;12:7–14.
17. Szczepaniak D, Treadwell PA. Acne therapy in primary care: Comprehensive review of current evidence-based interventions and treatments. *Adolesc Med* 2011;22:77–96.
18. Zaenglein AL, Thiboutot DM. Expert committee recommendations for acne management. *Pediatrics* 2006;118(3):1188–99.
19. Baldwin HE, Friedlander SF, Eichenfield LF, Mancini AJ, Jan AC. The effects of culture, skin color, and other nonclinical issues on acne treatment. *Semin Cutan Med Surg* 2011;30(3 Suppl):S12–5.
20. Krowchuk DP. Disorders of the skin. In: Greydanus DE, Patel DR, Pratt HD, eds. *Essential adolescent medicine.* New York: McGraw-Hill, 2006:411–43.
21. Haider A, Shaw JC. Treatment of acne vulgaris. JAMA 2004;292:726–35.
22. Layton AM. Optimal management of acne to prevent scarring and psychological sequelae. *Am J Clin Dermatol* 2001;2(3):135–41.
23. Dutil M. Benzoyl peroxide: Enhancing antibiotic efficacy in acne management. *Skin Therapy Lett* 2010;15:5–7.
24. Fakhouri T, Yentzer BA, Feldman SR. Advancement in benzoyl-peroxide-based acne treatment: Methods to increase both efficacy and tolerability. *J Drug Dermatol* 2009;8:657–61.
25. Thiboutot DM, Gollnick HP. Treatment considerations for inflammatory acne: Clinical evidence for adapalene 0.1% in combination therapies. *J Drugs Dermatol* 2006;5:785–94.
26. Eady EA, Cove JH, Joanes DN. Topical antibiotics for the treatment of acne vulgaris: A critical evaluation of their clinical benefit and comparative efficacy. *J Dermatol Treat* 1990;1:215–20.
27. Ozolins M, Eady EA, Avery AJ, et al. Comparison of five antimicrobial regimens for treatment of mild to moderate inflammatory acne vulgaris in the community: Randomized controlled trial. *Lancet* 2004;364:2188–95.
28. Monk E, Shalita A, Siegel DM. Clinical applications of non-antimicrobial tetracyclines in dermatology. *Pharmacol Res* 2011;63:130–45.
29. Garner SE, Eady EA, Popescu C, Newton J, Li WA. Minocycline for acne vulgaris: Efficacy and safety. *Cochrane Database Syst Rev* 2003;(1):CD002086.
30. Redmond GP, Olson WH, Lippman JS. Norgestimate and ethinyl estrodiol in the treatment of acne vulgaris: A randomized, placebo-controlled trial. *Obstet Gynecol* 1997;89:615–20.
31. Rosen MP, Breitkopf DM, Nagamani M. A randomized controlled trial of second versus third generation oral contraceptives in the treatment of acne vulgaris. *Am J Obstet Gynecol* 2003;188:1158–60.
32. Guerra-Tapia A, Sancho Pérez B. Ethinylestradiol/Chlormadinone acetate: Dermatological benefits. *Am J Clin Dermatol* 2011;12(Suppl 1):3–11.
33. Katsambas A, Dessinioti C. New and emerging treatments in dermatology: Acne. *Dermatol Ther* 2008;21:86–95.
34. Kim RH, Armstrong AW. Current state of acne treatment: Highlighting lasers, photodynamic therapy, and chemical peels. *Dermatol Online J* 2011;17:2–5.
35. Bowe WP, Logan AC. Acne vulgaris, probiotics and the gut-brain-skin axis – back to the future? *Gut Pathol* 2011;3:1–4.
36. Gold MH. Photodyamic therapy. *Curr Probl Dermatol* 2011;42:181–92.
37. Abel EA. Isotretinoin (Accutane) therapy for acne vulgaris for adolescents. *Adolesc Med* 1990;1(2):315–24.

38. Goldsmith LA, Bolognia JL, Callen JP. American Academy of Dermatology Consensus Conference on the safe and optimal use of isotretinoin: Summary and recommendations. *J Am Acad Dermatol* 2004;50:900–6.
39. Rigopoulos D, Larios G, Katsambas AD. The role of isotretinoin in acne therapy: Why not as first line therapy? Facts and controversies. *Clin Dermatol* 2010;28:24–30.
40. Krowchuk DP. Managing adolescent acne: A guide for pediatricians. *Pediatr Rev* 2005;26:250–61.
41. Hull PR, D'Arcy C. Isotretinoin use and subsequent depression and suicide: Presenting the evidence. *Am J Clin Dermatol* 2003;4:493–505.
42. Wysowski DK, Pitts M, Beitz J. An analysis of reports of depression and suicide in patients treated with isotretinoin. *J Am Acad Dermatol* 2001;45:515–9.
43. McGrath EJ, Lovell CR, Gillison F, Darvay A, Hickey JR, Skevington SM. A prospective trial of the effects of isotretinoin on quality of life and depressive symptoms. *Br J Dermatol* 2010;163:1323–9.
44. Yentzer BA, Hick J, Reese EL, Uhas A, Feldman SR, Balkrishnan R. Acne vulgaris in the United States: A descriptive epidemiology. *Cutis* 2010;86:94–9.
45. Smith JA. The impact of skin disease on the quality of life of adolescents. *Adolesc Med* 2001;12 (2):343–54.
46. Simić D, Situm M, Letica E. Psychological impact of isotretinoin treatment in patients with moderate and severe acne. *Coll Antropol* 2009;33(Suppl 2):15–19.
47. Uhlenhake E, Yentzer BA, Feldman SR. Acne vulgaris and depression: A retrospective examination. *J Cosmet Dermatol* 2010;9:59–63.
48. Féton-Danou N. Psychological impact of acne vulgaris. *Ann Dermatol Venereol* 2010;137(Suppl 2):S62–5.
49. Rapp DA, Brenes GA, Feldman SR, Fleischer AB Jr., Graham GF, Dailey M, et al. Anger and acne: Implications for quality of life, patient satisfaction and clinical care. *Br J Dermatol* 2004;15:183–9.
50. Mallon E, Newton JN, Klassen A. The quality of life in acne. *Br J Dermatol* 1999;140:672–6.
51. Yan AC. Current concepts in acne management. *Adolesc Med Clin* 2006;17:613–37.
52. Fried RG, Wechsler A. Psychological problems in the acne patient. *Dermatol Ther* 2006;19: 237–40.
53. Misery L. Consequences of psychological distress in adolescents with acne. *J Invest Dermatol* 2011;131:290–2.
54. Halvorsen JA, Stern RS, Dalgard F, Thoresen M, Bjertness E, Lien L. Suicidal ideation, mental health problems, and social impairment are increased in adolescents with acne: A population-based study. *J Invest Dermatol* 2011;131:363–70.
55. Saitta P, Keehan P, Yousif J, Way BV, Grekin S, Brancaccio R. An update on the presence of psychiatric comorbidities in acne patients, part I. Overview of prevalence. *Cutis* 2011;88:33–40.
56. Saitta P, Keehan P, Yousif J, Way BV, Grekin S, Brancaccio R. An update on the presence of psychiatric comorbidities in acne patients, part 2. Depression, anxiety, and suicide. *Cutis* 2011; 88:92–7.
57. Niemeier V, Kupfer J, Gieler U. Acne vulgaris – psychosomatic aspects. *J Dtsch Dermatol Ges* 2006;4:1027–36.
58. Niemeier V, Kupfer J, Gieler U. Acne vulgaris – psychosomatic aspects. *J Dtsch Dermatol Ges* 2010;8(Suppl 1):S95–104.
59. Greydanus DE, Calles J, Patel DR, eds. Pediatric and adolescent psychopharmacology. *A practical manual for pediatricians*. Cambridge, England: Cambridge University Press, 2008.
60. Greydanus DE, Calles JL, Patel DR, Nazeer A, Merrick J, eds. *Clinical aspects of psychopharmacology in childhood and adolescence*. New York: Nova Science Publishers, 2012.
61. Broniarczyk-Dyla G, Pajor A. Skin injuries in psychodermatological aspect. *Wiad Lek* 2011;64 (2):142–6.

62. Kent A, Drummond LM. Acne excoriée – a case report of treatment using habit reversal. *Clin Exp Dermatol* 1989;14:163–4.
63. Shama H. Psychogenic excoriation responding to fluoxetine: A case report. *J Indian Med Assoc* 2008;106:245–7.
64. Shah KN, Fried RG. Factitial dermatoses in children. *Curr Opin Pediatr* 2006;18:403–9.
65. Chuh A, Wong W, Zawar V. The skin and the mind. *Aust Fam Physician* 2006;35:723–5.
66. Dimoski A, Duricić S. Dermatitis artefacia, onychophagia and trichotillomania in mentally retarded children and adolescents. *Med Pregl* 1991;44:471–2.
67. Gupta MA, Gupta AK. Olanzapine may be an effective adjunctive therapy in the management of acne excorée: A case report. *J Cutan Med Surg* 2001;5:25–7.
68. Bowes LE, Alster TS. Treatment of facial scarring and ulceration resulting from acne excoriée with 585-nm pulsed dye laser irradiation and cognitive psychotherapy. *Dermatol Surg* 2004; 30:934–8.
69. Jansen T, Podda M. Therapy of acne scars. *J Dtsch Dermatol Ges* 2010;8(Suppl 1):S81–8.
70. Van Zuuren EJ, Kramer S, Carter B, Graber MA, Fedorowicz Z. Interventions for rosacea. *Cochrane Database Sys Rev* 2011;16;(3):CD003262.
71. Lazzeri D, Colizzi L, Licata G, Pagnini D, Proietti A, Ali G, Maseri P, et al. Malignancies within rhinophyma: Report of three new cases and review of the literature. *Aesthetic Plast Surg* 2012;36(2):396–405.
72. Scheinfeld N, Berk T. A review of the diagnosis and treatment of rosacea. *Postgrad Med* 2010;122:139–43.
73. Cribier B. The red face: Art, history and medical representations. *Ann Dermatol Venereol* 2011;138(Suppl 2):S116–23.
74. Chosidow O, Cribier B. Epidemiology of rosacea: Updated data. *Ann Dermatol Venereol* 2011;138 (Suppl 2):S124–8.
75. Léoni S, Mesplié N, Aitali F, Chamailliard M, Boralevi F, Marques da Costa C, et al. Metronidazole: Alternative treatment for ocular and cutaneous rosacea in the pediatric population. *J Fr Ophthalmol* 201;34(10):703–10.
76. Buechner SA. Rosacea: An update. *Dermatology* 2005;210:100–8.
77. Elsaie ML, Choudhary S. Updates on the pathophysiology and management of acne rosacea. *Postgrad Med* 2009;121:178–86.
78. Kennedy Carney C, Cantrell W, Elewski BE. Rosacea: A review of current topical, systemic and light-based therapies. *G Ital Dermatol Venereol* 2009;144:673–88.
79. Crawford GH, Pelle MT, James WD. Rosacea: I. Etiology, pathogenesis, and subtype classification. *J Am Acad Dermatol* 2004;51:327–41.
80. Jansen T. Clinical presentations and classification of rosacea. *Ann Dermatol Venereol* 2011;138 (Suppl 2):S138–47.
81. Cribier B. Physiopathology of rosacea. Redness, telangiectasia, and rosacea. *Ann Dermatol Venereol* 2011;138(2):S129–37.
82. McAleer MA, Lacey N, Powelll FC. The pathophysiology of rosacea. *G Ital Dermatol Venereol* 2009;144:663–71.
83. Forton FM. Papulopustular rosacea, skin immunity and Demodex: Pityriasis folliculorum as a missing link. *J Eur Acad Dermatol Venereol.* Epub 2011 Oct 24.
84. Schwab VD, Sulk M, Seelinger S, Nowak P, Aubert J, Mess C, et al. Neurovascular and neuroimmune aspects in the pathophysiology of rosacea. *J Investig Dermatol Symp Proc* 2011;15:53–62.
85. Yamasaki K, Gallo RL. Rosacea as a disease of cathelicidins and skin innate immunity. *J Investig Dermatol Symp Proc* 2011;15:12–5.
86. Steinhoff M, Buddenkotte J, Aubert J, Sulk M, Novak P, Schwab VD, et al. Clinical, cellular, and molecular aspects in the pathophysiology of rosacea. *J Investig Dermatol Symp Proc* 2011;15:2–11.

87. Bhat YJ, Manzoor S, Qayoom S. Steroid-induced rosacea: A clinical study of 200 patients. *Indian J Dermatol* 2011;56:30–2.
88. Gerber PA, Buhren BA, Steinhoff M, Horney B. Rosacea: The cytokine and chemokine network. *J Investig Dermatol Symp Proc* 2011;15:40–7.
89. Pfeffer I, Borelli C, Zierhut M, Schaller M. Treatment of ocular rosacea witih 40 mg doxycycline in a slow release form. *J Dtsch Dermatol Ges* 2011;9:904–7.
90. Del Rosso JQ, Bhatia N. Azelaic acid gel 15% in the management of papulopustular rosacea: A status report on available efficacy data and clinical application. *Cutis* 2011;88:67–72.
91. Kim MB, Kim GW, Park HJ, Chin HW, Kim SH, Kim BS, Ko HC. Pimecrolimus 1% cream for the treatment of rosacea. *J Dermatol.* Epub 2011 Sept 28.
92. Fowler J, Jarratt M, Moore A, Meadows K, Pollack, A, Steinhoff H, et al. Once-daily topical brimonidine tartrate gel 0.5% is a novel treatment of moderate to severe facial erythema of rosacea: Results of two multicenter, randomized and vehicle-controlled studies. *Br J Dermatol* 2012;166(3):633–641.
93. Jackson JM, Pelle M. Topical rosacea therapy: The importance of vehicles for efficacy, tolerability and compliance. *J Drugs Dermatol* 2011;10:627–33.
94. Levin J, Miller R. A guide for the ingredients and potential benefits of over-the-counter cleansers and moisturizers for rosacea patients. *J Clin Aesthet Dermatol* 2011;4:31–49.
95. Guerrero D. Dermocosmetic management of the red face and rosacea. *Ann Dermatol Venereol* 2011;138(Suppl 2):S163–6.
96. Park H, Del Rosso JQ. Use of oral isotretinoin in the management of rosacea. *J Clin Aesthet Dermatol* 2011;4:54–61.
97. Dahan S. Laser and intense pulsed light management of couperose and rosacea. *Ann Dermatol Venereol* 2011;138(Suppl 2):S167–70.
98. Sadick H, Riedel F, Bran G. Rhinophyma in rosacea: What does surgery achieve? *Hautarzt* 2011;62:834–41.
99. Iqbal M, Kolodney MS. Acne fulminans with synovitis-acne-pustulosis-hyperostosis-osteitis (SAPHO) syndrome treated with infliximab. *J Am Acad Dermatol* 2005;52(5 Suppl 1):S118–20.
100. DeSouza A, Solomon GE, Strober BE. SAPHO syndrome associated with hidradenitis suppurativa successfully treated with infiximab and methotrexate. *Bull NYU Hosp Jt Dis* 2011;69:185–7.
101. Azevedo VF, Dal Pizzol V, Lopes H, Coelho SP, Czeczko LE. Methotrexate to treat SAPHO syndrome with keloidal scars. *Acta Rheumatol Port* 2011;36:167–70.

Mohammad Jafferany

8 Psychogenic purpura (Gardner-Diamond syndrome)

Psychogenic purpura is a very rare syndrome noted typically in adult women with psychiatric comorbidity. It is also called autoerythrocyte sensitization syndrome or Gardner-Diamond syndrome. This condition is considered as an autoimmune vasculopathy that presents with spontaneous development of painful edematous skin lesions (isolated or multiple) that progress within 24 hours to eccymotic lesions. This syndrome typically occurs after severe stress, emotional trauma, or comorbidity with psychiatric disorders. Management includes psychotherapy and psychopharmacology for associated psychiatric disorders.

8.1 Introduction

Autoerythrocyte sensitization syndrome or Gardner-Diamond syndrome is an extremely rare syndrome noted typically in adult women with psychiatric comorbidity. It is regarded as an autoimmune vasculopathy with sensitization to phosphatidylserine, a component of erythrocyte stroma (1). It manifests by usually spontaneous development of painful edematous skin lesions, which could be isolated or multiple, progressing to ecchymoses in the following 24 hours. Autoerythrocyte sensitization syndrome usually develops after severe stress, emotional trauma, or comorbidity with certain psychiatric psychopathology. It most commonly occurs in adult women, but cases in men and adolescents have also been described (2,3).

8.2 History

The history of psychogenic purpura dates back to the early twentieth century. In 1927 the German psychiatrist Schindler described 16 patients with skin hemorrhages and suggested a possible link to hypnosis in causing or relieving these lesions (4). Later in 1928, another two cases were described with hysterical personality and delusions respectively, thus connecting these skin lesions with psychopathology. In 1955, Gardner and Diamond described in detail the cases of four women manifesting abnormal responses to bruises (4). These lesions were characterized by the development of areas of painful ecchymoses at the site of trauma followed by progressive erythema and edema. They suggested for the first time that this disorder was associated with autosensitization of patients to their own blood. They systematized the data, which was formally presented as the Gardner-Diamond syndrome. Since then about

200 cases of this syndrome have been reported in the literature. The term psychogenic purpura was coined by Ratnoff in 1989, who reported a series of 71 cases with autoerythrocyte sensitization syndrome (5).

8.3 Etiology and pathogenesis

The pathophysiology of Gardner-Diamond syndrome is poorly understood. Stress, hormonal changes, and local autoimmune reactions to patients' own erythrocytes are regarded as the main etiologic factors. Emotional stress can increase the hypothalamic-pituitary-adrenal axis and alters hemostatic mechanisms (6). Gardner and Diamond originally attributed the pathophysiology to autosensitization of erythrocytes, and they concluded that the causative agent resided in erythrocyte stroma. Later on it was confirmed by Groch et al that autosensitization to phosphatidylserine (phosphoglyceride of red blood cell membrane) is of pivotal importance in the pathogenesis of this syndrome (1).

Indirect immunoflourescence studies have suggested that 50% of enthrocyte phosphatidylserine of patients with Gardner-Diamond syndrome was found on the outer surface of the cell membrane (7,8). This finding was reproduced in an experiment after incubation of homologous erythrocytes from a healthy donor with an affected individual's plasma, which was found to contain specific IgE antibodies to cardiolipin and phosphatidylserine (9). Some authors have suggested an association with thrombocytosis, defective thrombocyte aggregation, increases in activated partial thromboplastin time, idiopathic thrombocytopenic purpura, and circulating fibrinolytic factors (10). There are several other mechanisms that have been suggested, including disturbances in the tone regulation of venous capillaries due to fluctuation in the kallikrein-kinin system and a disturbance of fibrin synthesis in the endothelium and formation of defective structures of capillary walls (11). Gardner-Diamond syndrome lesions have been noted as a reaction to stress in only 40–60% of cases, thus favoring the notion that other factors may also play a role in the production of these lesions (12).

It may be noted that the coagulation system or abnormalities in blood vessel development are not usually involved with the pathogenesis of Gardner-Diamond syndrome. However, some authors have suggested the presence of abnormal platelet responses during platelet aggravation studies (13). In addition, a number of immunological abnormalities have also been reported in patients with Gardner-Diamond syndrome, including positive anticardiolipin antibodies (14), decreased serum complement levels during the time of ecchymoses that return to normal when the lesions heal, vasculitis, angioimmunoblastic lymphadenopathy, lymphoid interstitial pneumonia, and association with multiple glomus tumors (15,16,17,18). Autoerythrocyte sensitization syndrome may also present as a primary manifestation of systemic lupus erythematosus (19).

8.4 Clinical features

There is always a prodromal phase characterized by malaise and fatigue. Initially, skin lesions are preceded by burning and itching or a stinging sensation or pain, followed by cutaneous indurations a few hours later. Later painful, edematous, pink or red plaques of variable sizes become visible. After a day or two these lesions may evolve into bluish ecchymoses with a yellowish shade. The lesions may become less tender as they regress and disappear completely in about a week. Extremities and trunk are common sites, but lesions may appear anywhere on the body. The lesions may be associated with fever, arthralgia, myalgia, headache, and dizziness.

Some patients report different gastrointestinal symptoms, such as epigastria pain, hemorrhages, nausea, vomiting, and diarrhea (17). Hematuria, epistaxis, and menorrhagia are also described in association with the Gardner-Diamond syndrome (20). Hormonal influences such as fluctuations in estrogen have also been reported (21). Some authors have suggested the development of lesions after intramuscular stimulation and stress (22). Lesions resembling child abuse lesions in children have been reported in a case report; the lesions had the form of intradermal hematomas, which turned out to be reddish, partly patterned, partly striped, and consisting of confluent punctate hemorrhages (23).

8.5 Differential diagnosis

Gardner-Diamond syndrome may be confused with several disorders, including disseminated intravascular coagulation, idiopathic thrombocytopenic purpura, Henoch-Schönlein purpura, Ehlers-Danlos syndrome, dermatitis artefacta, systemic lupus erythematosus, cellulitis, Munchausen's syndrome, compartment syndrome, Weber-Christian panniculitis, and polyarteritis nodosa.

8.5.1 Disease course

Overall prognosis is good, though in many patients relapses and remissions are common occurrences and may last for many years. The severity of the lesions may considerably fluctuate. The relief of acute stress and psychological factors are crucial in developing longer remissions.

8.5.2 Histopathology

Biopsies have revealed extravascular erythrocytes in the dermis as well as edema and non-specific lymphohistiocytic infiltration around the blood vessels. Macrophages may show pigment deposition.

8.5.3 Laboratory testing

There are no specific laboratory changes observed in the Gardner-Diamond syndrome. All hematological parameters are within normal limits, including hemoglobin, hematocrit, platelets, peripheral smear, erythrocyte sedimentation rate, electrolytes, prothrombin, thrombin, partial thromboplastin time, bleeding time, and coagulation factors. The reliable diagnostic test is intradermal injection of the patient's own washed erythrocytes, washed autologous lymphocytes, or heterologous and autologous DNA (24). Although Gardner and Diamond obtained a positive result in all four of their patients, Ratnoff called the response "erratic," noting positive findings only in 59%, and suggesting that a negative test result does not rule out the diagnosis (5).

8.5.4 Psychological disturbances

Association of psychological factors with the Gardner-Diamond syndrome is the mainstay for this diagnosis, and their presence is one of the essential diagnostic components of the syndrome. The first documented relationship between Gardner-Diamond syndrome and psychiatric symptoms was published by Agle and Ratnoff (25). Various psychopathologies were associated with this syndrome, including depression, anxiety, difficulty in addressing aggression and hostility, emotional instability, adjustment issues, hypochondriasis, abnormal guilt, sexual problems, masochism, histrionic as well as borderline personality disorders, conversion disorder, and obsessive disorder (20,25,26). Some studies, however, have suggested no apparent predisposing emotional distress, mental illnesses, or traumatic events (27).

A careful psychiatric history is often missed and not elicited until all medical tests, examinations, and treatments have been exhausted. This becomes the source of frustration on part of the treating provider, patient, and family alike. Also, frank discussion regarding the psychological nature of this disease further complicates the situation and increases the level of patient frustration and the family's denial. Communication issues develop and physician–patient rapport is severely affected. In many cases it is very hard on the part of the patient and family to accept the psychological nature of this disorder. In these circumstances it is advisable to avoid the term psychogenic purpura due to its stigmatization or autoerythrocyte sensitization syndrome due to the suggestion that it is an organic disorder (28).

8.6 Treatment approaches and recommendations

There is no specific treatment for the Gardner-Diamond syndrome. Several treatment approaches have been tried with variable success; these include antihistamines, corticosteroids, antidepressants, hormones, and vitamins. Psychotropic medications are used to treat comorbid psychiatric pathology such as depression or mood symptoms. Selective serotonin reuptake inhibitors (SSRIs) have been helpful in such cases (29). Some authors have suggested the role of medications affecting capillary tone or permeability of vessels in the treatment of Gardner-Diamond syndrome (30). Psychotherapy, both individual and family oriented psychodynamic psychotherapy, has been used in many cases with positive results in reducing the stress associated with production of these lesions (31,32).

8.7 Conclusion

Autoerythrocyte sensitization syndrome or Gardner-Diamond syndrome is a very rare syndrome noted typically in adult women with psychiatric comorbidity. It is also called psychogenic purpura and typically considered as an autoimmune vasculopathy that presents with spontaneous development of painful edematous skin lesions (isolated or multiple) that progress within 24 hours to eccymotic lesions. This syndrome typically occurs after severe stress, emotional trauma, or comorbidity with psychiatric disorders. Management includes psychotherapy and psychopharmacology for associated psychiatric disorders.

References

1. Grotch GS, Finch SC, Rogoway W, et al. Studies in the pathogenesis autoerythrocyte sensitization syndrome. *Blood* 1966;28:19–33.
2. Shustik C. Gardner-Diamond syndrome in a man. *Arch Intern Med* 1977;137:1621–2.
3. Kurczynski EM, Cassidy JT, Heyn RM. Autoerythrocyte sensitization in a young boy. *Lancet* 1973;1:424–5.
4. Gardner FH, Diamond LK. Autoerythrocyte sensitization: A form of purpura producing painful bruising following autosensitization to red blood cells in certain women. *Blood* 1955;10(7): 675–90.
5. Ratfnoff OD. Psychogenic purpura (autoerythrocyte sensitization): An unsolved dilemma. *Am J Med* 1989;87:16–21.
6. Panconesi E, Hautmann G. Stress, stigmatization and psychosomatic purpura. *Int Angiol* 1995;14(2):130–7.
7. Campbell AN, Freedman M, McClure PD. Autoerythrocyte sensitization. *J Pediatr* 1983;103: 157–60.
8. Kossard S, McGrath M, Finley G. Localized recurrent painful bruises. Gardner-Diamond syndrome of autoerythrocyte sensitization, psychogenic purpura. *Australas J Dermatol* 1993; 34: 37–8.
9. Silny W, Marciniak A, Czarnecka-Operaze M, et al. Gardner-Diamond Syndrome. *Int J Dermatol* 2010;US:1178–81.
10. Fey MF, Beck EA. Psychogenic purpura, idiopathic thrombocytopenic purpura and platelet dysfunction in the same patient. *J Clin Psychiatry* 1986;47:386–7.
11. Marlen JF. Echymotic patches of the fingers and Gardner-Diamond vascular purpura. *Phlebologie* 1987;40:473–87.

12. Ivanov OL, Lvov AN, Michenko AV, et al. Autoerythrocyte sensitization syndrome (Gardner Diamond Syndrome): Review of the literature. *J Eur Acad Dermatol Venereol* 2009; 23(5):499–504.
13. Puetz J, Fete T. Platelet function disorder in Gardner-Diamond syndrome: A case report and review of the literature. *J Pediatr Hematol Oncol* 2005;27(6):323–5.
14. Sudy E, Urbina F, Vasquez P. Autoerythrhrocyte sensitization syndrome with positive anticardiolipinantibodies. *Br J Dermatol* 1998;138:367–8.
15. Krain LS, Levin JM, Schultz B. Decreased serum compliment in the Gardner-Diamond syndrome: Immunoflouroscent findings and association with angioimmunoblastic lymphadenopathy. *Cutis* 1978;21:80–4.
16. Kennedy C, Sanderson KV, Spry C. Painful bruising syndrome with vasculitis treated by plasmapheresis. *Br J Dermatol* 1976;95(suppl 14):65–6.
17. DeCoteau WE, Tourville D, Ambrus JL, et al. Lymphoid interstitial pneumonia and autoerythrocyte sensitization syndrome. A case with deposition of immunoglobulin on the alveolar basement membrane. *Arch Int Med* 1974;134:519–22.
18. Pearson B, Mazza JJ. Gardner-Diamond syndrome with multiple glomus tumors. *Arch Dermatol* 1975;111:893–5.
19. Scott JP, Schiff DW, Githens JH. The autoerythrocyte sensitization syndrome as the primary manifestation of systemic lupus erythematosus. *J Pediatr* 1981;99:598–600.
20. Ratnoff OD. The psychogenic purpura: A review of autoerythrocyte sensitization, autosensitization to DNA, hysterical and factitial bleeding and the religious stigmata. *Semin Hematol* 1980;17:192–213.
21. Durmazlar SP, Atacan D, Cemil B, Eskioglu F. Is Gardner-Diamond Syndrome associated with hormonal influences along with psychosocial problems? A delayed diagnosis. *Eur J Dermatol* 2009;19(3):259–60.
22. Baek JO, Jee HJ, Kim TK. Case of Gardner Diamond Syndrome after intramuscular stimulation. *Dermatol* 2011;38(12):1197–9.
23. Hagemeir L, Schyma C, Zillhardt H. Gardner-Diamond Syndrome: A rare differential diagnosis of child abuse. *Br J Dermatol* 2011;164(3):672–3.
24. Spiera H., Schwartz AL. Autoerythrocyte sensitization reproducible by both autologous red cells and heterologous DNA. *Mt Sinai J Med* 1970;37:108–11.
25. Agle DP, Ratnoff OD. Purpura as a psychosomatic entity. A psychiatric study of autoerythrocyte sensitization. *Arch Intern Med* 1962;109:685–94.
26. Hallstrom T, Hersle K, Mobacken H. Mental symptoms and personality structure in autoerythrocyte sensitization syndrome. *Br J Psychiatry* 1969;115:1269–76.
27. Sudy E, Urbina F, Vasquez P. Autoerythrocyte sensitization syndrome with positive anticardiolipin antibodies. *Br J Dermatol* 1998;138:367–8.
28. Meeder R, Bannister S. Gardner-Diamond syndrome: Difficulties in the management of patients with unexplained medical symptoms. *Paediatr Child Health* 2006;11(7):416–19.
29. Settle EC. Autoerythrocyte sensitization successfully treated with antidepressants. *IAMA* 1983;250–1749.
30. Merlen JF. Ecchymotic patches of the fingers and Gardner-Diamond vascular purpura. *Phlebologie* 1987;40:473–87.
31. Lozano M, Avila JJ, Denia M, et al. Analysis of the family structure in a case of psychogenic purpura. *Gen Hosp Psychiatry* 1986;8:205–11.
32. Lindahl MW. Psychogenic purpura: Report of a case. *Psychosom Med* 1977;39:358–68.

Part III: PSYCHIATRIC DISORDERS WITH DERMATOLOGIC MANIFESTATIONS

Lucia Tomas-Aragones and Servando E. Marron

9 Body dysmorphic disorder in adolescents

Body dysmorphic disorder (BDD) in adolescents is a mental health disorder that is difficult to diagnose, causes much suffering as well as distress, and is a challenge to treat. These adolescents and adults alike take years before looking for help, and they often seek treatment for comorbid symptoms of depression, anxiety, or social phobia. Others go to dermatologists or plastic surgery surgeons to find a solution to their imagined or perceived defect in their appearance. Suicidal ideation and suicide attempts are frequent in individuals with BDD. Effective psychological and psychopharmacological treatments are now available, and although further study is needed to discover its etiology, probably the most pressing issue is to get health professionals who attend adolescents to ask specific questions about satisfaction with appearance in order to diagnose BDD at an early stage. Adolescents with BDD are high-risk patients, and early detection is very important.

9.1 Introduction

This chapter describes body dysmorphic disorder (BDD) in adolescents. In order to fully understand this condition, it is necessary to take into account theories of human development and psychological change. Adolescents usually become self-conscious – and sometimes anxious – about their physical changes. They often spend large amounts of time grooming themselves and worrying about how they look. They have a need to be accepted and liked; thus, it is quite normal for them to seek recognition from their peers (1).

According to Eric Erikson, the quest for identity is the principal developmental task confronting every individual throughout the lifespan – a quest that assumes a different form at each of the various developmental stages the individual passes through (2). Erikson believed that adolescence presents the most severe challenge to young people in their attempt to establish an individual identity. It is then that they are likely to experience an identity crisis that represents a period of confusion and low self-esteem.

It is a crisis because the post-puberty individual is simultaneously confronted by a changed body image, by the new pressures of sexuality, and by the need to make crucial choices, all giving rise to considerable emotional upheaval and making this a time of conflict and uncertainly (3). It is usually during adolescence that an inner image of oneself is formed, and this is sometimes very different to how others perceive them. This is especially true in BDD where most individuals have a normal appearance to others, yet their perception is totally different.

Body image affects our emotions, thoughts, and behaviors in everyday life. But, above all, body image influences our relationships. Furthermore, body image has the potential to dramatically influence our quality of life (see Chapter 4). Youngsters with BDD are at risk of being socially isolated or even housebound, and they also run more risk for suicide ideation. Therefore, we would like to stress the importance of identifying the suffering in adolescents who develop this disorder in order to be able to provide effective mental health support.

9.2 Definition

Body dysmorphic disorder is characterized by excessive concern and preoccupation with an imagined or a slight defect in bodily appearance that is not better accounted for by another mental disorder. The preoccupation has to cause clinically significant distress or functional impairment to satisfy the diagnostic criteria in the American Psychiatric Association's (APA) *Diagnostic and Statistical Manual for Mental Disorders* (DSM-IV) (4). See Table 9.1.

Body dysmorphic disorder (BDD) usually implies dissatisfaction with one's self. Asymmetry or lack of proportion can also be a concern. The repetitive thoughts in this disorder may resemble obsessions, and the person usually engages in extensive visual checking behavior. It is a chronic and distressing disorder that can lead to severe impairment in social, academic, and family functioning (5). Despite the repetitive thoughts and checking, BBD is different from obsessive compulsive disorder (OCD), being classified as a somatoform disorder in the DSM-VI and not as an anxiety disorder.

The main symptoms are the preoccupation with the perceived defect and the actions taken to reduce accompanying feelings of distress. Age of onset is usually during adolescence and the symptoms may appear either in a gradual or in an abrupt manner. BDD is a secretive and under diagnosed disorder that goes unidentified unless specific questions about satisfaction with appearance are asked. It is frequently accompanied by suicidal ideation or even suicide attempts. Individuals with BDD are high-risk patients, and early detection is very important.

Table 9.1: DSM-IV diagnostic criteria for BDD

The diagnostic criteria for BDD, according to DSM-IV (4), is:
A. Preoccupation with an imagined defect in appearance. If a slight physical anomaly is present, the person's concern is markedly excessive.
B. The preoccupation causes clinically significant distress or impairment in social, occupational, or other important areas of functioning.
C. The preoccupation is not better accounted for by another mental disorder (e.g., dissatisfaction with body shape and size in Anorexia Nervosa).

9.2.1 Epidemiology

Body dysmorphic disorder (BDD) is relatively common in both nonclinical and clinical settings, but it is often under diagnosed. This is due to the fact that many of these patients are too ashamed to talk about their symptoms. Thus, unless BDD is specifically asked about, it is easy to miss. For example, the prevalence of BDD is substantial in patients seeking surgical or dermatological interventions (6).

Studies indicate that the prevalence of BDD is between 0.7% and 1.1% in community samples, 2–13% in nonclinical student samples, and up to 13% in psychiatric inpatient settings. These figures, bearing in mind that BDD is a mental disorder, are even larger in dermatological clinics (9–12%) and in patients seeking cosmetic surgery (6–15%) (7). In a 2006 study conducted by W. Rief et al, the prevalence rate in the general population in Germany was 1.7%. The authors found slightly higher prevalence rates for women (1.4% for men versus 1.9% for women), although these differences were not significant. The base rate of BDD showed a trend to higher prevalence rates in adolescents (age <21 years; 2.3%) (8).

9.2.2 Clinical features

BDD usually begins during early adolescence, and it is typically a chronic disorder. Major depression is the most common comorbid disorder to BDD, while other comorbid conditions include substance use disorders, social phobia, obsessive compulsive disorders, and personality disorders (9).

Individuals with BDD worry about how they look and feel unattractive or even hideous. Most concerns are focused on the face or head but can include any body area or even the entire body. The appearance-related worry is difficult to control, and people with this disorder spend many hours a day worrying, mirror checking, and trying to hide the perceived defect or flaw. Most perform repetitive, compulsive behaviors aimed at examining, improving, or hiding the imagined or perceived defect. They also perform mirror checking, camouflaging, comparing with others, reassurance seeking, and skin-picking, among others (10).

Phillips KA et al conducted a study to describe BDD's clinical features in middle and late adolescence as well as to compare the clinical features of adults and adolescents with this disorder (11). Adolescents and adults did not differ significantly on most characteristics of BDD, and these researchers found that adolescents had similar lifetime rates of functional impairment and comorbidity, despite their younger age. However, adolescents had poorer insight and a higher rate of suicide attempts. The poorer insight probably reflects a lack of full development of cognitive skills (11).

Body dysmorphic disorder is characterized by poor insight, marked functional impairment, and high rates of suicidal ideation as well as suicide attempts. It is also thought that patients with this disorder are more aesthetically sensitive than the rest of the population (8). Although the onset of BDD is usually during adolescence, patients are usually diagnosed after many years of suffering. This is due to the fact that BDD usually goes unidentified, and many youngsters seek nonpsychiatric medical treatment, primarily from dermatologists and surgeons (12).

The “imagined ugliness” can lead adolescents with BDD to isolate themselves and therefore be deprived of social activities, which are so important during this developmental stage. In many cases, BDD causes impaired education, occupational, and social functioning. These patients suffer high levels of perceived stress and poor quality of life and self-esteem. Many adolescents with BDD also have ideas of delusions of reference and think that other people take special notice of the supposed defect and perhaps talk about it or mock them (13).

Youngsters with acne represent a danger group and should be screened for possible BDD by the dermatologist (see Chapter 7). It is important to remember that patients with BDD often go to the dermatologist. Skin picking is also a BDD symptom that is of particular relevance to dermatologists (see Chapter 11). However, the clinician must bear in mind that BDD patients generally feel misunderstood and are secretive about their symptoms because they think they will be viewed as being vain or narcissistic (12). Clinicians should ask appearance-specific questions in order to identify adolescents with BDD to offer them information about their condition and possible treatment options. The questions in Table 9.2 offer a guide on how to address the subject.

Finally, as with many other disorders, biological, psychological, and sociocultural factors probably play an important role in the etiopathogenesis of BDD. Its precise etiology remains unclear. The literature contains sparse references to biological correlates of BDD, and most studies are small and provide inconsistent findings (13).

9.2.3 Differential diagnosis

According to DSM-IV criteria, BDD diagnosis should not be made if the preoccupation is better accounted for by another mental disorder, such as anorexia nervosa, gender identity disorder, major depressive episode, avoidant personality disorder,

Table 9.2: Questions to help diagnose body dysmorphic disorder

Some people worry a lot about their appearance. Do you worry a lot about the way you look and wish you could think about it less?
What specific concerns do you have about your appearance? Do you think about them a lot and is it hard to stop thinking about them?
On a typical day, how many hours a day is your appearance on your mind? (More than 1 hour is considered excessive)
What effect does it have on your life?
Does it make it hard to go to school/college/work, or be with friends?

social phobia, or OCD. An additional diagnosis of delusional disorder, somatic type may be given if the preoccupation with the imagined defect in appearance is held with a delusional intensity (4). Other differential diagnoses to be considered and excluded before a definite diagnosis of BDD is made include psychotic disorders, adjustment disorders, hypochondriasis, psychogenic excoriation, and trichotillomania (see Chapter 12). Organic pathology as well as alcohol and substance misuse must also not be forgotten (13).

Misuse of alcohol and illegal substances are frequent in people suffering from BDD as it helps them cope with the associated distress and preoccupation. This can be an added problem in adolescence as a pattern of misuse can lead to more serious problems. A common diagnostic dilemma is with eating disorders because both disorders share a distorted body image and low self-esteem. Nevertheless, if the preoccupation is predominantly focused on being overweight, it does not meet criteria for BDD. Clinicians should also remember that patients with BDD usually seek help for other comorbid conditions, such as depression, social phobia, or OCD. Thus, it is important to screen for BDD symptoms in these already noted comorbid disorders.

9.3 Management

9.3.1 Preliminary considerations

There is a low level of awareness about BDD among health care professionals, and BDD is, thus, often overlooked. Direct questioning about appearance satisfaction is needed for the diagnosis as people with BDD are often too ashamed to reveal the true nature of their problem. When individuals with body dysmorphic disorder seek help, they either consult a dermatologist or cosmetic surgeon, or if they visit a doctor or mental health care professional, they usually present with other symptoms, such as depression or social phobia (14).

Many people with BDD have difficulty accepting a psychological or pharmacological intervention. Some prefer to either avoid or camouflage their appearance, and alternatively, they seek a cosmetic or dermatological procedure. On the other hand, too few mental health professionals have clinical experience in treating many patients with BDD. According to the National Clinical Practice Guideline on core interventions in the treatment of OCD and BDD, there is virtually no evidence based data for the treatment of BDD among children and adolescents (14). This guideline also recommends a stepped-care approach, meaning that the least intrusive intervention, such as education or self-help, should be used first. We should only move to more intense therapy when less intensive treatment has proved to be insufficiently effective (14).

We need to bear in mind that people with BDD are often ashamed and embarrassed by their condition and may find it very difficult to discuss their symptoms.

This is due to the fact that their condition often affects some of the most intimate aspects of a person's life. Therefore, health care professionals should be especially sensitive when exploring the hidden distress and disability commonly associated with this disorder. When treating adolescents with BDD, it is particularly important to develop and maintain a good therapeutic alliance with the patient as well as with the family, and if the symptoms of the disorder interfere with academic performance, it may be appropriate to liaise with the involved school professionals.

9.3.2 The clinical interview

Before the interview with the adolescent and the parents, it is useful to clarify the nature of the problem that has prompted the interview. It is important to ascertain who or what has prompted the need for the interview, and contact with the referral source can help the health professional sort out issues that need to be addressed during the interview.

If the adolescent comes accompanied by the family, it is good practice to begin the interview with all present, unless the patient wishes the contrary and the family agrees. A lot will depend on the age of the young patient (15). When working with adolescents in general, it is important to ask how they feel about their body and themselves in general. Two simple questions asked during the clinical interview can screen possible difficulties with body image and can give a lot of valuable information to work further:

1. On a scale of 1 to 10, how would you rate yourself regarding satisfaction with your appearance?
2. On a scale of 1 to 10, how would you rate yourself globally, regarding how you feel about yourself in general?

Depending on the answers given, we can continue prompting: What don't you like about your appearance/yourself? How do you think others feel about you? In what way would you like to change? Table 9.3 illustrates further issues to ask about and discuss during the interview.

It is important NOT to tell the adolescent with BDD that he/she has an "imagined defect" as the defect is very real to the person who suffers this disorder. Full information about the nature of BDD and treatment options should be discussed. Have information and resources ready to offer during the session. Information about support groups and suitable websites should also be available.

9.3.3 Assessment

Cognitive behavioral therapy (CBT) for adolescent BDD should begin with a good assessment. The therapist needs to evaluate the adolescent's concerns within a greater

Table 9.3: Issues to ask about and discuss during the interview

What don't you like about your appearance?
When did the preoccupation about the "defect" in appearance begin?
How does this preoccupation affect your life?
When you see photos where you appear, how do you see yourself?
At what age did you like the way you looked?
Try to remember things about your life at the time you became aware of your problem.
Did anyone tease you about your problem? Does anyone tease you now?
Have you shared your concern about your appearance with anyone?
Is your family aware of how this problem is affecting you?
What thoughts are associated with your problem?
Do you mirror check? How often?
Do you try in any way to camouflage or disguise your problem?
Tell me about your daily activities. What do you do during a normal day?
What type of social activities are you involved in?
Do you have a friend/friends?
How do you imagine your life without your problem?
Are there any positive aspects in your life? Tell me about them.

context, assessing for potential interference in daily life. It is also important to obtain information about the young person's strengths and interests. The evaluation should result in a list of goals for treatment (16).

While structured interviews are still considered to be the gold standard of classification for mental health problems, we must remember that patients with BDD tend to be very ashamed of their symptoms and thus are rather secretive. Therefore, in the case of BDD, it is possible that some individuals might be more comfortable acknowledging their symptoms in self-rating scales than in a personal interview. Computer-assisted assessment strategies might also be an option. Nevertheless, the question of which methods best classify individuals with BDD needs to be further investigated (8).

There are many rating scales and inventories available to help assess BDD and comorbid disorders. We offer an example of some that have been adapted for adolescents:

The Body Dysmorphic Disorder Diagnostic Module – Adolescent version is a reliable semi-structured diagnostic instrument based on DSM-IV criteria to diagnose BDD (17). *The Schedule for Affective Disorders and Schizophrenia for School-Age children – Present and Lifetime Version (K-SADS-PL)* is a semi-structured, integrated parent–child interview, assessing current and lifetime psychopathology. It includes mood, anxiety, and somatoform disorders and helps to provide diagnosis-specific impairment ratings and to generate a DSM-IV diagnosis (18).

The Yale-Brown Obsessive Compulsive Scale Modified for BDD – Adolescent Version (BDD-YBOCS-A) is a slightly modified version of the BDD-YBOCS, which has been developed for use with children and adolescents. It rates severity of BDD symptoms during the past week (19).
The Beck Depression Inventory (BDI-II) can be used to assess depressive symptoms. It is a 21-item self-report measure used in adolescents and adults (20). For assessing personality, either the *Millon Adolescent Clinical Inventory (MACI)* (21) or the *Adolescent Personality Questionnaire (16PF)* (22) can prove suitable for adolescents.

Also, self-esteem needs to be considered and assessed. Research is still needed on the domains on which individuals with BDD base their self-esteem (e.g. appearance, approval from others, academic competence). Hopefully, future research on self-esteem may also shed some light on the important question of whether poor self-esteem predisposes to BDD and/or is a consequence of the disorder (23). In order to assess self-esteem, *The Rosenberg Self-Esteem Scale (RSE)* is a 10 item self-report scale that is widely used and is suitable for adolescents (24).

Remember that parents of children and adolescents with BDD should be kept informed at every stage of the assessment and treatment.

9.3.4 Patient education

Psychoeducation is about educating people with BDD and their families about the symptoms of the disorder, possible origins of the condition, its evolution over time, and the various treatments available. It also includes education about the symptoms and treatment of any comorbid disorders, such as depression.

Most patients find it very helpful when they are informed about their problem, and some are greatly relieved to know that they are not alone in their suffering and that there are effective treatments available to them. Self-help books like *The Broken Mirror* (10) and *The BDD Workbook* (25) can also prove very useful for patients and families. Self-help and support groups are also possible options and information should be provided.

9.3.5 Treatment

Cognitive behavioral therapy (CBT), including exposure and response prevention (ERP), should be offered as first-line treatment. The treatment should ideally involve the family and be adapted to suit the developmental age of the patient. If the young person or the family decline psychological treatment or are unable to engage in treatment, a selective serotonin reuptake inhibitor (SSRI) should be considered with careful monitoring for adverse events (14).

When teaching ERP, the person is encouraged to confront the feared object, situation, or thought that provokes anxiety (exposure); also, they should be taught to resist engaging in the compulsive or other behavior that would rapidly reduce anxiety (response prevention) until the anxiety gradually reduces of its own accord. Through repeated exposure the person is said to habituate so that the object, situation, or thought no longer provokes anxiety, and the urge to engage in the compulsive behaviors is no longer present. The ERP program is usually conducted in a progressive way, starting with objects, situations, or thoughts that produce relatively low levels of distress. The technique can be used within structured therapy with the therapist present or with instructions from the therapist who is not present. It can also be used with support from a family member or other members of self-help groups, or alone as part of a pure self-help program.

In the treatment of BDD, CBT generally combines elements of behavior therapy, such as ERP, with elements of cognitive therapy, such as techniques to change beliefs about the things that patients find distressing. It usually involves reducing catastrophic thinking, too.

The key components of CBT are engagement and helping patients to develop a good psychological understanding of the factors that maintain BDD. This then leads to behavioral experiments or graded exposure tasks to situations or activities without the safety behaviors. Patients may require imagery rescripting for past traumas and cognitive restructuring for the idealized values they hold about the importance of appearance to the self (26). Although exposure and response prevention – together with cognitive therapy – seem to work best, little is still known about the optimum frequency of therapy sessions, the type or the duration of the therapy, or the rate of relapse in the long term (14).

David Veale et al propose a cognitive behavioral model of BDD that emphasizes factors such as selective attention on a distorted body image and behaviors such as mirror gazing that maintain processing of self as an aesthetic object (27). In a review of cognitive and behavioral treatment for BDD, the authors found no difference between the efficacy of one treatment strategy over another, nor the combination of cognitive and behavior therapy over behavior therapy. They conclude that further research is needed in this area (28).

As for pharmacologic treatment, K. Phillips reviewed the evidence on the efficacy of medication for BDD and concluded that serotonin reuptake inhibitors (SRIs) are often efficacious for this disorder. It also appears that higher SRI doses and longer treatment trials than those used for many other psychiatric disorders are often needed to treat BDD effectively (29).

Cognitive strategies help adolescents to identify and modify negative self-talk that leads to rituals and stops them from engaging in social activities. We need to bear in mind that cognitive distortions associated with BDD are likely to lead to a negative interpretation of social activities. Negative self-talk and predictions lead adolescents with BDD to time-consuming rituals in order to face social situations or to avoid them altogether (16).

Systematic problem solving should also be taught and modeled throughout the treatment as a way to generate and evaluate alternative solutions to a seemingly overwhelming problem. The treatment should also teach adolescents skills to improve social functioning. Systematic social skills training in which the therapist describes, models, and role plays various social skills is also useful (16).

Perceptual and mirror retraining should be used to teach adolescents how to see the "whole picture," enhancing their ability to describe themselves holistically in a neutral and non-judgemental manner (16). Suggestions on mirror use are given in Table 9.4 (30).

Finally, a treatment plan adapted to adolescents should include psychoeducation, motivation enhancement, parent training, cognitive interventions (cognitive restructuring), behavioral interventions (exposure and response prevention), mirror retraining, social skills building, and relapse prevention. It is wise to start with assessment and psychoeducation. Parents should be recommended or provided with reading materials about the disorder.

9.4 Other treatment techniques

9.4.1 Anxiety management training (AMT)

Individuals are taught a set of skills to help them manage their own anxiety and stress. These include:

Table 9.4: Dos and don'ts of mirror use

Use mirrors at a slight distance and use ones that are large enough to show most of the body.
Focus attention on the reflection in the mirror rather than on how you feel.
Use a mirror only for an agreed function (e.g. shaving, putting on make-up) and for a limited period of time.
Use a variety of different mirrors and lights rather sticking to one that you 'trust'.
Focus attention on the whole of your face rather than on selected areas.
Do not use mirrors that magnify.
Do not use ambiguous reflections (e.g. windows, the backs of compact disks or cutlery).
Do not use a mirror when you feel depressed: try to delay essential use until you feel happier or find other things to do until the urge to mirror-gaze has passed.

Taken from: David Veale. Cognitive-behavioural therapy for body dysmorphic disorder. Advances in Psychiatric Treatment (2001), vol 7, pp. 125–132.

1. *Relaxation training*: Consists of relaxing major muscle groups to decrease anxiety.
2. *Breathing retraining*: Slow abdominal breathing is taught and practiced to help avoid hyperventilation and the unpleasant physical sensations that accompany it.
3. *Positive thinking and self-talk*: Patients are asked to think of positive statements, to write them on cards, and to use them when negative thoughts appear during stressful experiences.
4. *Assertiveness training*: Patients are helped to express wishes, opinions, and emotions in a more appropriate way and without alienating others.

9.4.2 Eye movement desensitization and reprocessing (EMDR)

Although this technique was originally developed for the treatment of trauma, it may prove useful for some patients. Individuals are instructed to focus on a trauma-related image and its accompanying feelings, sensations, and thoughts while visually tracking the therapist's fingers as they move back and forth in front of the patient's eyes. After each set of approximately 20 eye movements, patients are instructed to let go of the memory and to discuss their reactions. This process is repeated, and includes focusing on different memories that come up in connection with the trauma. Once distress is reduced, patients are instructed to focus on the target image while rehearsing a positive thought connected to the image.

9.4.3 Family therapy

When a member of the family has a problem that is persistent, it can often dominate family life and impact significantly on family function, interaction, and communication. The aim of family therapy is to help family members recognize and understand how they function as a family and in particular how their patterns of interaction may have become organized around the symptoms or problems of one of their members. The family is helped to develop more functional patterns of organizing and interacting within the family.

9.4.4 Group therapy

In a group setting, patients are encouraged to understand their own and one another's difficulties with the goal of making changes. There are many different modalities of group therapy.

9.4.5 Metaphors

The use of metaphors for presenting information about BDD and treatment rationale and structure can be very illustrative as well as helpful in some patients.

9.4.6 Mindfulness

This is a meditation-based approach to treatment that has been developed in particular for relapse prevention. Mindfulness has been defined as "paying attention in a particular way: on purpose, in the present moment and non-judgementally." Mindfulness-based cognitive therapy aims to help patients make a shift in their relationship to thoughts, feelings, and sensations, learning to perceive them as "events in the mind" rather than as "self" or necessarily true.

Mirror retraining

This technique uses elements of mindfulness to help adolescents view and describe themselves in a neutral non-judgemental way, accepting what is there without trying to change it. Harth et al refer to other psychotherapy procedures in their book. Although they are not BDD specific, they provide a variety of treatment options for patients, some of these being Gestalt therapy, creative therapy, virtual reality therapy, hypnosis, neurolinguistic programming, transactional analysis, among others (31).

9.4.7 Intervention

We must bear in mind that poor insight, psychosocial impairment, and depression or suicide ideation can thwart motivation. Moreover, because adolescents do not usually present for treatment by choice, therapists need to find ways to make the treatment beneficial and even enjoyable. Finally, parents and adolescents should work together to set clear expectations for treatment attendance and practice assignments (16).

Self-esteem is a personal resource as well as a personality dimension that is affected by a person's interpretation of their world and the way they believe themselves to be perceived by others. Self-esteem is therefore closely associated with body image and should be worked on. Youngsters need to be helped to find and use their strengths so that they may cope more effectively with their lives. Effective therapy should result in improvement in mood, self-esteem, and overall quality of life (see Chapter 4). It is also likely that symptom improvement will facilitate improvements in self-esteem by enhancing adolescents' sense of self-efficacy (16).

9.4.8 Nonpsychiatric medical treatment

As mentioned earlier, many people with BDD seek non-psychiatric medical and surgical treatment to improve perceived defects in their physical appearance. Dermatological treatment is most frequently sought and received, followed by surgery. Such treatment rarely improves BDD, and thus, non-psychiatric medical treatments do not appear effective in its treatment (32).

However, dermatologists see young patients with BDD who would otherwise go untreated. They therefore play an important role in identifying, offering information, and being empathetic with these young patients. It is important to establish a relationship of trust before trying to refer these patients to a mental health specialist. If the patient refuses a referral, the dermatologist should continue giving appointments and provide the necessary support.

9.4.9 Final management considerations

When working with young people it is especially important to develop and maintain a good therapeutic alliance with both the patient and the family. Maintain optimism, enhance motivation, and reinforce desired behavior changes. Mental health professionals should work with cosmetic surgeons and dermatologists to ensure that young people are screened for BDD symptoms and referred to specialists for treatment. The risk of self-harm and suicide should be assessed in patients with BDD. All health care professionals offering psychological treatment to people of all ages with BDD should receive appropriate training in the interventions they are offering and receive clinical supervision.

9.5 Conclusions

BDD is a distressing and disabling disorder that is challenging to diagnose and to treat. Because BDD usually begins during early adolescence, it is particularly important to recognize its symptoms in this age group (33). Health care providers should screen for BDD symptoms more frequently, and treatment should be provided more systematically. The treatments should be offered more widely, and their availability should be brought to the attention of the general public (8).

A multimodal treatment approach is recommended, consisting of pharmacological and psychological treatment. It is advisable to engage family members in therapy and to intensify the sessions at the beginning of the psychological treatment as it seems to be more effective than weekly sessions. Adolescents are faced with developmental challenges such as pubertal development, emerging sexuality, and identity formation, to name just a few. The relationship between these development processes and BDD requires further study.

References

1. Meggitt C. Child development: An illustrated guide. Essex: Heinemann, 2006.
2. Erikson E. Identity: Youth and crisis. New York. Norton, 1968.
3. Schaffer HR. Key concepts in developmental psychology. London: Sage, 2006.

4. American Psychiatric Association. Diagnostic and Statistical manual of mental disorders, 4th edn. Washington, DC: Author, 1994.
5. Rachman S, De Silva, P. Obsessive-compulsive disorder, 4th edn. Oxford: Oxford University Press, 2009.
6. Phillips KA, Didie ER, Feusner J, Wilheim S. Body dysmorphic disorder: Treating an underrecognized disorder. Am J Psychiatry 2008;165:1111–8.
7. Phillips KA. Body dysmorphic disorder, in somatoform and factitious disorders. Washington, DC: American Psychiatric Publishing, 2001:67–94.
8. Rief W, Buhlmann U, Wilhelm S, Borkenhagen A, Brähler E. The prevalence of body dysmorphic disorder: A population-based survey. Psychol Med 2006;36:877–85.
9. Phillips KA. Body dysmorphic disorder: Recognizing and treating imagined ugliness. World Psychiatry 2004;3:12–17.
10. Phillips KA. The broken mirror: Understanding and treating body dysmorphic disorder. New York: Oxford University Press, 2005.
11. Phillips KA, Didie ER, Menard W, Pagano ME, Fay C, Weisberg RB. Clinical features of body dysmorphic disorder in adolescents and adults. Psychiatr Res 2006;141:305–14.
12. Phillips KA, Dufresne RG. Body dysmorphic disorder. In: Koo JYM, Lee CS, eds. Psychocutaneous medicine. New York: Marcel Dekker, 2003:153–67.
13. Veale D, Neziroglu F. Body dysmorphic disorder: A treatment manual. Oxford: Wiley-Blackwell, 2010.
14. National clinical practice guideline number 31. Obsessive-compulsive disorder: Core interventions in the treatment of obsessive-compulsive disorder and body dysmorphic disorder. Br Psychol Soc Royal Coll Psychiatr, 2006.
15. Cepeda C. The psychiatric interview of children and adolescents. Washington, DC: American Psychiatric Press, 2000.
16. Greenberg JL, Markowitz S, Petronko M.R, Taylor C.E, Wilhelm, S, Wilson GT. Cognitive-behavioral therapy for adolescent body dysmorphic disorder. Cogn Behav Pract 2010;17:248–58.
17. Phillips KA, Atala KD, Pope HG. Diagnostic instruments for body dysmorphic disorder. In: New Research Program and Abstracts of the 148th Annual Meeting of American Psychiatric Association; May 24, 1995; Miami Fla. Abstract NR 375:157.
18. Kaufman J, Birmaher B, Brent D, Rao U, Flynn C, Moreci P, Williamson D, Ryan N. Schedule for affective disorders and schizophrenia for school-age children-present and lifetime version (K-SADS-PL): Initial reliability and validity data. J Am Acad Child Adolesc Psychiatry 1997;36:980–8.
19. Phillips, KA, Hollander E, Rasmussen SA, Aronowitz BR, De Caria G, Goodman WK. A severity rating scale for body dysmorphic disorder: Development, reliability and validity of a modified version of the Yale-Brown obsessive-compulsive scale. Psychopharmacol Bull 1997;33:17–22.
20. Beck AT, Steer RA, Garbin MG. Psychometric properties of the Beck Depression Inventory: Twenty-five years of evaluation. Clin Psychol Rev 1988;8;77–100.
21. Millon T, Davis RD. The Millon Adolescent Personality Inventory and the Millon Adolescent Clinical Inventory. J Couns Dev 1993;71:570–4.
22. Schuerger JM. The Sixteen Personality Factor Questionnaire and its junior versions. J Couns Dev 1992;71:231–44.
23. Pillips KA, Pinto A, Jain S. Self-esteem in body dysmorphic disorder. Body Image I 2004:385–90.
24. Blascovitch J, Tomaka J. Measures of self-esteem. In: Robinson JP, Shaver PR, Wrightsman LS, eds. Measures of personality and social psychological attitudes. San Diego: Academic Press, 1991:116–60.
25. Claiborn J, Pedrick C. The BDD Workbook. Oakland, CA: New Harbinger, 2002.
26. Veale D. Advances in a cognitive behavioural model of body dysmorphic disorder. Body Image I 2004:113–25.

27. Veale D, Kinderman P, Riley K, Lambrou C. Self-discrepancy in body dysmorphic disorder. Br J Clin Psychol 2003;42:157–69.
28. Neziroglu F, Khemlani-Patel S. A review of cognitive and behavioural treatment for body Dysmorphic disorder. CNS Spectrums 2002;7:464–71.
29. Phillips KA. Pharmacologic treatment of body dysmorphic disorder: Review of the evidence and a recommended treatment approach. CNS Spectrums 2002;7:453–60.
30. Veale D. Cognitive-behavioural therapy for body dysmorphic disorder. Adv Psychiatr Treat 2001;7:125–32.
31. Harth W, Gieler U, Kusnir D, Tausk FA. Psychotherapy. In: Harth W, Gieler U, Kusnir D, Tausk FA, eds. Clinical management in psychodermatology. Berlin: Springer, 2009:231–8.
32. Crerand CE, Phillips KA, Menard W, Fay C. Nonpsychiatric medical treatment of body dysmorphic disorder. Psychosomatics 2005;46:549–55.
33. Dyl J, Kittler J, Phillips KA, Hunt JI. Body dysmorphic disorder and other clinically significant body image concerns in adolescent psychiatric inpatients: Prevalence and clinical characteristics. Child Psychiatr Hum Dev 2006;36:369–82.

Peter Lepping and Roland W. Freudenmann

10 Delusional infestation in childhood, adolescence, and adulthood

Delusional infestation (DI) is the fixed (false) belief that a person, or his or her immediate environment, is infested with living or inanimate pathogens. This belief is held despite a lack of medical evidence for such an infestation. Delusional infestation is rare in adolescents and may present in children as *Delusional Infestation by Proxy*. This chapter reviews principles of diagnosis and management. The core of pharmacologic management is with antipsychotics. Amisulpride is recommended as the first line agent; others include olanzapine, risperidone, perphenazine (or fluphenazine), haloperidol, or sulpiride. A positive response may occur within 3 to 10 weeks, and the recommended medication should be changed if no response is seen. Patients should be treated for at least 1 year for primary delusional infestation, while a shorter time may be needed for secondary delusional infestation.

10.1 Introduction

Delusional infestation is the fixed (false) belief that a person, or his or her immediate environment, is infested with living or inanimate pathogens. This belief is held despite a lack of medical evidence for such an infestation (1). Delusional infestation has had many different names in its long history, including Delusional Parasitosis, Ekbom's Syndrome, and Dermatozoenwahn (1,2,3,4,5,6). What all descriptions of the illness have in common is that patients have the belief that they have animate or inanimate objects on or underneath their skin, on their scalp or in their hair, in other orifices of their body, or in their immediate environment, such as their house or flat. Usually these imaginary pathogens are small in size, often microscopic.

These objects have changed themes over the years. It started with the belief about having scabies, later times saw a predominance of worms, and then newly discovered bacteria in the nineteenth century. This moved to viruses and parasites (primarily insects) in the twentieth century. In the twenty-first century, inanimate objects such as fibers, strands, or filaments (also called "morgellons" by some patients) became an increasingly common theme as the source of the alleged infestation, although insects are still the most commonly alleged pathogens (7,8,9).

In psychiatry, such changes of the delusional content within a set of well-known delusional themes are common. Such delusion themes include persecution, grandiosity, illness, jealousy, but also infestation. Delusions slightly vary in the way that they present, usually following fashions and scientific development. A similar phenomenon could be seen with delusional themes of persecution and paranoia. Various secret services have been the subject of accusations of persecution by people with such delusions, including the communists, the Nazis, the Mafia, the CIA, the KGB, Mossad, or other intelligence services, and more recently terrorists and pedophiles. This is an understandable contextualization of a perceived threat in any given society.

Similarly with delusional infestation, patients seem to favor objects of infestation that are currently spoken about or considered as harmful by wider society. What has never changed is the strong conviction with which the patient holds those beliefs despite the lack of evidence for the particular type of infestation claimed by the patient. However, even the intensity of a delusional belief can change. The same delusional belief can be held in various degrees of intensity (from an uncertain belief to an "overvalued idea" to an unshakable firm conviction of true delusional intensity), depending on current levels of distress and treatment success.

In other words, the same person may occasionally consider alternative explanations for their alleged infestation, such as a psychiatric explanation. However, at a different point during their illness, they may not be able to give such alternatives any consideration. For example, a patient with delusional infestation may very well be slightly less convinced of the infestation after seeing you in clinic and after hearing about the negative laboratory results. However, immediately afterwards, when the itching starts, they become much more convinced of the infestation again.

10.2 How to diagnose a delusion

The German psychiatrist and philosopher, Karl Jaspers (1883–1969), defined criteria for delusions in 1913 (10,11). A delusion is characterized by a belief that presents with an "extraordinary" or "incomparable, subjective conviction." This belief is held with conviction despite evidence to the contrary. Lastly, Jaspers suggested that the belief ought to be objectively impossible, but – as we will see – this criterion is problematic and can be a pitfall.

Modern psychiatrists use the former two criteria regularly. They would only consider the criterion of objective impossibility for the most severe delusions where the improbability of the belief is obvious. However, in reality we are not always able to verify the belief of a patient. We cannot usually ring Langley or other security organizations to get confirmation that someone is being followed by security agencies when the patient presents with paranoid and persecutory delusions. Neither can we ever be sure beyond doubt that the patient is definitely not infested (the history of medicine is full of newly identified infectious disorders where accepted medical knowledge was proven wrong!) if that happens to be the delusional belief of the patient (1).

However, we can make a judgment on the reasoning and explanations that the patient puts forward to justify that belief. If he is convinced he is being followed by government agents because he has seen a lot of black cars lately or because there were a lot of crime stories on the news, it is less likely to be a true belief. Equally, if the patient thinks his house is infested because he has heard noises he interpreted as rats running behind the floor boards, it is less convincing evidence than if he had found confirmed evidence of rats in the house.

In other words, we need to judge the probability and the rationale from the arguments the patients puts forward. Whether something is true or false is less of an issue for modern psychiatry. Thus, someone might be followed but still be delusional if the justification is delusional. Furthermore, the delusional intensity can be shifting and is only fixed in more severe cases. However, this should not deter us from making a diagnosis. Quite on the contrary, it is what we would expect because people's beliefs change with changing circumstances in normal life as well as within a delusional system.

10.3 Primary and secondary delusional infestation

Delusional infestation is neither a specific diagnosis nor a homogenous disorder. Like any other delusion, delusional infestation can occur as a mono-delusional disorder or in the context of other illnesses (1,4,5,12,13,14). If it occurs as a mono-delusional disorder, the patient would otherwise be free of any psychiatric symptoms. The only symptom they present with is the delusion about the infestation and consequences of this belief. This form is called *Primary Delusional Infestation*. The available case series in DI suggest that just fewer than 50% of cases are primary delusional infestation (DI) (14).

Secondary Delusional Infestation is the same delusion but occurring in the context of neurological, medical, or psychiatric illness, or as consequence of a medication or illicit drug use. Delusional infestation commonly occurs in medical illnesses, particularly those that have central nervous system (CNS) involvement (i.e. vascular encephalopathy, stroke, dementia, delirium, others) or produce a degree of pruritus or "pins and needles" sensations (i.e. diabetes, renal and liver failure, tumors, vitamin deficiencies). Any such unexplained sensation may be wrongly explained by the presence of alleged parasites, infections, or other pathogens, including inanimate particles in or under the skin (for review see [1,15]).

In psychiatric disorders DI can occur in the context of a psychotic depression, dementia, and schizophrenia. People who have a degree of sensory deprivation, particularly visual impairment, seem to have a higher risk of developing delusional infestation. Equally, older people and those who live alone seem to have a higher risk (5). Delusional infestation also occurs in the context of drug abuse, especially stimulants such as amphetamines or cocaine and, less frequently, tetrahydrocannabinol

(16,17,18,19). There are a number of case reports about medication causing delusional infestation, particularly antibiotics (20,21) or dopaminergic agonists used in Parkinson's disease or restless legs syndrome (22,23).

10.4 The context of children and adolescence

In the context of children and adolescents, it is important to look at the various forms in which delusional infestation can present to the clinician. The person presenting may be the person with the illness. Often, however, the person who has delusional infestation may induce similar delusions in a person close to them. In psychiatry, this is called "*folie à deux*" (literally, "madness by twos"), *Shared Psychotic Disorder* according to The American Psychiatric Association's (APA) *Diagnostic and Statistical Manual* (DSM-IV-TR) (297.3), or *Induced Psychotic Disorder* in the International Classification of Diseases (ICD-10: F24).

This means that the person with the original illness, the inducer, produces the same delusional ideas in a person close to them. These ideas are then shared by two people. Reports of up to five people or even whole families sharing the delusional belief exist in the DI literature (24,25,26). It is estimated from case series that the prevalence of Folie à Deux in delusional infestation is 14.4% (5). Our recent case selection found a rate of shared psychotic disorders of 11% (15), but reported frequencies range from 8% to 49% (1).

Another variant is a *delusional infestation by proxy*. In these cases the person who has the main illness thinks that somebody else close to them is infested, rather than the patient him- or herself. The infestation in delusional infestation by proxy is usually alleged to be in the patient's children (27), but there have been descriptions about patients' pets having an alleged infestation as well (28). Usually, the parent does not mention that he or she has the same symptoms and that he or she applies (unneeded) intensive skin cleaning measures to the child that cause the skin lesions.

This constellation of child abuse, "false stories and fabricated evidence," is the classic Münchhausen *by proxy*-constellation, as introduced by Roy Meadow in 1977 (29). The picture is characterized by the initiation of unnecessary, often harmful medical interventions in the child who is, in fact, healthy. The term has been adapted for delusional infestation as *delusional parasitosis by proxy* (27,30). In this case, unneeded trials with anti-microbiological agents or skin/body cleansing measures are requested by the parent "for" the child, although no such measure is really indicated.

The dilemma is that in small children, the physician usually has to rely on the parent's description of the child's symptoms, but in a *by proxy* situation such descriptions are misleading. Careful history taking, obvious discrepancies between abnormalities claimed by the parent, and objective evidence in a careful examination of the child may, at least in some cases, help to identify the real problem: the parent! If we imagine that we would genuinely believe that our children were infested with parasites or other animate or inanimate pathogens, this would cause us a high level of distress.

It is therefore not surprising that some parents try to get rid of the alleged infestation, particularly after they have consulted physicians who tell them that there is nothing to worry about. This can lead to significant impairment of the children's quality of life, including frankly dangerous procedures, such as being bathed in bleach or other pesticides. It is therefore very important to look for signs of the use of aggressive chemicals when children are presented with an alleged infestation.

It has been well described that patients with delusional infestation will go to quite some lengths to get rid of the alleged infestation, which, in the case of children, may very well represent a form of child abuse. It is important to remain alarmed to that possibility. Various internet sites and chat rooms on morgellons, unknown skin infestations, and conspiracy theories (that, in fact, just deal with forms of delusional infestation) are a pertinent and sad reminder of the efforts that patients will make to get rid of the alleged pests, including giving each other advice on the various pesticides to use.

10.5 Clinical pictures

10.5.1 Case one

In order to understand the suffering that is associated with delusional infestation, we need to understand the clinical picture of the disease (for details, see 1,5,16,31,32). There may be the 73-year-old near-sighted widow who lives alone and may suffer from the odd itching. As she is scratching the skin, she has the impression that she can see something moving underneath the skin. While she is able to put this thought to one side at the beginning, it becomes increasingly troublesome. Over a few weeks, she starts to think that there are living creatures underneath her skin, which explain her itching as well as her sensation of something moving. She has not seen anything move since, but the itching persists. She is starting to scratch harder to see whether she can dig out the parasites from her skin. The skin gets increasingly infected, which makes her believe even more strongly that she is infested with something. She starts to clean her house more often because the only reason she can think of why she might be infested is that the house may be infested.

After a few weeks, she cleans the house for about 5 to 6 hours every day. She is worried to let other people in the house in case the parasites are contagious. She is therefore increasingly isolated. Her hands are starting to suffer from the use of bleach. Eventually she sees her primary care physician, who decides to involve a dermatologist. She arrives at the dermatologist's clinic with a specimen in a little glass container that she says is evidence of the infestation. The dermatologist does a thorough investigation and finds evidence of excessive use of bleach on her hands and arms, as well as signs of excessive scratching and some super-infections all over her body, except for some areas on the back, which she was unable to reach with her hands.

During the next appointment, the dermatologist explains to her that the specimen showed no evidence of infestation but instead came back as showing skin scrapings. The dermatologist attempts to explain to her that there is no evidence of infestation and that quite possibly her distress and itching may be caused by other problems. She becomes very angry and accuses the dermatologist of not taking her seriously. Despite best efforts to resolve the impasse, she leaves the dermatologist's clinic without making another appointment. A day later she rings the pest control officer who is happy to disinfect her house but finds no evidence of any infestation. She becomes increasingly isolated and spends increasing amounts of time cleaning, but her symptoms do not get better, and she does not see another doctor for her problems.

10.5.2 Case two

Another example that starts to explain how children may be affected by delusional infestation is a 26-year-old divorced woman with two children, 2 and 6 years of age. One day, she sees what she thinks is probably a rat in the corner of one of the rooms in her house. She gets understandably upset about this and calls the city's environmental office who send an expert round to her house. They examine the house and tell her that they were unable to find any evidence of rats anywhere. However, she is so concerned that she buys rat poison, which she distributes around the house. She realizes that this may not be a good idea with a toddler and a 6-year-old in the house, so she restricts the children to the living room, where she has not put any rat poison.

Over the next 4 weeks she becomes increasingly convinced that there are rats in the house. She starts to hear creaking noises, which she interprets as evidence of the rats behind skirting boards and under the wooden flooring. She gets increasingly upset and does not want the children to live in the house. She takes them out to a café in town, where she sits all day with the children. When she comes back in the evening, she keeps the light on in the living room so that she can see the rats, should they appear. She feels that she has to protect her children from them. She also approaches the local authorities (i.e. Environmental Department) again, who come out to confirm that they cannot find any evidence of rats anywhere in the house. She gets the local press involved, who write a scathing article about the incompetence of the local Environmental Department.

She decides to seal all boxes for food storage because she thinks that the rats would be attracted by crumbs or other food remains in the house, and one day she wakes up to find that there are some particles of sand in her son's bed. She is convinced that these are rat droppings and takes them to be analyzed. The analysis confirms that they are in fact sand, but she is adamant that there are rats in the house. She considers ripping all trees out of her garden as she thinks that they may attract rats.

She eventually goes to her primary care physician as she feels increasingly distressed by all of this. The primary care physician manages to persuade her to see the local community mental health team in order to deal with her distress. After a difficult engagement period of several months, she is eventually willing to take an antipsychotic medication. In the first instance, she was persuaded to take it in order to deal with her distress. At a later stage, as she had gained insight, a full diagnosis was given to her with the full rationale for the antipsychotic medication. She improved within 2 weeks after starting on amisulpride. However, she still has a varying compliance. Eventually, she was persuaded to take the amisulpride regularly, and she fully recovered.

She gained insight to the point where she did no longer believe that there were rats in her house and that she questioned whether there had ever been rats in the house. However, she was not entirely sure about the past. She started to use her whole house again and got rid of the rat poison. The children started to sleep in their own bedroom again, and she stopped worrying about any infestation. About a year later, she stopped her medication and within a few weeks she started to get worried about infestations again. She was persuaded to restart amisulpride, and those worries subsided.

10.5.3 Case Three

A 43-year-old married man with two children aged 8 and 12 presents to the primary care physician complaining of parasites or objects that live underneath his skin. These have infested his whole house, as well as his wife and children. He has also read on the internet that there is a new disease called Morgellons, which he thinks he might have. He cleans the house for 3 hours every day and puts pressure on his wife to help him with the cleaning. He has also started to use bleach on his skin in order to get rid of the infestation, as this was suggested by various people on the internet.

The primary care physician refers him to a dermatologist, who investigates his skin, as well as the specimen that he provides in a matchbox. There is no sign of infestation, but there is some topical eczema from the use of bleach. The dermatologist tries to persuade him to take antipsychotic medication, as he makes a diagnosis of delusional infestation. However, this makes the patient as well as his wife very angry, and they refuse to try it. The dermatologist rings a consultant psychiatrist, who actually visits the family. Both parents are very distressed and are talking about using bleach on the children, as no professional is willing to take them seriously. Over some weeks, the parents can be dissuaded from using bleach on the children or themselves, but they continue to refuse a trial antipsychotic medication. Their symptoms persist, and they are now refusing follow-up appointments with the dermatologist as well as the community mental health team.

10.5.4 Commentary on these three cases

These three cases are real cases that have been changed somewhat to preserve anonymity. They exemplify the enormous pressure and distress that patients with delusional infestation are under. It also shows the persistent lack of insight that can be very difficult to overcome and that makes compliance with medication very unlikely. This is the reason why patients with delusional infestation very rarely present to psychiatrists and are unlikely to accept a diagnosis of delusional infestation from any other doctor such as their primary care physician, a dermatologist, or tropical medicine specialists. Children can themselves be patients, but this is exceedingly rare. They are much more likely to be involved through one or both of their parents being ill and fearing contamination or infestation in their children. This can lead to serious and damaging treatment attempts, which are usually pursued in desperation and because of the parents' delusional beliefs.

10.6 Delusional elaboration ("Wahnarbeit")

The before-mentioned German psychiatrist Karl Jaspers described how patients with delusions will try to make sense of the world around them by interpreting events, memories, and perceptions in a way that makes them fit with their delusional themes. He called this "Wahnarbeit," which literally means "delusional work" but is better translated as "delusional elaboration" (10,11). What he described is a process in which the patient reinterprets evidence that does not fit in with their fixed belief in order to make it fit. This happens even when, for an objective outsider, the patient makes associations and connections that are beyond reasonable probability. This can be called "errors in probabilistic reasoning" (14) as the patient favors unlikely explanations over likely ones.

In the case of delusional infestation, a patient may misinterpret normal house sounds as evidence that there are rats or vermin in the house. They may also misinterpret normal itching after the use of bleach as evidence of parasites underneath their skin. They may interpret super-infections on their skin as further evidence for the severity of their infestation. It becomes even more difficult for patients when they have to explain negative specimen results. Patients will often insist that the laboratory must have made an error, the biopsy was taken from the wrong place, or that generally the doctors just do not believe them and that is why they deliver "false" results. In more extreme cases, there can be a development of paranoia to explain these results. There has been one report where a delusional infestation patient eventually attacked his family physician (33).

Because the delusional elaboration has to be seen in the context of the patient's life experience and environment, the content of the delusions is likely to change over time. In the twenty-first century, it is much more common than it was in the last century that patients will think they are infested with viruses or inanimate pathogens (1,7,34). The overall spectrum is vast and covers big vermin like rats as well as lice or microscopic fibers.

It is interesting to look at the new phenomenon of so-called Morgellons Disease, which is no accepted medical diagnosis. It was first mentioned by a lay person in 2002. It was described by a woman who felt that her children were infested with a hitherto unknown fiber. After some research on the internet, she connected her children's symptoms to an outbreak of a mysterious disease called morgellons in the south of France in the nineteenth century.

Since then a few papers have been published. All published papers in favor of a true existence of morgellons can be traced back to a handful of authors who offer little actual scientific data but managed to publish their assertions in peer reviewed papers (35,36,37,38,39). These authors firmly reject any insinuation that people with self-diagnosed "morgellons" may suffer from delusional infestation. The vast majority of the scientific community, however, believe that morgellons is *not* a new entity, but rather a new form of delusional infestation (for review see 1,8,35,40,41,42,43,44,).

However, the morgellons supporters' very public campaign has somehow captured the imagination of a lot of people who suffer with what they consider to be unexplained infestations with fibers and filaments. They organized themselves well and started a campaign to research this new "disease." They even managed to get Hillary Clinton, in her then capacity as an American senator, to lobby on their behalf. In the end, they succeeded in getting United States CDC (Centers for Disease Control and Prevention) funding for a big study on the alleged phenomenon, which they consider to be a new illness (a recent publication did not confirm the existence of a new pathogen [45]). This was to the point that the CDC actually took the category "delusional parasitosis" off their website and replaced it with a much more morgellons friendly phrase ("unexplained dermopathy").

Thousands of people are registered to the so-called Morgellons Research Foundation's (MRF) website without any evidence that it exists as an illness. Some authors have suggested that one of the main proponents of the morgellons cause, Mary Leitao, may have experienced delusional infestation by proxy, as she believed that her son was infested (30).

In a high profile 2011 study, a group around Hylwa et al from the Mayo Clinic in Rochester, Minnesota, published findings of specimen results in people who were thought to have delusional infestation or suffered from an infestation with such fibers (34). They found that neither skin biopsies nor examination of patient-provided specimens provided objective evidence of skin infestation. The authors, in our opinion correctly, concluded that the search for an inanimate source of infestation in these patients was yet another variant of the delusional theme of infestation. But how big is the risk that we may miss a real infestation? Research of large samples with delusional infestation would suggest that the number of patients who subsequently are found to have some form of infestation is in the region of less than 1% (1). This means that by and large the investigations that preclude diagnoses of delusional infestation appear rather robust, but it is obviously always necessary to keep an open mind.

10.7 Prevalence of delusional infestation

It is very difficult to estimate the real prevalence of delusional infestation because most patients do not present to physicians. In the cases that they do present to physicians, they do often not return for follow up once being told that their skin or their specimens show no signs of infestation. A diagnosis of delusional infestation in these circumstances is often not made. In most health systems it is therefore very unlikely to be computerized in an easily accessible manner. The available evidence comes from estimates and surveys, as well as case series.

The German psychiatrist Wolfgang Trabert published estimated prevalence figures for the year 1988 in Germany (46,47). He tried to capture all possible services where delusional infestation patients may present, including primary care physicians, public health clinics, and tropical medicine institutions, as well as dermatologists and psychiatrists. These figures are based on survey estimates, but still the figures are likely to be an underestimation because of the patients' tendency to lose confidence in professional medicine. His corrected *prevalence* estimate based on outpatients visits was 83.23 patients per 1 million. His prevalence estimate based on hospitals and public health departments was 5.58 per million (47). According to Trabert, this equates to an annual *incidence* rate of 17 per 1 million inhabitants per year (47).

Our own research in the United Kingdom calculated a prevalence figure from a survey of UK dermatologists covering more than half of the UK population and suggests a figure of 5 patients per 1 million in the UK, if we take only those who present to dermatologists (48). Given that prevalence estimates based on analyses from psychiatric units and clinics show much lower figures, it confirms that dermatologists are much more likely to see delusional infestation patients than psychiatrists.

Trabert's investigations of large case series with $N = 1{,}223$ patients with DI published until 1995 have also shown a clear age distribution in the presenting patients (5). In essence, the risk of developing delusional infestation rises with age with a female preponderance in the region of about 3:1. In this large case series, there were literally only a handful of patients under 18 years of age. Various other case series from France and Britain have confirmed this distribution (32,49). These figures show that, by and large, delusional infestation is not an illness of the young. However, children and adolescents can be directly affected through ill parents or grandparents as well as shared psychotic disorders and DI by proxy. Furthermore, the diagnosis of DI cannot be entirely dismissed in adolescents, given that there have been cases in the literature that show children under the age of 18 being diagnosed with delusional infestation.

10.7.1 Treatment

There is reasonable evidence to suggest that antipsychotic medication is effective in the treatment of delusional infestation (1,4,5,15,50,51). There is, however, a dearth of data from randomized control trials for both primary (4) and all other forms of this disorder. This is because patients with delusional infestation usually lack insight into their illness and, if a psychotic disorder is mentioned in any research protocol, patients are not inclined to participate. Recruitment is therefore virtually impossible if modern standards of patient information are being maintained. Any such attempt in recent years has failed (48,52).

The only available placebo-controlled data is from a small Swedish study by Hamann and Avnstorp from 1982 with $N = 11$ cases (5 of these primary DI) (53) and a small Hungarian study from Ungvari and Vladar with 10 primary DI cases (54), suggesting efficacy of pimozide as compared to placebo. Notably, these trials lack true randomization and are limited by small samples as well as other methodological flaws (for review see reference 1).

Still, pimozide, an ultra-high potency first generation antipsychotic, became the first line substance in delusional infestation in the 1980s and 1990s, based on the two studies mentioned and larger retrospective case series (31,32). This has very much changed due to concerns about drug safety with pimozide (e.g. prolongation of the QTc interval, extrapyramidal side effects, high risk of drug–drug interactions). Today, pimozide is at best a third-line substance in any indication. A Cochrane review has found that pimozide has a higher liability to cause Parkinsonian symptoms than other first generation antipsychotics in the treatment of schizophrenia and that there is no high-level evidence for or against its use in delusional disorder in general (55).

In view of this lack of recommendations for antipsychotic treatment in primary and other forms of DI, our group has used a specific systematic review methodology that allowed us to estimate treatment effects by pooling data from standardized case reports (4,15). These have shown that remission rates are good when compliance can be established. Response rates for second generation antipsychotics are in the region of 75%, and response rates with first generation antipsychotics are in the region of 60% to 100%, provided that regular medication intake can be achieved. In naturalistic samples the rates are usually lower.

First generation antipsychotics achieved more full remissions, with second generation antipsychotics achieving more partial remissions. On the basis of this evidence, as well as considerations of adverse effects and transmitter profiles, we have already published treatment guidelines for dermatologists (50). As first line treatments for delusional infestation we suggest the use of second generation antipsychotics such as amisulpride, olanzapine, risperidone (in alphabetical order), or, among first generation antipsychotics, low doses of haloperidol, sulpiride, or phenothiazines (1).

However, the necessity to use an antipsychotic very much differs for the different forms of DI. For example, in a case of cocaine intoxication, symptoms of DI may resolve within hours or days, making antipsychotic treatment dispensable in many cases. By contrast, in a classic patient who suffers from primary delusional infestation for several years and holds his or her delusional belief with high intensity, antipsychotic treatment is very much needed, yet often not possible due to lack of cooperation. If the patient agrees to use an antipsychotic, the available low-level evidence suggests that the doses can be lower than the doses used for the treatment of schizophrenia (15). It is not clear whether primary delusional infestation responds better or worse than secondary delusional infestation to antipsychotic treatment, as results are slightly variable. However, there is consensus that, in secondary delusional infestation, the underlying illness needs treatment in its own right (for further details see 1,15,50).

There is also good practical experience from various liaison psycho-dermatology clinics suggesting that it is always important to treat the skin of the affected patient, as well as treating the delusional illness with antipsychotics. In such specialized settings, up to 81% of patients accept psychiatric medication, but still many of them are lost to follow-up (56). In most clinics, it would be common to use emollients as topical treatment against dry skin (resulting from excessive cleansing), with a possibility of adding antibiotics if there are super-infections. It is *not* recommended to give in to any, even perseverant, requests by the patients to prescribe pesticides, antiviral agents, or the like outside a proven infestation with any of the respective pathogens just in order to please the patient. Referrals to psychiatry are rarely successful, because the patients do not turn up. It is therefore important to use the trustful relationship that the dermatologist has with his or her patient to initiate antipsychotic treatment, even though this may be outside the dermatologist's usual expertise.

10.7.2 Which antipsychotic in DI?

The current evidence for the use of antipsychotics in delusional infestation is relatively robust, but of a low level. The evidence comes largely from systematic reviews of case series and case reports. We have introduced systematic reporting criteria for such case reports. In one large study, we looked at cases of primary delusional infestation (4). For first generation antipsychotics, remission rates were between 60% and 100%. These were primarily cases treated with pimozide, but also fluphenazine, trifluoperazine, and haloperidol. In another study looking at second generation antipsychotics (such as risperidone, olanzapine, or amisulpride), the average remission rate was 75% (15). This was the final outcome after therapy switches. The results for quetiapine were disappointing despite its strong antihistaminic action. The rates of full remission were slightly higher with first generation antipsychotics, where they reached almost 50%, while they were in the region of 25% for second generation antipsychotics. However, it is clear that, when patients are compliant with medication, the vast majority get better.

It is difficult to make firm recommendations of the best antipsychotic to use. However, it is clear that pimozide should not be the drug of choice, although it has been widely used for delusional infestation in the 1980s and thereafter. The reason is its unfavorable side effect profile. In accordance with the hypothesis that delusional infestation originates from problems with dopaminergic frontal-striatal pathways, it would be logical to use dopaminergic antipsychotics. This is why we have previously recommended amisulpride as first line treatment; alternatives would be perphenazine or sulpiride. In cases in which extra-pyramidal side effects such as stiffness, muscle aches, or restless legs are a problem, it would be possible to choose olanzapine as an alternative with fewer potential extra-pyramidal side effects.

The evidence with modern medication is most robust for olanzapine and risperidone because most cases have been treated with those two medications. In essence, it would probably be best for a non-psychiatrist to choose the antipsychotic they are most familiar with. Should they not be familiar with any antipsychotic, we would recommend amisulpride as the first choice. Doses are by and large smaller than doses used in schizophrenia. It is often possible to treat delusional infestation successfully with what in schizophrenia would be considered a starting dose (i.e. amisulpride at 200 mg, olanzapine 5 mg, risperidone 2 mg, and haloperidol 5 mg).

We have also shown that changing medication in unsuccessful cases is useful. The patient will often respond to a different antipsychotic. It is good to know that the time to onset of effect of the antipsychotics is quite short. It is in the region of 10 days. On average, maximum effects can be expected after 6 weeks, with earlier remission within 10 days in secondary delusional infestation and 3 weeks in primary delusional infestation. We therefore do not have to wait very long for an effect to occur. The maximum effect is reached 6 weeks to after 3 months.

In a paper published in 2011, British dermatologists Wong and Bewley point out that 25% of patients may relapse on stopping treatment, with the greatest risk being within the first few months of discontinuation (56). They recommend that those patients may require longer treatment courses. Their patients had taken medication for 9 months to 2.5 years, which is roughly in keeping with recommendations for treatment continuation after a first psychotic episode.

10.7.2.1 Management of pediatric patients

In the case of children and adolescents, it will be rare that the adolescent is the actual patient with the delusional belief. It is more common that a child is presented to a physician by a parent. In cases of delusional infestation by proxy as well as shared delusions (Folie à Deux), it needs to be established whether the child is at risk from measures against the alleged infestation. Child protection procedures may have to be initiated. This obviously depends on the level of risk to the child. Cases where there is a direct risk to the patient or a patient's relative may also necessitate an involuntary admission in the United Kingdom under the UK's Mental Health Act legislation. Cases of delusional infestation by proxy are even more difficult to treat. The main challenge is to approach the parent's false belief and eventually achieve compliance with medication, which may require involuntary treatment in some rare cases. Dermatologists are unlikely to be able to solve such cases without a psychiatrist.

10.7.2.2 Steps to successful treatment

In order to achieve maximum benefit in managing patients with DI, these steps are recommended:

1. Take the patient's story seriously and investigate for somatic explanations, including investigations of any specimen the patients may bring.
2. Perform a physical examination that carefully looks at the patient's skin. Be mindful of evidence of excessive cleaning in children as well.
3. Explore the patient's reasoning for their belief that they are infested.
4. Treat skin problems dermatologically, and introduce antipsychotics to reduce the distress that people experience and their preoccupation, indicating that such medication has helped many others of your patients with similar problems.
5. At follow up, explain the results of the specimen or biopsies.
6. Avoid challenging confrontations about the patient's delusional beliefs, but do not agree with their beliefs. Sometimes it is necessary to agree to disagree.
7. Try and persuade the patient to be compliant with antipsychotic medication. It may be necessary to tell the patient that they have nothing to lose giving it a try, as nothing else seems to have worked.
8. Rapport with the patient and a trusting relationship will be essential and is difficult to establish with delusional infestation patients. However, good rapport improves compliance.

10.8 Antipsychotics

The main pillar of any treatment of delusional infestation is to persuade the patient to take antipsychotic medication. This is difficult to achieve because of the patient's lack of insight, and a stepwise approach has been put forward by most authors in this area. It is important to take time at the first meeting, to take a careful history including the tropical medicine history, and to examine the patient thoroughly. All specimens should be analyzed routinely and properly. The critical point is usually when the patient returns and the specimen biopsies and other investigations have all proven not to show any infestation. At this point it is important to find a compromise between keeping the patient in care by offering more investigations, but equally not to over diagnose the patient with too many investigations.

At some point, you have to approach the question of diagnosis, and it is at that stage that the patient will either remain engaged or not. The patient will never be reassured by the absence of pathogens but will rather question the quality of the biopsy, the laboratory, your competence, or the examination. Certain things will help to be successful in maintaining rapport with the patient and achieving compliance with medication (adjusted from 1):

- Acknowledge the patient's suffering, show empathy, and offer to help to reduce the patient's distress.
- Paraphrase the symptoms as the patient presents them ("you are itching," "the crawling," etc.) rather than reinforcing or questioning them.
- Indicate that you are familiar with the problem and that you have been able to help other patients before, but that this may take a little while.
- Answer that you did not find any pathogens so far, but you believe the patient's symptoms.
- Indicate that the symptoms may be due to an over-activity in the nervous system. This may help to give a more somatic explanation.
- Try to introduce antipsychotics as the only substances that are helpful against these processes, as suggested by current research.
- If the patient asks for a diagnosis, try to use more descriptive terms such as "unexplained dermopathy." Only introduce the diagnosis delusional infestation when the patient has regained a reasonable amount of insight.
- Introduce antipsychotics as helpful against the patient's distress and itching. Many patients may also need additional antihistamines.
- Do not try to convince the patient or question their beliefs directly.
- Never attempt an immediate psychiatric referral, and do not try to approach the possibility of antipsychotic medication too soon. Do not use words like delusional or psychiatric, which may indicate a non-somatic diagnosis. Equally, do not try to reassure the patient by offering a psychogenic explanation.
- Prescribe according to the type of delusional infestation. Secondary delusional infestation requires treatment of the underlying illness, as well as an antipsychotic.
- Do not prescribe antibiotics without evidence for a real infection, as it can further reinforce the delusion.
- Do not overlook frank aggression against other health care professionals. It may be necessary to evaluate the risk that the patient may pose to those professionals.

Consider the possibility that the patient's despair may lead to suicidal ideation, which has to be evaluated, monitored, and treated.

It is always useful when trying to explain delusional disorders to acknowledge to the patient the possibility that an infestation cannot be identified at present, but that we will continue to analyze any specimen that the patient hands in. Equally, this would be an opportunity to introduce a second etiological possibility to the patient: that there is a possible over-sensitivity and over-activity in the peripheral and central nervous system, which is indeed a common cause for feelings of crawling or itching. It may be useful to explain this with other analogies in other disorders, such as pain or anxiety in which central nervous system problems can cause physical symptoms. The clinician could explain that many chronic symptoms cause adaptive reactions in the responsible neuronal networks.

Should this not lead to a better understanding, the other way of trying to persuade the patient to take medication would be to argue that, while you are still trying to establish whether there is an infestation, you acknowledge the patient's distress about their current situation. This distress and the associated itching could be treated with anxiolytic medication, such as an antipsychotic. You will have to explain that antipsychotics are normally used for schizophrenia, but in the case of the patient, it would be used to treat distress and itching. You could use the analogy of aspirin being used for pain as well as a cardiac medication. This often helps to persuade the patient to start medication without giving inaccurate information.

10.9 Conclusion

Delusional Infestation is the fixed (false) belief that a person, or his or her immediate environment, is infested with living or inanimate pathogens. This belief is held despite a lack of medical evidence for such an infestation (1). A number of recommendations are provided to help in the management of delusion infections:

- Choose an antipsychotic you are familiar with, preferably a dopaminergic agent.
- We recommend amisulpride first line. Other reasonable options include olanzapine, risperidone, perphenazine (or fluphenazine), haloperidol, or sulpiride.
- Use low doses of the respective medication.
- Expect a response within 3 to 10 weeks depending on the type of DI.
- Change medication if no response is seen and compliance is assured.
- Treat patient for at least 1 year in the case of primary DI; in cases secondary to reversible causes, shorter treatment will often suffice.
- A minority of patients may relapse after discontinuing medication and may have to restart medication.

References

1. Freudenmann RW, Lepping P. Delusional infestation. *Clin Microbiol Rev* 2009;22(4):690–73
2. Ekbom KA. Der praesenile Dermatozoenwahn. *Acta Psychiatr Neurol Scand* 1938;13:227–59.
3. Ekbom KA, Yorston G, Miesch M, Pleasance S, Rubbert S. The pre-senile delusion of infestation. *Hist Psychiatry* 2003;14(54(Pt2):229–56.
4. Lepping P, Russell I, Freudenmann RW. Antipsychotic treatment of delusional parasitosis: Systematic review. *Br J Psychiatry* 2007;191:198–205.
5. Trabert W. 100 years of delusional parasitosis. Meta-analysis of 1,223 case reports. *Psychopathology* 1995;28(5):238–46.
6. Trabert W. 100 Jahre Dermatozoenwahn [100 years of delusional parasitosis]. *Medizinische Welt* 1997;48:33–7. [German]
7. Freudenmann RW, Kölle M, Schönfeldt-Lecuona C, Dieckmann S, Harth W, Lepping P. Delusional parasitosis and the matchbox sign revisited: The international perspective. *Acta Derm Venereol* 2010;90(5):517–9.
8. Fair B. Morgellons: Contested illness, diagnostic compromise and medicalisation. *Sociol Health Illn* 2010;32(4):597–612.
9. Vila-Rodriguez F, Macewan BG. Delusional parasitosis facilitated by web-based dissemination. *Am J Psychiatry* 2008;165(12):1612.
10. Jaspers K. *General psychopathology*, 4th edn. Manchester, UK: Manchester University Press, 1963.
11. Jaspers K. *Allgemeine psychopathologie*. 9 unveränderte Auflage edn. Berlin: Springer, 1973.
12. Musalek M, Bach M, Passweg V, Jaeger S. The position of delusional parasitosis in psychiatric nosology and classification. *Psychopathology* 1990;23(2):115–24.
13. Arnold LM. Psychocutaneous disorders (Chapter 25.7). In: Sadock BI, Sadock VA, eds. *Kaplan and Sadock's comprehensive textbook of psychiatry*, 7th edn, CD-ROM. Philadelphia, PA: Lippincott Williams Wilkins, 2000.
14. Dunn J, Murphy MB, Fox KM. Diffuse pruritic lesions in a 37-year-old man after sleeping in an abandoned building. *Am J Psychiatry* 2007;164(8):1166–72.
15. Freudenmann RW, Lepping P. Second-generation antipsychotics in primary and secondary delusional parasitosis: Outcome and efficacy. *J Clin Psychopharmacol* 2008;28(5):500–8.
16. Skott A. *Delusions of infestation. Dermatozoenwahn – Ekbom's Syndrome.* Report from the Psychiatric Research Center. Goteborg: St. Jörgen Hospital, University of Goteborg. Sweden 1978. Report No.: Nr.13.
17. Elpern DJ. Cocaine abuse and delusions of parasitosis. *Cutis* 1988;42(4):273–4.
18. Hanisch F, Wustmann T, Piro J, Röttig S. Successful treatment of methamphetamine-induced delusional parasitosis with sertindole and sertralin. *Br J Psychiatry* 2009;eLetters (http://bjp.rcpsych.org/cgi/eletters/191/3/198).
19. Siegel RK. Cocaine hallucinations. *Am J Psychiatry* 1978;135(3):309–14.
20. Steinert T, Studemund H. Acute delusional parasitosis under treatment with ciprofloxacin. *Pharmacopsychiatry* 2006 Jul;39(4):159–60.
21. Tse KC, Li FK, Tang S, Lam MF, Chan TM, Lai KN. Delusion of worm infestation associated with clarithromycin in a patient on peritoneal dialysis. *Perit Dial Int* 2001;21(4):415–6.
22. Kölle M, Lepping P, Kassubek J, Schönfeldt-Lecuona C, Freudenmann RW. Delusional infestation induced by pirepidil add-on in Parkinson's disease. *Pharmacopsychiatry* 2010;43(6):240–2.
23. Flann S, Shotbolt J, Kessel B, Vekaria D, Taylor R, Bewley A, et al. Three cases of delusional parasitosis caused by dopamine agonists. *Clin Exp Dermatol.* 2010 Mar 19.
24. Musalek M, Kutzer E. The frequency of shared delusions in delusions of infestation. *Eur Arch Psychiatry Neurol Sci* 1990;239(4):263–6.
25. Trabert W. Shared psychotic disorder in delusional parasitosis. *Psychopathology* 1999;32(1):30–4.

26. Mercan S, Ögütcen Ö, Altunay IK, Karamustafalioglu O. Folie à famille ve Delüzyonel Parazitoz: Olgu Sunumu ve Literatürün Gözden Gecirilmesi. *Klinik Psikofarmakoloji Bülteni* 2005; 15:71–8.
27. Sarkar S, Ghosal MK, Bandyopadhyay D, Ghosh SK, Guha P. Delusional parasitosis by proxy. *Clin Exp Dermatol* 2009;34(7):e487–8.
28. Nel M, Schoeman JP, Lobetti RG. Delusions of parasitosis in clients presenting pets for veterinary care. *J S Afr Vet Assoc* 2001;72(3):167–9.
29. Meadow R. Munchausen syndrome by proxy. The hinterland of child abuse. *Lancet* 1977;2 (8033):343–5.
30. DeVita-Raeburn E. The Morgellons mystery. *Psychol Today Magazine* 2007 Mar 01. http://www.psychologytoday.com/articles/200702/the-morgellons-mystery(Mar).
31. Reilly T, Batchelor D. The presentation and treatment of delusional parasitosis: A dermatological perspective. *Int Clin Psychopharmacol* 1986;1:340–53.
32. Lyell A. Delusions of parasitosis (The Michelson lecture). *Br J Dermatol* 1983;108(4):485–99.
33. Bourgeois ML, Duhamel P, Verdoux H. Delusional parasitosis: Folie a deux and attempted murder of a family doctor. *Br J Psychiatry* 1992;161:709–11.
34. Hylwa SA, Bury JE, Davis MD, Pittelkow M, Bostwick JM. Delusional infestation, including delusions of parasitosis: Results of histologic examination of skin biopsy and patient-provided skin specimens. *Arch Dermatol* 2011 May 16.
35. Bransfield RC. Morgellons disease. *Psychiatr News* 2007;42(11):24.
36. Harvey WT. Morgellons disease. *J Am Acad Dermatol* 2007;56(4):705–6.
37. Harvey WT, Bransfield RC, Mercer DE, Wright AJ, Ricchi RM, Leitao MM. Morgellons disease, illuminating an undefined illness: A case series. *J Med Case Reports* 2009;3:8243.
38. Robles DT, Romm S, Combs H, Olson J, Kirby P. Delusional disorders in dermatology: A brief review. *Dermatol Online J* 2008;14(6):2.
39. Savely VR, Leitao MM, Stricker RB. The mystery of Morgellons disease: Infection or delusion? *Am J Clin Dermatol* 2006;7(1):1–5.
40. Accordino RE, Engler D, Ginsburg IH, Koo J. Morgellons disease? *Dermatol Ther* 2008;21(1):8–12.
41. Davis JL. Rare Skin Problem Baffles Experts. CDC Launches Investigation of Morgellons Disease. *MedicineNetcom WebMD Health News*. 2008 Jan 17, 2008;Sect. http://www.medicinenet.com/script/main/art.asp?articlekey=86523.
42. Harth W, Hermes B, Freudenmann RW. Morgellons in dermatology (Morgellons in der Dermatologie). *J Dtsch Dermatol Ges* 2009 Oct 29.
43. Molyneux J. AKA Morgellons. *Am J Nurs* 2008 May;108(5):25–6.
44. Paquette M. Morgellons: Disease or delusions? *Perspect Psychiatr Care* 2007;43(2):67–8.
45. Pearson ML, Selby JV, Katz KA, Cantrell V, Braden CR, Parise ME, Paddock CD, Lewin-Smith MR, Kalasinsky VF, Goldstein FC, Hightower AW, Papier A, Lewis B, Motipara S, Eberhard ML; Unexplained Dermopathy Study Team. Clinical, epidemiologic, histopathologic and molecular features of an unexplained dermopathy. *PLoS One*. 2012: 7(1):e29908. Epub 2012 Jan 25.
46. Trabert W. Epidemiologie des Dermatozoenwahns [Epidemiology of delusional ectoparasitic infestation]. *Nervenarzt* 1991;62(3):165–9.
47. Trabert W. *Der Dermatozoenwahn. Untersuchungen zur Häufigkeit, Klassifikation und Prognose* [Delusional parasitosis. Studies on frequency, classification and prognosis] [Habilitationsschrift]. Homburg/Saar: Universität des Saarlandes; 1993.
48. Lepping P, Baker C, Freudenmann RW. Delusional infestation in dermatology in the UK: Prevalence, treatment strategies, and feasibility of a RCT. *Clin Exp Dermatol* 2010;35(8):841–4.
49. Bourgeois M, Rager P, Peyre F, Nguyen-Lan A, Etchepare JJ. Fréquence et aspects du syndrome d'Ekbom enquête auprès des dermatologues francais (A propos de 150 cas). *Ann Med Psychol* (Paris) 1986;144(6):659–68.

50. Lepping P, Freudenmann RW. Delusional parasitosis: A new pathway for diagnosis and treatment. *Clin Exp Dermatol* 2008 Jan 16;33(2):113–7.
51. Ungvari G. Behandlung des Dermatozoenwahns durch Neuroleptika [Treatment of a dermatozoon delusion with neuroleptics]. *Psychiatr Prax* 1984;11(4):116–9. [German]
52. Healy R, Taylor R, Dhoat S, Leschynska E, Bewley AP. Management of patients with delusional parasitosis in a joint dermatology/liaison psychiatry clinic. *Br J Dermatol* 2009;161(1):197–9.
53. Hamann K, Avnstorp C. Delusions of infestation treated by pimozide: A double-blind crossover clinical study. *Acta Derm Venereol* 1982;62(1):55–8.
54. Ungvari G, Vladar K. Pimozide treatment for delusion of infestation. *Activitas Nervosa Superior* (Praha) 1986;28(2):103–7.
55. Rathbone J, McMonagle T. Pimozide for schizophrenia or related psychoses. *Cochrane Database Syst Rev* 2007(3):CD001949.
56. Wong S, Bewley A. Patients with Delusional Infestation (Delusional Parasitosis) often require prolonged treatment as recurrence of symptoms after cessation of treatment is common: An observational study. *Br J Dermatol* 2011 May 23. [Epub ahead of print]

Helen D. Pratt

11 Dermatitis artefacta, skin picking, and other self-injurious behaviors: A psychological perspective

One third of young patients seen for dermatologic problems also present with comorbid psychiatric/psychological problems. These youth are vulnerable to chronic self-injurious behavior; in severe cases, they are at risk for suicidal behavior. The majority of youth who self-injure do not intend to commit suicide. Instead, they use their self-injurious behavior as a non-verbal form of communication. Dermatitis artefacta (also called factitious dermatitis or factitious skin disorder) is the deliberate self-harm (DSH) of the tissue of one's own body tissue such as cutting, carving, skin picking (SP), and other self-injurious behaviors, such as self-mutilation behavior (SMB). The psychological literature employs some of the same terms but includes some slightly different terms: self-destructive behavior, self-injurious behavior (SIB), and non-suicidal self-injurious (NSSI) behavior. This chapter focuses on understanding and treating NSSI and includes information that is general and specific to dermatitis artefacta, skin picking, and other self-injurious behaviors. NSSI is often a chronic problem that is associated and comorbid with affective disorders and sometimes with psychosis. Empirically supported treatments (EST) for children and adolescents who engage in NSSI are behavior therapy (BT), cognitive behavior therapy (CBT), and interpersonal behavior therapy (IPT). Teamwork is essential for effective treatment. Referring physicians should serve as the team leader of the medical home and employ consultants as treatment team members; this may include other medical specialists (dermatology and psychiatry), psychologists, social workers, occupational therapists (for youth with tactile issues), parents, and the patient/client when appropriate.

11.1 Introduction

The medical literature refers to deliberate self-injurious behavior as dermatitis artefacta (factitious dermatitis), skin picking, and other self-injurious behaviors (self-mutilation). These behaviors are classified in the psychiatric literature as factitious skin disorders. The psychological literature employs some of the same terms (i.e. deliberate self-harm [DSH], skin picking [SP], and self-mutilation behavior [SMB]) but also includes some slightly different terms, such as self-destructive behavior and self-injurious behavior (SIB). This chapter focuses on non-suicidal self-injurious behavior (NSSI) and includes information that is general and specific to dermatitis artefacta, skin picking, and other self-injurious behavior.

All terminology may include different forms of self-inflicted skin damaging behavior, such as biting, bruising, burning, carving, cutting, gouging, lacerating, scratching, as well as suicidal attempts and completions. Skin picking is classified as unconscious self-injury that is compulsive, repetitive, and habitual. Other self-injurious behaviors may include amputation, castration, and other body modifications. All forms of self-injurious behavior are thought to occur in response to physical pain, psychological pain, chronic medical problems, psychiatric distress, severe mental illness, or psychosis.

Youth who present to their physician's office with symptoms of SIB may be referred to dermatology when their SIB continues or lesions expand, become infected, do not heal, or if they initially appear to be dermatitis artefacta. A significant number (30%) of young patients seen for dermatologic problems also present with comorbid psychiatric/psychological problems; as a result these youth are vulnerable to suicidal behavior (see Table 11.1) (1,2,3,4,5,6,7,8,9). The risk of suicidal attempts and completions increase with comorbid severe mental illness, psychosis, and a history of DSH (10–14). Those youth who engage in SIB with the intent of suicide represent the highest level of psychopathology (3,11,12,15). The most extreme form of SIB is suicide.

Table 11.1: Behaviors, cognitions, psychiatric disorders that are associated or comorbid with NSSI (1,2,3,4,5,6,7,8,9)

Determatitis Artefacta (4) and NSSI	Skin Picking	Other Self-Injurious Behavior
Associations	**Associations**	**Associations**
Depression	Anxiety	Depression
Anxiety	Inattention	Depression and dissociation
Substance use	Oppositional attitude	Self-burning with self-cutting
Poor family function	Developmental functioning	Self-mutilating behavior
Unstable body image	Quality of life issues	Traumatic events
Family history (1st degree relatives) of psychiatric disorders		
Neuropsychological trauma		
Individual Psychosocial factors		
Poor coping mechanisms		
Victim of child abuse		
Comorbidity	**Comorbidity**	
Personality disorders – borderline	PWS ritualistic behaviors	
Personality disorder	Food-related and non-food-related	
Delusional disorders	hoarding excessive cleaning	
Dissociative disorders	Ordering	
Eating disorders	Arranging	
Bulimia nervosa		
Binge eating		

(Continued)

Table 11.1: Behaviors, cognitions, psychiatric disorders that are associated or comorbid with NSSI (1,2,3,4,5,6,7,8,9) (*Continued*)

Determatitis Artefacta (4) and NSSI	Skin Picking	Other Self-Injurious Behavior
Purging Mood disorders Chronic pain syndromes Chronic dermatological disorders, specifically: Acne Alopecia (ie, alopecia areata, androgenic alopecia) Atopic dermatitis Chronic idiopathic urticaria Psoriasis Rosacea Vitiligo	Needing to ask or tell Self-mutilating behavior	

11.2 Epidemiology

Prevalence for specific SIB varies widely (7.5–61%) depending on the population and comorbid disorders (see Table 11.2) (1,2,3,4,5,6,7,8,9,10,11,12,13,14,15,16,17,18). The lifetime prevalence of SIB for Japanese students was reported as 9.9% in one study (15). A review of the literature on dermatitis artefacta concluded that the incidence for youth in the United States is 1 in 23,000 (4). While the data did not identify specific demographic variables (i.e. ethnic, racial, or economic factors) that described those affected by NSSI, gender predominance was female.

Other studies include populations such as the following: (a) European and Euro, Hispanic, and African Americans; (b) youth from other countries and cultures whose ethnicity was not defined; (c) youth diagnosed with mental illness (eating disorders [ED], major depression [MDD], psychosis, substance abuse), (d) developmental disabilities (autism spectrum disorders [ASD], Down syndrome [DS]), and (e) intellectual disabilities (ID; i.e. mental retardation [MR] and Prader-Willi syndrome [PWS]).

These study subjects were evaluated in academic settings (middle school, high school, and early college), psychiatric hospitals, outpatient clinics, juvenile detention centers, and community centers; these subjects were randomly selected. These subjects lived in several countries and regions of their countries, including Finland, Germany, Hong Kong (China), Japan, Mexico City (Mexico), Northwest United Kingdom, Switzerland, southeastern and midwestern regions of the United States, and Western Australia (1,2,3,4,5,19,20,21). Females showed a significant increase in their rates of NSSI during adolescence as compared to males (22).

The highest incidences of dermatitis artefacta are between the ages of 11–14 years (2,4,10,11,12). Research providing prevalence data are limited for children and

Table 11.2: Studies reviewed for age range, populations, gender, incidence and prevalence

Authors	Year	Ages	Population/Setting	Gender	Incidence and Prevalence
Baetens, Claes, Muehlenka, Grietens, Onghena (10)	2011	12–18	1,417		13.71%
Cloutier, Martin, Kennedy, Nixon, Muehlenkamp (11)	2010	12–17 yrs	468 youth emergency crisis services	63.5% Female	50% self harmed most within 24 hours of admission
Hankin, Abela (12)	2011	11–14	103 community sample 2½-yr study		18%
Hilt, Cha, Nolen–Hoeksema (2)	2008	10–14 years	94 49% Hispanic; 25% African American 6th, 7th, and 8th graders questionnaire survey of community sample	Female	Overall 7.5%
Maclean (13)	2010	<6 yrs Mean age 42.7 mos.	Developmental delays Cerebral Palsey Autism Seizure disorders		32%
MatsumotoT, Yamaguchi, Chiba, Asami, Iseki, Hirayasu (14)	2005		201 Japan Juvenile Detention Center Questionnaire		33 (16.4%) had cut their wrists or forearms at least once 35.8% burned self at least once
Tang, Yu, Wu, Du, Ma, Zhu, et al. (15)	2011	10–24	Chinese/Han adolescents and college students	912 female 1,101 males	15.5%,
Mitrou, Gaudie, Lawrence, Silburn, Stanley, Zubrick (16)	2010	4–16 to 18–31	2,736 Western Australian random sample		37 (1.4%)
You, Leung, Fu, Lai (17)	2011		6,374 17-yr study Hong Kong Chinese adolescents secondary school students	67.6% female	15%

(Continued)

Table 11.2: Studies reviewed for age range, populations, gender, incidence and prevalence (*Continued*)

Authors	Year	Ages	Population/Setting	Gender	Incidence and Prevalence
			Eating Disorders		
Peebles, Wilson, Lock (8)	2011	10–21,	1,432 Diagnosed with eating disorders (ED) in an academic center	Female	40.8%
			Dermatitis Artefacta		
Koo (4)	2009	≤6	Children and adolescents	Female 4.7:7.1	1 case in 23,000
			Self-Mutilation		
Ross, Heath, Toste (18)	2009	440		Female	13.9%
			Skin-Picking		
Morgan, Storch, Woods, Bodzin, Lewin, Murphy (5)	2010	15–19	67 subjects Internet-based survey of parents about their child		95.5% of youth in study 49.3% on hands

adolescents diagnosed with dermatitis artefacta. The epidemiological data is most often offered for other forms of NSSI, such as skin picking (SP), which is a very common problem (86–95.5%) among youth with Prader-Willi syndrome, severe mental retardation, and psychosis (6,23).

11.3 Etiology

The causes of NSSI, dermatitis artefacta, SP, and other SIB are multifactorial, poorly understood, and the range varies widely depending on the study population (4). Causes of all NSSI are "probable causes and associations" (i.e. genetics, personal or family history of psychiatric illness, and other psychosocial factors) (3,4,5,12, 13,14,21,24). One explanation for the development of NSSI among children and adolescents is that they are responding to stresses of growth and development. As youth matriculate through the stages of adolescence toward adulthood, they experience many significant changes (i.e. biological, cognitive, emotional, hormonal, physical, and psychosocial) and experience increasing demands on their abilities to meet personal, interpersonal, and public expectations (coaches, college admissions committees, employers, family, intimate partners, parents, peers, and teachers) (2). Younger children and adolescents are less equipped to cope with all the factors of change (contextual features, frequency, intensity and complexity) (4).

All of these changes and demands may produce distress in some youth and result in NSSI. Reactions to emotional, physical, mental, and comorbid affective disorders are often manifested in the dermis. The interconnectedness among mind, body, nervous system, and the dermis may result in itching skin, acne, rashes, and hives (see Chapter 2). This may originally begin with scratching until damage to the skin occurs (4).

Some researchers suggest that the act of producing skin lesions and the visual stimulus of the lesions can serve as powerful, self-expressive, non-verbal messages. When an individual engages in SIB, the visual and proprioceptive stimuli produced in the brain may cause them to feel relief, escape, or reduce the discomfort. A maladaptive response set develops:

a. The adolescent becomes distressed and engages in SIB;
b. He or she experiences relief or stress reduction;
c. The distress, SIB, relief cycle develops;
d. Repeated instances of this cycle strengthens the behavior of SIB;
e. This results in stronger ties between the SIB, stress reduction, psychological pain reduction, and, sometimes, the elimination of these aversive/negative stressors.

In cases of severe comorbid mental disorders, individuals may report psychological feelings of euphoria or other strong emotions when they self-injure (2,5). No one knows how this almost automatic reaction to irritants to the skin then morphs into the individual engaging in NSSI (i.e. burning, cutting [See Figure 11.1], stabbing, carving, puncturing, or scratching).

The onset, duration, frequency, intensity, and severity of the self-inflicted harm are triggered, exacerbated, and maintained by the individual factors, social factors, and environmental factors (see Tables 11.3 and 11.4).

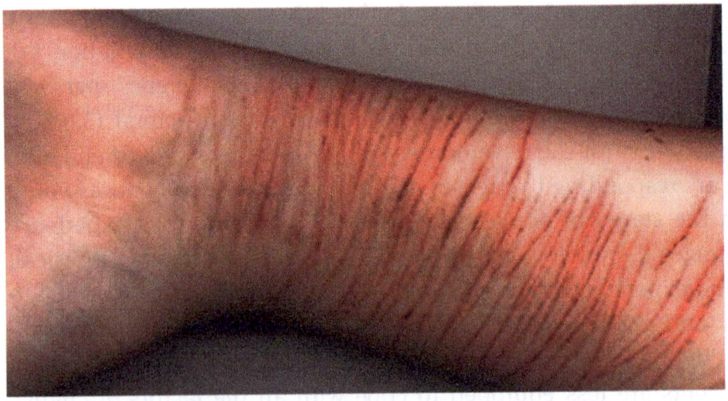

Figure 11.1: Self-cutting.

Table 11.3: Risk factors for SIB in childhood and adolescence (1,2,3,4,5,6,7,8,9,10,11,12,13,14,15,16,17,18,23,24,25,26,27,30,31)

Bully victim	Poor relationship quality (parents, peers, friends, at school)
Bulimia nervosa	Previous body customization
Cognitive vulnerabilities	Previous over dose
Co-morbid mood disorder	Previous psychiatric treatment
Diagnosis of borderline personality disorder	Previous self-mutilation
Excessive reassurance seeking	Previous self-injury
Extensive psychotherapy	Previous suicide attempts
Extreem intoxication + psychotic disorder	Severe or chronic mental illness (affective disorders, psychotic disorders)
History of binge eating, purging	Severe mental illness
Intellectual disability (ID)	Social isolation
Prader Willi syndrome	Substance use, or abuse
Down syndrome	Suicidal attempts
autism spectrum disorders	Stressors
Interpersonal vulnerabilities	Temperament (difficult anxious, attachment issues)
Mothers' depression	Youth with sensory impairments and intellectual disabilities
Multiple visits to the emergency or crisis rooms	Youths' depression

Risk factors (see Table 11.3) for developing NSSI and reasons why youth say they engaged in NSSI are varied and most often involve mental illness, affective states, and social conditions (see Table 11.4) (1,2,3,4,5,6,7,8,9,10,11,12,13,14,15,16,17,18,19,20,21,22,23,24,25,26,27,28,29,30,31,32,33,34). Individuals who engage in SIB often deny responsibility for their wounds, and this denial often makes detection of NSSI difficult (4). In some cases where there is comorbid mental illness, the adolescent may wear the NSSI as a "badge of courage" and do it to control stimuli in the affected youth's life or to manipulate contingencies (even people) in their environment. In the medical environment, damage to a person's body usually receives immediate attention, intervention, and follow-up. Such attention may serve to reward NSSI, thus increasing this maladaptive behavior and serving to undermine the benefits of treatment. Youth who have repeated NSSI combined with suicide attempts and/or psychiatric illness may develop a lifelong pattern of NSSI (7). Youth diagnosed with intellectual disability and have chronic repetitive NSSI are at the highest risk of NSSI when they are agitated. Chronic NSSI usually continues into adulthood (5,14,22,23,29).

11.4 Clinical features

Episodes of NSSI can be acute or episodic, and chronic SIB may result in permanent scaring of the body tissue (4,35). The characteristics of NSSI are generally stable across cultures (1,2,3,4,5,20,21). Most data from empirical studies on interventions

Table 11.4: Reasons for nonsuicidal self-injury (1,2,3,4,5,6,7,8,9,10,11,12,13,14,15,16,17,18,23,24,30,31,34)

Cognitive Control
To resist suicidal thoughts
To influence others
To resolve times of dissociation
To use as a practiced ritual
To escape or avoid unwanted cognitions
Interpersonal Relationship Control
To display affection for a current boyfriend, girlfriend, or significant other
To address interpersonal distress (peer victimization)
To regulate the social environment
To reduce social conflict
To suppress an unwanted social stimulus
To reduce emotional conflict with in self
To suppress self-threatening cognitions
To reduce or eliminate psychological numbness
To retaliate being jilted by a boyfriend or disciplined by a parent
To reduce distressing symptoms of posttraumatic stress as a social strategy
To seek help from others
To escape or avoid an unwanted interpersonal interaction
Emotional Regulation
To suppress negative affect
To express self-anger
To express disgust
To act out feelings of rage
To express sadness
To alleviate chronic depression
To suppress feelings of emptiness
To suppress feelings of hurt
To suppress feelings of rejection
To suppress feelings of loss
To respond to a sense of increasing tension
To escape or avoid an unwanted situation
Environmental Stressors
To being laughed at
To being teased
To being alone
Habituation
To needing sensory stimulus to reduce or eliminate boredom

for SIB are published in the behavioral literature and focus on individuals with developmental disability and intellectual disability. Although research on NSSI is limited, studies that do exist are based on retrospective data from surveys or reviews of hospital or institutional records. Another form of data gathering comes from serial case reviews of youth who engage in SIB, and NSSI data was often culled from that data. Longtitudinal studies of NSSI and outcomes provide another avenue for retrospective and outcome data. Still, few empirical studies exist.

Youth diagnosed with Down syndrome engage in more significant NSSI than those with Prader-Willi syndrome (i.e. head hitting and may focus on their eyes, ears, or mouths or bang their heads on walls); those diagnosed with autistic spectrum disorders more often hit and bite themselves, targeting their heads, hands, and legs (30). Youth with profound intellectual disabilities are particularly vulnerable to SIB and often have chronic behavioral patterns of injury; once a pattern is well-established, there is a relative lack of effective treatment (3,22,29). Consequently, most experts call for early and intensive intervention at many levels to prevent the accumulation of psychological problems (3,22).

The families of youth who inflict significant damage to their bodies from engaging in NSSI (especially those with developmental disabilities, intellectual disabilities, and profound mental retardation) may experienced marked distress over the damage to their children (26). A review of the empirical literature on NSSI supports that youth engage in this behavior for multiple reasons that may serve to allow the affected individuals

a. to control their internal feelings (stress reduction);
b. to escape or avoid aversive conditions, situations, tasks, or stimuli;
c. to control social contact either that will make people go away so that he or she can be alone, or so that he or she will get the attention of others or access to wanted tangible objects or events (i.e. food, music, ability to watch television); or
d. to generate sensory reinforcement as a means to change boring sensory stimuli (7,9,13,31,32,33).

11.4.1 Dermatitis Artefacta

In *dermatitis artefacta* youth produce cutaneous lesions on their body and engage in self-injury consciously and deliberately in order to satisfy an unconscious psychological or emotional need (4). Affected youth generally focus their SIB on easily accessible body parts (i.e. arms, face, hands, legs, and stomach) mostly on the nondominant side of the body. Cutting and scratching occur most often in youth of normal intellectual functioning, while severe skin picking, biting, and gouging occur most often in youth with developmental disability, Down syndrome, intellectual disability, and mental retardation (26).

Youth may use their digits, finger nails, teeth, objects (i.e. razor blades, knives, pencils, pens, safety pins, paper clips, broken glass, or other sharps), or chemical means to injure themselves. Lesions are generally symmetric or linear, and the shapes vary according to the method used (see Figure 11.1) (4,6,21). Examination of the limbs, stomach, inner thighs, breasts, and the face on the non-dominant side of the body may reveal (a) superficial lesions in about half of presenting youth, and (b) hyper-pigmented macules or purpura in one third (4). Some adolescents may also present with self-inflicted tattoo-like scars.

Three fourths of youth will engage in one type of SIB on one or two areas of the body. Three or more lesions or damaged body parts increases the likelihood the individual will have disfiguring scars on exposed body areas. This also indicates serious pathology and increased risk of suicidal behavior (5,10,12,15,16,18). Self-injurers who engage in repetitive NSSI will have more emotional and impulse-control problems than episodic self-injurers (1,25).

11.4.2 Skin picking

Skin picking (SP) is characterized by repetitive, ritualistic, or impulsive skin picking that leads to tissue damage and causes significant distress or impairment in daily functioning. It may be maintained by contingent arousal reduction (5). Common areas of picking also include nail cuticles, scalp, and picking at scabs on the skin (see Figure 11.2) or in the nose, in addition to those areas listed for NSSI. Skin picking is associated with obsessive compulsive disorders, anxiety disorders, body dysmorphic disorder, impulse control disorders, trichotillomania, and other repetitive or ritualistic behaviors (i.e. head banging) (4,5). Skin picking is a compulsive behavior in 70% of adolescent patients diagnosed with Prader-Willi syndrome and is significantly increased in frequency when these youth are agitated.

In most cases skin picking primarily has non-social functions and may be targeted toward existing blemishes, imaginary flaws, or areas of the skin that are irritated. The picking behavior can involve picking, pulling, poking, prodding, scratching, squeezing, or tearing of the skin on any part of the body. Skin picking (80% to 90%) occurs when the adolescent is at school, waiting on something, watching TV, in the car, or lying in bed. Affected youth (30% to 40%) pick while they are reading, taking a shower, while sleeping, when denied food, while on the phone, or when looking in a mirror. The consequences of skin picking for the individual (46–80%) include developing minor sores, scars, or infections (20).

11.4.3 Self-mutilation behavior

SMB is the deliberate and impulsive alteration or destruction of body tissue without conscious suicidal intent. SMB includes two broad categories labeled as

(a)

(b)

(c)

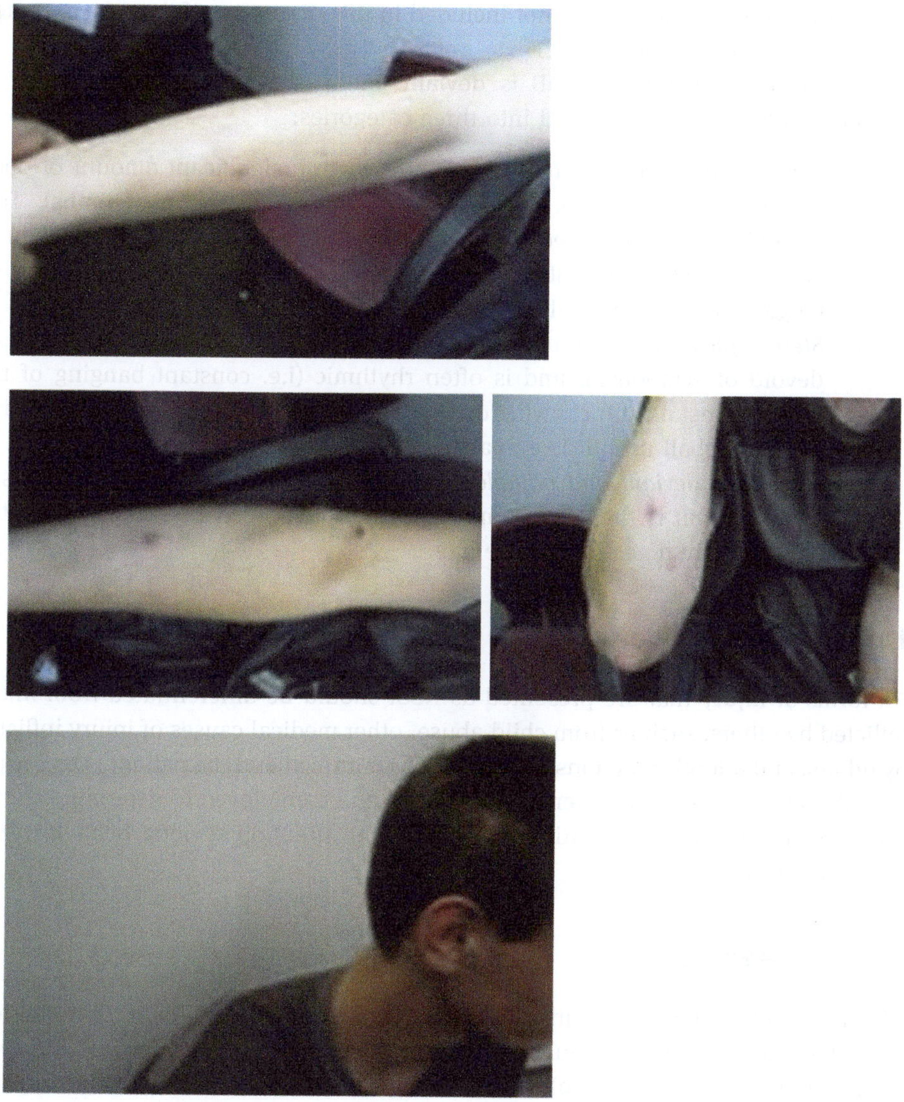

Figure 11.2: (a) Skin Picking; (b) Scarring from repeated skin-picking over 6 months in a 16 year old male; (c) Accompanying acne.

culturally sanctioned rituals and practices as well as deviant and pathological behaviors (21).

1. The first category includes culturally sanctioned rituals and practices (i.e. ear piercing and genital circumcision, scarification, and other rituals) that are the custom of the individual's group or culture or to signify rites of passage.

Scarification and tattoos are not included in this discussion if they are executed by professional artists (1,20,21).

2. The second category of SMB is deviant and pathological self-injury that is self-mutilation and is divided into three categories:

   a. *Major SMB* involves infrequent acts in which a significant amount of body tissue is destroyed (i.e. self-castration or self-amputation of limbs). This form of SMB is associated with organicity and usually occurs while the individual is extremely intoxicated or suffering from psychosis (including religious or demonic delusions).
   b. *Stereotypic deviant and pathological SMB* has fixed patterns of expression, is devoid of symbolism, and is often rhythmic (i.e. constant banging of the head against a wall, chewing on fingers that destroys the tissue, or pressing on the eyeball until it is damaged or destroyed).
   c. *Superficial deviant and pathological SMB* includes repetitive and ritualistic behavior that is the most common form of compulsive behavior and often occurs many times in a single day.

11.5 Differential diagnosis

All forms of injury that are presented as NSSI should be differentiated from injury inflicted by others, such as from child abuse, other medical causes of injury inflicted by others, and allergic reactions. Once NSSI is confirmed and the patient is medically and physically stable, the differential process can be employed to determine causation (i.e. stress, anger, retaliation, retribution, or attention seeking behavior) (see Table 11.5) (4,27,35).

11.6 Management

All adolescents who present with behavioral or mental health problems that interfere with their daily function should be screened for (a) suicidal behavior (ideation, intent, attempts, and plans), (b) any tissue damage, (c) a combination of eating disorders and NSSI, and (d) previous SIB of any kind. The index of suspicion is highest for severe SIB combined with psychosis.

Treatment of NSSI, SP, and SMB present many challenges (ethical, methodological, and practical). Reasons for ethical issues involve delivering treatments for severe SIB that are unacceptable to many members of our society, such as electroconvulsive shock therapy (ECT). ECT is highly controversial and has had many legal challenges. However, it is one option for treating children and youth who engage in stereotypic SMB (destroying their eyes, lip tissue, fingers, skulls, and brain matter).

The use of helmets to protect the brains of youth who head bang and physical restraints to keep youth who gouge their eyes out, tear off their ears, or bite off their

Table 11.5: Differential diagnoses for dermatitis artefacta

Rule Out Other Causes	
Medical or Mental Causes (4)	**Mimics and Associations** (4)
Hypochondriasis	Pyoderma gangrenosum
Substance abuse disorder	Acquired hemophilia
Psychotic disorders	T-cell lymphoma
Neurotic excoriation (conscious compulsive nature)	Hepatitis C virus–associated porphyria Cutanea tarda.
Not a factitious disorders	**Plants that produce similar symptoms** (36)
Delusional disorders	Four main plant families:
Malingering	1. Umbelliferae (hogweed, cow parsley, wild parsnip, celery, wild carrots)
Münchhausen syndrome (except Münchhausen syndrome by proxy)	2. Rutaceae (rue bergamont, citrus fruits),
Dermatitis neglecta	3. Moraceae (figs)
Painful bruise syndrome	4. Leguminosae (scurf pea)
Alopecia areata	Self-mutilation (18)
Anagen effluvium	**Comorbidity**
Atopic dermatitis	Delusional disorders
Bedbug bites	Neurotic excoriation (conscious compulsive nature).
Contact dermatitis, allergic	Psychotic disorders
Contact dermatitis, irritant	Substance abuse
Delusions of parasitosis	Extreme intoxication
Friction blisters	
Impetigo	
Insect bites	
Onycholysis	
Prurigo nodularis	
Pruritus and systemic disease	
Telogen effluvium	

digits have also faced ethical and legal challenges. One major issue with the use of helmets and other "protective" wear is in the mental health realm. United States federal, state, and local governments and their entities regulate the use of "restrictive equipment interventions for special populations" (youth, mental health recipients, prisoners, etc.); use of such equipment has to be approved by behavior management boards and monitored to ensure appropriate and correct use. The use of helmets falls under these guidelines. Reasons for challenging the use of ECT and restrictive interventions include the following:

1. A clear understanding of causation is not available.
2. Effective treatment design is problematic because identifying specific characteristics and correlates of self-injurious behavior is difficult as the use of typical components of research design (control groups, wait lists, with holding treatment,

and matched pairs) that allow researchers to identify clinical and cost effective components of treatment are unacceptable with this population.
3. Data on empirically based effective interventions are sparse. The behavior of self-injury is not the focus of treatment interventions. The literature supports that the focus of treatment is usually on underlying causes (i.e. anxiety, depression, stress, and compulsive behaviors).
4. Access to clinicians with essential knowledge and skills to design ethical, cost effective, and clinically effective treatment is limited. Clinicians require specialized training and specific skills to work with children and adolescents who have mental illness, behavioral problems, and NSSI.
5. Interventions designed to eliminate or reduce NSSI usually employ extinction as a part of the contingency plan. Once stimuli that maintain a person's NSSI are removed, the behavior undergoes an "extinction burst," which is a brief time where the NSSI behavior increases; because of the increased NSSI, more serious/intense and frequent damage may occur. Although this outcome is brief and expected, most observers cannot tolerate this increase in SIB. The use of extinction procedures also presents ethical challenges due to the transient increase in self-injury.
6. When youth are required to wear personal protective equipment (PPE), their mobility might be restricted.
7. Youth who must wear helmets to prevent brain damage may be embarrassed to be seen in public wearing their personal protective equipment. This is a serious concern for many members of behavior management boards and for some parents. (27,32,33,34)

Medical treatment of wounds is necessary but may not be sufficient for children and adolescents who engage in NSSI, SIB, and SMB. Youth who self-injure need assistance in correcting their maladaptive responses to aversive stimuli in their lives. Their parents also need support to help their children develop adaptive and functional behavior to matriculate to adulthood. Psychopharmacological management and psychotherapy are two choices for treatment options for affected youth. Basic office counseling is the first intervention, but if the NSSI continues or increases, further evaluation is necessary. Those youth who engage in SMB, suicidal behavior, or are experiencing psychosis (hallucination or delusions) require referral to a psychiatrist. A referral to a skilled clinician/therapist for psychotherapy is more relevant in the absence of psychosis.

Prior to any referrals, the referring clinician should gather background information on premorbid functioning, physical health, family mental and physical health histories, social and emotional functioning, hospitalization history, personal mental status, academic function, cognitive and intellectual functioning, and any previous mental health treatments. This detailed background information will enhance the evaluation process for all subsequent referrals. Along with the referral letter, a signed release of information (by the parents or legal guardians of the youth) will allow the referral clinician to return the results of the evaluation. Mental health clinicians cannot send any information to a referring physician without a release. If a release accompanies the referral, the clinician receiving the referral can contact the referring physician if the youth cancels or does not show.

11.6.1 Pharmacological Treatment

One empirical study systematically examined the evidence for the pharmacological management of severely disruptive and noncompliant behavior and SIB with youth diagnosed with pervasive developmental disorders (PDD), such as autism spectrum disorders (26). Treatment consisted of parent training combined with administration of risperidone (over 6 months) and showed greater reduction in behavioral problems (such as irritability, tantrums, and impulsiveness) (26).

Researchers in a separate systematic review of the PubMed database found 21 English language biomedical articles on clinical trials with medication in autism spectrum disorders (27). Their efforts yielded five medications that produced significant improvement as compared to placebo, including tianeptine, methylphenidate, risperidone, clonidine, and naltrexone. However, only risperidone and methylphenidate demonstrated results that have been replicated across at least two studies. They concluded that although many medications have been studied under placebo-controlled conditions, few produced significant improvement, and they called for additional research.

Psychopharmacological treatments are directed at treating the underlying causes of NSSI or for healing wounds. Reduction or elimination of maladaptive behavior in NSSI is a by-product of addressing those causes. No empirical studies or reviews of the literature reported approved uses of medication for the treatment of NSSI. Psychopharmacological interventions are for treatment of the underlying mental health issues of NSSI.

11.6.2 Psychotherapy

Psychotherapy is an umbrella term for the use of “talk” therapy. Clinicians can be counselors, psychiatrists, psychologists, or social workers. These clinicians obtain special training to develop skills and competency in the delivery of specific treatment techniques based on a particular theoretical orientation (see Chapter 23). Clinicians/therapists generally approach therapy based on their personal theoretical orientation, knowledge of treatment interventions, and skill. All clinicians/therapists conduct an assessment of the client’s/patient’s needs and then select a type of treatment designed to attain the client’s/patient’s goal(s).

These clinicians/therapists work with patients and their parents (guardians) to help them understand personal and family strengths as well as weaknesses. Clinicians/therapists then help patients and parents (a) develop strategies to minimize the negative impact of the youth's disorder, (b) develop and implement strategies to resolve or minimize their problems, (c) evaluate outcomes, and (d) make adjustments to unsuccessful strategies until the goals of therapy are met.

In all forms of psychotherapy, therapists help clients/patients identify upsetting thoughts and feelings, explore self-defeating patterns of behavior, identify difficult and potentially toxic situations as well as people, and learn alternative ways to handle their emotions surrounding these issues (37). Psychotherapy is appropriate for adolescents who have normal intellectual development and well developed executive functioning. Therapy involves addressing cognitive skills (i.e. thinking, problem solving, planning, and executing), coping skills, and in-depth psychological counseling.

Psychotherapy is divided into modalities (e.g. individual, group, family) and multiple theoretical approaches to treatment (e.g. behavior therapy (BT), cognitive behavior therapy (CBT), interpersonal psychotherapy (IPT), psychoanalytic, etc.; see Table 11.6) (36,37). Three specific types of therapies were identified as having

Table 11.6: Modalities of psychotherapy (37)

Individual Therapy
Psychotherapy is most effective with individuals who are of average to above average intelligence and who have well developed abstract thinking (understanding and processing complex information from its parts, logical thinking, executive functioning), and communication skills (receptive and expressive listening, reflective listening skills).
Family Therapy
This form of therapy involves immediate family members or careproviders and the affected patient and it focuses on improving interpersonal and group dynamics; communications affect the function of family members to help them modify problem dynamics within the family. Positive changes can be made to improve the family's ability to be a positive environment for its members, and especially the member who engages in NSSI. Interventions from BT, CBT (conflict management, anger management, self control), psychoanalysis (resolve psychic distress), and social psychology (social skills, child management training) are adapted to address the family issues and problems.
Group Psychotherapy
This modality provides patients/clients with access to youth who have common problems. In this type of treatment, youth learn from structured interventions delivered by clinicians/therapists. In most groups, professionals guide patients/clients through problem solving and conflict resolution exercises. In some groups, the patient/client's peers deliver challenges and advice under the guidance of the therapist. Most groups are homogeneous and offer a supportive environment. The groups generally meet at a specific time, in a specific place, and for a specific length of time. The groups are either open (members are allowed to attend at will and new members are allowed) or closed (a certain number of patients/clients are allowed to participate and no new members are allowed after the first session).

well established research to support that they are efficacious in treating children and adolescents who exhibit symptoms of underlying psychological/psychiatric issues associated and/or comorbid with NSSI (see Table 11.7) (37,38). Readers who would like to review treatments that were identified as "probably efficacious," and "possibly efficacious" are referred to URL: http://www.effectivechildtherapy.com/sccap/ for detailed information (37).

Table 11.7: Types of Psychotherapy (37)

Behavior Therapy (BT)

Behavior therapy employs: (a) problem identification; (b) identifying the target behavior for intervention; (c) contingency management; (d) training of change agents (i.e., therapists, teachers, parents, and care providers) (e) implementation of interventions; (f) evaluating outcomes to determine if the intervention is effective by seeking feedback from all participants; and (g) modifying parts of the intervention program that are not effective.

Experts in behavior analysis agree that conducting a functional analysis is an essential part of a successful treatment. This analysis will strengthen the analyst's ability to use contingency management. This step has 5 major components:

1. Functional analysis allows analysts to identify the controlling variables (establishing operations, antecedents, behavior, and consequences). (36)

   a. The establishing operations (EO) are those environmental stimuli or conditions that set the stage for the antecedent stimuli, and alter the effect of rewards and aversive consequences of the target behaviors.

   b. Antecedents are stimuli (like anxiety or stress) that cue the individual to engage in the target behavior

   c. Target behavior (NSSI) is the maladaptive behavior.

   d. The consequence of this maladaptive behavior is the relief or reduction of feelings of the anxiety.

2. The analyst the looks to identify which environmental conditions or stimuli occur that cause the individual to "feel" anxious or distressed. Typically, the antecedent-behavior-consequence triad is what most analysts address when writing behavior management interventions to control NSSI. Many interventions fail if they do not address the appropriate target: the conditions under which the antecedent occurs. The target of the analyst's efforts, when directed at eliminating or reducing the antecedent versus focusing on the NSSI, is appropriate. The correct target of change is the reason why individuals experience anxiety or distress. Once identification of the cause of the distress occurs, the analyst can design an intervention that changes environmental conditions that result in the patient/client experiencing anxiety or distress.

3. The next step is to meet with the parents, teachers, care providers and the patient/client invested in affecting positive change in the clients/patients behavior. The information gathered allows the design of an acceptable intervention.

4. All individuals involved in the clients/patients' lives should receive specific training on program implementation or support.

5. Implementation of the program occurs.

(*Continued*)

Table 11.7: Types of Psychotherapy (37) *(Continued)*

6. Monitoring of the program and involved family or staff is essential to ensure success of the interventions. Monitoring helps, the analyst identify problems, and implement changes that can reduce or avert difficulties with maintaining positive changes in the target behavior. It is highly advisable for program designers and all interested parties meet often to monitor the program and make appropriate adjustments to the program. (36)
Habit Reversal Therapy (HRT) is a form of BT that treats maladaptive compulsive and repetitive behaviors. (20,33) Youth who engage in NSSI (especially SP) learn to engage in behaviors that are incompatible with self-injury. Most studies show that the following techniques are successful in reducing or extinguishing self-injurious skin picking: (a) awareness training, (b) competing response training, (c) relaxation training, (d) contingency reinforcement, (e) emotional regulation training, and (f) anger and/or stress management training. Habit reversal is good for automatic reinforcement (i.e., self stimulating behavior). (38) HRT is also effective in treating lip and mouth biting and self-choking, but research with general NSSI populations is limited. HRT is effective with youth with limited cognitive function as well as those with normal cognitive function.
Cognitive-Behavioral Therapy (CBT)
This is a structured and directive method of therapy designed to help youth work on immediate issues and change his or her maladaptive behavior. CBT combines components of psychotherapy (challenging assumptions, didactic discussion, cognitive processing, problems solving, and behavior therapy (problem solving, planning, relaxation training, social skills training, stress management, systematic desensitization, and time management), support groups, parent training, teacher training, and peer mediation. Adolescents learn to use the Socratic Method to improve their ability to think through their problems and employ induction to challenge assumptions that result in negative feelings [guilt, hopelessness, self-blame, and thoughts of worthlessness] with rational thinking. This form of therapy is appropriate for addressing the underlying psychological problems that are associated and comorbid with NSSI.
Interpersonal Psychosocial Therapy (IPT)
Youth who engage in NSSI have significant psychological problems. ITP focuses on helping youth address issues with personality characteristics, behavior, interpersonal and social relationships, and depression. The effects of poor or problematic communication skills plays a major role in the adolescent's part of those interactions and plays a major role in the development inter- and intra-personal relationships. Youth learn to address distressful and problematic issues related to growing up and struggling to attain independence. Youth who successfully complete treatment learn how to manage their feeling of loss by helping them effectively mourn perceived or real losses and prepare for role transitions.

The well established empirically based treatments for specific disorders are as follows (37):

1. CBT was effective in treating symptoms of generalized anxiety disorders using individual therapy and group therapy (with and without parents present).
2. CBT was effective in treating symptoms of depression using group therapy (child or adolescent groups and child and parents groups).

3. IPT was effective in treating symptoms of depression using individual therapy.
4. BT (using parent management training) was effective in treating disruptive behavior problems, such as those exhibited by youth diagnosed with oppositional behavior disorder (ODD) and conduct disorder (CD).
5. CBT was effective in treating symptoms of posttraumatic stress disorder (PTSD) using trauma-focused interventions.
6. CBT was effective in treating youth with symptoms of substance abuse using group therapy.

11.6.3 Issues with Treatment

Effective treatment interventions with children and adolescents suffering from mental health problems are limited. A review of the literature on well-established effective psychological treatments based on empirical and studies published in peer reviewed journals yielded no additional interventions. A number of issues plague the use of psychotherapy with youth:

1. One major controversy regarding treatment of children and adolescents focuses on the use of empirically supported treatments (EST) to determine which mental health psychotherapies are best for working with youth.
   a. There are problems with only using empirically based treatments; clinicians charge that the use of research subjects in contrived environments limits the utility of outcomes from the studies. Replication of research methods and obtaining similar treatment results are difficult to produce in community settings, treatment facilities, and private offices.
   b. A number of practicing clinicians caution clinicians and researchers against only embracing treatments that are "empirically based." They argue that this approach is ignoring that these types of treatments have little to no relevance to the realities of treating clients/patients in the offices of clinicians in practice.
   c. A number of "promising and probably" efficacious treatment interventions are reported in the literature. The movement toward promoting "proven" and evidence-based treatments for mental health problems is following the medical model of clinical research and trials. Most clinicians support efforts to ensure that all youth receive clinical and cost-effective treatments. However, these clinicians counter that ESTs are not the only treatment interventions that work with youth. They cite such issues as culture, ethnicity, religion, gender, family structure, and socioeconomic status as each affecting the types of therapies that work with different populations.

2. A different empirical study examined the use of group therapy to treat NSSI in adolescents using a structured treatment program (manualized program: 6 weekly sessions plus a booster). This treatment package was specifically designed for adolescents (12–17 years) who (a) had harmed themselves at least two times and (b) were not psychotic or institutionalized. Researchers concluded that individuals who completed this type of group therapy did not have fewer episodes of NSSI, nor was the treatment therapeutic or cost effective (24).
3. Although CBT and IPT are effective with treating the underlying symptoms of NSSI, they are not effective with youth diagnosed with mental retardation, developmental disabilities, intellectual disabilities, or with youth who suffer from other severe impairments. This population does best with BT and a BT intervention program called Habit Reversal Training (HRT). These treatment interventions are good for addressing scratching and chronic skin picking, but if the target behavior is maintained because the client/patient engages for escape or avoidance, the HRT should not be used.
4. Psychotherapy is not effective with very young children as their cognitive skills are limited (i.e. abstract and deductive reasoning).
5. Play therapy works best for young children. However this type of therapy is not listed as "efficacious with children" but is identified as "probably efficacious." It is one form of intervention for youth who are very concrete in their thinking skills and learn best when exposed to visual stimuli plus oral stimuli. Skilled clinicians/therapists address problems by using directed play therapy where they present structured and guided activities designed to address problems and process emotions.

   The use of pretend and interactive activities between the therapist and child and between the therapist, child, and parent allows parents to teach and reward adaptive behaviors. Children can make mistakes and correct their actions based on parental feedback. The child is taught how to handle personal pain and distress as well as how to deal with the cognitive and behavioral challenges they face. Patients/clients are taught to engage in alternative behaviors instead of NSSI. For example, instead of biting, cutting, hitting, or scratching themselves, the child learns to squeeze a ball, hit a pillow, draw, run, or talk to a trusted person.

   Parents are taught to help their child learn these skills through play. Clinicians who use a form of directed play therapy called parent interaction therapy use the process as follows: they (a) train parents how to employ techniques designed to teach adaptive play, (b) monitor them through two way mirrors, and (c) provide feedback (corrective and praise) as the parents play with their children. Parents learn how to interact with their children to produce adaptive socially acceptable behavior and how to maintain growth in therapy.

6. An additional barrier to treatment of NSSI is financial. The cost of psychotherapy is a major financial issue for many families in the United States. Few individuals

or families can afford long term psychotherapy in the absence of insurance coverage. Many insurance policies in the United States do not cover psychotherapy, and those carriers that do pay for psychotherapy place strict limits on the number and type of sessions, have life time use limits, and have laborious and time consuming reauthorization processes for clinicians. This is a critical problem because youth with any form of NSSI and mental illness will need long term care.

11.7 Conclusions

Dermatitis artefacta, skin picking, and other self-injurious behaviors (SMB) are defined by the self-inflicted damage to ones body tissue. Youth are at high risk for suicide if they have any combination of comorbid severe mental illnesses, psychosis, developmental disabilities, intellectual disabilities, mental retardation, or histories of previous suicidal attempts. Most youth who engage in NSSI do not kill themselves and have no intention of committing suicide when they self-injure; their actions are more likely non-verbal expressions of their emotional distress.

Teaching these children and adolescents to communicate with others in order to get their emotional needs met is an essential part of any therapy they receive. Youth with severe forms of NSSI and a diagnosis of severe developmental disabilities, intellectual disabilities, mental retardation, or psychosis will respond best to BT. Chronic NSSI is very treatment resistant, which seems to indicate the need to have effective treatment early in the lives of all youth who engage in NSSI.

Clinicians in the medical home of a patient/client and who encounter youth who present with NSSI will need to use a team approach to intervention. Teamwork is essential for effective treatment of youth who engage in NSSI. The referring physician usually serves as the team leader, and consultants for treatment may include other medical specialties (dermatology and psychiatry), psychologists, social workers, occupational therapist (for youth with tactile issues), parents, and the patient/client when appropriate.

Acknowledgments

A special thank you to my editorial team. Your contributions to this chapter are greatly appreciated:

Michigan State University/Kalamazoo Center for Medical Studies

Elizabeth Cary, BA, Psychology Intern, Behavioral Developmental Pediatrics Division, Pediatrics Program

Jan Minges, BA, Program Coordinator, Pediatrics Program
Sherry Pancost, MA Temporay limited Licensed Psychologist, Behavioral Developmental Pediatrics Division, Pediatric Program
Aaron Roberts, MD Medicine/Pediatrics Resident PGY I
LaSondra Wayne, BA, Psychology Intern, Behavioral Developmental Pediatrics Division, Pediatrics Program
Katie White, MA Temporay limited Licensed Psychologist, Behavioral Developmental Pediatrics Division, Pediatric Program

Germany

Robin Stier, Medical Student, Freiburg, Germany

References

1. Bolognini M, Plancherel B, Laget J, Stéphan P, Halfon O. Adolescents' self-mutilation – Relationship with dependent behaviour. *Swiss J Psychol* 2003;62(4):241–9.
2. Hilt LM, Nock MK, Lloyd-Richardson EE, Prinstein MJ. Longitudinal study of nonsuicidal self-injury among young adolescents: Rates, correlates, and preliminary test of an interpersonal model. *J Early Adolesc* 2008; 28(3):455–69.
3. Kohlboeck G, Quadflieg N, Fichter MM. Acting out and self-harm in children, adolescents and young adults and mental illness 18 years later: The Longitudinal Upper Bavarian Community Study. *Eur J Psychiatry* 2011; 25(1):32–40.
4. Koo JYM, Dermatitis artefacta treatment & management. *Medscape* 2009. http://emedicine.medscape.com/article/1121933
5. Morgan JR, Storch EA, Woods DW, Bodzin D, Lewin AB, Murphy T K. A preliminary analysis of the phenomenology of skin-picking in Prader-Willi syndrome. *Child Psychiatry Hum Dev* 2010; 41:448–63.
6. Saez-de-Ocariz M, Orozco-Covarrubias L, Mora-Magaña I, Duran-McKinster C, Tamayo-Sanchez L, Gutierrez-Castrellon P, et al. Dermatitis artefacta in pediatric patients: Experience at the national institute of pediatrics. *Pediatr Dermatol* 2004;21(3):205–11.
7. Wilkinson P, Kelvin R, Roberts C, Dubicka B, Goodyer I. Clinical and psychosocial predictors of suicide attempts and nonsuicidal self-injury in the Adolescent Depression Antidepressants and Psychotherapy Trial (ADAPT). *Am J Psychiatry* 2011;68(5):495–501.
8. Peebles R, Wilson JL, Lock JD. Self-injury in adolescents with eating disorders: Correlates and provider bias. *J Adolesc Health* 2011; 48(3):310–3.
9. Iwata BA, Dorsey MF, Slifer KJ, Bauman KE, Richman GS. Toward a functional analysis of self-injury. *J Appl Behav Analysis* 1994; 27(2):197–209.
10. Baetens I, Claes L, Muehlenkamp J, Grietens H, Onghena P. Non-suicidal and suicidal self-injurious behavior among Flemish adolescents: A web-survey. *Arch Suicide Res* 2011; 15(1):56–67.
11. Cloutier P, Martin J, Kennedy A, Nixon MK, Muehlenkamp JJ. Characteristics and co-occurrence of adolescent non-suicidal self-injury and suicidal behaviours in pediatric emergency crisis services. *J Youth Adolesc* 2010; 39(3):259–69.
12. Hankin BL, Abela JR. Nonsuicidal self -injury in adolescence: Prospective rates and risk factors in a 2 ½year longitudinal study. *Psychiatr Res* 2011; 186(1): 65–70.

13. MacLean WE Jr, Tervo RC, Hoch J, Tervo M, Symons FJ. Self-injury among a community cohort of young children at risk for intellectual and developmental disabilities. *J Pediatr* 2001; 157(6): 979–83.
14. Matsumoto T, Yamaguchi A, Chiba Y, Asami T, Iseki E, Hirayasu Y. Self-burning versus self-cutting: Patterns and implications of self-mutilation: A preliminary study of differences between self-cutting and self-burning in a Japanese juvenile detention center. *Psychiatry Clin Neurosci* 2005;59(1):62–9.
15. Tang J, Yu Y, Wu Y, Du Y, Ma Y, Zhu H, et al. Association between non-suicidal self-injuries and suicide attempts in Chinese adolescents and college students: A cross-section study. *PLoS ONE* 2011;6(4):e17977.
16. Mitrou F, Gaudie J, Lawrence D, Silburn SR, Stanley FJ, Zubrick SR. Antecedents of hospital admission for deliberate self-harm from a 14-year follow-up study using data-linkage. *BMC Psychiatry* 2010;10:82.
17. You J, Leung F, Fu K, Lai CM. The prevalence of nonsuicidal self-injury and different subgroups of self -injurers in Chinese adolescents. *Arch Suicide Res* 2011; 15(1):75–86.
18. Ross S, Heath N. A study of the frequency of self-mutilation in a community sample of adolescents. *J Youth Adolesc* 2002;31(1), 67–77.
19. Lucassen MFG, Merry SN, Robinson EM, Denny S, Clark T, Ameratunga S, Crengle S, Rossen FV. Sexual attraction, depression, self-harm, suicidality and help-seeking behaviour in New Zealand secondary school students. *Aust NZ J Psychiatry* 2011;45(5):376–83.
20. Bohne A, Wilhelm S, Keuthen NJ, Baer L, Jenike MA. Skin picking in German students. Prevalence, phenomenology, and associated characteristics. *Behav Modif* 2002;26 (3):320–39.
21. Bolognini M, Plancherel B, Laget J., Stêphan P, Halfon O. Adolescents' self-mutilation – relationship with dependent behavior. *Swiss J Psychol* 2003;62(4):241–9.
22. Taylor L, Oliver C, Murphy G. The chronicity of self-injurious behaviour: A long-term follow-up of a total population study. *J Appl Res Intellect Disabil* 2011;24(2):105–17.
23. Didden R, Korzilius H, Curfs LMG. Skin-picking in individuals with Prader-Willi Syndrome: prevalence, functional assessment, and its comorbidity with compulsive and self-injurious behaviours. *J Appl Res Intellect Disabil* 2007;20(5):409–19.
24. Nock MK, Prinstein, MJ, Sterba SK. Revealing the form and function of self-injurious thoughts and behaviors: A real-time ecological assessment study among adolescents and young adults. *J Abnorm Psychol* 2009;118(4):816–27.
25. Boxer P. Variations in risk and treatment factors among adolescents engaging in different types of deliberate self-harm in an inpatient sample. *J Clin Child Adolesc Psychol* 2010;39(4): 470–80.
26. Aman MG, McDougle CJ, Scahill L, Handen B, Arnold LE, Johnson C, et al. Medication and parent training in children with pervasive developmental disorders and serious behavior problems: Results from a randomized clinical trial. *J Am Acad Child Adolesc Psychiatry* 2009; 48(12):143–54. http://www.nimh.nih.gov/science-news/2009/
27. Parikh MS, Kolevzon A, Hollander E. Psychopharmacology of aggression in children and adolescents with autism: A critical review of efficacy and tolerability. *J Child Adolesc Psychopharmacol* 2008;18 (2):157–78.
28. Muehlenkamp JJ, Williams KL, Gutierrez PM, Claes L. Rates of non-suicidal self-injury in high school students across five years. *Arch Suicide Res* 2009;13(4):317–29.
29. Denis Jo, Van den Noortgate W, Maes B. Self-injurious behavior in people with profound intellectual disabilities: A meta-analysis of single-case studies. *Res Dev Disabil* 2011;32(3): 911–23.
30. Buono S, Scannella F, Palmigiano MB. Self-injurious behavior: A comparison between Prader-Willi syndrome, Down syndrome and autism. *Life Span Disabil* 2010;13(2):187–201.

31. Nock, MK, Prinstein MJ, Sterba SK. Revealing the form and function of self-injurious thoughts and behaviors: A real-time ecological assessment study among adolescents and young adults. *Psychol Violence* 2010; 1(S): 36–52.
32. Lerman DC, Iwata BA, Wallace MD. Side effects of extinction: Prevalence of bursting and aggression during the treatment of self-injurious behavior. *J Appl Behav Anal* 1999;32(1):1–8.
33. Iwata BA, Pace GM, Dorsey MF, Zarcone JR, Vollmer TR, Smith RG, et. al. The functions of self-injurious behavior: An experimental-epidemiological analysis. *J Appl Behav Anal* 1994; 27(2): 215–40.
34. Green JM, Wood AJ, Kerfoot MJ, Trainor G, Roberts C, Rothwell J, et al. Group therapy for adolescents with repeated self harm: Randomised controlled trial with economic evaluation. *BMJ* 2011;342(d7802).
35. Mehta AJ, Statham BN. Phytophotodermatitis mimicking non-accidental injury or self-harm. *Eur J Pediatr* 2007; 166:751–52.
36. Smith RG, Iwata BA, Han-Leong G, Shore BA. Analysis of establishing operations for self-injury maintained by escape. *J Appl Behav Anal* 1995;283(4):515–35.
37. Association for Behavioral and Cognitive Therapists, Society of Clinical Child and Adolescent Psychology. Evidenced-based mental health treatments for children and adolescents. http://www.abct.org/sccap/?m=sPro&fa=pro_ESToptions
38. Nicholson AA, Adams MA, Miltenberger RC. Habit Reversal Training. In: O'Donohue WT, Fisher JE, eds. *Habit reversal training. Cognitive behavior therapy: Applying empirically supported techniques in your practice.* Hoboken, NJ: John Wiley, 2008:245–52.

Arthur N. Feinberg

12 Trichotillomania

This chapter reviews the normal hair growth cycle, defines as well as identifies trichotillomania, develops a differential diagnosis, and considers the assessment of trichotillomania with particular emphasis on its comorbidities. Concepts of current management are presented with inclusion of recent articles. Finally, consideration of future directions is provided.

12.1 Introduction

All humans have hair follicles from birth. Hair then grows in a cyclic fashion. There are three phases: *anagen*, the growth phase, lasting about 3 years; *catagen*, the involutional phase; and *telogen*, the resting phase. At any given time, approximately 90% of follicles are in anagen, about 2% are in catagen, and about 10% are in telogen. Not all hair follicles undergo these phases in unison; otherwise humans would have periods of extensive hair loss and alopecia.

Contributing to this is the fact that anagen lasts up to 3 years, catagen up to 3 weeks, and telogen up to 4 months. Thus, typically, one sheds approximately 75 hairs per day at the end of telogen, as an equal number of follicles are entering into the anagen phase. Shed hairs during the telogen phase appear club-shaped under the microscope (1).

12.2 Definition

Trichotillomania (TTM) is self-induced, non-scarring, hair pulling affecting about 1–3.5% of adults and late adolescents (2). It may also manifest itself as trichoteiromania (hair pulling), trichotemnomania (hair cutting), and trichodaganomania (hair biting) (3). It characteristically leaves behind patchy areas of alopecia with varying lengths of hair.

According to the American Psychiatric Association's (APA's) *Diagnostic and Statistical Manual of Mental Disorders'* (DSM-IV-TR), the diagnostic criteria for TTM include the following:

- Recurrent pulling out of one's hair resulting in noticeable hair loss;
- An increasing sense of tension immediately before pulling out the hair or when attempting to resist the behavior;
- Pleasure, gratification, or relief when pulling out the hair;

- The disturbance is not better accounted for by another mental disorder and is not due to a general medical condition (e.g. a dermatological condition); and
- The disturbance causes clinically significant distress or impairment in social, occupational, or other important areas of functioning.

Unfortunately, the incidence or prevalence among children is not well known (4).

Although there is evidence associating TTM with other psychiatric comorbidities in adolescents and adults (such as anxiety, obsessive compulsive disorder [OCD], mood disorder, tics, eating disorder, and personality disorder), there are no prospective studies to date assessing long range mental health outcomes in children who pull out their hair. Thus, it is not clear whether hair pulling in childhood is a predictor of subsequent psychopathology (5), or in some cases a developmental phase that is self-limited. Nor is it clear if psychological factors can be the underlying cause of trichotillomania in this age group.

Hair pulling has been classified into "automatic" (unconscious) and "focused" (affective triggers), but no studies have been done to delineate the natural course of each. However, studies have shown that there are differences in treatment selection for the two types (6).

Other physical complications of TTM include skin irritation, infection, and repetitive overuse injuries of the hand (6). Another interesting sequel is the Rapunzel Syndrome, or the swallowing of so much hair as to cause a trichobezoar resulting in intestinal obstruction (7).

12.3 Differential diagnosis

Differential diagnosis of non-scarring alopecia includes tinea capitis, alopecia areata, telogen effluvium, anagen effluvium, androgenetic alopecia, infectious causes (such as syphilis), connective tissue disorders (specifically systemic lupus erythematosus), and various toxic-metabolic causes (such as hyperthyroidism, hypervitaminosis A, and deficiencies in zinc and biotin) (8). A thorough history and physical examination will help arrive at the correct diagnosis. Observation of the child pulling his/her hair is of paramount help, especially at night or during times of stress. Often the child will pull the hair while spinning it around his/her fingers and sucking the thumb.

On physical examination, patchy baldness with varying lengths of hair is the hallmark of TTM (Figure 12.1) (9). In tinea capitis, there is invariably scaling, and the remaining hairs appear stubbly. Sometimes an inflammatory "kerion" will be present (Figures 12.2 and 12.3). There is often a history of exposure to a "ringworm" infection. KOH prep may reveal hyphae and spores.

In alopecia areata, the hair loss is complete with a smooth underlying bare scalp appearing in small circles (Figure 12.4; see Chapter 14). On rare occasion, the hair

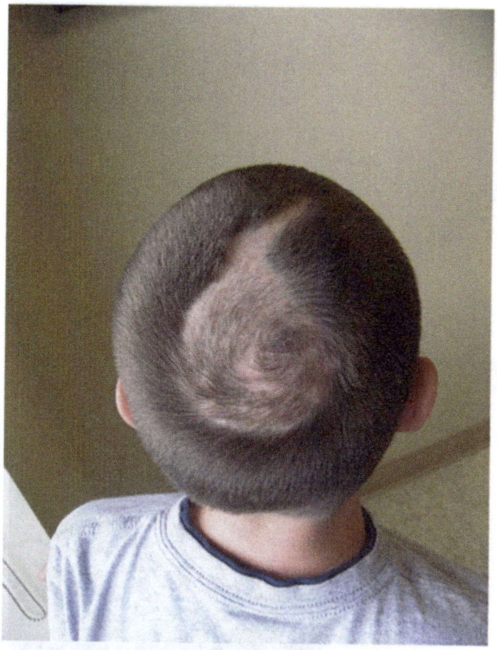

Figure 12.1: Trichotillomania, note varying hair length.

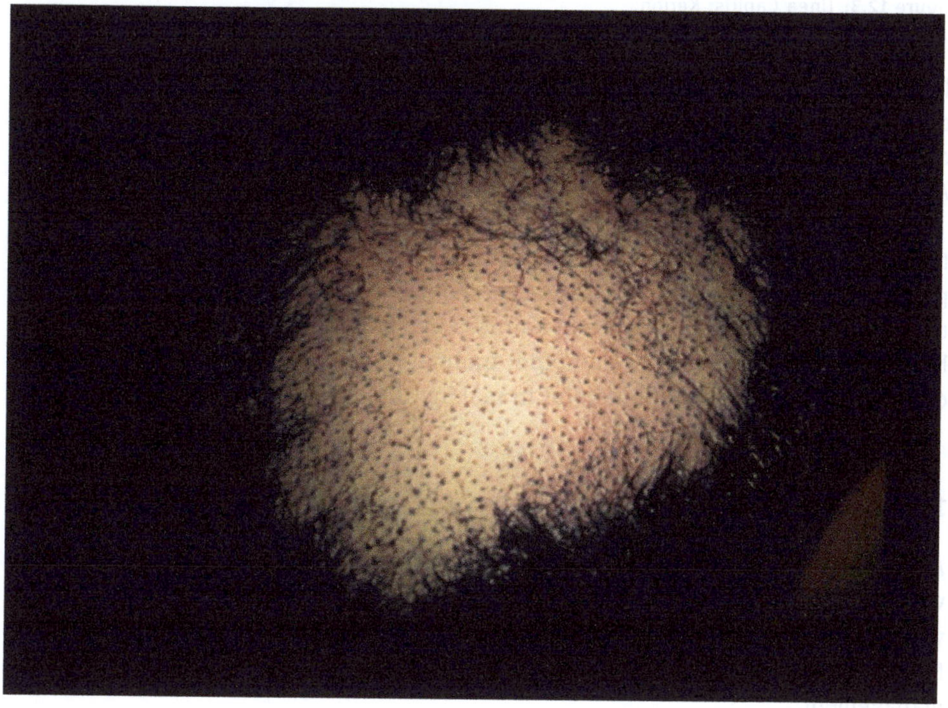

Figure 12.2: Tinea Capitis, note stubbles of hair.

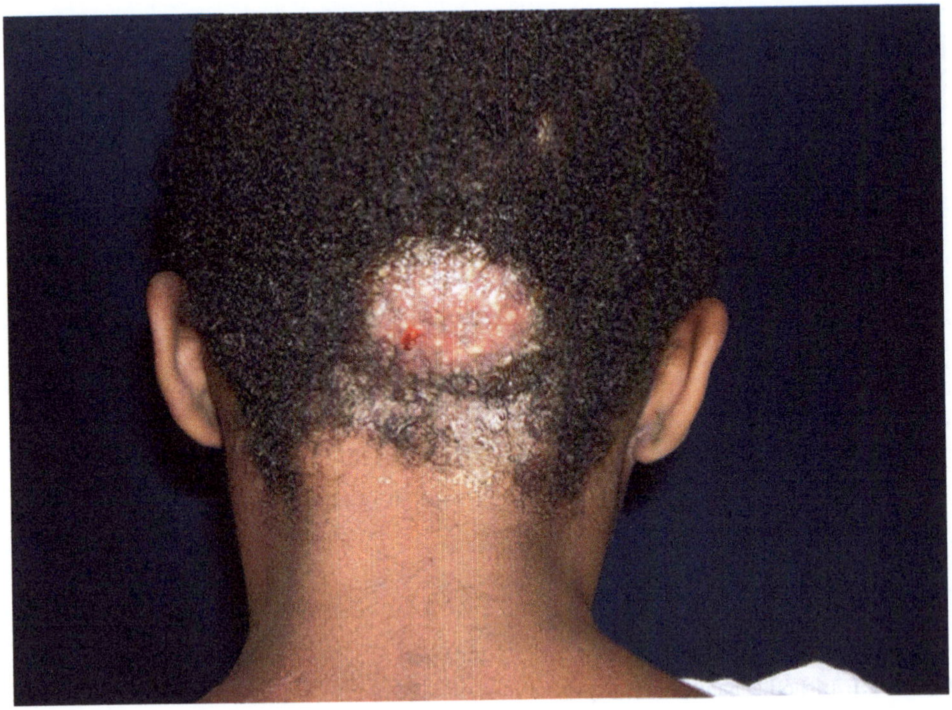

Figure 12.3: Tinea Capitis: Kerion.

loss may spread to the point of alopecia totalis. Anagen effluvium is due to an arrest of anagen phase. The most common cause for this condition is a side effect of cancer chemotherapy, resulting in a rapid loss of 90% of hair in about a 2-week period. After the cycle of chemotherapy is completed the hair regrows.

Telogen effluvium is due to increased loss of mature hairs more rapidly during the telogen phase, often associated with pregnancy, acute medical conditions, or psychological trauma. It is diffuse and reversible and sheds club-shaped hairs. Traction alopecia is a common cause of hair loss in children resulting from stretching of hair with curlers or barrettes and other trauma. A careful history of the location of curlers and barrettes will be helpful in making this diagnosis (8,9).

12.4 Assessment

As discussed previously, the medical diagnosis is made purely on clinical grounds with a thorough history and physical examination. However, although it is unclear whether psychological comorbidities are a cause or a result of TTM, it is paramount to assess these objectively and correctly as this will play a critical role in future management.

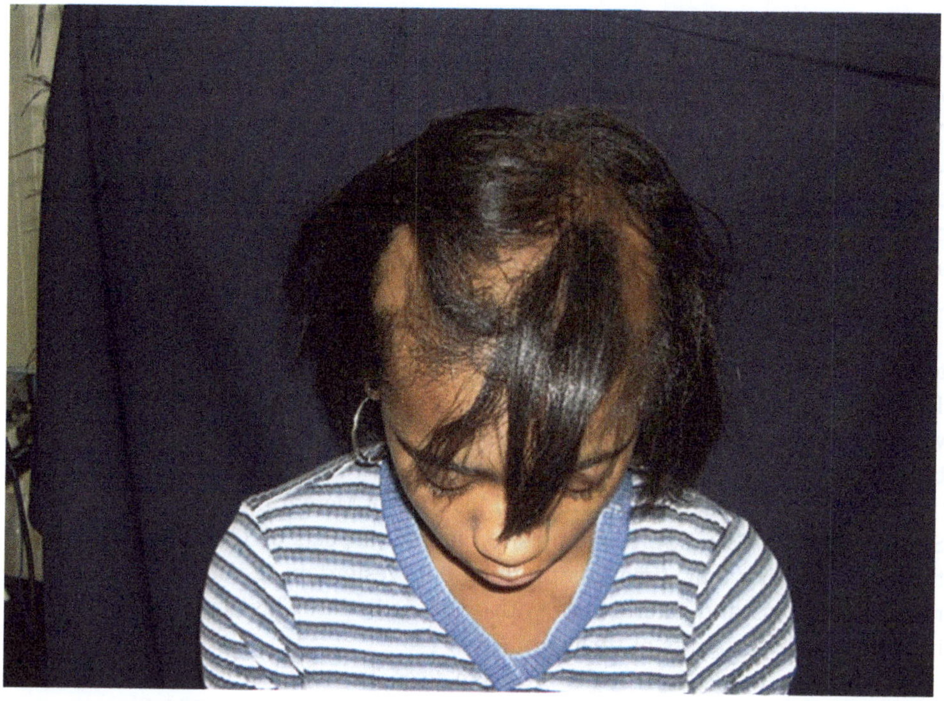

Figure 12.4: Alopecia Areata, note bare scalp and varying sizes of affected areas.

Adults with TTM report difficulties with school and work (10). Older children and adolescents are more vulnerable to ostracism and bullying, and it is important to assess the degree of this as well as their response to it (e.g. shame, anger, and fear), their subsequent behavior (retaliation, violence, isolation, concealment of symptoms), and specific psychiatric diagnoses (depression, mood disorders, eating disorders, anxiety, and substance abuse). In addition to assessing the individual patient, it is important to view him/her in the context of their various environments such as school, work, peers, and family (11). The clinician should ask about their academic and social progress.

The actual assessment consists of a thorough interview and administration of standardized validated tests. The interview should be geared toward the individual particularly in the context of his/her need. For example, a small child may require the presence of a parent to obtain more factual information. Moreover, both parents, whether together or separated, may have different views of the situation and should be included in the interview phase. Throughout this encounter it is important to observe the interaction between the patient and the parent(s) as this can provide some interesting insights into family dynamics.

As children become older and enter adolescence, it is important to interview the adolescent alone at first to respect his/her privacy and to determine how much parental involvement the patient wants. If the patient at first refuses any parental involvement, respect that at first and try to work toward obtaining information with the permission of the patient. Differences of opinion may well exist between parent and child, and it is important for the clinician to assess the dynamics of the situation. It can be challenging to the clinician to develop a feel not only for the interpersonal dynamics, but for patient and parents' awareness and perceptions of the symptoms. Is either of them concealing information to "save face"? How aware is everyone of the extent of the problem? Could any of them be overestimating or underestimating this?

Thus, in spite of a thorough interview, it is also necessary to perform objective testing. There are objective tests that are both valid and reliable. As an example, the Trichotillomania Diagnostic Interview (TDI) is a semi-structured interview that provides a three-point clinician rating for each DSM-IV-TR criterion for TTM; this can be administered easily and quickly.

Other tests include the U.S. National Institute of Mental Health Trichotillomania Severity Scale (NIMH-TIS). It attempts to quantify aspects of TTM, such as average time spent pulling hair, time spent pulling hair yesterday, resistance to urges, and resulting distress and interference with daily activities. This scale is also helpful in following the progress of treatment (6).

The Premonitory Urge Scale, although used for other disorders, has demonstrated internal validity and reliability and may be applied to TTM for assessing urges in patients over 9 years of age (6). Other objective tests include the Massachusetts General Hospital Hair pulling Symptom Severity Scale (MGH-HS), which assesses seven items, including frequency, urgency, resistance to urges, distress, and more. The Milwaukee inventory of Subtypes of Trichotillomania (MIST) assesses the style of hair pulling (6).

A truly objective measurement of TTM is a photograph. A still photo can quantify the actual amount of hair loss. A video will demonstrate openly patient behavior. Of course, any photography or videos must be obtained with full knowledge and written consent. This may be very enlightening if a patient is minimizing, denying, or truly unaware of the extent of the TTM.

12.5 Management

Treatment of TTM should be multifaceted (psychological, pharmacologic) as no one method has demonstrated clear superiority. More studies need to be done to determine if these two modalities of treatment may have additive effects. Unfortunately, there are few data that are prospective and randomized, although recent studies will be cited later in this section. Also, very few reports have been published on young children, and there is a need for more longitudinal studies in this group.

12.5.1 Psychotherapy

Flessner, Lochner, Stein, et al attempted to correlate outcomes with age of onset (very early, early, and late) of hair pulling and were unable to determine any significant differences in psychological outcomes, but found some significant differences in the sites of hair pulling (12). However, all subjects of this study had current hair pulling, and some with early onset were symptomatic for a long period of time. Thus, the study was cross-sectional.

Neal-Barrett, Flessner, Franklin, et al performed a demographic study comparing differences between Caucasians and minorities regarding interference with normal activities and found minorities had more difficulties in the home in distinction to the Caucasian group, which experienced more academic difficulties in school (13). Caucasians reported higher levels of stress. Response to treatment was similar in both groups.

Cognitive behavioral training (CBT) has demonstrated effectiveness in adults, although relapse can be a problem. The essence of CBT is, first, the recognition of symptoms, specifically awareness of the symptom as well as awareness of the premonitory urge. A second aspect of CBT is stimulus control, or training patients to set up their own roadblocks to hair pulling once the urge is recognized. The third aspect of CBT is habit-reversal, or competing response training, which is applying techniques to make it difficult to pull hair (e.g. sitting on hands), or perhaps other psychological responses such as relaxation training and developing competing thoughts to counteract the urge to pull hair (6).

Another form of therapy, dialectical behavior therapy (DBT), has been shown to be effective. Recent studies have demonstrated its effectiveness in treating focused hair pulling, whereas CBT is more effective for treating automatic pulling (13). At present, the duration of success for this treatment has extended for 3–6 months (14).

12.5.2 Medication

Presently, the use of selective serotonin reuptake inhibitors (SSRI) have proven disappointing for hair pulling in and of itself, although it does treat other comorbid conditions such as depression and OCD. Golubchik, Sever, Weitzman, et al demonstrated that the use of methylphenidate was helpful in treating ADHD symptoms in a patient diagnosed with trichotillomania and ADHD, but they were not able to demonstrate any significant changes in hair pulling using the MGH-HS as the measuring tool (15).

A double-blind placebo-controlled study regarding the use of N-acetylcysteine, a glutamate modulator, showed promising results in 50 adults. Fifty-six percent of subjects were significantly improved as compared to 16% in the placebo group, using the MGH-HS as the measuring tool (16).

A case report demonstrated effectiveness in treating trichotillomania with oxcarbazepine in a 43-year-old obese woman with comorbid binge-eating disorder and trichotillomania (17).

Van Ameringen, Mancini, Patterson, et al studied 25 participants in a randomized double-blind, placebo-controlled fashion in a trial of oplanzapine, a dopaminergic medication used in Tourette syndrome (18). In the 13 patients who were in the treatment group, 11 of them improved significantly, employing the Yale-Brown Obsessive Compulsive Scale for Trichotillomania and the Clinical Global Impressions-Severity of illness scale. In the control group, 2 of 12 improved.

Another study involving dopamine (D2) agonist aripiprazole was a small ($n = 12$) open label flexible-dose study using the MGH tests for hair pulling as a measuring tool. There was a significant reduction of hair pulling based on actual test scores as well as percent reduction of scores. The authors conceded that larger double blind placebo studies are needed (19).

12.6 Conclusions: Future directions

The present state of the art of trichotillomania raises more questions than answers. Trichotillomania is easy to identify clinically, but its classification into mental disorders can be elusive. It stands by itself as a diagnosis in the DSM-IV-TR (i.e. not explained by other disorders, such as obsessive compulsive disorder (OCD) or Tourette syndrome). Also one cannot diagnose OCD based solely on trichotillomania. However, if OCD or Tourette syndrome is diagnosed based on its criteria, then trichotillomania, if it exists, can be considered as comorbid. However, the converse is unclear. It would seem that if trichotillomania is associated with OCD, trichotillomania cannot be considered a primary diagnosis unless the clinician knows that it occurred first.

There are no good prospective studies that follow the natural course of trichotillomania starting in children. Thus, it is not clear at this time how to differentiate the "chicken from the egg." Of all children who pull their hair, how many of them resolve this symptom spontaneously? Do any of them recur, and how many of those subsequently develop other diagnoses? For those that do not recur, how many of them develop other diagnoses without trichotillomania? Can trichotillomania in childhood be considered a harbinger for other psychiatric conditions? Are there any indicators that can help prognosticate whether a child with trichotillomania will resolve spontaneously, recur, or incur other mental health diagnoses in the future? All of these questions need to be addressed to determine how much of trichotillomania is stand-alone and how much of it is tag-along with other psychiatric conditions.

Recent studies regarding management indicate that SSRIs are of no benefit in reducing trichotillomania in patients responding well to co-existing diagnoses, such as OCD. Also, stimulants such as methylphenidate will ameliorate symptoms of attention deficit hyperactivity disorder (ADHD) but will not reduce hair pulling. Other medications involving the neurotransmitter system have demonstrated improved scores in objective tests such as the Massachusetts General Hospital or the Yale-Brown tests. In some studies with olanzapine, there was improvement in both hair pulling and OCD symptoms. More studies need to be done to validate early findings and to determine which symptoms each drug addresses best.

Psychotherapy, specifically CBT and DBT, have demonstrated efficacy. Future studies should be done to delineate further which treatment will benefit which patients. Most likely combinations of psychotherapy and pharmacotherapy will be employed in the future, and it is important to assess these outcomes.

The author is grateful to Dr. Tor Shwayder for providing the illustrations for this chapter.

References

1. Price VH. Treatment of hair loss. *N Engl J Med* 1999;341:964.
2. Christenson GA, Pyle RI, Mitchell JE. Estimated lifetime prevalence of trichotillomania in college students. *J Clin Psychiatry* 1991;52:415–17.
3. Jafferany M, Feng J, Hornung RL. Trichodaganomania: The compulsive habit of biting one's own hair. *J Am Acad Dermatol* 2008;60(4):689–91.
4. Tolin DF, Franklin ME, Diefenbach GJ, et al. Pediatric trichotillomania: Descriptive psychopathology and an open trial of cognitive-behavioral therapy. *Cogn Behav Ther* 2007;36:129–44.
5. Christenson GA, Mackenzuie TB, Mitchell JE. Characteristics of 60 adult chronic hairpullers. *Am J Psychiatry* 1991;148 365–70.
6. Franklin ME, Zagrabbe K, Benavides KL. Trichotillomania and its treatment: A review and recommendations. *Expert Rev Neurother* 2011;11(8):1165–74.
7. Bege T, Desjeux A, Coquet-Renier B, et al. The Rapunzel syndrome: A hard to swallow tale. *J Gastrointestinal Surg* 2011;15(8):1486–7.
8. Goldstein BG and Goldstein AO. Nonscarring hair loss. http:www.uptodate.com/contents/nonscarring-hair-loss?view=print.
9. Greydanus DE, Feinberg AN, Patel DR, Homnick DN. *The pediatric diagnostic examination.* New York, NY: McGraw-Hill, 2008.
10. Seedat S, Stein DJ. Psychosocial and economic implications of trichotillomania: A pilot study in a South African sample. *CNS Spect* 1998;3:40–3.
11. Moore PS, Franklin ME, Keuthen NC, et al. Family functioning in pediatric trichotillomania, behavioral and interpersonal sequelae. *Clin Fam Behav Ther* 2009;31:265–9.
12. Flessner CA, Lochner C, Stein DJ, et al. Age of onset of trichotillomania symptoms: Investigating clinical correlates. *J Nerv Ment Dis* 2010;198(12) 896–900.
13. Keuthen NJ, Rothbaum BO, Welch SS, et al. Pilot trial of dialectical behavior therapy-enhanced habit reversal for trichotillomania. *Depress Anxiety* 2010;27:953–9.
14. Keuthen NJ, Rothbaum BO, Falkenstein MJ, et al. DBT-enhanced habit reversal treatment for trichotillomania: 3- and 6-month followup results. *Depress Anxiety* 2011;28:310–13.

15. Golubchik P, Sever J, Swetzman A, et al. Methylphenidate treatment in pediatric patients with attention-deficit/hyperactivity disorder and comorbid trichotillomania: A preliminary report. *Clin Neuropharmacol* 2011;34(3):108–10.
16. Grant JE, Odlaug BL, Kim SW. N-acetylcysteine, a glutamate modulator, in the treatment of trichotillomania: A double-blind, placebo controlled study. *Arch Gen Psychiatry* 2009;66(7):756–63.
17. Leombruni P, Gastaldi F. Oxcarbbazpine for treatment for trichotillomania. *Clin Neuropharmacol* 2010;33(2):107–8.
18. Van Ameringen M, Mancinc C, Patterson B, et al. A randomized double-blind placebo-controlled trial of olanzapine in the treatment of trichotillomania. *J Clin Psychiatry* 2010;71(10):1336–43.
19. White MP, Koran LM. Open-label trial of aripiprazole in the treatment of trichotillomania. *J Clin Psychopharmacol* 2011;31(4):503–6.

Adam Reich and Jacek C. Szepietowski

13 Psychogenic pruritus with particular emphasis on children and adolescents

This chapter considers psychogenic pruritus with special application to the pediatric population. The topic is defined and then various features covered, including its epidemiology, clinical features, differential diagnosis, and principles of management. It is important to address the underlying factors precipitating the pruritis. Management consists of psychotherapy and/or psychotropic drugs in addition to general measures as use of emollients and avoidance of factors that worsen the condition. Recommended medications include doxepin, serotonin re-uptake inhibitors (e.g. paroxetine, sertralin), or benzodiazepines (e.g. escitalopram) in standard doses; if this fails, mirtazapine can be tried. Local pruritis may be improved with use of local anesthetics.

13.1 Introduction

Pruritus is defined as an unpleasant sensation provoking a desire to scratch (1). It could be acute (i.e. lasting less than 6 weeks) or chronic (i.e. with a duration longer than 6 weeks). According to the newest pruritus classification proposed by the International Forum for the Study of Itch (IFSI) (1), based on the underlying cause, itching could be classified to one of six categories: "dermatologic," "systemic," "neurologic," "psychogenic," "mixed," or "other" pruritus. Although the term "psychogenic pruritus" is the most popular one, a number of other descriptors were used to define this type of pruritus, such as "functional itch disorder," "pruritus sine materia," "pruritus without underlying origin," "psychosomatic pruritus," "non-organic pruritus," or "somatoform pruritus."

According to IFSI, psychogenic pruritus can be defined as a somatoform pruritus with a comorbidity of psychiatric or psychosomatic diseases (1). A more accurate definition was proposed by the French Psychodermatology Group (FPDG), which defined psychogenic pruritus as "an itch disorder, where itch is at the center of symptomatology, and where psychological factors play an evident role in the triggering intensity, aggravation or persistence of the pruritus" (2). Importantly, based on the clinical presentation, psychogenic pruritus may be accounted for with two groups of pruritus: "pruritus on primarily normal, non-inflamed skin" and "pruritus with chronic secondary scratch lesions" (1).

13.2 Epidemiology

The exact prevalence of itching in the general population has been poorly investigated; however, recent studies have indicated that about 8% to 17% of Caucasians have been suffering from chronic itch (3,4,5). It seems that the frequency of chronic itch among adolescents is similar; Halvorsen et al. observed that nearly 9% among 4,744 of studied adolescents reported chronic pruritus (6). The prevalence of itching in other ethnic populations, except some small, limited studies (4), was not well assessed until now.

The frequency of psychogenic pruritus is far more less defined. In one study on a consecutive sample of 109 inpatients with chronic itch, more than 70% had psychiatric comorbidity with the most frequent diagnosis (46.8%) being "psychological impact on or psychosomatic cofactor in itch" (7). In another retrospective study including 139 outpatients with chronic itch, 31 (22.3%) subjects had concomitant psychiatric disorder, but psychogenic pruritus could only be confirmed in 17 of them (8). On the other hand, pruritus was commonly noted in psychiatric patients. In one Israeli study on 111 mentally ill patients, 32% out of them suffered from itching (9). In a pilot study by our group on individuals with depression, psychogenic pruritus was found in 17.5% of study participants (10).

The prevalence of psychogenic pruritus in children and adolescents is completely unknown and difficult to be estimated. On one hand, the literature data on psychogenic pruritus in people less than 18 years old are very limited (11,12). Furthermore, in a study by Rajalakshmi et al on lichen simplex chronicus of anogenital region, a skin condition provoked by chronic rubbing or scratching due to pruritus, only 1 out of 105 patients was less than 15 years old (13). Based on this it could be assumed that psychogenic pruritus is rather an uncommon phenomenon in the pediatric population.

On the other hand, however, in the study by Halvorsen et al. (6) including 4,744 adolescents and showing the prevalence of chronic itch as high as nearly 9% of all analyzed subjects, mental distress was the major factor contributing to the presence of itch in this population. The prevalence of itching in individuals with mental distress was 17.3% (95% CI: 14.9–19.7%), while in subjects without mental distress it was 5.9% (95% CI: 5.0–6.8%); also, crude bivariate analysis demonstrated that mental distress was associated with itch at an odds ratio (OR) of 3.9 (95% CI: 2.9–5.1) (6).

In addition, it is well known that psychological factors are of great importance in atopic dermatitis, a very common itchy allergic dermatosis of children and adolescents, and psychological interventions seem to be a promising adjunctive of pruritus therapy in this group of patients (14) (see Chapter 5). Therefore, the frequency of psychogenic pruritus in the children population might be much more common than suggested if based only on literature data; thus, prospective studies on that issue are urgently needed for the near future.

13.3 Clinical features

According to the definition of pruritus, itching is a subjective sensation that cannot be seen. However, as it produces an urge to scratch, this mechanical response (namely scratching, rubbing, or even stroking) can be frequently and easily observed, confirming the diagnosis of pruritus. Furthermore, if itching is lasting sufficiently long, secondary scratch lesions (excoriations, lichenification, prurigo nodules, scars) may be found on the skin. Psychogenic itch can be generalized or localized, with the genital or anal region being most commonly affected (15).

Psychogenic pruritus is a diagnosis of exclusion as other causes of pruritus must be carefully sought and excluded. Importantly, chronic pruritus of any cause is a very unpleasant and bothersome symptom, significantly reducing the quality of life, and as a consequence these patients may frequently demonstrate a number of secondary (to the itching) psychological or psychiatric disturbances (16). Therefore, identifying psychological or psychiatric problems in patients with chronic itch does not necessarily mean that a patient is suffering from psychogenic pruritus.

In order to facilitate the proper diagnosis, the French group (FPDG) lead by Laurent Misery from Brest, has recently proposed diagnostic criteria for psychogenic pruritus (2). Three major (compulsory) and seven minor (optional) criteria have been suggested (Table 13.1). According to FPDG recommendation, all major and at least 3 out of 7 minor criteria must be fulfilled to make the diagnosis of psychogenic pruritus (2,17). However, based on FPDG, chronic pruritus (i.e. lasting over 6 weeks) can only be considered a psychogenic one. In our opinion, acute itching may also be of psychogenic origin, as it was already reported (11,12,18), and, therefore, the criterion "chronic course of itch" does not necessarily have to be handled as an obligatory one.

Table 13.1: Criteria for Psychogenic Pruritus (2)

Criteria	Description	Frequency (acc. to 17)
Major	– Localized or generalized pruritus without primary skin lesions	100%
	– Chronic course of pruritus (>6 weeks)	100%
	– No somatic cause of pruritus	100%
Minor	– A chronological relationship of pruritus with one or several life events that could have psychological repercussion	46%
	– Variations in pruritus intensity associated with emotional stress	46%
	– Nocturnal variations of itch	69%
	– Predominance during rest or inaction	57%
	– Associated psychological disorder	74%
	– Pruritus that could be improvement with psychotropic drugs	60%
	– Pruritus that could be improved by psychotherapy	14%

In clinical practice, following additional features may be helpful in the diagnosis of psychogenic pruritus; these include the presence of psychological problems that are important with respect to the occurrence, intensity, elicitation or sustaining of itching; great suffering or detriment to social or professional life; preoccupation with the pruritus or the state of the skin; and a search for medical help (15).

13.4 Differential diagnosis

Psychogenic pruritus should be differentiated with a long list of other itchy conditions listed in Table 13.2. In daily practice the most important differential diagnoses include atopic dermatitis, various forms of eczema, urticaria and cutaneous infestations, such as scabies or lice. The other conditions are rather uncommon or quite rare.

Table 13.2: Differential diagnoses of psychogenic pruritus in children and adolescents

13.7 Type of pruritus	13.8 Diseases
Dermatologic	– Xerosis (skin dryness) – Eczema (all forms) – Dyshydrosis – Cutaneous drug reactions – Urticaria – Atopic dermatitis – Psoriasis – Palmoplantar pustulosis – Lichen planus – Seborrheic dermatitis – Polymorphic light eruptions – Autoimmune blistering diseases (pemphigoid, linear IgA bullous dermatosis, acquired epidermolysis bullosa, dermatitis herpetiformis) – Autoimmune connective tissue diseases (dermatomyositis, systemic sclerosis) – Skin infections (herpes simplex, varicella, herpes zoster, tineas, candidal intertrigo, *Malassezia* folliculitis) – Skin infestations (scabies, lice, cutaneous larva migrans) – Insect bites and arthropod reactions – Mastocytosis – Primary cutaneous amyloidosis – Cutaneous lymphomas (mycosis fungoides and its variants, Sezary's syndrome)

(Continued)

Table 13.2: Differential diagnoses of psychogenic pruritus in children and adolescents (*Continued*)

13.7 Type of pruritus	13.8 Diseases
Systemic	– Liver diseases (primary biliary cirrhosis, primary sclerosing cholangitis, extrahepatic cholestasis, hepatitis) – Chronic kidney insufficiency – Lymphoproliferative diseases (Hodgkin's disease, Non-Hodgkin's lymphomas and leukemias, myeloma multiplex, systemic mastocytosis, hypereosinophilic syndrome, myelodysplastic syndromes) – Iron deficiency – Endocrine disorders (hyperthyroidism, hypothyroidism, hyperparathyroidism, diabetes) – Parasitic infections – HIV infection/AIDS – Drug-induced pruritus
Neurologic	– Brain injury/tumor (frequently unilateral pruritus) – Sclerosis multiplex – Small fiber neuropathy – Brachioradial pruritus – Notalgia paresthetica

13.5 Management

The initial management of the patient with psychogenic itch does not differ from that which is done in subjects with other types of chronic pruritus; this is because it is crucial to exclude other possible causes of itching to be able to make the diagnosis of pruritus with purely psychogenic origin. Therefore, every patient with itching should undergo a careful history and full physical examination that includes a dermatological assessment. A detailed history of itching episodes should begin with the inquiries into onset, location, diurnal rhythm, and alleviating or aggravating factors surrounding an itching period. The patient history should also include details about concomitant diseases, medicines taken by the patient, symptoms of pruritus in the close relatives, history of traveling, presence of skin lesions, and potential allergens at home or at places where the patients is living.

During the physical examination any signs of a rash should be sought on the skin (see Chapter 1). It is important to palpate lymph nodes, the thyroid gland, and the abdomen. Close inspection of the hair and nails may provide important clues for systemic disease (see Chapter 14). If no primary skin symptoms can be found, basic laboratory investigations listed in Table 13.3 should be performed. If psychogenic pruritus is suspected, psychological and/or psychiatric consultation would be of help.

Table 13.3: Basic laboratory investigations recommended in pruritic patients without primary skin lesions

Blood smear with differential blood count
C-reactive protein level or erythrocyte sedimentation rate
Serum iron level (in patients with anemia)
Serum urea and creatinin level
Liver function tests (total bilirubin, free bilirubin, serum aminotransferase activity, serum alkaline phosphatase activity)
Serum glucose level
Thyroid gland function tests (TSH, fT3, fT4)
Stool examination for parasite detections

Once the diagnosis of psychogenic pruritus is established, the patient should receive proper medical care. To date, the data on the effectiveness of various treatment options in psychogenic pruritus are limited, and no treatment guidelines for psychogenic pruritus in children and adolescents exist. If pruritus is a symptom of underlying psychiatric disease (e.g. depression, schizophrenia), then the causative disorder should be appropriately treated under the leadership of a psychiatrist. If pruritus is only related to psychological problems, then the treatment may be guided by a dermatologist with the psychodermatological skills or other adequately educated specialist with the help of a psychologist or psychiatrist, if needed.

The treatment should consist of psychotherapy and/or psychotropic drugs. The patient and his/her parents should be made aware of the connection between psychological problems and itching. This alone often contributes to considerably better coping with pruritus (15). Among the psychotherapy techniques, psychodynamic psychotherapy, cognitive behavior therapy, and relaxation techniques seem to be beneficial (15).

Among the medicines, the use of antihistamines, preferably sedating ones, is the first line therapy (15). Non-sedating antihistamines may be tried, too, but usually they are not very efficacious. If antihistamines are not helpful, neuroleptics with antihistaminic action, antidepressants, or benzodiazepines may be tried (15,19,20,21,22). In our practice we prefer doxepin, serotonin re-uptake inhibitors (e.g. paroxetine, sertralin), or benzodiazepines (e.g. escitalopram) in standard doses. If this fails, mirtazapine is worth a trial (23). If pruritus is localized, lignocaine or other local anesthetics may be tried to break the vicious itching-scratching-itching cycle. However, it must be remembered that local anesthetics are frequent contact allergens and may cause contact eczema, especially if used for a longer time.

We would like also to underline that the treatment of any type of chronic pruritus should consist not only of directed antipruritic therapies, but also of general measures (24). Therefore, during treatment every patient and her/his parents have to be instructed about the necessity of wearing sheer clothes as well as avoiding hot baths, alcohol, and spicy foods; it is also important to keep proper humidity of rooms and avoid contact with wool and animal furs.

Irrespective of the cause of itching, skin dryness worsens each type of pruritus. Thus, all patients should regularly moisturize their skin – a twice daily application of an emollient is recommended. A large number of various formulations are currently available. Among them, those containing 5–10% of urea or others enabling the regeneration of epidermal lipids can be prescribed. The patient should have the possibility to test several preparations to choose the optimal one. Oil-baths, both with natural or mineral oils, may also help to decrease xerosis. Furthermore, localized pruritus also may be diminished with cold wet dressings. Keeping the nails short in patients with severe pruritus may prevent excoriations and other secondary scratch lesions (24,25).

13.6 Conclusion

Pruritus is defined as an unpleasant sensation provoking a desire to scratch. It could be acute (lasting less than 6 weeks) or chronic (with a duration longer than 6 weeks). According to the newest pruritus classification proposed by the IFSI (1), based on the underlying cause, itching could be classified to one of six categories: "dermatologic," "systemic," "neurologic," "psychogenic," "mixed," or "other" pruritus. The prevalence of psychogenic pruritus in children and adolescents is completely unknown and difficult to estimate.

Psychogenic pruritus is a diagnosis of exclusion, as other causes of pruritus must be carefully sought and excluded (Table 13.2). Psychogenic itch can be generalized or localized, with the genital or anal region being most commonly affected. Once the diagnosis of psychogenic pruritus is established after a careful evaluation, the patient should receive proper medical care.

Currently the data on the effectiveness of various treatment options in psychogenic pruritus are limited, and no treatment guidelines for psychogenic pruritus in children and adolescents exist. Recommended treatment consists of psychotherapy and/or psychotropic drugs. Among the psychotherapy techniques, psychodynamic psychotherapy, cognitive behavior therapy, and relaxation techniques seem to be beneficial. A number of medications may be helpful as noted in this discussion; these include antihistamines (especially the sedating ones), neuroleptics with antihistaminic action, antidepressants, or benzodiazepines. The authors recommend doxepin, serotonin re-uptake inhibitors (e.g. paroxetine, sertralin), or benzodiazepines (e.g. escitalopram) in standard doses; if this fails, mirtazapine can be tried. In chronic conditions localized pruritis may be improved with lignocaine or other local anesthetics. General measures are helpful such as use of emollients and avoiding factors that worsen the condition, such as exposure to wool, animal furs, and others.

References

1. Ständer S, Weisshaar E, Mettang T, Szepietowski JC, Carstens E, Ikoma A, et al. Clinical classification of itch: A position paper of the International Forum for the Study of Itch. *Acta Derm Venereol* 2007;87:291–4.
2. Misery L, Alexandre S, Dutray S, Chastaing M, Consoli SG, Audra H, et al. Functional itch disorder or psychogenic pruritus: Suggested diagnosis criteria from the French psychodermatology group. *Acta Derm Venereol* 2007;87:341–4.
3. Dalgard F, Svensson A, Holm JO, Sundby J. Self-reported skin morbidity in Oslo. Associations with sociodemographic factors among adults in a cross-sectional study. *Br J Dermatol* 2004; 151:452–7.
4. Weisshaar E, Dalgard F. Epidemiology of itch: Adding to the burden of skin morbidity. *Acta Derm Venereol* 2009;89:339–50.
5. Ständer S, Schäfer I, Phan NQ, Blome C, Herberger K, Heigel H, Augustin M. Prevalence of chronic pruritus in Germany: Results of a cross-sectional study in a sample working population of 11,730. *Dermatology* 2010;221:229–35.
6. Halvorsen JA, Dalgard F, Thoresen M, Thoresen M, Bjertness E, Lien L. Itch and mental distress: A cross-sectional study among late adolescents. *Acta Derm Venereol* 2009;89:39–44.
7. Schneider G, Driesch G, Heuft G, Evers S, Luger TA, Stander S. Psychosomatic cofactors and psychiatric comorbidity in patients with chronic itch. *Clin Exp Dermatol* 2006;31:762–7.
8. Ferm I, Sterner M, Wallengren J. Somatic and psychiatric comorbidity in patients with chronic pruritus. *Acta Derm Venereol* 2010;90:395–400.
9. Mazeh D, Melamed Y, Cholostoy A, Aharonovitzch V, Weizman A, Yosipovitch G. Itching in the psychiatric ward. *Acta Derm Venereol* 2008;88:128–31.
10. Pacan P, Grezesiak M, Reich A, Szepietowski JC. Is pruritus in depression a rare phenomenon? *Acta Derm Venereol* 2009;89:109–10.
11. Robinson P, Szewczyk M, Haddy L, Jones P, Harvey W. Outbreak of itching and rash. Epidemic hysteria in an elementary school. *Arch Intern Med* 1984;144:1959–62.
12. Halvorson H, Crooks J, Lahart DA, Farrell KP. An outbreak of itching in an elementary school: A case of mass psychogenic response. *J Sch Health* 2008;78:294–7.
13. Rajalakshmi R, Thappa DM, Jaisankar TJ, Nath AK. Lichen simplex chronicus of anogenital region: A clinico-etiological study. *Indian J Dermatol Venereol Leprol* 2011;77:28–36.
14. Chida Y, Steptoe A, Hirakawa N, Sudo N, Kubo C. The effects of psychological intervention on atopic dermatitis. A systematic review and meta-analysis. *Int Arch Allergy Immunol* 2007; 144:1–9.
15. Harth W, Gieler U, Kusnir D, Tausk FA. Other undifferentiated somatoform disorders (cutaneous sensory disorders). In: Harth W, Gieler U, Kusnir D, Tausk FA (eds.). *Clinical management in psychodermatology*. Springer-Verlag, Berlin, Heilderberg 2009;67–71.
16. van Os-Medendorp H, Eland-de Kok PC, Grypdonck M, Bruijnzeel-Koomen CA, Ros WJ. Prevalence and predictors of psychosocial morbidity in patients with chronic pruritic skin diseases. *J Eur Acad Dermatol Venereol* 2006;20:810–7.
17. Misery L, Wallengren J, Weisshaar E, Zalewska A. French Psychodermatology Group. Validation of diagnosis criteria of functional itch disorder or psychogenic pruritus. *Acta Derm Venereol* 2008;88:503–4.
18. Fjellner B, Arnetz BB. Psychological predictors of pruritus during mental stress. *Acta Derm Venereol* 1985;65:504–8.
19. Meyers C, Vranckx C, Elgen K. Psychosomatic disorders in general practice: Comparisons of treatment with flupenthixol, diazepam and sulpiride. *Pharmatherapeutica* 1985;4:244–50.

20. Biondi M, Arcangeli T, Petrucci RM. Paroxetine in a case of psychogenic pruritus and neurotic excoriations. *Psychother Psychosom* 2000;69:165–6.
21. Shaw RJ, Dayal S, Good J, Bruckner AL, Joshi SV. Psychiatric medications for the treatment of pruritus. *Psychosom Med* 2007;69:970–8.
22. Pukadan D, Antony J, Mohandas E, Cyriac M, Smith G, Elias A. Use of escitalopram in psychogenic excoriation. *Aust N Z J Psychiatry* 2008;42:435–6.
23. Davis MP, Frandsen JL, Walsh D, Andresen S, Taylor S. Mirtazapine for pruritus. *J Pain Symptom Manage* 2003;25:288–91.
24. Szepietowski J, Reich A. *Pruritus: Pathomechanism, clinics, treatment.* Poznan, Poland: Termedia, 2010.
25. Reich A, Ständer S, Szepietowski JC. Pruritus in the elderly. *Clin Dermatol* 2011;29:15–23.

Part IV: DERMATOLOGIC DISORDERS PREDISPOSING TO PSYCHIATRIC DISORDERS

Dilip R. Patel

14 Disorders of hair loss

Normal hair growth cycle is divided into anagen, catagen, and telogen phases. Normally approximately 50–100 hairs are shed daily. Hair loss can cause significant psychological distress in children and adolescents. Causes of hair loss are numerous; the most common causes of hair loss in children and adolescents include tinea capitis, telogen effluvium, androgenic alopecia, alopecia areata, and traumatic alopecia. This chapter reviews the epidemiology, diagnostic approach, and management of common causes of hair loss in children, adolescents, and young adults.

14.1 Introduction

The human scalp is estimated to have 100,000 hairs on average, and the terminal hair typically grows at a rate of 1 cm/month (1,2). The hair shaft itself is not living structure; the hair follicle is the active portion of the hair responsible for hair growth. The human hair follicle goes through three phases during a complete growth cycle (2). During the initial *anagen* phase, which typically lasts between 2 and 6 years, the active hair growth occurs. During the second phase, the *catagen* phase, which typically lasts about 3 weeks, the hair goes through involution. This is followed by the *telogen* phase or resting phase, which lasts about 3 months. At the end of the telogen phase, new hair grows from the hair follicle pushing out the hair. Eighty to ninety percent of hair in a healthy scalp is generally in the anagen phase at any given time. Normally approximately 50–100 hairs are shed daily.

14.2 Causes of hair loss

Causes of hair loss are numerous and can be broadly divided into congenital (Table 14.1) and acquired (Table 14.2) (1,2,3,4,5,6,7,8,9). Depending on the specific cause, hair loss patterns can be circumscribed or diffused, and may or may not be associated with scarring. In pediatric populations, most cases of acquired hair circumscribed hair loss are due to tinea capitis, alopecia areata, or traumatic alopecia (2). Overall, telogen effluvium is the most common cause of alopecia in children and adolescents (2,4).

Table 14.1: Causes of Congenital Alopecia

Circumscribed hair loss
Birth marks
Conradi disease
Incontinentia pigmenti
Triangular alopecia of frontal scalp
Goltz syndrome
Diffuse hair loss
Hair shaft defects
Ectodermal dysplasias
Congenital hypothyroidism
Progeria

Table 14.2: Causes of Acquired Alopecia

Circumscribed hair loss
Tinea capitis
Kerion
Varicella
Lichen planus
Darier disease
Systemic lupus erythematosis
Alopecia areata
Traction alopecia
Trichotillomania
Diffuse hair loss
Hypothyroidism
Hyperthyroidism
Diabetes mellitus
Androgenic alopecia (male pattern baldness)
Telogen effluvium
Anagen effluvium
Zinc deficiency
Malnutrition
Iron deficiency anemia
Drug induced
Chemotherapy
Radiation therapy
Hypervitaminosis A

14.3 Diagnostic approach to hair loss

14.3.1 History

When a child or adolescent presents with hair loss, a careful history is the most useful tool in narrowing the diagnosis into one of the categories of hair loss – congenital or acquired, and diffuse or local (4). Inquire about the onset and progression of hair loss and determine if the hair loss is congenital or acquired. Ascertain the general health status of the patient as many medical conditions and therapeutic drugs used in these conditions may contribute to hair loss. Some of the conditions in which hair loss is seen include Down syndrome, hypothyroidism, systemic lupus erythematosus, and diabetes mellitus (2). Medications implicated in hair loss are numerous and include anticoagulants, antimetabolites, and high dose vitamin A.

Exposure to children with tinea capitis as well as to animals such as dogs and cats provide settings for the child acquiring tinea capitis. Tinea capitis is spread from person-to-person or from animal-to-person depending on the type of the organism. Most cases in the United States are caused by *Trichophyton tonsurans* (2).

Behaviors or mannerisms of the child are also important to note, such as playing with hair, habitual twisting, or pulling the hair. Traumatic hair loss can result from persistent pulling of the hair, while hair braiding practice can also result in traction on hair roots with resultant hair loss. History of hair hygiene habits is also important. Use of different hair dressing chemicals and shampoos may contribute to acquired hair loss. Nutritional history of the child is also important. For example, general malnutrition, zinc deficiency, or iron deficiency can contribute to hair loss. Inquire about psychological or physical stress or illnesses during the preceding 6 months. Telogen effluvium, for example, results from recent stressful experiences. Family history of hair loss is reported in about 10–20% of cases of alopecia areata (4,5,6).

14.3.2 Examination

General physical examination should be directed to detect signs of systemic diseases or infections. Specifically note for abnormalities of nails and teeth; also, assess the growth and nutrition of the patient. Determine the pattern of hair loss based on examination of the scalp – circumscribed or diffuse. A circumscribed area of hair loss present since birth may suggest specific congenital causes of alopecia. In tinea capitis characteristic circumscribed lesions are noted with areas in which hair are broken off, giving the "black dot" appearance (2,3). Scaly, patchy areas of hair loss are seen in tinea capitis, atopic dermatitis, or traumatic alopecia. Pustules are seen in infectious folliculitis. In telogen effluvium hairs have a tapered shaft and are easily pulled. The hair pull test is useful in determining if alopecia is active. Hair in the affected area are grasped between the thumb and forefinger and gently pulled; removal of six hairs indicates a positive hair pull test (2).

14.3.3 Laboratory investigation

Microscopic examination of hair can be helpful in ascertaining the etiology; for example, in telogen effluvium, the root is non-pigmented and bulb shaped (4). Microscopic examination requires a certain level of skill and experience on the clinician's part. Fungal infection of the scalp is common in children. A fungal culture is the gold standard to identify the specific etiological agent. The specimen for culture should be obtained by using a soft sterile brush or curette. Hair long enough to be plucked is likely not infected, and, therefore, plucked hair may give a false negative result. Wood light examination is useful only to identify infections with *Microsporum crosporum canis* and *M. audouinii* with hair fluorescing yellow-green, and for *Trichophyton schoenleinii*, with hair fluorescing pale green (2). *Trichophyton tonsurans* does not cause fluorescence with Wood light examination (2). If the room is not dark, Wood light examination may be false negative. False positive Wood light examination may be due to fluorescence caused by hair scale, lint, or petrolatum ointments.

14.4 Tinea capitis

Tinea capitis is a dermatophyte infection of scalp hair most commonly caused by *Trichophyton tonsurans* and less commonly by *Microsporum canis* as well as other species (2). It is a common infection that is most prevalent in the 4–14 year age group. *Trychophyton tonsurans* infects the hair shaft (endothrix infection), whereas other species infect the sheath around the hair (ectothrix infection) (2). *Trychophyton tonsurans* infection is more chronic, and the infection in most cases is spread via direct contact with infected hair or epithelial cells. In addition to direct contact with scalp hair, infected material can also be acquired by contact with theater seats, hats, and combs. Rarely the infection is spread via air borne spores.

The hair loss in tinea capitis is characterized by small, circular patches with hairs broken close to hair follicles. Tinea capitis can result in chronic or permanent alopecia. Kerion can result in scarring. Tinea capitis is treated with oral griseofulvin microcrystalline, 20 mg/kg/day for 8–12 weeks. The treatment should be continued for 4 weeks following negative culture to prevent recurrence. Other medications used include itraconazole (3–5 mg/kg/day for 4–6 weeks) and terbinafine (3–6 mg/kg/day for 4–6 weeks).

14.5 Telogen effluvium

Telogen effluvium describes excessive hair loss of telogen hair due to abnormal hair cycling and is the most common cause of alopecia in children (1,2,3,4). The exact prevalence of telogen effluvium is not known, and the hair loss can range from mild to severe. The child or adolescent presents with a history of hair loss that is more than usual and describes hair loss in handfuls. The alopecia is diffuse and non-scarring, while the pull test is positive. The onset is usually sudden and generally preceded by a stressful event within the past 3 months. The progression of hair loss can be either acute or chronic.

Acute telogen effluvium can result following acute severe illness, especially febrile illness, major surgical procedure, or traumatic event. In adolescents and young women it can result following childbirth. *Chronic* telogen effluvium can be associated with iron deficiency, hyper- or hypothyroidism, disordered eating, celiac disease, zinc deficiency, or other chronic illnesses. Some of the medications implicated include oral contraceptive pills, isotretinoin, or anticonvulsants. Once the underlying inciting event resolves, normal hair growth resumes and, in most cases, no further treatment is necessary. In chronic cases the recovery may be prolonged with an intermittent course.

14.6 Alopecia areata

Alopecia areata is characterized by abrupt onset of patchy, nonscarring hair loss (4,5,6). It is a common disorder with an estimated prevalence of 1 in 1,000 in the population (4). The lesion can be an isolated patch of hair loss or can be multifocal. Severe cases may result in total scalp hair loss (alopecia totalis) or total loss of all body hair (alopecia universalis). At the periphery of the patch of hair loss the broken hair has tapered proximal ends (the “exclamation-mark hairs”) and the pull test is positive (4,5). In a pattern called the ophiasis pattern, the hair is lost in bands at the lower periphery of the scalp (2).

The exact pathogenesis of alopecia areata is not elucidated; however, it is believed to be immune-mediated. In most cases of alopecia areata, the hair regrows within a year (6). In some cases the course is unpredictable and can be characterized by multiple remissions and relapses over many years. Childhood onset and more extensive hair loss at the onset are poor prognostic features. Although there is no cure for alopecia areata, pharmacological agents have been used to shorten the course and prevent the relapses. Such treatment modalities include intralesional corticosteroid injections, high potency or ultra-potency topical steroids, and topical minoxidil (2,4,10). In more resistant and severe cases, potent sensitizers such as squaric acid dibutyl ester (SADBE) or diphencyprone (DCP) have been used.

14.7 Male pattern hair loss

Male pattern hair loss is an androgen-dependent hereditary disorder in which dihydrotestosterone acts on genetically susceptible hair follicles resulting in the characteristic pattern of hair loss (1,4,7,8,9). The anagen phase of the hair cycle is reduced, and large hair follicles are transformed into small follicles. The hair is finer and shorter and no longer covers the scalp as well. Androgenic alopecia often begins in adolescence and is the most common type of hair loss in adults. The main age of onset is reported to be as early as 15 years.

In men, the thinning and hair loss is more pronounced in the frontal and vertex regions with some temporal recession. The patient usually does not present with complaint of hair loss, rather the patient is first concerned about thinning and decreased density of hair. Other symptoms and signs suggestive of endogenous or exogenous androgen excess should be ascertained in the evaluation of androgenic alopecia. Family history of similar hair loss in parents is often positive. Androgenic alopecia is a progressive disorder.

The goal of treatment is to slow the progression of hair loss and regrow hair. Minoxidil (2% or 5%) applied to the scalp, 1 ml for 1 hour daily for at least 12 months, is found to be effective. Progression of hair loss occurs when the minoxidil is discontinued. Finasteride oral treatment is approved for age 18 years of age and older.

14.8 Hair Loss due to Chemotherapy

Hair loss in children and adolescents is psychologically distressing and has a negative impact on the quality of life. Long term hair loss such as that associated with chemotherapy and some medical disorders can be especially difficult to cope with leading to considerable distress. Children and adolescents with hair loss can suffer from low self-esteem, depression, and social withdrawal. In many cases there is no effective treatment available, and regrowth of hair may take a long time in those whose hair loss is due to reversible causes. In these children and adolescents hair prosthetics can be used. The cost of professionally fitted prosthetic hairpieces in the United States is between $3,000 and $6,000 (11). The not-for-profit organization Locks of Love in the United States has been providing hair prosthetic hairpieces to individuals between 6 and 18 years of age who are not able to afford them (11).

14.9 Psychiatric aspects

Though it is well known that hair loss can induce various behavioral sequelae, data is limited on the incidence or prevalence of psychiatric disorders in children and adolescents with major hair loss disorders. Prevalence rates of cormorbid psychiatric disorders in patients with alopecia areata varies between not finding any association at all (12) to as much as three quarter of patients having comorbid psychological factors (13). The differences could be due to the different methodological approaches used, the number of subjects enrolled, selection of the research population, and the nature of psychometric measures employed.

The prevalence of psychiatric comorbidity was reported to be much higher by the study conducted by Colon et al when they used the Diagnostic Interview Schedule to interview patients with alopecia areata (13). They reported that 74% of patients with alopecia areata had one or more psychiatric disorders over the course of their lifetime. They reported that both depression and anxiety were very common in their population as 39% of the patients reported the symptomatology meeting the criteria of major depression disorder and generalized anxiety disorder. There was a preponderance of generalized anxiety disorders in patients developing patchy alopecia over the ones with non-patchy hair loss. They also reported a higher degree of familial predisposition for psychiatric disorders in patients with alopecia areata. About 58% of these patients had a first degree relative with generalized anxiety disorder, and 35% of them had a first-degree relative afflicted with depressive disorders and some type of substance abuse disorders (13).

Psychological stress plays a two-fold role in cases of children afflicted with alopecia. There appears to be a temporal relationship between alopecia areata and stress. Liakopoulou et al reported that children who developed alopecia areata had fewer positive events in the year predating the onset of alopecia areata. On the other hand, having a disorder such as alopecia areata significantly impacts the self-image of children and adolescents, giving rise to secondary psychiatric disorders.

Children with disorder of hair loss, such as alopecia areata, attending a pediatric clinic were assessed with several validated psychometric scales (14). The children with alopecia areata were found to have significant psychiatric issues, including feeling depressed and anxious. They also showed more behavior problems, such as being aggressive and delinquent, as well as other internalizing and externalizing behaviors in comparison to the age matched controls. These children displayed more somatic focus and appeared socially withdrawn. Attention and concentration problems are also reported in association with AA. (14)

A Polish study also reported very high levels (62% to 80%) of occurrence of major stressful life events in patients with AA (15). This study also found that about 73% patients with alopecia areata were likely to have personality traits that could predispose them to alopecia areata, and about 62% of these patients suffered from some kind of attachment loss (15). The same kind of association with attachment loss, avoidance behaviors, and avoidant personality traits along with alexithymia was also reported by other studies (16). A high incidence of other anxiety disorders, such as simple phobia, in children has also been reported (17).

14.9.1 Psychological treatment approaches

Patients with alopecia areata develop a significant psychological burden that, if overlooked while planning the treatment strategies, can lead to poor prognosis. Hair loss causes significant obstacles, especially for children and adolescents as they do not have fully developed coping skills to deal with an illness that impacts their self-esteem and body image in a profound way. In this age, when peer acceptance is important, they may feel that peers are looking at them differently or making fun of their appearance, leading them to withdraw and isolate themselves, adversely impacting the psychiatric well-being and, thus, worsening the overall prognosis.

Empathic and supportive approaches are necessary with these patients as they may have significant life stresses to deal with along with their illness. Being aware of these stressors is important for the clinician, and they may play a major role in relapses of the hair disease. Psychoeducation, taking in account the age of the child, should be considered as part of all treatment plans as this will increase awareness of the psychological factors playing a part in their disease cycle, correct the faulty perception about their disease, and improve compliance with treatment recommendations. Attempts should be made to identify faulty perceptions impacting their self-esteem and how to intervene so that it will not result in lifelong patterns of psychological distress. Studies have shown that poor adjustment to life is associated with development of a personality disorder or a comorbid depression and anxiety in patients with alopecia areata (18).

The National Alopecia Areata Foundation (NAAF) is an organization that was started by a young patient herself about 30 years ago (19). Today NAAF has grown steadily to the extent that it now has a network of about 80 patient support groups in the United States, Canada, and other countries (19). NAAF provides resources not only for patients but also for parents and families, such as annual family conferences in addition to informative publications both in written and online format; there is also a comprehensive website (http://www.naaf.org) with a message board that provides an opportunity to engage with other patients online. Information about resources in general and about local support groups can also be requested by emailing info@naaf.org (19). Children and adolescents are likely to take advice from their peers or role models, and if such forums or support groups can be arranged locally, at these meetings they can learn about their illness, what coping skills to employ, and how to respond assertively to the teasing and bullying that occurs because of their appearance. Psychoeducation for parents and families may also be necessary when the psychosocial factors relate to specific family situations; interpersonal interactions and parenting styles are thought to be the perpetuating factors in these situations.

Various alternative and psychotherapeutic modalities have been utilized in management of recalcitrant alopecia, including progressive muscle relaxation, meditation, acupuncture, visual imagery, and systemic desensitization with varied results, but none of these have been conducted in children and the adolescent population (20). Individual, interpersonal, and cognitive behavioral therapy all have shown efficacy in patients with chronic medical illness who have comorbid psychiatric conditions (21). Interpersonal therapy and cognitive behavioral therapy have shown efficacy in treatment of chronic dermatologic conditions including alopecia (22). Hypnosis and post-hypnotic ego strengthening and positive suggestion were also found to be effective (23).

Given the significant comorbidity of psychiatric disorder with alopecia areata, attempts have been made to utilize antidepressants as part of the treatment regimen in alopecia areata with promising results (24). The tricyclic antidepressant imipramine was shown to be effective in treating alopecia areata in a small double blind placebo controlled study (25). Five out of 7 patients who were treated with imipramine for 6 months showed hair regrowth that was significantly better than the patients on placebo who did not show any regrowth (25). More recently, a double-blind, randomized, placebo-controlled trial utilized paroxetine, a selective serotonin reuptake inhibitor (SSRI), in 13 patients with alopecia (26). Two of the patients treated with paroxetine showed complete regrowth of hair, while four patients showed partial regrowth; in comparison, only one patient in the placebo group showed regrowth of hairs (26). Early resolution of alopecia was also reported when paroxetine was used in combination with triamcinolone (27).

It is to be noted that all of these studies were conducted in the adult population. Another thing to keep in mind when dealing with alopecia and comorbid psychiatric disease is that alopecia can also be a rare adverse drug reaction (ADR) of SSRIs (see Chapter 22). A review of reported cases of alopecia as an ADR in the Swedish registry from the time SSRIs were marketed until 2004 revealed about 27 cases of alopecia. This should be noted in the context that cumulative SSRIs use amounted to 2.8 million patients per year or 10.25 million defined daily doses (DDDs) in the same registry (28).

14.10 Conclusion

Normal hair growth cycle is divided into anagen, catagen, and telogen phases. Hair loss can result in considerable psychological distress in the pediatric population. Common causes of hair loss in this group include tinea capitis, telogen effluvium, androgenic alopecia, alopecia areata, and traumatic alopecia. Management is variable and dependant on the underlying cause. Clinicians should be sensitive to hair loss disorders in their pediatric patients and provide medical as well as behavioral support. Alopecia is a dermatologic condition that has significant psychiatric comorbidity. A multidisciplinary approach may be the best way to approach these disorders, especially when disease can be recalcitrant and affect the quality of life. Patients with alopecia may respond to psychotherapeutic interventions in a way that may improve not only the symptomatology of their psychiatric disorder but also the course and outcome of these hair loss disorders.

References

1. Krowchuk DP. Disorders of the skin, In: Greydanus DE, Patel DR, Pratt HD, eds. *Essential adolescent medicine*. New York: McGraw Hill, 2006:411–43.
2. Paller A, Mancici AJ. Disorders of hair and nails, In: Paller A, Mancici AJ. *Hurwitz Clinical Pediatric Dermatology*, 4th edn. Philadelphia: Elsevier Saunders, 2011:130–66.
3. Mounsey AL, Reed SW. Diagnosing and treating hair loss. *Am Fam Physician* 2009;80(4):356–62.
4. Bedocs LA, Bruckner AL. Adolescent hair loss. *Curr Opin Pediatr* 2008;20:431–5.
5. Nanda A, Al-Fouzan AS, Al-Hasawi F. Alopecia areata in children: A clinical profile. *Pediatr Dermatol* 2002;19:482–5.
6. Tosti A, Bellavista S, Iorizzo M. Alopecia areata: A long term follow-up study of 191 patients. *J Am Acad Dermatol* 2006;55:438–41.
7. Olsen EA, Messenger AG, Shapiro J, Bergfeld WF, Hordinsky MK, Roberts JL, Stough D. Evaluation and treatment of male and female pattern hair loss. *J Am Acad Dermatol* 2005;52:301–11.
8. Price VH. Androgenic alopecia in adolescents. *Cutis* 2003;71:115–21.
9. Kim BJ, Kim JY, Eun HC, Kwon OS, Kim MN, Ro BI. Androgenic alopecia in adolescents: A report of 43 cases. *J Dermatol* 2006;33:696–9.
10. Georgala S, Benton A, Maniatopoulou E, Georgala C. Topical minoxidil in children and systemic side effects. *Dermatology* 2007;214:101–2.
11. Silverberg NB. Helping children cope with hair loss. *Cutis* 2006;78:333–6.
12. Gülec AT, Tanriverdi N. Dürü Ç. The role of psychological factors in alopecia areata and the impact of the disease on the quality of life. *Int J Dermatol* 2004; 43:352–6.
13. Colón EA, Popkin MK, Callies AL. Lifetime prevalence of psychiatric disorders in Patients with alopecia areata. *Comprehen Psychiatry* 1991;32:245–51.
14. Liakopoulou M, Alifieraki T, Katideniou A. Children with alopecia areata: Psychiatric symptomatology and life events. *J Am Acad Child Psychiatr* 1997;36:678–84.
15. Wygledowska-Kania M, Bodanowski T. Psychic factors in case histories of patientswith alopecia areata – preliminary report. *Psychiatr Pol* 1996;30:669–84.
16. Picardi A, Pasquini P, Cattaruzza MS. Psychosomatic factors in first-onset alopecia areata. *Psychosomatics* 2003;44:374–81.
17. Reeve EA, Savage TA, Bernstin GA. Psychiatric diagnoses in children with alopecia areata. *J Am Acad Child Psychiatry* 1996;35:1518–22.
18. Ruiz-Doblado S, Carrizosa A, García-Hernández MJ. Alopecia areata: Psychiatric comorbidity and adjustment to illness. *Int J Dermatol* 2003;42:434–37.
19. Kalabokes VD. Alopecia areata: Support groups and meetings – how can it help your patient. *Dermatologic Ther* 2011;24:302–4.
20. Stowe JE, Goldenberg E. Systematic desensitization as a component for treatment of alopecia areata: A case study. *Psychologic Rep* 1980;46:875–81.
21. Bolan R. Cognitive-behavioral therapy, psychotherapy, and psychosocial interventions in the medically ill. *Psychother Psychosom* 2009;78:261–64.
22. Fried RG, Hussain SH. Nonpharmacological management of common skin and psycho-cutaneous disorders. *Dermatol Ther* 2008;21:60–8.
23. Shenefelt PD. Complementary psychocutaneous therapies in dermatology. *Dermatol Clin* 2005;23:723–34.

24. Gregoriou S, Kazako C, Rigopoulos D. Treatment options for alopecia areata. *Ext Rev Dermatol* 2011;6:537–48.
25. Perini G. Zara M, Cipriani R. Imipramine in alopecia areata. *Psychother Psychosom* 1994; 61:3–4.
26. Cipriani R, Perini G. Rampinelli S. Paroxetine in alopecia areata. *Int J Dermatol* 2001; 40:600–1.
27. Ricciardi A, Ruberto A, García-Hernández MJ. Alopecia areata with comorbid depression; early resolution with combined paroxetine-triamcinolone treatment. *J Eur Acad Dermatol Venerol* 2006;40:100–1.
28. Hedenmalm K, Sundström A, Spigse O. Alopecia associated with treatment with selective serotonin reuptake inhibitors (SSRIs). *Pharmacoepidemiol Drug Saf* 2006;15:719–25.

Dilip R. Patel

15 Disorders of skin pigmentation

Melanin is the pigment responsible for the color of the skin and hair. Melanin is formed and stored in the melanosomes. The intensity of skin pigmentation depends on the size and number of melanosomes present in the keratinocytes, the rate of melanin synthesis, and the rate of transport of melanin within keratinocytes. Changes in skin pigmentation, especially on the visible parts of the body, can contribute to social withdrawal and psychological distress in children, adolescents, and their parents. This chapter also reviews common disorders of skin pigmentation, including vitiligo, albinism, postinflammatory changes, tinea versicolor, and different medical disorders that are associated with changes in skin pigmentation. Psychosocial complications of skin pigmentation disorders and principles of management are considered as well in pediatric patients with skin pigmentation disorders.

15.1 Introduction

Melanin is the pigment responsible for the color of the hair and skin. Melanin present in the epidermis of the skin serves a protective function against ultraviolet radiation-induced changes that may lead to skin cancer. Melanin is synthesized in the melanocytes, which are embyrogenically derived from the neural crest (1,2). Melanin is formed from the amino acid tyrosine. Tyrosine is converted to dihydroxyphenylalanine (DOPA) by tyrosinase. DOPA is then oxidized to dopaquinone and finally to melanin (2). In addition to the presence of melanin in the epidermis, other factors contribute to the color of the skin that include the thickness of the stratum corneum and local blood flow (2,3,4).

Skin pigmentation largely depends on the formation and packaging of melanin in the melanosomes of the epidermal cells. The intensity of the skin pigmentation depends on the size and number or density of melanosomes present in the keratinocytes, the rate of melanin synthesis, and the rate of transport of melanin within keratinocytes (2). Sex steroids (estrogen and progesterone) and peptide hormones (alpha- and beta-melanocyte stimulating hormone [MSH], and adrenocorticotropin hormone [ACTH]) also affect skin pigmentation. Skin pigmentation is also influenced by genetic factors. Typically the dorsal and extensor surfaces are relatively darker than the ventral surfaces. Numerous conditions can cause either hypopigmentation (Tables 15.1 and 15.2) or hyperpigmentation of the skin (Table 15.3) (1,2,3,4,5,6).

Table 15.1: Causes of Generalized Hypopigmentation

Vitiligo
Albinism
Pheylketonuria
Homocysteinuria
Histidinemia
Griscelli syndrome
Elajalde syndrome
Menkes syndrome
Copper deficiency
Selenium deficiency

Table 15.2: Causes of Localized Hypopigmentation

Vitiligo
Piebaldisim
Waardenburg syndrome
Nevus anemica
Tuberous sclerosis
Postinflammatory hypopigmentation
Lichen sclerosis
Pityriasis alba
Tinea versicolor

15.2 Disorders of hypopigmentation

15.2.1 Vitiligo

Vitiligo is characterized by loss of skin pigmentation typically resulting in oval or irregular ivory-white patches of skin with well-demarcated convex borders (1,2,7). The underlying cause of vitiligo is genetically determined – autosomal dominant trait of variable penetrance – and its prevalence is estimated to be 2% in the population (2). Approximately 30% of individuals with vitiligo have a positive family history of vitiligo, halo nevi, traumatic depigmentation of the skin, or markedly premature graying of the scalp hair (2).

Although the onset of vitiligo is most common during young adult age, it can begin at any age, and approximately half of the cases are reported to have onset before age 20 years (1,2,3). About 20% of cases have been reported with onset before age 10 years (1). Rare cases of congenital vitiligo have been reported.

Table 15.3: Causes of Hyperpigmentation

Postinflammatory hyperpigmentation
Melasma
Riehl melanosis
Poikiloderma
Erythema dyschromicum perstans
Familial progressive hyperpigmentation
Nevoid hypermelanosis
Adrenal insufficiency
Hyperpituitarism
Cushing syndrome
Hemochromatosis
Ochronosis
Argyria – silver toxicity
Chrysiasis – gold toxicity
Drug-induced hyperpigmentation
Fixed drug eruptions
Café-au-lait spots
Lentigines

In three quarters of the cases the initial lesions at presentation are noted on the exposed areas such as dorsal surfaces of the hands, face, and neck. Other sites that are relatively more prone to develop depigmentation include the axillae, groin, around the eyes, nostrils, mouth, navel, areolae, genitals, perianal regions, and bony prominences around joints of the extremities (3,4,5,6). The lesions vary in size and shape and can be partially or fully depigmented. Individual depigmented areas can be just a few millimeters in size to total body involvement.

The patient typically presents with concerns about hypopigmented areas of the skin following a recent sun exposure. Often the patient initially attributes the lesion to effects of sunburn. Some patients present following a period of severe psychological or physical stress. The diagnosis of vitiligo is clinical based on the history and characteristic morphology of the skin lesions. Wood light examination may help differentiate normal skin from depigmented lesions, especially in fair skinned individuals.

Lesions of vitiligo should be differentiated from other common conditions. These include postinflammatory hypopigmentation, albinism, and hypopigmented macules seen in tuberous sclerosis, pityriasis alba, and tinea versicolor. The mainstay of differentiation is the morphologic characteristics of the lesions in different conditions.

There is no cure for vitiligo. The clinical course of vitiligo is variable with intermittent periods of exacerbations and partial improvement. Often physical or psychological stress seems to exacerbate the condition. Although complete remission of lesions is rare, partial improvement is often noted during summer months. Repigmentation is a very slow process and seen in areas with relative abundance of hair follicles because the migration of melanocytes from the hair bulbs to epidermis is believed to contribute to the repigmentation.

Treatment of vitiligo is difficult, and long term and patients should be referred to a dermatologist for long term care. The options for treatment include use of topical corticosteroids, topical tacrolimus, topical pimecrolimus, and administration of psoralen compounds followed by gradually increasing exposure to sunlight or long-wave ultraviolet light. In addition, different cosmetic makeup can be used to mask small lesions (1,2,7).

15.2.2 Albinism

Albinism is an uncommon inherited disorder affecting synthesis of melanin. Patients present with areas of complete lack of pigmentation affecting the skin, hair, and eyes at birth. Two types of albinism are described: *oculocutaneous*, involving both the skin and the eyes; and *ocular*, involving only the eyes (2). Oculocutaneous albinism is an autosomal recessive disorder affecting 1 in 17,000 individuals in the United States (2). The lesions are characterized by irregular reduction in pigmentation affecting the skin and hair, translucent irides, and hypopigmented ocular fundi. Often there is associated nystagmus.

The clinical findings in whites with oculocutaneous albinism include milk-white skin, white to yellow or brown hair, pink pupils, and gray or blue irides (2,3). Photophobia and photosensitivity are also common. In blacks the findings may include tan colored skin, freckles, blond or red colored hair, and blue or hazel eyes. Because of photophobia and central scotomas, patients develop habitual squinting and nystagmus.

Patients with ocular albinism have translucency of the iris, photophobia, nystagmus, and head nodding mannerisms. There is decreased pigmentation of the irides and posterior fundus, and stippling of the retina. There is no effective treatment of albinism. Contact lenses and tinted spectacles may help ameliorate photophobia. Some types of oculocutaneous albinism are associated with bleeding diathesis, while others are fatal. All cases of albinism should be referred to specialists for further evaluation and management.

15.2.3 Postinflammatory hypopigmentation

Postinflammatory decrease in pigmentation is common and can be associated with a number of inflammatory conditions affecting the skin. Areas of hypopigmentation are noted following resolution of inflammatory conditions such as burns, local infections, eczema, psoriasis, and pityriasis rosea. It is also seen in secondary syphilis and pityriasis lichenoides. Although the exact mechanism of postinflammatory hypopigmentation is not clear, it is postulated that the keratinocytes affected by inflammation are transiently not able to accept melanosomes from the melanocyte dendrites. It is important to recognize postinflammatory hypopigmentation because it is common and it improves with time so that the patients can be reassured and relieved of distress.

15.2.4 Pityriasis alba

Pityriasis alba is a common disorder characterized by scaly hypopigmented patches on the face, neck, upper trunk, arms, and shoulders (1,2,4). In young children it may also affect the lower trunk and extremities. Individual lesions can vary in size from very small to extensive. The margin of lesion is typically sharply delineated. It is seen most commonly in pediatric patients between 3 and 16 years of age. The exact cause is not known. The course is variable with most resolving over time. Application of topical corticosteroid for 2–3 weeks reduces inflammation. Repigmentation eventually occurs in most cases; however, patients should be counseled that it may take up to 1 year for this to occur.

15.2.5 Tinea versicolor

Tinea versicolor is a common disorder that causes irregular areas of hypopigmentation affecting mainly the trunk and neck regions (1,4). Lesions have well defined borders and are round or oval with fine scales, while individual macules may coalesce to form large patches. It is believed to be caused by *Pityrosporum orbiculare (Malassezia* furfur), an organism that is a normal component of skin flora (1,5). Tinea versicolor is seen most commonly in adolescents and young adults.

Diagnosis is apparent from history and morphology of the lesions but can be confirmed by potassium hydroxide (KOH) preparation on scales obtained from the lesion. Spores and hyphae of the organisms can be seen on the KOH preparation. Wood light examination often reveals a yellow-orange to blue-white fluorescence (2).

Tinea versicolor is treated with topical selenium sulfide 2.5% lotion. The lotion is applied to affected areas for 10 minutes once daily for 7 days (1,2). In order to prevent recurrences, selenium sulfide is applied for 8–12 hours every 1–2 months for a period of 4–6 months (2). Stinging and unpleasant odor are common side effects of selenium sulfide. Another treatment used is ketoconazole shampoo applied for 5 minutes daily for 1–3 days. In more persistent cases topical imidazome has been used. Other treatments used in such cases include oral ketoconazole, itraconazole, or fluconazole. Patients should be counseled that it will take several months for repigmentation to occur.

15.3 Disorders of hyperpigmentation

15.3.1 Postinflammatory hyperpigmentation

Postinflammatory hyperpigmentation is the most common cause of hyperpigmentation in children and adolescents. It is due to an increased synthesis of melanin following skin inflammation. Some of the causes for postinflammatory hyperpigmentation include skin trauma, friction, application of skin irritants, eczema, lichen simplex chronicus, pityriasis rosea, psoriasis, drug reactions, skin infections, and sunburns. Individuals with dark complexions and who tan easily tend to have more intense postinflammatory hyperpigmentation. The hyperpigmentation resolves over time, and fading is facilitated if further exposure to ultraviolet light is avoided. In cases with more extensive, severe, or persistent lesions, topical low-potency corticosteroid may be used.

15.3.2 Melasma

Melasma is characterized by patchy, dark-brown hyperpigmentation predominantly affecting the cheeks and the forehead (2,8). Lesions can also affect the temples, upper lip, and neck. It is reported in women taking contraceptive pills and also in pregnant women. Sun exposure often triggers the hyperpigmentation, and the disorder is more prominent during summer. Melasma is also reported to be triggered by some drugs, such as phenytoin. Melasma typically persists for several months, and there is no effective treatment. Often the resolution occurs following removal of the triggering factors.

15.3.3 Hyperpigmentation associated with medical disorders

Various medical conditions are associated with hyperpigmentation (2). In some of these hyperpigmentation is the presenting sign of the underlying disease. In patients with chronic liver disease a diffuse hyperpigmentation is often seen. Blotchy areas of brown hyperpigmentation occasionally may be seen. In adrenal insufficiency hyperpigmentation results from increased production of MSH and is most prominent in flexural areas, sites of pressure or friction, in the creases of palms and soles, around genitalia, areolae, and in sun-exposed areas. Oral mucosa can also be affected.

Hyperpigmentation is seen in some cases of primary thyrotoxicosis. There is usually a diffuse pattern of hyperpigmentation. Similar hyperpigmentation can also be seen in hyperpituitarism and Cushing syndrome.

15.3.4 Café-au-lait spots

Café-au-lait spots are hyperpigmented, sharply demarcated macules seen in many disorders, of which neurofibromatosis type 1 is the most common. The lesions vary widely in age of onset, size, and distribution. One to three lesions are common in many children and are considered normal without indicating any underlying condition. The lesions may be present at birth or develop later in childhood and adolescence. Some of the disorders in which café-au-lait lesions are seen include neurofibromatosis type 1 and 2, MaCune-Albright syndrome, Russell-Silver syndrome, tuberous sclerosis, Boom syndrome, Hunter syndrome, Turner syndrome, and Chediak-Higashi syndrome (2,3,4). Therefore, presence of café-au-lait lesions should prompt further evaluation for possible underlying disorders, including various syndromes.

15.3.5 Lentigines

Lentigines are small, round, dark brown macules that affect any region of the body. These lesions are permanent and do not change with sun exposure. It is important to recognize that in most cases these lesions are benign and permanent. Lentigines are also seen in LAMB syndrome (lentigines of the face and vulva, atrial myxoma, mucocutaneous myxomas, and blue nevi) and in LEOPARD syndrome (lentigines, electrocardiogram abnormalities, ocular hypertelorism, pulmonary stenosis, abnormal genitals, growth retardation, and sensorineural hearing loss). Hyperpigmented macules are also a feature of Peutz-Jeghers syndrome (2,3).

15.4 Psychological aspects of disorders of pigmentations

The disorders of skin that cause some form of disfigurement can impact a person's life in a profound way, and disorders of pigmentations are one of these disorders. Psychological stress is proposed in the pathogenesis of vitiligo, suggesting a psychoneuroimmunologic factor via hypothalamo-pituitary-adrenal (HPA)-axis stimulation along with the genetic predisposition and autoimmune etiology. In a study of patients with vitiligo, a stressful life event was cited as leading to the skin change; major stressors that were reported included personal injury or illness, major changes in health or behavior of a family member, death of a friend or family member, and change in residence (9). Another study conducted in Tehran also reported that this same kind of belief was held by about 60% of patients diagnosed with vitiligo in that psychological stressors played a role in their disease (10). This same study also reported that about half of the patients noted that vitiligo exerted major consequences on their lives and that their illness has strongly impacted their self-esteem (10).

Although vitiligo is a relatively rare skin condition, it is still one of the most common skin conditions leading to disfigurement and has a significant impact on self-esteem as well as reduced quality of life (11). About half of the cases of vitiligo start before age 20, leading to a profound impact on the self-esteem and body image of children, adolescents, and young adults (12). First, qualitative description of the psychosocial impact of vitiligo was presented by Porter et al who surveyed patients with vitiligo in 1978 and discovered that the majority of these patients felt self-conscious in social situations, even embarrassed by their appearance, preventing them from establishing relationships with new people; these patients considered vitiligo as a significant difficulty when approaching intimate physical relationships (13). Patients also reported that people gawked at them, made rude remarks, and treated them differently (13).

The burden on quality of life as measured by the dermatology quality of life index (DQLI) in patients with vitiligo was assessed and compared with another skin disease with high psychosocial comorbidity – psoriasis. It appears that QoL impact of vitiligo was lower than what was experienced by patients with psoriasis, overall; however, when asked about impact of symptoms and treatment on QoL, patients with vitiligo and psoriasis scored equally on items such as feelings of embarrassment, choice of clothing (in an attempt to hide lesions), and impact on social, leisure, and daily routines (14). Women with vitiligo were more likely to report these issues and were more likely to avoid certain activities, choose certain types of clothing, and be more embarrassed about their appearance than their male counterparts (14). It was also noted that patients who reported high on the DQLI were more likely to frequently visit their dermatologist. In another similar study, vitiligo patients were found to have better psychosocial adjustment than the patients with psoriasis (15).

Schmid-Ott et al studied the level of stigmatization in patients with vitiligo and their utilization of coping skills. Three psychometric scales were used: Experience with Skin Complaints (QES), Sense of Coherence (SOC) questionnaires, and Adjustment to Chronic Skin Disorders (ASC). This study reported that these patients experienced a higher level of stigmatization in participants with visible lesions (16). In responding to the general health questionnaire (GHQ), 35% of patients with vitiligo reported a sense of stigmatization and subsequently avoided certain social situations and activities that impacted their overall sense of general well-being (17). Children and adolescents are especially more vulnerable to the negative impact of a skin disease such as vitiligo during their formative years of their life when their psychological profile is still under development.

One study examined children and adolescents between ages 8–18 years with vitiligo and found that those with vitiligo reported higher scores on psychometric testing for depression; however, the scores for state and trait anxiety were comparable to the control group (12). When the adolescent group between ages 13–18 years of age were reviewed, no significant differences were observed on depression and anxiety scales when compared to the control group. However, the severity of vitiligo was found to be negatively correlated with psychosocial scores as measured by pediatric quality of life-psychosocial subset (Peds QL-P) (12). One interesting finding of this study was that girls reported more impact on health-related quality of life (HRQoL) when the vitiligo lesions were located on feet, legs, and genitalia in comparison to lesions on head, face, and neck; boys, however, scored worse if they had lesions affecting head, neck, and face (12).

It has been suggested that this difference could be explained by the observation that girls are more likely to hide or camouflage the lesions on the face and neck area with make-up than boys, while the lesions on hidden parts of the body generally are not camouflaged with makeup and can cause significant difficulties in sexual identity (12). Other studies also have reported significant psychiatric comorbidity with vitiligo, although most studies are conducted in the adult population.

15.4.1 Psychosocial management of disorders of pigmentation

Patients with disorders of pigmentation often have misconceptions about their illness. The overall prognosis can be improved over the long term by providing psychoeducation regarding the nature and course of this illness, along with the available treatment options, including complimentary and psychosocial therapies. Vitiligo and other disorders of pigmentation can impact psychosocial aspects of a person's life in a significant way, as described earlier.

When treating patients with vitiligo it should be kept in mind that many start early in life with their disease, and the condition is likely to run a chronic, pervasive, and progressive course. Attempts should be made to assess QoL issues early on so that they can be appropriately addressed. Many QoL scales are available and can be easily administered in office settings including self reported scales such as the general health questionnaire (GHQ) and dermatology quality of life scale (DQLI). When QoL issues are so significant that they are predisposing this patient to a psychiatric illness (i.e. depression or anxiety), prompt referral for a psychiatric evaluation and management may result in an improved course and prognosis for the disorders of pigmentations; therapy and, if indicted, psychotropic medication can be very beneficial to these patients.

Patients may use makeup to conceal the lesions of vitiligo due to the disfigurement and stigma attached to these visible depigmented lesions. The use of makeup to camouflage these lesions on visible skin areas was studied and patients reported significant improvement in QoL issues, such as feelings of embarrassment, self consciousness, and choice of clothing (18). When patients were trained to use camouflage makeup and continued to use it to conceal visible depigmented lesions, they reported improvement in quality of life issues 1 month after this education (19).

Psychotherapeutic approaches have been used and were found to be effective. Cognitive behavioral therapy (CBT) was used in 16 patients for 8 consecutive weeks focusing on helping patients understand their negative thought processes; therapy revealed that this negativity was impacting their mood and psychological well-being, which in turn was causing worsening of their skin condition (i.e. vitiligo) (20). These patients were taught to identify their faulty thought patterns and to change these negative thought patterns, replacing them with a positive frame of mind. They were also encouraged to use better coping skills when faced with stigmatizing social conditions. The vitiligenous lesions were photographed before and after CBT along with assessment of the level of psychiatric disability via psychometric measures (20). Prior to the start of CBT, participants reported significant distress related to their body image, self-esteem, and quality of life issues. Psychometric testing showed improvement in scores of the patients who received CBT immediately after completion of treatment and at a 5 month follow up; there was no change in scores in the control group (20) Also, improvement in the size of lesions was also noted in some patients (20).

Other therapeutic interventions have shown success when used in treating disfiguring psychodermatologic diseases; these treatment modalities include supportive therapy, interpersonal therapy, peer support groups, family therapy, guided imagery, and medical hypnotherapy. Also utilized was behavioral therapy that involved techniques such as biofeedback, gradual muscle relaxation, and graded exposure to social situations, which are anxiety provoking and tend to be avoided (21,22,23). All of these reports are from studies carried out in the adult population, and there is no reported study specifically conducted in the pediatric population in regard to treating psychological aspects of pigmentation disorders. Similarly, there is no available data examining the benefit of using antidepressants and anxiolytics in treating psychiatric comorbidity in children and adolescents who have vitiligo and other disorders of pigmentations.

15.5 Conclusion

Melanin is the pigment responsible for the color of the hair and skin. Melanin that is present in the epidermis of the skin serves a protective function against ultraviolet radiation-induced changes that may lead to skin cancer. Melanin is synthesized in the melanocytes, which are embyrogenically derived from the neural crest. Skin pigmentation largely depends on the formation and packaging of melanin in the melanosomes of the epidermal cells. The intensity of the skin pigmentation depends on the size and number or density of melanosomes present in the keratinocytes, rate of melanin synthesis, and the rate of transport of melanin within keratinocytes. Numerous conditions affect skin pigmentation; some are self limited and benign, whereas others are chronic and associated with medical disorders.

For most primary skin pigmentation disorders, the treatment is not curative but can provide symptomatic amelioration and contribute to improved self-esteem as well as psychosocial adjustment in children and adolescents. Psychosocial complications of skin pigmentation disorders and principles of management are considered as well in pediatric patients with skin pigmentation disorders. Clinicians should be aware that these young patients not only have to deal with the burden of a chronic disease and its treatment but also have to deal with stigmatization, teasing, bullying, and quality of life issues, which can complicate the course and prognosis of the disorders of pigmentations.

References

1. Krowchuk DP. Disorders of the skin. In: Greydanus DE, Patel DR, Pratt HD, eds. *Essential adolescent medicine*. New York: McGraw Hill, 2006:411–43.
2. Paller A, Mancici AJ. Disorders of pigmentation. In: Paller A, Mancici AJ. *Hurwitz clinical pediatric dermatology*, 4th edn. Philadelphia, PA: Elsevier Saunders, 2011:234–67.
3. Tey HL. A practical classification of childhood hypopigmentation disorders. *Acta Derm Venereol* 2010;90:6–11.
4. Van der Veen JP. Pigmentary disorders in Western countries. *Dermatol Clin* 2007;25(3):449–55.
5. Rudikoff D. Differential diagnosis of round or discoid lesions. *Clin Dermatol* 2011;29(5):489–97.
6. Treat J. Patterned pigmentation in children. *Pediatr Clin North Am* 2010;57(5):1121–9.
7. Lotti T, Gori A, Zanieri F, Colucci R, Moretti S. Vitiligo: New and emerging treatments. *Dermatol Ther* 2008;21(2):110–7.
8. Achar A, Rathi SK. Melasma: A clinic-epidemiological study of 312 cases. *Indian J Dermatol* 2011;56(4):380–2.
9. Papadopoulos L, Bor R, Legg C. Impact of life events on the onset of vitiligo in adults: Preliminary evidence for a psychological dimension in aetiology. *Clin Exp Dermatol* 1998;23(6):243–8.
10. Firooz A, Bouzari N, Fallah N. What patients with vitiligo believe about their condition. *Int J Dermatol* 2004;43:811–4.
11. Finlay AY, Ryan TJ. Disability and handicap in dermatology. *Int J Dermatol* 1996;35(5):305–11.
12. Bilgiç Ö, Bilgiç A, Akiş HK, Eskioğlu F, Kiliç EZ. Depression, anxiety and health-related quality of life in children and adolescents with vitiligo. *Clin Exp Dermatol* 2011;36(4):360–5.
13. Porter JR, Beuf AH, Nordlund JJ, Lerner AB. Personal responses to vitiligo. *Arch Dermatol* 1978;114:1348–85.
14. Ongenae K, Van Geel N, De Schepper S, Naeyaert JM. Effect of vitiligo on self-reported health-related quality of life. *Br J Dermatol* 2005;152(6):1165–72.
15. Porter JR, Beuf AH, Lerner A, Nordlund J. Psychosocial effect of vitiligo: A comparison of vitiligo patients with "normal" control subjects, with psoriasis patients, and with patients with other pigmentary disorders. *J Am Acad Dermatol* 1986;15(2 Pt 1):220–24.
16. Schmid-Ott G, Künsebeck H-W, Jecht E, Shimshoni R. Stigmatization experience, coping and sense of coherence in vitiligo patients. *Dermatology* 2005;210(4):279–85.

17. Kent G, Al Abedie M. Psychologic effects of vitiligo: A critical incident analysis. *J Am Acad Dermatol* 1996;35(6):895–8.
18. Ongenae K, Dierckxsens L, Brochez L, van Geel N, Naeyaert JM. Quality of life and stigmatization profile in a cohort of vitiligo patients and effect of the use of camouflage. *Dermatology* 2005;210 (4):279–85.
19. Tanioka M, Yamamoto Y, Kato M, Miyachi Y. Camouflage for patients with vitiligo vulgaris improved their quality of life. *J Cosmet Dermatol* 2010; 9(1):72–5.
20. Papadopoulos L, Bor R, Legg C. Coping with the disfiguring effects of vitiligo: A preliminary investigation into the effects of cognitive behavioral therapy. *Psychol Psychother* 1999;72:385–96.
21. Rumsey N, Clarke A, White P, Wyn-Williams M. Altered body image: Appearance-related concerns of people with visible disfigurement. *J Adv Nurs* 2004;48(5):443–53.
22. Shenefelt PD. Complementary psychocutaneous therapies in dermatology. *Dermatologic Clinics* 2005;23:4:723–34.
23. Shenefelt PD. Psychodermatological disorders: Recognition and treatment. *Int J Dermatol* 2011; 50(11):1309–22.

Ladan Mostaghimi

16 Skin adnexal disorders

This chapter will help the reader have a good understanding of hidradenitis suppurativa (HS), a chronic and painful dermatology disorder, other skin adnexal disorders, such as hyperhidrosis, anhidrotic ectodermal dysplasia, and nevus sebaceous. The chapter briefly reviews these disorders and current available treatments and focuses on psychocutaneous problems related to these disorders. All of these chronic disorders require a holistic approach to help these patients cope with their dermatological conditions. Physicians need to help their patients have a better understanding of their disease and ways to control its symptoms. The physician's most important mission in chronic diseases is to help patients have the highest quality of life possible. Holistic evaluation of patients while having an age-appropriate bio-psycho-social approach in mind will help physicians accomplish this important mission.

16.1 Hidradenitis suppurativa (HS)

16.1.1 Introduction

Hidradenitis is a misnomer. The name was proposed due to distribution in areas containing apocrine glands prior to discovery of the primary problem being in the pilosebaceous unit; it is also known as Acne inversa and Verneuil disease. Hidradenitis suppurativa (HS) is a chronic, recurrent, inflammatory skin disease that causes a fair amount of scarring. It involves flexor parts of the body, such as axillary, groin, anogenital and inframammary areas. HS is a debilitating disease that impacts a patient's life in a most profound way, not only physically but also emotionally. Like any chronic disorder specially associated with pain, HS needs a holistic approach to help patients cope with this condition.

16.1.2 Diagnosis

Hidradenitis suppurativa can go undiagnosed for years. It is frequently misdiagnosed as boils. Early diagnosis is important to have appropriate treatment and prevent progression to a chronic disabling stage with a severe negative effect on the quality of life.

Hurley stages of HS is the first classification system proposed that emphasized extent of involvement:

Stage I: abscess formation, single or multiple without sinus tracts and cicatrization.
Stage II: recurrent abscesses with tract formation and cicatrization, single or multiple widely separated lesions.
Stage III: diffuse or near-diffuse involvement, or multiple interconnecting tracts and abscesses across entire area.

In order to have more dynamic and precise scoring for diagnosis and treatment, Karin Sartorius, during the Second International HS Research, proposed the following variables to be used in all reports (1):

1. Anatomic regions involved (axilla, groin, gluteal, or other region or infra-mammary region left or right);
2. Number and scores of lesions involved (nodules and fistula);
3. The longest distance between two relevant lesions (i.e. nodules and fistulas in each region or size if only one lesion present); and
4. The presence of normal skin in between lesions (i.e. are all lesions clearly separated by normal skin?).

She also proposed to add a visual analogue scale (VAS) to evaluate pain.
The symposium adopted the following diagnostic criteria (1,2):

1. Typical lesions: either deep seated painful nodules (blind boils) in early primary lesions or abscesses, draining sinuses, bridged scars, and tombstone open comedones in secondary lesions;
2. Typical topography: axillae, groin, genitals, perineal, and perianal region, buttocks, infra- and intermammary folds;
3. Chronicity and recurrences.

The prevalence is between 1% to 4% depend on the criteria used(2). HS usually starts after puberty, it's most frequent in 3rd decade of life and sometimes continues into old age(3).

16.1.3 Etiology

HS is multifactorial and genetic factors play a role; 35% to 40% of patients have positive family history, and in some patients, an autosomal dominant inheritance has been noted (2,4). Various infection agents can be cultured from HS lesions, but it is generally agreed that the role of bacteria is indirect. The super infection of lesions may be responsible for part of the destruction of tissue in stage III. Hormonal factors (especially androgens) play a role since the disease usually starts after puberty. Also, HS is more frequent in women and aggravates around menstrual periods; it improves after menopause.

The anti-androgens are effective in HS patients (5). Local innate immunity plays a role in causing the inflammation around the ruptured follicles, but there is no general inflammation, such as fever or lymphadenopathy; cultures are usually sterile.

Some factors can trigger or cause a flare in HS: medications such as lithium (6), sirolimus (7), and medroxyprogesterone acetate (2). Obesity is a risk factor, and patients with obesity have more severe disease (8). Nicotine may have a role in pathogenesis of the disease, and many patients with HS are smokers (9).

16.1.4 Clinical features

HS is a follicular disease and can be differentiated from other problems such as furunculosis (large boils) and epidermal cysts by presence of recurrent blind boils (round and deep) with opening under the skin and formation of sinus tracts. It causes a fair amount of scarring in the involved areas. Early lesions are usually sterile and can get secondary infections.

16.1.4.1 Psychiatric features and quality of life issues

Pain and suppuration as well as foul odor of the lesions cause considerable morbidity and impairment of quality of life (see Chapter 4). Patients complain of a non-ending cycle of stressful life events leading to acute relapses, which in turn impacts efficiency in their occupational roles, self-esteem, ability to make relationships, satisfaction with role fulfillment, and depressive symptomatology.

An online survey was conducted on the website of a major support organization for HS patients known as HS-USA Organization (10). At the time of accessing this information on October 05, 2011, this survey was taken by 4,436 patients (10). Following are some of the important findings of the survey:

- 3% of their patients were unemployed due to HS.
- In 5% of cases the disease started under age of 10 and in 50% between age 11 to 20; in 28% it was between ages 21–30.
- Groin/labia/scrotum was the most frequent affected site (45%) followed by armpits (37%) and other areas; about 6% had symptoms in head and neck area.
- Interestingly 44% of patients had normal weight when HS appeared but at the time of survey 54% were either overweight or slightly overweight and only 18% reported normal weight.
- 38% of respondents had stage 3 and 51% stage 2 HS.
- 33% of respondents felt that stress definitely makes their HS worse, while 40% felt it does make the HS worse but they were not sure. Only 3% did not feel that stress has a negative effect on their HS.
- 52% of patients never had a period of remission more than 3 months.
- 49% reported that they are often tired.
- 33% of patients reported having acne/chloracne/rosacea and 13% had pilonidal cysts.
- 25% of patients had the diagnosis of depression and were under treatment, 11% had the diagnosis but were not under treatment, and 27% felt they have

depression but they have not been officially diagnosed. About 33% of patients denied depression.
- Pain is a frequent problem and only 41% of patients never took pain pills for HS; in this group only 9% noted that pain is not a problem for them, and some reported that the doctor did not think they need pain medication. Also, 38% would use over the counter pain pills, and about 6% of patients have used narcotic pain medications for their HS.

As this survey of the patients indicates, depression is a problem for many patients; therefore, it is important to screen the patients for depression. Depression decreases the pain threshold and increases the number of doctor visits and rate of disability; thus, appropriate treatment and referral is very important.

Also, young patients in their formative years, when affected by this type of chronic, painful problem, may develop social anxiety and start to avoid social situations. They may also lose days of school, which in turn affects their academic achievements and aggravates the situation. Prompt evaluation for potential problems and therapies to improve patients' coping skills with the chronic problems created by HS is another important part of the comprehensive management.

16.1.5 Differential Diagnosis

This includes infections, tumors, cysts, Crohn's disease, and anal or vulvo-vaginal fistulae.

16.1.5.1 Complications

Long standing HS is associated with formation of fistulae (anal and perianal are the most common), arthropathy, lymphedema, recurrent cellulitis, secondary infections, and rarely septicemia. Similar to other chronic illnesses, HS can cause anemia and hypoproteinemia; it rarely causes amyloidosis. Squamous cell carcinoma is another late and uncommon complication (2,3). Also, low self-esteem, interpersonal withdrawal, depression, and suicidality are serious complications that need to be identified and treated.

16.1.5.2 Dermatologic Management

Treatment depends on severity of illness and includes topical agents, systemic treatments, and surgical management (2,11) (see Chapter 7). Topical treatments include topical application of antimicrobial agents, while systemic treatments include oral antibiotics, zinc gluconate, combination of antibiotics, isotretinoin (with limited efficacy), antiandrogens, immunosuppressives (including topical steroid injections), and TNF α inhibitors. Surgical options include unroofing of lesions, wide excision, and laser treatments. Other options include blue light treatment, dietary and metabolic management, including diets with no dairy products (due to hormones in dairy products), as well as low glycemic diets (2,11).

16.1.5.3 Psychiatric management

The psychological effects of HS on quality of life depend on age of onset, severity of the illness, and individual factors such as coping style and support systems (see Chapter 4). A severe illness with an early age of onset has detrimental effects on self-esteem and interpersonal relationships. When the disease is active, in addition to pain, there is a problem with foul odor of the lesions. Using topical antibacterial washes and topical antibiotics such as clindamycin gel can sometimes help with the odor.

A great resource center for patients is HS-USA, a nonprofit organization for support of patients with HS. In addition to the latest information on the disease and its treatment, they have patient surveys with invaluable information on patients who are affected by HS and their most bothersome symptoms.

Different techniques of stress reduction (i.e. cognitive behavioral therapy, mindfulness, and biofeedback) will lead to better coping skills (see Chapter 23). Also, interpersonal relationship training in the case of young patients with avoidance of social situations is helpful. Techniques such as mindfulness meditation (Buddhist meditation) are routinely used in pain clinics, are effective techniques, and may reduce use of pain medications. In a busy dermatology practice, the use of simple screening questionnaires to help identify patients with anxiety or depression is helpful. The self-screening questionnaires are usually easy to fill by patients and can be scored by office staff. They help to start the conversation on psychological effects of chronic skin problems. They also help patients and parents to be more receptive of mental health referrals. The following site from Massachusetts General Hospital department of psychiatry has a comprehensive list of validated and useful questionnaires for children and adolescents: http://www2.massgeneral.org/schoolpsychiatry/screeningtools_table.asp

Once the psychological effects of HS on individual patients is acknowledged, referral to the appropriate mental health providers will help to improve the quality of life of these patients (see Chapter 23). Psychotropic medications have restrictions for use in young patients as well as a U.S. Food and Drug Administration (FDA) black box warning and are best managed by child psychiatrists.

16.2 Hyperhidrosis

16.2.1 Definition

Hyperhidrosis is excessive production of sweat by sweat glands. Humans have two principal types of sweat glands: eccrine and apocrine glands. In 1987, Soto et al described a third type of these glands called "apoeccrine" glands that are found on the axillae of adults (12). All of these glands are innervated by cholinergic neurons of the sympathetic nervous system:

- *Eccrine glands* play a role in thermoregulation, as well as hyper- and hypohidrosis (13).
- *Apocrine glands* are associated with terminal hair follicles and help olfactory communication. They have a pathogenic role in follicular apocrine Fox-Fordyce disease (13).
- *Apoeccrine glands* participate in thermoregulation, axillary hyperhidrosis, and non-follicular Fox Fordyce disease (13).

Sweating is mostly produced by eccrine glands and is part of the normal physiologic function of skin that helps adjust the body temperature. Sweating becomes a problem when individuals sweat excessively in response to heat or stress and/or in conditions that would not cause sweating in most individuals, such as after eating or in air-conditioned rooms (14).

16.2.2 Epidemiology

The prevalence of hyperhidrosis is about 3% of the population (14), and this varies in different studies from 2.8% in the United States (15) to 4.6% in some parts of China (16).

16.2.3 Etiology

Sweating is a reflex controlled by the sympathetic nervous system. Neuronal impulses that cause hyperhidrosis can be generated from the cortex (emotional trigger), hypothalamus (thermal regulation), medulla (gustatory type), spinal cord, and local axonal reflexes. Hyperhidrosis is either primary or secondary. It causes important morbidity, including significant social, functional, and emotional problems.

Primary hyperhidrosis usually starts in early childhood and worsens until puberty and may or may not improve afterwards (14). Patients usually have a family history of hyperhidrosis. It typically affects palms and soles and sometimes axillae; sweating is triggered by intense emotions and stress. This type of hyperhidrosis is due to increased stimulus of eccrine glands by the cerebral cortex and is also called "cortical" hyperhidrosis (13).

Secondary hyperhidrosis usually accompanies an underlying condition and can be localized or generalized. It can be due to fever and infection, endocrine and metabolic problems (i.e. diabetes, thyroid problems, pheochromocytoma, menopause, acromegaly), neurologic disorders (i.e. Parkinson's disease, cerebrovascular accidents, tumors, autonomic nervous system dysfunction), cardiovascular problems (i.e. congestive heart failure), medication side effects (i.e. anticholinesterases, serotonin reuptake inhibitor antidepressants, anti-glaucoma agents, bladder stimulants, opioids) (17), substance abuse (i.e. alcohol or opioid withdrawal), toxins (i.e. mercury and arsenic toxicity), spinal cord problems (i.e. tabes dorsalis and syringomyelia), cancer (i.e. lymphoma, carcinoid syndrome), disorders of cornification and genodermatosis (i.e. palmoplantar keratodermas, Epidermolysis bullosa, etc.), and compensatory hyperhidrosis (i.e. post sympathectomy). More exhaustive lists of causes of hyperhidrosis can be found in dermatology textbooks (13).

16.2.4 Clinical features

Patients with hyperhidrosis suffer from excessive sweating ranging from moist palms and soles to visible droplets of sweat or dripping of sweat; axillary sweating causes stains on clothing. Excessive sweating usually causes embarrassment and emotional stress that in turn aggravates the sweating. Severe episodes can lead to electrolyte imbalance and dehydration.

Hyperhidrosis causes irritation and maceration; it also facilitates infections and growth of yeast. Overgrowth of bacteria and maceration can cause a foul odor (eccrine bromhidrosis). The foul odor also exists in metabolic disorders and ingestion of certain medications or foods. Sweating from apocrine sweat glands can manifest with foul odor (bromhidrosis) and staining (chromhidrosis) of clothing. Hyperhidrosis affects different aspects of the patient's life, from simple hand shaking to intimate relationships. Performing activities such as writing or playing a musical instrument could become very difficult (18,19).

In secondary hyperhidrosis patients may have additional findings that help with the diagnosis, such as increased sweating after meals in gustatory hyperhidrosis. Sweating can be tested by the starch-iodine test (20), or it can be quantitated by gravimetric assessment (21). These tests are not routinely performed in the clinical setting but are useful research tools and also help measure the response to different treatments.

16.2.5 Differential diagnosis

Different diseases causing secondary hyperhidrosis are all in the differential diagnosis. Establishing the correct diagnosis starts with a good history and physical examination. The family history is important, especially in primary hyperhidrosis. When suspecting secondary hyperhidrosis, laboratory testing should be performed to rule out renal disease, diabetes mellitus, hyperthyroidism, infections such as tuberculosis, underlying cancer, connective tissue diseases, and pheochromocytoma. The tests are decided based on clinical findings and may include complete blood count, erythrocyte sedimentation rate, blood glucose levels, blood urea nitrogen, creatinine, serum electrolytes, PPD (purified protein derivative), chest x-ray, antinuclear antibodies, and, if suspecting pheochromocytoma, urinary catecholamines.

16.2.6 Management

An important part of the treatment of hyperhidrosis is to evaluate and address its impact on the quality of life. Onset in childhood can affect self-esteem as well as social activities and be a source of stress and embarrassment. Later on hyperhidrosis may cause social anxiety and avoidance of many situations. It also affects the choices of activities in young patients and choices in career and hobbies in adults. Similar to other chronic medical problems, management should include both medical treatment and psychological support. Education of patients and family members is very important.

Since emotional stress worsens hyperhidrosis, training on coping with stress and relaxation techniques is helpful (see Chapter 23). Coaching the patient on dealing with different situations and prevention of avoidance of social situations is important. Strategies such as keeping the environment cool, having loose clothing, and wearing clothings that do not show the stain of sweat are helpful. Screening of patients for anxiety as well as depression and proper treatment will improve their quality of life. Biofeedback and behavioral modification are effective in some patients with chronic hyperhidrosis (22).

A few informative sources to help educate and support patients with hyperhidrosis include the following:

- www.hyperhidrosisuk.org
- www.hyperhidrosis.org

The International Hyperhidrosis Society (www.sweathelp.org) has information in different languages. It is a non-profit, independent, global organization that provides patients with information and resources. Nevertheless, information on the web needs to be scrutinized for commercial ties.

Medical treatments depend on the severity of the problem. It is best to start with lower risk topical treatments such as aluminum chloride hexahydrate (20–25% solution) or 6.25% aluminum tetrachloride. These have limited efficacy and can be irritating. It's important to dry the area thoroughly to prevent irritation; application is usually nightly. Mild topical steroids may reduce the irritation. Once the symptoms are controlled, the frequency of maintenance applications is adjusted to the minimum number of applications that will control symptoms (23). *Second steps* in treatment are as follows:

- Topical anticholinergics such as glycopyrrolate (1.5 to 2% cream or pad) (13).
- Iontophoresis with tap water works for palmo-plantar and axillary hyperhidrosis. It is used 3 times a week for 20 minutes until the sweating is under fair control

and then the frequency is reduced. It is contraindicated in patients with a pacemaker or metal implants and in pregnancy (23). Sometimes if the tap water iontophoresis fails, the anticholinergic medications (such as glycopyrridium bromide) may be delivered through iontophoresis; however, there is risk of systemic absorption and side effects. There are also reports in small samples of patients on delivering botulinum toxin via iontophoresis. Based on some reports, this method is effective and causes less pain than local injections (24). Side effects of tap water iontophoresis include tingling and discomfort during the session.
- Botulinum toxin A injections every 4–6 months prevents release of acetylcholine and causes long periods of relief. However, the injections are painful and cause weakness of the muscles. Botulinum toxin B is also effective in treating hyperhidrosis (23).
- Oral therapy:
  - Oral anticholinergics produce symptom relief that is dose related. This limits their efficacy due to side effects such as dry mouth, constipation, and tachycardia. The most commonly used are glycopyrronium bromide (Robinul) at 1–2 mg x 3/day or propantheline at 15 mg x3/day. Robinul is not indicated for children under age 12. Sometimes temporary use of an oral anticholinergic at the beginning of topical treatment with aluminum chloride increases the efficacy and decreases the irritation.
  - Other oral therapies are based on anecdotal case reports and have not had double blind placebo control trials. These treatments include
  - Calcium channel blockers such as diltiazem (No U.S. Food and Drug Administration (FDA) approval for use in children), alpha 2-adrenergic agonist clonidine, and tricyclic antidepressants have been reported to help in small number of patients. Their use is limited due to side effects.
  - Clonazepam (0.25 to 0.5 mg twice daily) is an anxiolytic that may help with hyperhidrosis, but it causes drowsiness and is habit forming.

The *third step* in treatment includes local excision (causes scarring) and sympathectomy. These methods produce permanent results. However, sympathectomy can cause compensatory hyperhidrosis and Horner's syndrome (drooping eyelid, decreased pupil size, and decreased sweating on the affected side of the face). Liposuction has also been reported for treatment of axillary hyperhidrosis (25). Destruction or excision of eccrine nevus, and syringomas are other methods of treatment in patients suffering from eccrine nevus or multiple syringomas. Complementary and alternative medicine may help some of the patients, and there are reports of acupuncture being effective in some patients (26).

Finally, hyperhidrosis is a chronic disease, and more research in different coping strategies will help to find high risk maladjusted patients and plan special psychological treatments that will help improve patients' quality of life. This type of research is well recognized in chronic diseases such as diabetes mellitus (27).

16.3 Anhidrotic ectodermal dysplasia

16.3.1 Definition

Anhidrotic ectodermal dysplasia is also known as hypohidrotic ectodermal dysplasia (HED) and Christ-Siemens-Touraine syndrome. Anhidrotic/Hypohidrotic ectodermal dysplasia is one of the ectodermal dysplasias (ED). EDs are a group of heterogenous disorders due to defects in development of at least two tissues derived from ectodermal embryonic tissue. When they are accompanied by other organ defects, they are called ED syndromes. These are genetic congenital problems that affect skin, hair, nails, teeth, sweat glands, sebaceous glands, and mucous glands. The most frequent ED is hypohidrotic ectodermal dysplasia (HED). HED is most frequently an X-linked recessive disorder (28), but both autosomal dominant and autosomal recessive forms have been reported. Also, an X-linked recessive form associated with immune defects (HED-ID) has been reported (13).

16.3.2 Epidemiology

The x-linked recessive form of HED happens in about 1/100,000 boys in all racial and ethnic groups; the other forms are much less common (13).

16.3.3 Clinical features

Newborns have scaly skin and may have a collodion membrane. Hair is usually sparse, thin, and light in color, but it may darken later around puberty. They have teeth problems with absence teeth and misshapen teeth (peg-shaped). Saddle nose and frontal bossing are other features; lips are turned inside out (13). Children have absence or decreased sweating that causes an inability to maintain body temperature, and episodes of hyperpyrexia. Many patients have eczema. They may have sebaceous hyperplasia of their face as well as periorbital hyperpigmentation and excessive wrinkling (29). They also have thickened mucosal secretions and frequent respiratory infections. Female carriers may have variable degrees of symptoms.

16.3.4 Differential diagnosis

The differential diagnosis includes other ectodermal dysplasias. Classifications are based on affected ectodermal structures, inheritance, and presence or absence of sweating. At birth, if a collodion membrane is present, HED should be differentiated from congenital ichthyosis. The diagnosis of autosomal dominant or recessive forms is based on the family history. The form with immunodeficiency has additional features, immune defects, and occasional lymphedema as well as osteoporosis (13).

16.3.5 Management

As in any other inherited disease, genetic counseling is important. Control of the environmental temperature is important to prevent episodes of hyperpyrexia. Air-conditioning, a cooling vest, and wet clothing to bring down the temperature are all important. Help with the cosmetic aspects of this disease, including dental reconstruction, is very important to help normal psychological development in children. Regular psychological evaluation and evaluation of coping styles helps to prevent future mood problems.

As in other chronic disorders, it is very important to evaluate patients within a bio-psycho-social model and take care of the problems in all three spheres to help patients achieve their highest potential. This approach is especially important in children while they are forming their personalities and self-esteem. The National Foundation for Ectodermal Dysplasias (NFED) is an important resource that has publications for patients and physicians. Their website is http://www.nfed.org

16.4 Nevus sebaceous

16.4.1 Definition

Nevus sebaceous is a congenital hamartoma; other names include nevus sebaceous of Jadassohn (described by Jadassohn in 1895) and organoid nevus.

16.4.2 Epidemiology

It occurs in less than 1% of newborns (30).

16.4.3 Clinical features

Nevus sebaceous is usually located on the head (scalp, face) and neck; location on the trunk is rare. It usually is located along the lines of Blaschko, and at birth it is subtle and hardly visible. With age it takes a more verrucous appearance with a yellow to orange color. There is no hair growth on the lesion, and placement on the scalp causes a patch of alopecia that gets bigger with age and extension of the skin. In the past people used to believe that there was a 10% risk of malignancy in this nevus, but recent studies show a much lower rate. However, this nevus is a base for many secondary adnexal tumors. An 18 year follow up study showed the incidence of basal cell carcinoma to be 0.8% and incidence of syringocystadenoma papilliferum was 1.1% (a tumor with potential for malignant transformation) (30). Old, neglected sebaceous adenomas rarely may develop secondary sebaceous carcinoma or apocrine carcinoma (13).

16.4.4 Differential diagnosis

Sometimes nevus sebaceous may look similar to an epidermal nevus.

16.4.5 Management

Management includes complete conservative excisional removal not only due to risk of multiple other benign adnexal growths and small risk of carcinomas, but also due to problems with the appearance of the nevus that makes it hard for patients to cope with. Earlier excision in childhood before further development of verrucous changes has a reduced scarring outcome and prevents further psychological hardship for children. If parents decide against excision in childhood, the child's psychological well-being and coping with a visible nevus should be evaluated periodically; also, the nevus should be observed closely for development of other tumors. In making a decision for surgical removal of the nevus, it is important to ask the children how they feel about having the nevus and if their peers make any negative remarks about the lesion. Surgical intervention is even more important if the nevus causes shame or embarrassment for children. Detailed discussion with parents on how they perceive the problem and pros/cons of the surgery will help parents on their decision making process.

16.5 Conclusion

This chapter has reviewed some of the common disorders of skin appendages affecting children, adolescents, and young adults. Conditions discussed are hidradenitis suppurativa, hyperhidrosis, anhidrotic ectodermal dysplasia, and nevus sebaceous. This chapter has provided an overview of the management of these disorders, while paying special attention to the psychological and psychosocial issues complicating the prognosis of these disorders. All of these chronic disorders require a holistic approach to help these patients cope with their dermatological conditions. A bio-psycho-social approach will allow physicians help their patients achieve a better quality of life.

References

1. Abstracts from The Second International HS Research Symposium March 5, 2009, San Francisco, CA, HS foundation 2009. http://www.hs-foundation.org/pdf/2009_HSF_SympProgram.pdf
2. Danby FW, Margesson LJ. Hidradenitis suppurativa. *Dermatol Clin* 2010;28(4):779–93.
3. Revuz J. Hidradenitis suppurativa. *J Eur Acad Dermatol Venereol* 2009;23(9):985–98.
4. Gao M, Wang PG, Cui Y, Yang S, Zhang YH, Lin D, et al. Inversa acne (hidradenitis suppurativa): A case report and identification of the locus at chromosome 1p21.1–1q25.3. *J Invest Dermatol* 2006;126(6):1302–6.
5. Kraft JN, Searles GE. Hidradenitis suppurativa in 64 female patients: Retrospective study comparing oral antibiotics and antiandrogen therapy. *J Cutan Med Surg* 2007;11(4):125–31.
6. Gupta AK, Knowles SR, Gupta MA, Jaunkalns R, Shear NH. Lithium therapy associated with hidradenitis suppurativa: Case report and a review of the dermatologic side effects of lithium. *J Am Acad Dermatol* 1995;32(2 Pt 2):382–6.
7. Mahe E, Morelon E, Lechaton S, Sang KH, Mansouri R, Ducasse MF, et al. Cutaneous adverse events in renal transplant recipients receiving sirolimus-based therapy. *Transplantation* 2005;79(4):476–82.
8. Yazdanyar S, Jemec GB. Hidradenitis suppurativa: A review of cause and treatment. *Curr Opin Infect Dis* 2011;24(2):118–23.
9. Konig A, Lehmann C, Rompel R, Happle R. Cigarette smoking as a triggering factor of hidradenitis suppurativa. *Dermatology* 1999;198(3):261–4.
10. HS-USA. Patient survey results. 2011. http://www.hs-usa.org/survey/static/StaticResultsSurvey2.htm
11. Lebwhohl Mark G, Heymann Warren R, Berth-Jones J, Coulson Ian. *Treatment of Skin Disease*, 3rd edition. Philadelphia: Elsevier, 2010:97-Gregor BE Jemec; 309–10.
12. Sato K, Leidal R, Sato F. Morphology and development of an apoeccrine sweat gland in human axillae. *Am J Physiol* 1987;252(1 Pt 2):R166–80.
13. Dermatology, 2nd edition, Bolognia JL, Rapini R, Jorizzo JL, eds. *Dermatology*, 2nd edition. Mosby: London
14. Callejas MA, Grimalt R, Cladellas E. [Hyperhydrosis update]. *Actas Dermosifiliogr* 2010;101 (2):110–8.
15. Strutton DR, Kowalski JW, Glaser DA, Stang PE. US prevalence of hyperhidrosis and impact on individuals with axillary hyperhidrosis: Results from a national survey. *J Am Acad Dermatol* 2004;51(2):241–8.
16. Lin TS, Kuo SJ, Chou MC. Uniportal endoscopic thoracic sympathectomy for treatment of palmar and axillary hyperhidrois: Analysis of 2000 cases. *Neurosurgery* 2002;51(5 Suppl):S84–7.
17. Cheshire WP, Fealey RD. Drug-induced hyperhidrosis and hypohidrosis: Incidence, prevention and management. *Drug Saf* 2008;31(2):109–26.
18. Halford J, Hunt L, Millington G. Hyperhidrosis. *BMJ* 2009;338:b1166.
19. Sumner J. How recovery helped me to recover. Experiences of hyperhydrosis. *Br J Theatre Nurs* 1993;3(5):17–9.
20. Swinehart JM. Treatment of axillary hyperhidrosis: Combination of the starch-iodine test with the tumescent liposuction technique. *Dermatol Surg* 2000;26(4):392–6.

21. Hund M, Kinkelin I, Naumann M, Hamm H. Definition of axillary hyperhidrosis by gravimetric assessment. *Arch Dermatol* 2002;138(4):539–41.
22. Duller P, Gentry WD. Use of biofeedback in treating chronic hyperhidrosis: A preliminary report. *Br J Dermatol* 1980;103(2):143–6.
23. Lebwhohl Mark G, Heymann Warren R, Berth-Jones J, Coulson Ian. *Treatment of Skin Disease*, 3rd edition. Philadelphia: Elsevier, 2010: 100- James AA Langtry, 317–320.
24. Kavanagh GM, Oh C, Shams K. BOTOX delivery by iontophoresis. *Br J Dermatol* 2004;151(5):1093–5.
25. Lillis PJ, Coleman WP, 3rd. Liposuction for treatment of axillary hyperhidrosis. *Dermatol Clin* 1990;8(3):479–82.
26. Wang WZ, Zhao L. Acupuncture treatment for spontaneous polyhidrosis. *J Tradit Chin Med* 2008;28(4):262–3.
27. Bazzazian S, Besharat MA. An explanatory model of adjustment to type I diabetes based on attachment, coping, and self-regulation theories. *Psychol Health Med* 2011:1–12.
28. Kara N, Shah M, Elston DM, et al. Ectodermal dysplasia. *Emedicine/Medscape*. 2009. http://emedicine.medscape.com/article/1110595-overview.
29. Bhargava A, Sharma A, Popli S, Bhargava R. Prosthodontic management of a child with ectodermal dysplasia: A case report. *J Indian Prosthodont Soc* 2010;10(2):137–40.
30. Rosen H, Schmidt B, Lam HP, Meara JG, Labow BI. Management of nevus sebaceous and the risk of Basal cell carcinoma: An 18-year review. *Pediatr Dermatol* 2009;26(6):676–81.

Part V: SYSTEMATIC DISEASES WITH PSYCHODERMATOLOGIC MANIFESTATIONS

Zeba Hasan Hafeez

17 Neurocutaneous disorders

The skin and the nervous system are both derived from the ectoderm, and congenital conditions involving the skin and nervous system are classified as neurocutaneous disorders. Many of these diseases manifest variable phenotypes (observable characteristics or traits) due to different mutations in a single gene. This chapter focuses primarily on neurofibromatosis and tuberous sclerosis complex, which are the more common genodermatoses conceptualized as neurocutaneous disorders. Principles of management are presented.

17.1 Introduction

The skin and the nervous system are both derived from the ectoderm, and congenital conditions involving the skin and nervous system are classified as neurocutaneous disorders. Many of these diseases manifest variable phenotypes (observable characteristics or traits) due to different mutations in a single gene. Neurocutaneous disorders substantiate many disease conditions, as represented in Table 17.1; however, this discussion focuses primarily on neurofibromatosis and tuberous sclerosis complex, which are the more common genodermatoses conceptualized as neurocutaneous disorders.

17.2 Neurofibromatosis

Neurofibromatoses are autosomal dominant disorders of the nervous system that mainly affect the growth and development of nerve cell tissue. The disorders are known as neurofibromatosis type 1(NF1), which is the more common type, and *neurofibromatosis type 2* (NF2). NF1, also known as Von Recklinghausen's neurofibromatosis, is a chronic progressive genetic disease that affects about 1 in 3,000 subjects (1). It has been mapped to the proximal long arm of chromosome 17 (2,3). The gene locus has been cloned (4) and prenatal diagnosis is possible (5). About one half of the affected persons inherit the gene from a parent, and one half develop NF1 as the result of a spontaneous mutation.

Table 17.1: Neurocutaneous disorders

Neurofibromatosis type 1
Neurofibromatosis type 2
Tuberous sclerosis complex
Von Hippel-Lindau disease
Neurocutaneous melanosis
Basal Cell Nevus syndrome
Epidermal Nevus syndrome
Multiple endocrine neoplasia type 2
Ataxia-telangiectasia
Incontinentia pigmenti
Hypomelanosis of Ito
Cowden disease
Pseudoxanthoma elasticum
Ehlers–Danlos syndrome
Progeria E.
Blue Rubber Bleb Nevus syndrome
Hereditary hemorrhagic telangiectasia (Osler-Weber-Rendu)
Hereditary neurocutanous angiomatosis Richard LeBlanc
Cutaneous hemangiomas: vascular anomaly complex
Sturge–Weber syndrome
Lesch–Nyhan syndrome
Multiple carboxylase deficiency
Homocystinuria due to cystathionine-synthase (CBS) deficiency
Fucosidosis
Menkes Kinky Hair syndrome/Menkes disease
Xeroderma pigmentosum, Cockayne syndrome, and trichothiodystrophy. Cerebrotendinous xanthomatosis
Adrenoleukodystrophy
Peroximal disorders
Familial dysautonomia
Fabry disease
Giant axonal neuropathy
Chediak–Higashi syndrome
Encephalocraniocutaneous lipomatosis
Cerebello–Trigemino–Dermal dysplasia
Coffin–Siris syndrome
Lipoid proteinosis
Macrodactyl-nerve fibrolipoma

17.2.1 Clinical features

17.2.1.1 Dermatological diagnostic criteria

At least two of the following clinical features must be present in order to establish the diagnosis of NF1:

1. Six or more café-au-lait macules. These are often seen at birth, are greater than 5 mm in diameter in a prepubertal patient, and are 1.5 cm in a postpubertal patient.
2. Axillary or inguinal freckling was first described by Crowe (Crowe's sign). These are usually 1 to 3 mm in diameter, occurring in clusters in skin folds of the neck or under the breasts in women.
3. Two or more neurofibromas or one plexiform neurofibroma.
4. An optic pathway tumor.
5. Two or more Lisch nodules of the iris.
6. Characteristic bone lesions.

Neurofibromatosis type 2 (NF2), also called bilateral acoustic neurofibromatosis (BAN), is much less common compared to NF1. It has an estimated prevalence of 1/50,000. NF2 does not usually manifest in childhood, and the mean age of onset of symptoms for acoustic neuromas has been estimated to be about 20 years of age (6). The criteria for NF2 includes:

A. bilateral eighth nerve masses, occurring in 95% of cases, and diagnosed with appropriate imaging techniques (i.e. computed tomography or magnetic resonance imaging); or
B. a first degree relative with type 2 and either (a) unilateral eighth nerve mass or (b) two of the following: neurofibroma, meningioma, glioma, schwannoma, and juvenile posterior subcapsular lenticular opacity.

17.2.2 Neuropsychiatric aspects of neurofibromatosis type 1

Academic difficulties and learning disabilities appear to be common manifestations of NF1. In a population-based study in Wales, 8% of all subjects required remedial class education or had a specific learning difficulty (1). According to another study, 77% of the parents involved said that NF1 had caused issues for their child at school (7). These included learning difficulties, trouble in forming friendships, and behavioral problems. Thirty-two percent of the parents reported the involvement of an educational psychologist (7). It was noted that children with NF1 had a significantly lower full scale IQ, although well within the normal range. However, a visual-perceptual disability was noted significantly more often than in control subjects.

This pattern of cognitive strength and weakness was significantly dissimilar compared to non-NF1 children with learning disabilities (8,9).

Psychiatric comorbidity is well documented in patients with neurofibromatosis (10,11).

In their study, Samuelsson and Axelson reported that 18% of the children had behavioral disorders (12). Several studies have documented an association of NF1 with attention deficit disorder (10). Concomitant occurrence of neurofibromatosis and autistic disorder has been described (13,14), as well as comorbid depressive syndrome, anxiety state with vegetative dysfunction, and organic brain syndrome (10). The association of seizures with NF1 is well-documented. Seizures, especially those arising from the temporal lobe, can be associated with psychiatric symptoms, including psychosis (10). The prevalence of seizures in NF1 (4%) was noted to be approximately twice that in the general population (15). Dissociative-like spells in a 10-year-old boy with NF1 with paroxysms of auditory and visual hallucinations, assaultiveness, and amnesia have been reported (16).

17.2.3 Management

There is no specific treatment for neurofibromatosis types 1 and 2, and most complications are managed symptomatically. NF1 has varied disease complications, and patients may consult many different specialists during their life time. Although many complications are individually rare, it is likely that patients are not diagnosed sufficiently early, nor receive appropriate follow up and counseling. According to the Welsh study (1), many parents were told that the café-au-lait spots were "just birth marks" and were unaware that subsequent problems were related (e.g. educational difficulties, scoliosis).

The NIH Consensus Development Conference addressed these problems and recommended that NF1 sufferers should have an annual clinical assessment to monitor for complications (17). Screening investigations, such as cranial computed tomography, may not be justified unless there were clinical indications. Huson recommended biannual review for children as disease complications develop in childhood (17).

Examination should be geared toward monitoring for the development of complications, therefore paying particular attention to examination of the spine and nervous system (especially for signs of an optic glioma). It is important for patients to have a detailed cutaneous and slit lamp examinations.

A preschool psychological assessment is appropriate as educational problems are so frequent. Plexiform neurofibromas (diffuse ill defined swellings often with overlying skin hypertrophy or pigmentation) are rarely seen as isolated lesions; they are one of the most frequent complications and present a difficult management problem. As their margins are ill defined, complete surgical removal is often impossible.

Therefore, unless these lesions cause severe cosmetic problems or are localized bony overgrowth, conservative management is advisable. Mast cells constitute a major component of both discrete peripheral and plexiform neurofibromas. Riccardi postulated that they may play an integral role in the pathogenesis of these lesions and described possible control of the growth of aggressive plexiform neurofibromas and neurofibroma-associated pruritus with ketotifen, which blocks mast cell secretions (18).

Patients with NF2 do have café-au-lait spots (but always fewer than six) or peripheral neurofibromas more frequently than the general population. In the past, the two forms of the disease were not clearly distinguished. Cases have been reported with an earlier presentation, and the diagnosis should be considered in children presenting with meningeal or Schwann cell tumors in any location. In these cases, the finding of lens opacities on slit lamp examination would make the diagnosis of neurofibromatosis type 2 a strong possibility.

Genetic counseling is also important for NF1 and NF2 patients and their families. A closely linked chromosome 22 DNA marker has been identified for neurofibromatosis type 2 (19). As most gene carriers develop acoustic neuromas, screening for their development is justified as surgery on small tumors at an early stage is associated with the preservation of hearing in some cases, and a noticeable decrease in other complications (20). There is a 50% risk of transmission to offspring, and approximately 50% of all cases of NF1 are new mutations.

Informing families about the varied complications of NFI is a difficult counseling task, and there is a fine balance between providing adequate information without causing unnecessary alarm. Individuals with NF1 are vulnerable to pitfalls with intellectual, academic, and social skills; thus, it will often be necessary to ensure that they are able to make optimal use of academic and vocational programs. Management of comorbid psychiatric conditions can be accomplished by referral to clinicians for therapy or a combination of medications and therapy, as indicated. Symptoms such as seizures should be thoroughly investigated as neurosurgical relief is sometimes the treatment of choice.

NF1 is associated with a high frequency of psychiatric morbidity due to its cosmetic impact (21). Reducing deformity with dermatological and/or plastic surgery should not be neglected by physicians as it could lessen the implications of NF1 on patients' mental health and improve their well-being. The more disfiguring lesions, if not diffuse, should be excised. Carbon dioxide laser surgery is a treatment modality for cutaneous neurofibromas (22).

Several centers in the United States have now established multidisciplinary neurofibromatosis clinics, with a view toward improved coordination of care, particularly for NF1 patients. This would enable expertise to be developed in treating some of the more problematic complications that are individually rare (e.g. facial plexiform neurofibromas), the assessment of unusual cases, and the application as well as evaluation of new developments. Support and general resources for parents and patients include the following:

- Children's Tumor Foundation
- Neurofibromatosis, Inc.
- Genetic Science Learning Center at the Eccles Institute of Human Genetics
- Neurofibromatosis (Medline Plus)
- Neurofibromatosis type 1 (Genetics Home Reference)
- Understanding NF1 (Harvard University)

17.2.4 NF1 summary

During the past two decades, there has been an increasing awareness of the problems encountered in the diagnosis and management of the different forms and manifestations of neurofibromatosis. In addition to medical complications, individuals with NF1 may have cognitive and psychiatric comorbidities; also, the knowledge obtained from studies of children and adults with NF1 can be applied meaningfully in genetic counseling. It can also be used to acquire better understanding of cognitive and behavioral development in unaffected subjects.

Clinical research and laboratory investigations have resulted in the mapping of the genes for type 1 and type 2 neurofibromatosis to chromosomes 17 and 22, respectively (17). Subsequently, prenatal diagnosis and the cloning of the actual genes have assisted greatly in the pathogenesis and possible treatment options for the two main types of neurofibromatosis. Lastly, the insights gained from studying the molecular biology of the neurofibromatosis type 1 gene have had a direct impact on other biologic processes, such as neoplasia, cellular differentiation, and growth factor-mediated signal transduction, as well as potential applications for improved treatments for NF1 and cancer (23).

17.3 Tuberous Sclerosis Complex (TSC)

17.3.1 Introduction

This is an autosomal dominant genetic disorder that affects the brain, skin, heart, lungs, kidneys, and other organs. It has a birth incidence of 1 in 6,000. The term "complex" emphasizes the multisystem involvement and highly variant expression of the disease. Lesions are usually present at birth. While classically identified as Vogt's triad of facial angiofibromatosis, mental retardation, and intractable epilepsy, only about 30% to 40% of affected individuals have all three of these features (24).

17.3.2 Clinical features of TSC

17.3.2.1 Skin lesions

These include hypomelanotic macules (ash leaf spots) that are seen in 90% of patients in addition to the shagreen patch (often on the back or flank), facial angiofibromas (adenoma sebacceum), and ungula fibromas. Poliosis of the scalp hair or eyelids occurs less often. Subungual and periungual fibromas (Koenen tumors) are firm, flesh-colored fibromas in the nail matrix or bed that result in destruction of the nail plate.

17.3.2.2 Systemic lesions

Retinal lesions include hamartomas that can cause visual impairment or loss due to retinal detachment, vitreous hemorrhage or hamartoma enlargement. Cardiac lesions are seen in about two thirds of patients and include cardiac rhabdomyomas, which are often multiple; most of the patients who develop cardiac dysfunction have cardiac failure soon after birth. Renal angiomyolipomas occur in about three fourths of TSC patients. Most of these lesions are histologically benign tumors with varying amounts of vascular tissue, fat, and smooth muscle. Bilateral or multiple tumors typically occur in each kidney and tend to grow as the person ages. Complications include bleeding and renal failure. Patients can present with polycystic kidney disease due to the presence of single or multiple renal cysts. At least 1% of TSC patients develop significant lung disease due to lymphoangiomatosis (LAM); pulmonary dysfunction is more common in females (25).

17.3.3 Neurologic lesions

Cortical tubers are characteristic of tuberous sclerosis. These are potato like nodules of glial proliferation occurring anywhere in the cortex, ganglia, or ventricle walls. Other central nervous system findings include mental retardation, subependymal hamartomas, paraventricular calcifications, and giant cell astrocytomas (26,27). Symptoms include mental retardation, epileptic seizures, behavioral abnormalities, and sleep disorders. However, individuals with minimal or no neurological impairment are common. Also, 10% of children with infantile spasms have tuberous sclerosis (28).

17.3.4 Psychiatric symptoms

TSC is associated with significant, variable psychiatric comorbidities. The prevalence of psychiatric comorbidities reported in TSC ranges from 19% to 43% for depressive disorders, 5% to 56% for anxiety disorders, 26% to 86% for ADHD, 13% to 56% for aggressive and disruptive behaviors, and 21% for autistic like conditions (29,30) Other comorbidities reported less frequently include schizophrenia, capgras' syndrome, psychosis, auditory hallucinations, anorexia nervosa, alcoholism, bipolar disorder, and expressive language disorder (25,30,31,32,33,34,35).

17.3.5 Management

Many of the complications of TSC can be managed or their effects at least minimized. The NIH-sponsored Tuberous Sclerosis Consensus Conference (25) recommended the following measures in the evaluation and management of TSC: neurodevelopmental testing, ophthalmologic evaluation, electroencephalogram (if seizures are present), echocardiography (if cardiac symptoms are present), chest computed tomography (CT) scanning (for pulmonary symptoms), renal ultrasonography, and cranial CT scanning or MRI for renal and central nervous system symptoms, respectively. With reference to family members, consider cranial computed tomography (CT) scanning, renal ultrasonography, and genetic testing (25).

17.3.6 Treatment of neuropsychiatric problems

17.3.6.1 Epilepsy

Individuals with TSC benefit from use of aggressive antiepileptic treatment that seek the highest possible degree of seizure control. Medications such as topiramate, zonisamide, and acetazolamide can aggravate preexisting cognitive impairments (24). Oxcarbazepine, phenytoin, and levetiracetam allow more rapid titration and may be better tolerated than lamotrigine. Felbamate, a potent antiepileptic agent with primarily antiglutamatergic properties, can lead to potentially irreversible hepatic failure and aplastic anemia in approximately 1:5,000 to 1:10,000 individuals (24).

Infantile spasms associated with TSC have traditionally been treated with corticosteroids and various antiepilepsy medications such as benzodiazepines. However, recent reports suggest that sedating anticonvulsants (such as barbiturates and benzodiazepines) have a limited role in TSC and should be avoided (24). Vigabatrin (an inhibitor of GABA degradation) has been found effective in the treatment of infantile spasms in TSC (36). Valproate or topiramate have efficacy in treating infantile spasms and may be added to vigabatrin if the condition is refractory to vigabatrin monotherapy (24).

Focal symptomatic cortical lesions occurring in patients failing medical treatment have been treated surgically. Surgical removal or resection of the cortex containing epileptogenic tubers has been successfully used in the treatment of refractory symptomatic epilepsy in some cases (37). Vagal nerve stimulation was found to be effective for controlling refractory partial-onset seizures (38). Oral rapamycin therapy can induce regression of astrocytomas, angiofibromas, and angiomyoliomas, as well as improved pulmonary function in persons with TSC (39,24).

17.3.6.2 Autism symptoms and treatment of epilepsy

It has been reported that two preadolescent boys with moderate to severe autism and probable TSC improved after epilepsy surgery with respect to autism symptoms such as abnormal social interaction, echolalia, and extreme insistence on routine (40). This included scores on standardized autism rating scales and observed behavioral symptoms, such as attention difficulties, peer interaction, aggression, and self-injurious behavior (40). Another case report involved a toddler who underwent bilateral resective epilepsy surgery who demonstrated significant gains in language and motor skills 24 months after the procedure, in addition to a reduction in seizure frequency by 90% (41).

17.3.6.3 Behavior problems

There is no curative treatment for the core symptoms of autism involving deficits in interpersonal interaction, language development, and attention deficit issues; symptomatic therapy, such as a combination of psychosocial interventions and medication can be beneficial. Reinforcing prosocial behaviors and assisting the development of verbal as well as nonverbal communication skills can be addressed with educational and behavioral methods.

Psychotropic agents can be useful for the treatment of aggression, impulsivity, low level of tolerance for frustration, self-injurious behaviors, hyperactivity, and obsessive compulsive symptoms. Mood disorders (such as depression) and anxiety (obsessive compulsive and stereotyped behaviors) can be treated with serotonin reuptake inhibitors. These medications can lower seizure threshold in individuals with TSC but, overall, are considered safer than bupropion, which has a greater incidence of this side effect and should be avoided. Use of serotonin reuptake inhibitors (such as venlafaxine) and antipsychotics (such olanzapine, quetiapine, and risperidone) also have a low incidence of seizures at therapeutic doses (27). However, use of these medications can be problematic; there is the possibility of psychotropics causing seizures at therapeutic doses, issues of overdosage, and pharmacodynamic effects between psychotropic and antiepilepsy drugs that can contribute to worsening of seizures and decreasing the effectiveness of treatment (27).

17.3.6.4 Sleep disorders

Sleep disorders have been reported to occur frequently in TSC children with epilepsy and can be associated with a high level of daytime behavioral disturbance.

In a small randomized double-blind placebo-controlled crossover trial, melatonin (5 mg) improved total sleep time (42). Melatonin deficiency has not been described in the TSC population; however, factors, such as hyperactivity, seizures, and anticonvulsant therapy can contribute to disrupted sleep (27).

Significant progress in the understanding of TSC has been made since the identification of the TSC genes and their protein products, TSC2 (tuberin) in 1993 and TSC1 (hamartin) in 1997. The use of newer imaging technology, such as positron emission tomography (PET) and magnetic resonance spectroscopy, can facilitate correlation of developmental brain abnormalities with biologic markers. Serum markers, such as neurotrophins and neuropeptides, can also serve as developmental markers and are helpful considering that the neuropsychiatric problems of TSC, such as autism, are now considered a developmental brain disorder. Family screening as well as genetic counseling should be carried out, and referral should be made to a clinical genetics service. DNA testing can be done in 85% of cases and should be discussed. Prenatal diagnosis is not an option for the 60–70% of cases who represent new mutations (23).

17.4 Conclusion

During the past 20 years there have been significant advances in the therapeutics for TSC, particularly the understanding of its molecular pathophysiology (24). It has gone from being perceived as a neurologic disorder with little hope of improvement to one in which specified medical therapies are undergoing clinical trials for the management of the neurologic, pulmonary, and renal manifestations of the disease. Diagnostic studies play an important role in the assessment of TSC patients and help both to confirm its diagnosis and identify clinically significant complications in newly diagnosed patients. These can also provide evidence of TSC in asymptomatic relatives of children with this disease. For those with an established diagnosis of TSC, these studies can identify treatable complications in their early stages when therapies can be more effective.

References

1. Huson SM, Harper PS, Compston DAS. Von Recklinghausen neurofibromatosis. A clinical and population study in South-East Wales. *Brain* 1988;111:1355–81.
2. Barker D, Wright E, Nguyen K, et al. Gene for von Recklinghausen neurofibromatosis is in the pericentromeric region of chromosome 17. *Science* 1987;236:1100–2.
3. Seizinger BR, Rouleau GA, Ozelius U, et al. Genetic linkage of von Recklinghausen neurofibromatosis to the nerve growth factor receptor gene. *Cell* 1987;49:589–94.
4. Wallace MR, Marchuk DA, Andersen LB, et al. Type 1 neurofibromatosis gene: Identification of a large transcript disrupted in three NF1 patients. *Science* 1990;249:181–6.

5. Upadhyaya M, Fryer A, MacMillan J, et al. Prenatal diagnosis and presymptomatic detection of neurofibromatosis type 1. *J Med Genet* 1992;29:180–3.
6. Kanter WR, Eldridge R, Fabricant R, Allen JC, Koerber T. Central neurofibromatosis with bilateral acoustic neuroma: Genetic, clinical and biochemical distinctions from peripheral neurofibromatosis. *Neurology* 1980;30(8):851–9.
7. Huson SM, Harper PS, Compston DAS. Von Recklinghausen neurofibromatosis. A clinical and population study in South-East Wales. *Brain* 1988;111:1355–81.
8. Benjamin CM, Colley A, Donnai D, et al. Neurofibromatosis type 1 (NFl): knowledge, experience, and reproductive decisions of affected patients and families. *J Med Genet* 1993;30:567–74.
9. Eliason MJ. Neurofibromatosis: Implications for learning and behavior. *Dev Behav Pediatr* 1986;7:175–9.
10. Eliason MJ. Neuropsychological patterns: Neurofibromatosis compared to developmental learning disorders. *Neurofibromatosis* 1988;1:17–25.
11. Mouridsen Sørensen SA. Psychological aspects of von Recklinghausen neurofibromatosis (NF1). *J Med Genet* 1995;32:921–4.
12. Samuelsson B, Riccardi VM. Neurofibromatosis in Gothenburg, Sweden. III. Psychiatric and social aspects. *Neurofibromatosis* 1989;2:84–106.
13. Samuelsson B, Axelsson R. Neurofibromatosis. A clinical and genetic study of 96 cases in Gothenburg, Sweden. *Acta Derm Venereol Suppl (Stockh)* 1981;95:67–71.
14. Gillberg C, Forsell C. Childhood psychosis and neurofibromatosis – more than a coincidence? *J Autism Dev Disord* 1984;14: 1–8.
15. Mouridsen SE, Andersen LB, Sorensen SA, et al. Neurofibromatosis in infantile autism and other types of childhood psychoses. *Acta Paedopsychiatr* 1992;55:15–18.
16. Kulkantrakorn K, Geller TJ. Seizures in neurofibromatosis 1. *Pediat Neurol* 1998;19:347–50.
17. Singleton GM, Lagges AM, Meighen KG. Dissociative-like spells in a child with neurofibromatosis (type 1). *Jefferson J Psychiatr* 2007;21(1).
18. Huson SM. Recent developments in the diagnosis and management of neurofibromatosis. *Arch Dis Childhood* 1989;64:745–9.
19. Riccardi VM. Mast-cell stabilization to decrease neurofibroma growth. *Arch Dermatol* 1987; 123:1011–6.
20. Wertelecki W, Rouleau GA, Superneau DW, et al. Neurofibromatosis 2: Clinical and DNA linkage studies of a large kindred. *N Engl J Med* 1988;319:278–83.
21. Martuza RL, Eldridge R. Neurofibromatosis 2 (bilateral acoustic neurofibromatosis). *N Engl J Med* 1988;318:684–8.
22. Wolkenstein P, Zeller JE. Visibility of neurofibromatosis and psychiatric comorbidity. *Arch Dermatol* 2003;139:103–4.
23. Irvine AD, Mellerio JE. Genetics and genodermatoses. In: Burns T, Breathnach S, Cox N, Griffiths C, eds. *Rook's textbook of dermatology*, vol. 1, 8th edn. Oxford: Blackwell, 2010:15.
24. Krueger DA, Franz DN. Current management of tuberous sclerosis complex. Paediatr Drugs2008;10(5):299–313.
25. Roach ES, DiMario FJ, Kandt RS,Northrup H. Tuberous sclerosis consensus conference: recommendations for diagnostic evaluation. National Tuberous Sclerosis Association. *J Child Neurol* 1999;14(6):401–7.
26. Harper JI, Trembath RC. Genetics and genodermatoses. In: Burns T, Breathnach S, Cox N, Griffiths C, eds. *Rook's textbook of dermatology*, 7th edn. Oxford: Blackwell, 2008:12.
27. Roach E. Tuberous sclerosis complex. In: Roach MV, Miller VS, eds. *Neurocutaneous disorders.* Cambridge: Cambridge University Press, 2004:60–5.
28. Asato MR, Hardan AY. Neuropsychiatric problems in tuberous sclerosis complex. *J Child Neurol* 2004;19(4):241–9.

29. Gillberg IC, Gillberg C, Ahlsen G. Autistic behavior and attention deficits in tuberous sclerosis: A population-based study. *Dev Med Child Neurol* 1994;36:50–6.
30. Muzykewicz DA, Newberry P, Danforth N, Halpern EF, Thiele EA. Psychiatric comorbid conditions in a clinic population of 241 patients with tuberous sclerosis complex. *Epilepsy Behav* 2007;11:506–13.
31. Zia Ul Haq M, Dubey I, Christoday RJ Khess, Das U, Kumar R. Bipolar disorder and tuberous sclerosis complex: Is it a mere coincidence? *CNS Spectr* 2009;14(11):643–7.
32. Khanna R, Borde M. Mania in a five-year-old child with tuberous sclerosis. *Br J Psychiatry* 1989;155:117–9.
33. Hagenah U, Coners H, Kotlarek F, et al. Tuberous sclerosis and organic bipolar disorder in a 15-year-old adolescent. *Z Kinder Jugendpsychiatr Psychother* 1999;27:283–9.
34. Chopra VK, Cintury Y, Sinha VK. Bipolar disorder associated with tuberous sclerosis: Chance association or aetiological relationship? *Indian J Psychiatry* 2006;48:66–8.
35. Raznahan A, Joinson C, O'Callaghan F, Osborne JP, Bolton PF. Psychopathology in tuberous sclerosis: an overview and findings in a population-based sample of adults with tuberous sclerosis. *J Intellect Disabil Res* 2006;50:561–9.
36. Hancock E, Osborne JP. Vigabatrin in the treatment of infantile spasms in tuberous sclerosis: Literature review. *J Child Neurol* 1999;14(2):71–4.
37. Guerreiro MM, Andermann F, Andermann E, Palmini A, Phwang, et al. Surgical treatment of epilepsy in tuberous sclerosis: Strategic and results in 18 patients. *Neurology* 1998;51:1263–9.
38. Parain D, Penniello MJ, Berquen P, Delangre T, Billard C, Murphy JV. Vagal nerve stimulation in tuberous sclerosis complex patients. *Pediatr Neurol* 2001;25:213–6.
39. Franz DN, Leonard J, Tudor C, Chuck G, Care M, Sethuraman G, Dinopoulos A, Thomas G, Crone KR. Rapamycin causes regression of astrocytomas in tuberous sclerosis complex. *Ann Neurol* 2006;59(3):490–8.
40. Gillberg C, Uvebrant P, Carlsson G, Hedstrom A, Silfvenius HJ. Autism and epilepsy (and tuberous sclerosis?) in two pre-adolescent boys: Neuropsychiatric aspects before and after epilepsy surgery. *J Intellect Disabil Res* 1996;40(Pt 1):75–81.
41. Romanelli P, Weiner H, Najjar S, Devinsky O, et al. Bilateral resective epilepsy surgery in a child with tuberous sclerosis: Case report. *Neurosurgery* 2001;49(3):732–5.
42. O'Callaghan FJ, Clarke AA, Hancock E, et al. Use of melatonin to treat sleep disorders in tuberous sclerosis. *Dev Med Child Neurol* 1999;41:123–6.

Manmohan K. Kamboj and Ruqiya Shama Tareen

18 Collagen vascular disorders: Psychiatric and dermatologic manifestations

Collagen vascular diseases include complex multisystemic disorders of varying underlying etiopathogenic mechanisms with significant cutaneous manifestations. Many of these conditions are associated with significant psychiatric manifestations and hence are of psycho-dermatologic importance. These disorders may not be diagnosed early because of significantly varied clinical presentations. Many times the psychiatric symptoms may be pre-emptive to an underlying systemic collagen vascular disorder. Therefore, it is very important to keep a high index of suspicion for these complex disease conditions and to be able to diagnose these disorders in a timely manner to minimize systemic and psychiatric morbidity. This chapter discusses the psychodermatologic aspects of some of these disease conditions, including systemic lupus erythematosus, dermatomyositis, and rheumatoid arthritis.

18.1 Lupus erythematosus (LE)

Lupus erythematosus (systemic lupus erythematosus [SLE]) is a multisystemic spectrum of conditions characterized by chronic inflammation due to autoimmunity against ribonucleoproteins and nucleosomes (1). The underlying pathophysiology is complex and still not clear. Several underlying etiopathologic processes have been implicated in LE, including immunogenetic, environmental, hormonal, and infectious factors (2).

18.1.1 Epidemiology

The exact prevalence of LE (SLE) is not known, and a prevalence of 5–10/100,000 is estimated (3,4). About 25% of LE starts in the first two decades of life. Sex distribution for males and females is about 3:4 until puberty; however, this ratio becomes 1:9 after puberty (5). Racial differences exist with much higher incidence in African Americans, Hispanics, and Asians as compared to Caucasians (4,6).

18.1.2 Clinical features

A wide spectrum of clinical presentation is seen in LE primarily because of multisystemic involvement, variable onset, and unpredictable course of the disease. The typical presentation may be modified significantly with early institution of therapy.

Table 18.1: Constitutional and systemic features of LE

Constitutional Symptoms • Fatigue • Fever • Weight changes: weight gain or weight loss **Dermatological Features: Discussed Later** **Musculoskeletal Features** • Arthralgia • Arthritis • Myalgias **Renal Features** • Edema o Periorbital o Peripheral o Anasarca • Renal failure • Hematuria • Hypertension Underlying pathology: • Acute or chronic renal failure • Nephritic syndrome • Nephrotic syndrome **Pulmonary Features** • Dyspnea • Hemoptysis • Pleuritic chest pain Lung parenchyma involvement • Pleurisy, pleural effusion • Pulmonary embolism • Chronic lupus interstitial lung disease • Lupus pneumonitis • Pulmonary hypertension-with right sided heart failure	**Cardiovascular Features** • Positional chest pain (improves on leaning forward) • Heart failure symptoms • Angina • Pericardia effusions • Arrhythmias • Systemic murmurs Underlying pathology: • Pericarditis • Myocarditis • Coronary vasculitis • Ischemic heart disease **Gastrointestinal Features** • Nausea, vomiting, diarrhea, dyspepsia • Abdominal pain • Jaundice Underlying pathology • Peritonitis • Pancreatic • Bowel infarction • Mesenteric vasculitis • Autoimmune hepatitis **Hematologic Features** • Cytopenia- • leukopenia, lymphopenia, anemia • Thrombocytopenia • Low complement levels • Anti-phospholipid antibody syndrome **Neuropsychiatric Features** Discussed later in the chapter

The general and systemic clinical presentations are listed in Table 18.1 (7). A high index of suspicion for LE should be maintained for females in the child bearing age group presenting with fever, rash, and joint pains.

18.1.3 Cutaneous manifestations

There are three main dermatologic features in the diagnostic criteria as per the 1982 revised criteria for the classification of SLE (7). These include the following:

- *Malar rash*: This is an erythematous rash over the cheeks and bridge of the nose, spares the naso-labial folds, and has been typically referred to as the classic butterfly rash of SLE or acute cutaneous lupus erythematosus (ACLE) as well. These lesions may last for variable periods of time, ranging from hours to weeks, sometimes even longer. Generally these lesions do not leave any scarring on healing.

- *Photosensitivity*: This is another prominent feature of SLE as well, so much so that sometimes the generalized form of ACLE is also referred to as photosensitive lupus dermatitis. This is typically precipitated or exacerbated by sun exposure. The malar rash and photosensitivity of SLE both portray waxing and waning during the course of the disease.
- *Discoid rash*: This is the cutaneous manifestation seen in the subacute cutaneous type of LE (SCLE), also referred to as disseminated lupus erythematosus (DLE). These lesions are also photosensitive and, therefore, observed in generally the sun-exposed areas such as the neck, shoulders, arms, upper back, and also, less commonly, the face. Initially these present as erythematous, maculopapular lesions, which may transition to hyperkeratotic, papulosquamous lesions, annular plaques, or polycyclic plaques (1).
- *Other nonspecific cutaneous lesions:* Other cutaneous lesions may be seen that are otherwise not specific for LE. These include (a) alopecia, generally involving the temporal area of the scalp and exhibiting patchy hair loss; (b) Raynaud's phenomenon; (c) panniculitis, also referred to as lupus profundus; (d) livido reticularis; (e) bullous, erythema multiforme-like lesions; and (f) vasculitic purpura or telangiectasia. Urticaria has also been reported with SLE. Lupus may be considered in cases of oral, vaginal, and, even more specifically, palatal ulcers (1).

18.1.4 Neuropsychiatric systemic lupus erythematosus (NPSLE)

SLE in children is more likely to present with early central nervous system involvement. Varied prevalence rates ranging from 20–95% for NPSLE have been reported in the pediatric population. However, this may be more reflective of lack of a unified process of NPSLE characterization (8,9,10,11). Also, 70% of children may manifest features of NPSLE in the first year of illness (10).

The manifestations of NPSLE may be due to different pathophysiological processes, including (a) the primary autoimmune and inflammatory attributes of the underlying disease, (b) complications of the main disease process, (c) unintended side effects of the medications being used to treat the primary disease process, or (d) due to the psychosocial and emotional burden as well as stigma of the disease (8).

After a multispecialty collaborative effort with input from rheumatologists, neurologists, psychiatrists, hematologists, and other specialists, the American College of Rheumatology (ACR) proposed 19 NPSLE syndromes in 1999, with guidelines for diagnostic and therapeutic evaluation (12). Although these are mainly based on the NPSLE data in adults, they are adopted for pediatric populations as well.

According to the ACR report, NPSLE can manifest in many ways, but the most common manifestations include cerebrovascular accidents, aseptic meningitis, seizure disorder, demyelinating syndrome, Guillain-Barré syndrome, cranial and peripheral neuropathy, and movement disorder like chorea (12). Psychiatric symptoms of NPSLE include an acute confusional state, cognitive disturbances, and anxiety, as well as mood disorders and frank psychosis (12).

An alternative classification process for NPSLE is based on the specific neurologic manifestations, such as diffuse central nervous system (CNS) involvement, focal CNS involvement, and peripheral nervous system (PNS) involvement. This classification, however, is somewhat arbitrary, as about 20% of patients have more than one type of neuropsychiatric presentation (8). The markers of disease activity include complement C3/C4 levels, antiphospholipid antibodies, anticardiolipin antibodies, and anti-dsDNA antibodies titer; however, these markers do not correlate very well with the NPSLE events. NPSLE predicts a higher mortality rate when compared to patients with SLE who do not have NPSLE (13). Figure 18.1 lists different manifestations of NPSLE.

Cognitive dysfunction has been reported with a variable prevalence rate of 21–66%, again depicting the diagnostic variability. Hanly et al reported a 13% prevalence rate of cognitive impairment after a 5 year follow-up of 70 patients; only 4% of these patients demonstrated ongoing cognitive impairment, while the others showed improvement over time (8). Several neurologic symptoms may be seen in NPSLE, with headaches being the most common and affecting about 66–75% of patients. However, true lupus headaches associated with other intracranial manifestation of NPSLE are relatively uncommon and may occur in about one quarter of the patients (10).

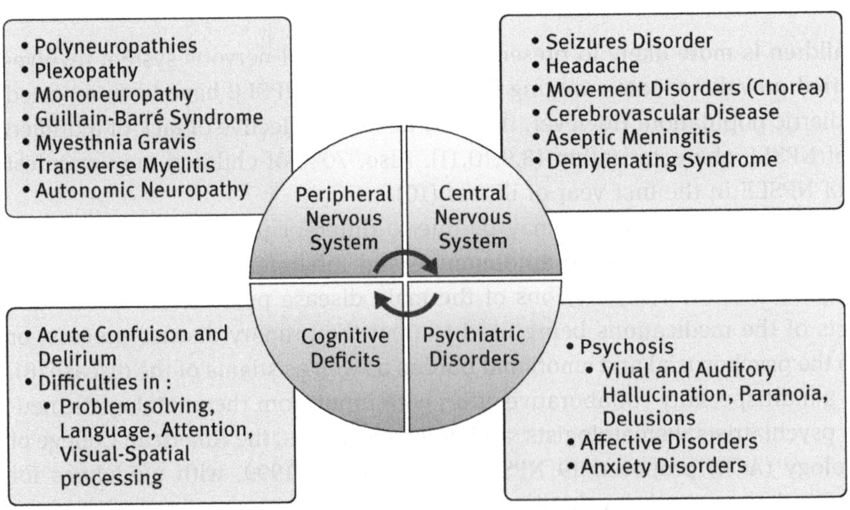

Figure 18.1: Different manifestations of NPSLE.

Seizures may be seen in about 20% of children and may result in a lifelong seizure disorder, along with significant impact on neurocognitive function (10). Cerebrovascular disease is seen in approximately 25% of pediatric SLE patients; this most commonly manifests as small vessel vasculitis leading to microthromboembolic events. In the pediatric population involvement of larger vessels can cause venous thrombosis, hemorrhage, and stroke, although very rarely (10).

Peripheral nervous system involvement occurs in about 5–15% of children with NPSLE and usually presents as transverse myelitis, peripheral neuropathy, and aseptic meningitis; autonomic instability is very rarely seen in pediatric NPSLE (10). Psychiatric symptoms are common and seen early on in the course of pediatric NPSLE. Sibbitt et al followed 75 children with SLE over the course of 6 years and found that, at any given time, a cross section of this cohort showed high prevalence of NPSLE, including mood disorders in 57%, acute confusional state in 35%, anxiety in 21%, and psychosis in about 12% of the cohort (11).

A retrospective chart review of 10 adolescents between ages of 10–19 years with acute psychiatric presentation and hospitalization in a psychiatric hospital revealed that paranoid delusions were the most common presentation followed closely by visual and auditory hallucinations (14). Children with psychotic disorders may present with illogical thought processes and flat affect; also, they can be very guarded, especially about disclosing the full nature of the psychotic symptoms (14). This could be due to the frightening nature of visual hallucinations and commanding or persecutory auditory hallucinations. Since young children often have difficulty reporting these symptoms to the medical caregivers and parents, involvement of psychiatric expertise will be helpful to illicit and treat such symptoms (10).

Affective disorders mostly present as depressive episodes affecting more than half of the pediatric patients with symptoms such as insomnia, psychomotor retardation, slow speech, and depressed as well as blunted affect. The pathogenesis of depression in SLE patients is thought to be multifactorial. It is postulated to be a direct reflection of the severity of SLE itself, related to the degree of the CNS involvement, or dependent on the severity of pain and discomfort associated with the disease process. However, there is evidence indicating that depression and SLE may have a completely parallel course with no correlation with the SLE severity as measured by disease severity markers (13).

This can be explained most likely due to the impact of “illness intrusiveness” and associated psychosocial stressors (15). Illness intrusiveness is defined as severity of the impact of a chronic debilitating illness on a patient’s life and lifestyle. It encompasses various aspects of a person’s perception about self and others in their world, including negative self-image, low self-esteem, self-criticism, subjective sense of distress, mood disturbances, pessimism, dissatisfaction with life, interpersonal difficulties in close relationships, and global symptoms of psychopathology.

Patients with SLE face ongoing challenges of dealing with the emotional and physical aspects of their disease, its unpredictable course, and side effects of treatment (15,16). Mania has been reported much less commonly in the pediatric population, and one case described in a 17-year-old girl was thought to be associated with initiation of methylprednisolone infusion. Manic symptoms such as euphoria, grandiose delusions, illogical thought pattern, hypersexuality, and agitation were reported (15). Factitious lupus has been reported in a 15-year-old girl who was noted to develop unexplained fever, facial erythematous rash, and hair loss after severe psychosocial stress. Lab work revealed ANA negative SLE unresponsive to 6-methyleprednisolone therapy; however, rapid improvement in her clinical condition was noted after closely supervised hospitalization, therefore, establishing the factitious nature of the disease (17).

18.1.5 Differential diagnosis

SLE has a wide spectrum of clinical manifestations and, therefore, a very broad differential diagnosis. The common diagnoses to consider in the differential are listed in Table 18.2 (1,18).

18.1.6 Clinical diagnosis

The diagnosis of LE is challenging for clinicians for many reasons, including the wide spectrum of clinical presentations ranging from very mild presentations of localized skin lesions as in discoid LE, to the very serious presentations with multisystemic involvements, which may even be fatal. Also, LE is a slowly evolving condition, with intermittent flare-ups and exacerbations; therefore, it is important that there be ongoing follow-up and a high index of suspicion over time. Diagnostic guidelines have been facilitated by the American College of Rheumatology and are listed in Table 18.3 (3,7). The simultaneous or serial presence of any 4 or more of the 11 diagnostic criteria makes the official diagnosis of SLE (3,7).

Table 18.2: Differential diagnosis of lupus erythematosus

Drug effects: Common drugs implicated are: chlorpromazine, hydralazine, procainamide, isoniazid, quinidine, methimazole, beta blockers, carbamazepine, and many other drugs
Infectious Conditions: infectious mononucleosis, syphilis, lyme disease, infective, endocarditis, acute pericarditis, rheumatic fever, septicemia with arthritis
Connective Tissue Disorders: rheumatic arthritis, mixed connective tissue disorders, anti-phospholipid syndrome, fibromyalgia
Malignancies: B cell Lymphoma

Table 18.3: Diagnostic criteria for lupus erythematosus

Dermatologic

- **Malar rash:** Fixed erythema, sparing nasolabial folds
- **Discoid rash:** Erythematous raised patches, keratotic scaling, follicular plugging; atrophic scarring
- **Photosensitivity:** Skin rash as a result of unusual reaction to sunlight
- **Mucosal ulcers:** Oral or nasopharyngeal ulceration, usually painless

Musculoskeletal

- **Arthritis:** Non-erosive arthritis involving 2 or more peripheral joints, characterized by tenderness, swelling, or effusion

Renal

- **Proteinuria:** Greater than 0.5 grams per day or greater than 3+ (if quantitation not performed) **OR**
- **Cellular cast:** Either red cell, hemoglobin, granular, tubular, or mixed

Neuropsychiatric

- **Seizures OR**
- **Psychosis-**in the absence of offending drugs or known metabolic derangements

Hematologic disorders

- **Hemolytic anemia with reticulosytosis OR**
- **Leukopenia-**less than 4,000/mm3 total on two or more occasions **OR**
- **Lymphopenia** -less than 1,500/mm3 on two or more occasion **OR**
- **Thrombocytopenia-**less than 100,000/mm3 in the absence of offending drugs

Immunologic

- **Positive antiphospholipid antibody OR**
- **Anti-DNA -antibody to native DNA in abnormal titer OR**
- **Anti-Sm -presence of antibody to Sm nuclear antigen OR**
- **False positive serologic test for syphilis confirmed by Treponema pallidum immobilization or fluorescent treponemal antibody absorption test**
- **Antinuclear Antibodies:** An abnormal titer of antinuclear antibody by immunofluorescence or an equivalent assay at any point in time and in the absence of drugs known to be associated with "drug-induced lupus" syndrome

Serositis

- **Pleuritis:** convincing history of pleuritic pain or rub or evidence of pleural effusion **OR**
- **Pericarditis:**documented by EKG, rub or evidence of pericardial effusion

18.1.7 Diagnostic workup

The diagnosis of LE may be straightforward if the clinical presentation and laboratory workup meet the diagnostic criteria as currently used per recommendations of the ACR. However, because of the extremely broad spectrum of presentation and findings in LE, the diagnosis may not be as straightforward. A systematic approach for workup will be helpful in establishing the diagnosis as summarized in Figure 18.2 (19).

18.1.8 Management

The spectrum of clinical presentation of LE is quite variable, and therefore, the treatment modalities need to be individualized to the manifestations of the disease seen in a particular patient. Many different groups of medications are used depending on the specific needs. The main therapeutic agents used include the following:

- Nonsteroidal anti-inflammatory drugs (NSAIDs): these include ibuprofen, naproxen, ketoprofen, and diclofenac. Fever, rash, serositis, and musculoskeletal manifestations respond quite well to NSAIDS. These drugs work by inhibition of prostaglandin synthesis.
- Antimalarials (e.g. hydroxychloroquine): these are useful in the treatment of cutaneous lupus lesions (20). They also relieve arthralgias as well as arthritis and prevent flare-ups of the disease.

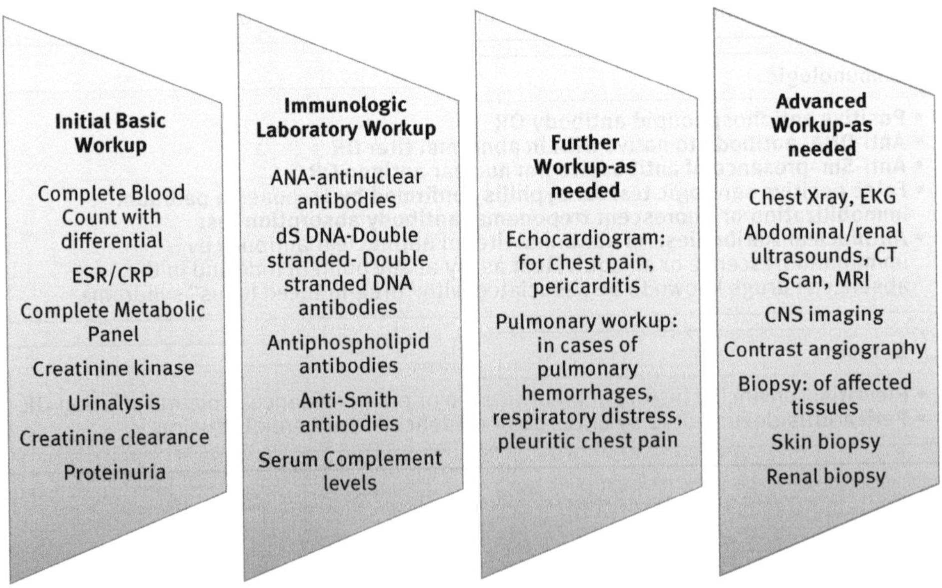

Figure 18.2: Diagnostic workup for systemic lupus erythematoses.

- Immunosuppressant medications: these medications act as immunosuppressive agents, anti-inflammatory agents, and cytotoxic agents as well. Methotrexate is generally used in the management of chronic arthritis and cutaneous lesions. Cyclophosphamide and azathioprine are used in severe SLE with multisystemic involvement. Intravenous immunoglobulin may be used. Mycophenolate is used as maintenance therapy for lupus nephritis and also in other serious SLE conditions (21,22).
- Belimunab: an immunomodulator that acts by inhibiting the biologic activity of the B-lymphocyte stimulator and is used in active, acute, antibody positive patients in conjunction with other medications.
- Corticosteroids, including prednisone and methylpredinisolone: they are used for their acute anti-inflammatory and immunosuppressant function. The advantage of these drugs is that they can be administered via different routes: oral, intravenous, intramuscular, topical, or intra-articular.

18.1.9 Treatment of cutaneous lupus lesions

The aim of treatment is to prevent skin lesions, prevent long term sequelae of the dermatologic lesions, and to minimize skin exposure to UVA and UVB, which minimizes photosensitivity. This may be achieved by the use of protective barriers, sunscreens with sun protective factor (SPF) ≥ 30, and protective clothing with SPF ≥ 30. Vitamin D deficiency may be more prevalent with all these barriers. Therefore, these patients should be tested and treated for vitamin D deficiency. Additional medications include the following:

- Topical therapy for skin lesions: these include topical glucocorticoids and fluorinated steroid topical preparations for use in thicker skin lesions (23).
- Topical immunosuppressant creams: tacrolimus and pimecrolimus (24).
- Topical retinoids: e.g. tretinoin and tazarotene.
- Systemic treatment options that may be helpful in treating cutaneous lesions are
  Antimalarials, such as hydroxychloroquine, chloroquine, and quinacrine;
  Glucocorticoids and other immunosuppressive agents; and
  Other systemic medications, including gold compounds, dapsone, IV immune globulin, and interferon alpha.

18.1.10 Treatment of NPSLE

Children and adolescents presenting with acute confusion, severe mood disorders, and psychotic symptoms may require hospitalization and specialist psychiatric care either as a psychiatric consultation or by transferring to a psychiatric unit.

Use of oral, intravenous, or intramuscular haloperidol may be indicated if the patient is presenting with severe disturbance of orientation, agitation, and aggression. Compazine is another typical neuroleptic, which can be used in such acute situations; however, it does not provide the flexibility of administration route as haloperidol does.

Extrapyramidal symptoms (EPS), such as dystonia and akathesia, may be seen and limit the use of such agents. More recently atypical neuroleptics have been used with success in pediatric cases of NPSLE and are preferred over older medications because of the concern about EPS. Risperidone has potent action on dopamine 2 receptors and may cause EPS, although generally it is well tolerated in low doses, such as 0.25 to 0.5 mg once or twice daily. Olanzapine, quetiapine, and aripiprazole have been used with good success in such patients (14,25). Complete resolution of all psychotic symptoms is usually seen with no persistence of such symptoms, thus long term management with antipsychotic medications is not required.

Treatment of depression and anxiety, however, may require long term treatment in some patients; this is especially noted when psychosocial stressors are not modifiable and continue to aggravate illness intrusiveness and negative self-appraisal. In such cases individual, cognitive, behavioral, and interpersonal psychotherapies may prove to be the mainstay of treatment with adjunctive use of psychotropic medications such as serotonin reuptake inhibitors (SSRIs) as indicated.

18.2 Dermatomyositis

Dermatomyositis belongs to the heterogeneous group of autoimmune disorders that are included in the group of idiopathic inflammatory myopathies. Most of the disorders in this group have in common their effect on skeletal musculature and skin, giving rise to skeletal muscle weakness and the hallmark cutaneous inflammatory disease. The underlying etiology is not clear, but it is believed to be caused by a combination of autoimmune reactions targeted toward muscle tissues, probably in response to environmental triggers on top of an underlying genetic predisposition. There are many subtypes of dermatomyositis and polymyositis disease conditions in this category of illnesses (26). However, for the purposes of this review, classic dermatomyositis is used as the prototype.

18.2.1 Epidemiology

The prevalence of idiopathic inflammatory myopathies is about 1:100,000. The rate in females is twice that in males, and the peak incidence is seen in adults in the 5th decade of life (27). Cutaneous involvement is seen in a majority of children with the disease (95%) and in about 30–40% of adults (26).

18.2.2 Clinical features

Dermatomyositis may involve multiple organ systems. Systemic features of dermatomyositis are summarized in Table 18.4 (26,27).

18.2.3 Cutaneous manifestations

A broad range of cutaneous features are seen in dermatomyositis. The common cutaneous findings are summarized here (27):

Table 18.4: Systemic non-cutaneous manifestations of dematomyositis

System	Manifestations
Malignancy	• High risk of malignancy
Pulmonary	• Interestitial lung disease • Aspiration pneumonia • Respiratory failure/weak musculature
Cadrdiovascuar	• Cardiomyopathy • Myocardiits • Conduction defects
Musculoskeletal	• Proximal muscle weakness • Distal muscle weakness (rare) • Myalgias • Polyarthritis • Muscle atrophy and contractures
Gastrointestinal	• Pharygeal and oesophageal muscle weakness • Dysphagia and regurgitaiton • Bowel infarction and perforation
Others	•Retinopathy •Raynaud's Phenomenon

- *Gottron's sign*: This presents as a symmetrical, erythematous, scaly lesion seen over the interphalangeal and metacarpophalangeal joints of the hands, elbows, and knees.
- *Heliotrope rash*: This is the classic violaceous rash on the upper eyelids with periorbital edema and swelling.
- *Erythroderma*: These are erythematous, violaceous, and symmetrical skin lesions noted on the malar areas of the forehead and around the "shawl area" of the neck and shoulders.
- *Poikiloderma vasculare atrophicans*: This commonly affects the neck, chest, shoulders, and buttocks. The characteristic lesions are characterized by a circumscribed rash with various levels of hyper and hypopigmentation, telangiectasia, and superficial atrophy (27).
- *Mechanic's hands*: This is the characteristic appearance of hands of manual laborers with symmetric, confluent, hyperkeratotic lesions on both hands (27).
- *Peri-ungual abnormalities*: These include telangiectasias, dystrophic cuticles, and bleeding cuticles.
- Other skin lesions: Other skin lesions noted in SLE include psoriasis-like lesions in the scalp, calcinosis cutis, and flagellate erythematous lesions on the trunk.
- Histopathologically these lesions are indistinguishable from lesions of lupus erythematosus and reveal hyperkeratosis, atrophy of the epidermis, thickening of the basement membrane, effacement of the rete ridges, and perivascular lymphocytic infiltration (27).

18.2.4 Psychiatric manifestations

The pain, fatigue, and overall disability associated with dermatomyositis, along with an uncertain and fluctuating course of illness, are reasons for symptoms of anxiety. It is likely that a patient may simultaneously suffer from more than one anxiety spectrum disorder such as panic disorder, obsessive compulsive disorder, and phobic anxiety. In comparison to myasthenia gravis, another severe debilitating neuromuscular disease, panic disorder is less common in dermatomyositis. Patients with dermatomyositis reported severe anxiety and depression as measured by various psychometric scales, irrespective of the severity of the disease, and chronicity of the disease course (28).

Patients with dermatomyositis also reported symptoms such as psychoticism, interpersonal sensitivity, paranoia, hostility, and somatization (28). Juvenile dermatomyositis is highly associated with sleep fragmentation and poor quality of sleep, which results in increased discomfort and pain. Fatigue was noted to profoundly impact the quality of life in these children (29). Sleep disturbances, pain, and disease severity were found to be directly correlated with mood disturbances (29).

Quality of life (QoL) issues have been studied in various rheumatologic diseases, including dermatomyositis (see Chapter 4). Alsanafi et al queried patients with dermatomyositis and found that pruritus was the most troublesome symptom, impacting the quality of life significantly; this was even more than noted with some of the other skin conditions associated with pruritus (30,31). Pruritus not only interfered with sleep but also caused embarrassment in social situations leading to social isolation. Most patients with dermatomyositis who complained of depression, anxiety, and emotional distress stated their concerns with various issues; these included being labeled with a chronic disease and its treatment, social embarrassment caused by skin lesions, inability to participate in any social activity involving sun exposure (which can exacerbate skin lesions), constant pruritus, and fragmented sleep. There are also feelings of insecurity because of the dependency on their caregivers, most commonly in parents in the case of juvenile dermatomyositis (30).

Research on the impact of juvenile dermatomyositis as the patient transitions to adulthood reveals the significant impact of prolonged school absences and presence of physical disabilities on the long term education outcomes in about half of these patients. The ability to initiate and sustain relationships as well as getting married was also significantly affected at about 50% compared to 84% in the general population. In terms of employability, the overall employment rate was a high 83% (72% full-time), but most were involved in sedentary jobs (32).

18.2.5 Management

18.2.5.1 Medical management

The main therapeutic agents used for dermatomyositis are listed in Table 18.5 (33,34). Glucocorticoids are the mainstay of treatment, and glucocorticoid-sparing medications may be used as well; resistant cutaneous lesions of dermatomyositis may need additional medications (33,34).

18.2.5.2 Management of psychiatric issues

Early assessment of QoL in the course of dermatomyositis in children and adolescents with this debilitating illness is very important (see Chapter 4). It provides the opportunity not only to allow more targeted treatment of the physical symptoms, but also to identify the emotional factors causing a significant decline in QoL. Short Form (SF)-36 is a QoL study tool that has been used to assess QoL issues in various diseases. It inquires about QoL issues such as limitations in physical activity and its impact on social activities, role related activities, and emotional distress. Skindex-29 is another QoL survey specific to skin diseases that can also be used in these patients to assess QoL issues. The Dermatology Life Quality Index (DLQI) is a valid test with

Table 18.5: Main therapeutic agents used for treatment of dermatomyositis

Therapeutic Agents for Treatment of Dermatomyositis

- Glucocorticoids
- Glucocorticoid sparing medications:
  - Azathioprine
  - Methotrexate
  - Antimalarials

Cutaneous Lesions of Dermatomyositis

General measures:

- Protection from photosensitivity
- Use of anti-pruritic agents

For resistant cutaneous lesions:

- Mycophenolate mofetil
- Intravenous immunoglobulin
- Dapsone
- Rituximab
- Immunosuppressants
- TNF alpha inhibitors
- Anti-estrogens

only 10 questions that can be efficaciously used to reliably assess QoL. However, the difficulty in interpreting the scores hinders its use in busy clinical practices. A score change of 5 or more indicates a significant change in patients' QoL. Implementation of routine QoL assessment in dermatologic practices can enhance the clinical decision making and may improve the overall outcome measures (35,36).

18.3 Rheumatoid Arthritis

Rheumatoid arthritis (RA) is a chronic, systemic, inflammatory, autoimmune disease that characteristically involves symmetrical polyarthritis and significant, non-articular manifestations causing progressive disability. If the onset is under 16 years of age, terms that are used include juvenile idiopathic arthritis (JIA) and juvenile rheumatoid arthritis (JRA).

18.3.1 Epidemiology

There is a significant variation in the prevalence of RA worldwide. The prevalence in North America is about 1% of the adult population. Peak incidence is noted after age 50 with a 2–3 times predominance in females versus in males (37).

18.3.2 Etiopathogenesis

The exact underlying pathogenesis is not clear. A combination of factors are postulated to exert a role, including genetic factors (HLA DR1 and HLA DR4 gene associations), mechanical factors, trauma, autoimmune (via B cells), and non-autoimmune (via T cell activation) (38,39).

18.3.3 Clinical features

The clinical features of RA may be considered under the following 3 sub-headings:

1. Non-specific symptomatology: These are general constitutional signs and symptoms that may be seen earlier in the condition, but the diagnosis is generally delayed because of the symptomatology being non-specific. These include fever, fatigue, loss of appetite, general weakness, and nonspecific musculoskeletal aches and pains.
2. Articular manifestations: The presentation of joint involvement may be variable. The typical presentation involves the small joints of the hands and feet; characteristically the proximal interphalangeal and metacarpophalangeal joints may be spared. There is usually symmetric, synovial inflammation of joints with characteristic morning stiffness. Other larger joints of upper and lower limbs are progressively involved (40). Episodic joint involvement described as palindromic rheumatism may be seen (41). Joint involvement may start with monoarthritis involving a simple large joint persistently progressing to involve more joints.
3. Systemic/Non-articular manifestations in RA: These are summarized in Table 18.6 (42).

18.3.4 Cutaneous manifestations

A wide range of dermatologic findings may be seen in RA. Overall, systemic and dermatologic findings are found in RA patients with severe disease. The main dermatologic findings are as follows:

- *Rheumatoid nodules (RN):* The most common skin lesions seen are rheumatoid nodules, which are generally seen in seropositive RA patients, overall occurring in about 25% of RA patients. Rheumatoid nodules are generally benign and occur most commonly over pressure surfaces such as the olecranon, Achilles tendon, and forearm extensor (43). Histopathologically, these lesions reveal palisaded granulomas with fibrinoid degeneration of collagen, neutrophils, fibrosis, and proliferation of vessels (44). Complications in these nodules may occur in the form of infections, ulcerations, fistulas, and joint effusions (43).

Table 18.6: Systemic non-articular manifestations of rheumatoid arthritis

Renal
- Focal glomerulonephrits
- Drug induced nephrotoxicity

Pulmonary
- Pleuritis
- Parenchymal disease

Neurologic
- Cerebrovascular accidents
- Neuropathy
- Radiculopathy

Opthalomologic
- Episceleritis
- Scleritis
- Keratoconjuctivitis Siccca

Musculoskeletal
- Osteopenia
- Myosisitis
- Synoviositis
- Drug induced myopathy

Cardiovascular
- Vasculitis
- Pericarditis
- Myocarditis
- Corornary artery disease
- Cardiac failure

Hematologic
- Anemia
- Felty's syndrome
- Lymphoproleferative disease
- Large Granular lymphocytesyndrome

- *Rheumatoid vasculitis*: The vasculitis generally involves small and medium sized vessels. There is associated neuropathy, digital ulcerations as well as gangrene, nail fold infarcts as well as telangectasias, petechiae, and purpura (43). The presence of vasculitis in RA is generally a reflection of severe disease and poor outcome. The presentation of vasculitis varies with the size of vessels and areas of the body involved. Lower limbs are more commonly involved, presenting with leg ulcers. The annual incidence overall of vasculitis is less than 1% and is noted to be more common in seropositive RA and in males (45). Histologically the lesions reveal leukocytoclastic vasculitis, infiltration of the vessel wall with neutrophils, fibroid necrosis, and hemorrhage; no palisaded granulomatous reaction is seen (46).

- *Rheumatoid neutrophilic dermatosis*: These chronic skin lesions are also seen in severe RA and are very rare. The lesions are generally described as erythematous, popular or plaque-like urticarial lesions (44). Histologically these lesions are characterized by a dense infiltrate of neutrophils, mixed infiltrate, and papillary edema; however, there is no leukocytosis (46).
- Other dermatologic lesions that may be seen in RA include erythema elevatum diutinum, livedo vasculitis, palmar erythema, epidermolysis bullosa acquista, erythema multiforme, and erythema nodosum (44).

18.3.5 Psychiatric manifestations

Juvenile rheumatoid arthritis (JRA) affects the patient's life in multiple ways similar to other chronic debilitating diseases. The illness intrusiveness is an important determinant of the psychological impact of a chronic disease like JRA. The disease engulfs all aspects of a child or adolescent's life at the time when he or she is also going through multiple developmental tasks as well as figuring out themselves and their place in their world. Chronic diseases are known to impact personal perceptions of self, interpersonal relationships, and the ability to make social connections; it also impacts on academic and professional areas. The higher the rate of illness intrusiveness, the higher the likelihood of developing psychiatric disorders (15). Figure 18.3 reviews psychiatric conditions in JRA.

The evidence for psychosocial impact resulting in established psychiatric disorders is conflicting. While many studies point toward significant psychiatric issues, some studies state that there was no significant difference noted between children and adolescents suffering from JRA and the control groups. This finding was attributed to "psychological hardiness," the resilience they may have developed to better deal with their disease (45). Psychiatric comorbidity is reported to be quite significant in JRA by other studies (46,47). Children and adolescents with JRA suffer from generalized growth failure not only because of destruction of joint space and early epiphyseal closure, but also due to the long term use of corticosteroids (48). This gives rise to negative self-perception and psychosocial maladjustment, which leads to chronic depressive syndromes.

Although major depressive disorder has also been reported by several studies, chronic depressive symptoms meeting the American Psychiatric Association's

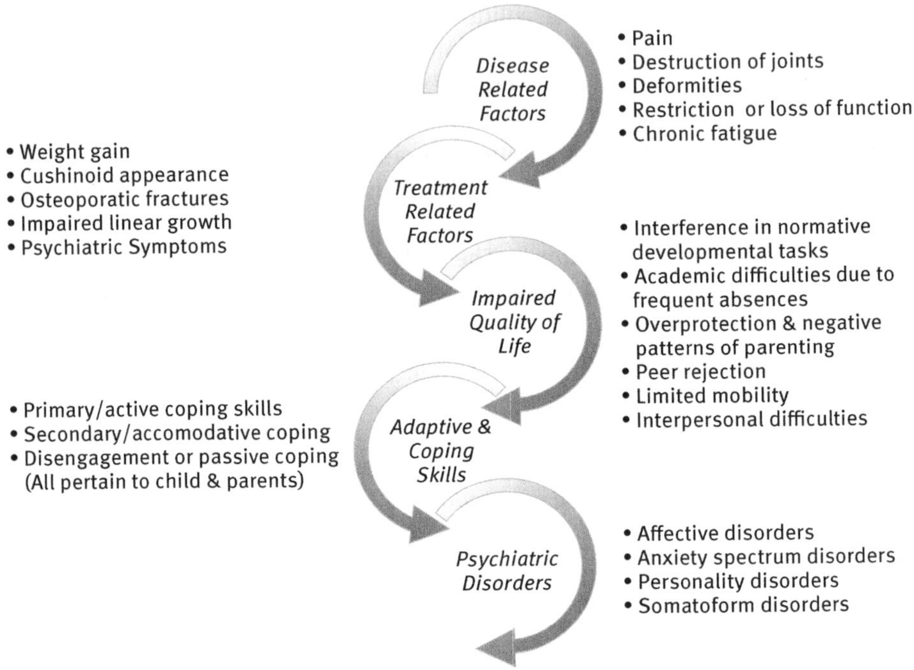

Figure 18.3: Development of psychiatric conditions in juvenile rheumatoid arthritis.

(APA's) *Diagnostic and Statistical Manual of Mental Diseases'* (DSM-IV-TR) criteria of dysthymic disorder is also common. Erdogdu et al reported depressive disorders in 31% and anxiety disorder in 17.7% in a cohort of 45 children with JRA. The depression and anxiety were not correlated to the severity of pain level (47). Vandvik et al used structured psychiatric interviews with children admitted to the hospital with JRA and reported that about 51% had some type of emotional difficulties, while 64% reported social difficulties. Most children displayed more internalizing behaviors (46). Alexithymia is defined as the inability to perceive one's own feeling or distinguishing between different feelings and a sense of blunted emotional response to everything. Patients with JRA are reported to have higher levels of alexithymia, which may cause them to misinterpret their feeling and project their anger inwardly, resulting in somatoform disorders such as chronic pain syndromes (49).

Several studies have looked into whether developing such a debilitating illness earlier in life impacts the patient's personality in any predictable way. Some personality traits were reported by several studies, although no particular personality disorder was noticed consistently with JRA. Common personality traits noticed were reflective of internalization of anxiety and hostility, such as being a perfectionist, rigid, over moralistic, over conscientious, self-limiting, and self-sacrificing. Externalizing behaviors are uncommon in JRA, and if patients display anger or hostility, they tend to be very remorseful and self-punishing about it. Feelings of inadequacy are often mentioned in children with JRA, leading to shyness and difficulties in interpersonal relations with peers and others. Rangel et al reported that when comparing the chronic fatigue syndrome to juvenile idiopathic arthritis, about 78% of patients in this cohort displayed only certain personality traits but did not have any personality disorder meeting specific diagnostic criteria (50).

One relationship that is most affected in JRA is the child–parent dyad. The relapsing remitting nature of disease, residual pain, chronic disability, and discomfort make the psychosocial adjustment very difficult not only for the child but also for parents (51). This relationship is critical in a child achieving a level of psychological adaption and developing good coping skills to overcome such a chronic illness. Perceived uncertainty of illness in children is a predictor of higher levels of parental maladjustment, leading to parental distress and over-protectiveness that in turn negatively impacts the child's psychosocial adjustment, child–parent relationship, and mood (51).

Chronic pain associated with RA affects children and adolescents profoundly. Research has shown that coping skills that are useful in dealing with other stressors are not effective when children are trying to cope with pain (52). The multidimensional construct of pain makes it a unique stressor for young children with pain as the emotional factors influence the subjective perception of pain. Girls were more likely to have higher perception of pain than boys (53).

Sleep disturbances are common in JRA along with nocturnal pain, which may play a major role in an overall sense of well-being. Sleep quality is an important predictor of disease severity, academic performance, and the parent–child relationship; also, it may result in disturbance of mood, emotional dysregulation, and behavioral problems. Chronic sleep deprivation can also give rise to inattention, easy distractibility, and paradoxical hyperactivity, at times mislabeling these children with attention deficit hyperactivity disorder (54).

Long term follow up studies have shown that up to 56% of children suffering from JRA develop severe functional difficulties. Physical activity and mobility is a key component in the life of any child and adolescent as most of their social activities revolve around sports and active participation in social events. Decline in physical activity can give rise to significant problems in social, emotional, and cognitive development. Depression was found to be correlated with physical abilities and sense of well-being in these children (55).

18.3.6 Laboratory findings

The common laboratory testing aims to support the diagnosis of RA and to differentiate it from other conditions with similar symptomatology. These are listed in Table 18.7 (56). The ACR/EULAR (European League against Rheumatism) criteria for diagnosis of rheumatoid arthritis are summarized in Figure 18.4 (57).

Table 18.7: Common laboratory tests for rheumatoid arthritis

Initial testing	Erythrocyte sedimentation rate (ESR) C-Reactive protein (CRP) Rheumatoid factor Anticyclic citrullinated peptide (CIP) antibodies
Testing to rule out other underlying diagnosis	Antinuclear antibody (ANA) testing Anti-Smith and anti-double stranded DNA antibody Serum uric acid Testing to rule out underlying infectious etiology
Testing to establish underlying status	Complete blood count Comprehensive metabolic panel with liver function tests
Imaging studies	Imaging of the involved joints with radiography, CT scans, and MRI

18.3.7 Management

The therapeutic measures available to treat RA need to be individualized to the specific manifestations of the condition in each patient. The therapy selection needs to consider the underlying clinical status, cost of therapy, and potential of adverse reactions. Sequential or combination use of drug agents available may determine

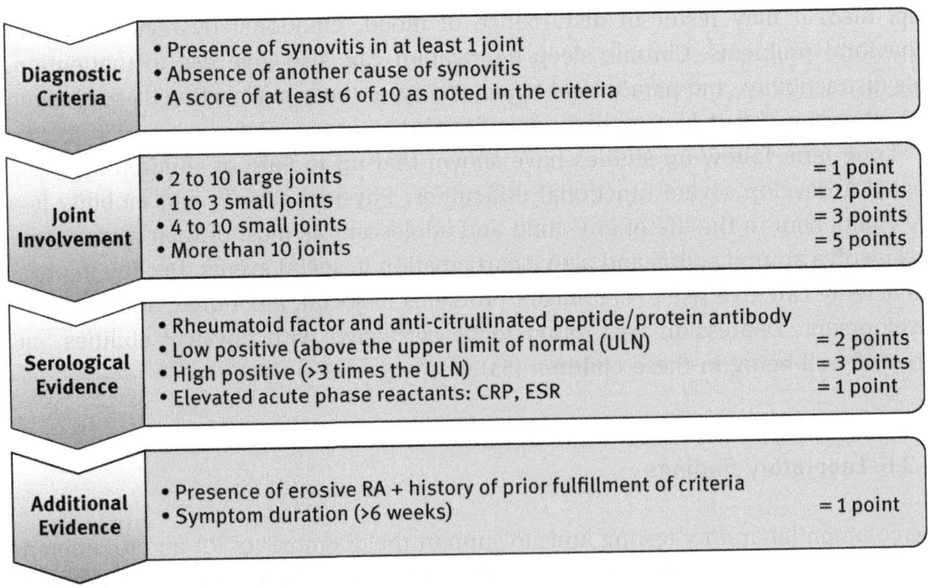

Figure 18.4: American College of Rheumatology (ACR) 2010/European League against Rheumatism (EULAR) criteria for diagnosis of rheumatoid arthritis.

successful treatment of the disease activity. These are listed in Table 18.8 (44,58). Management of systemic RA as well as the cutaneous manifestations needs to be coordinated between the rheumatologist and dermatologist. The cutaneous lesions usually need aggressive treatment of not only the underlying systemic manifestations but also of the particular dermatologic conditions as well (see Table 18.8).

Table 18.8: Options for management of rheumatoid arthritis

Non Pharmacologic, Preventive, and Supportive Measures
- Rest, exercise
- Nutrition and diet therapy
- Physical therapy
- Occupational therapy
- Bone protection measures
- Modification of atherosclerotic risk factors
- Vaccinations
- Patient education and counseling

Pharmacologic Agents

Analgesics – Drugs used to control pain and inflammation:
- Oral: acetaminophen, propoxyphene, tramadol, oxycodone hydrocodone
- Local: diclofenac, capsaicin
- Nonsteroidal anti-inflammatory drugs (NSAIDS) -Anti-inflammatory/Analgesics
- Glucocorticoids: Anti-inflammatory/Analgesics; More effective but have more side effect

Disease-Modifying Anti-rheumatic Drugs (DMARDS): Recommended Much Earlier on in the Disease Process

Non-biologic DMARDS:
- Hydroxychloroquine
- Sulfasalazine
- Methotrexate
- Leflunomide
- Minocycline

Biologic DMARDS: (Anti-cytokine medications)

TNF a inhibitors (Tumor necrosis factor 1)
- Etanercept
- Infliximab
- Adalimumab
- Golimumab
- Certolizumab pegol
- Interleukin (IL) 1 receptor antagonist
- Anakinra

IL-6 receptor antagonist
- Tocilizumab

Other biologic response modifiers
- Abatacept (CTLA4-Ig)
- Anti-CD20 B-cell depleting monoclonal antibody
- Rituximab

18.3.8 Management of psychiatric issues

Identifying and treating psychiatric disease should be part of a comprehensive treatment plan. Depression is often associated and is highly correlated with noncompliance with recommended treatment of RA (59). It is of the utmost importance to differentiate between fully established psychiatric disorders meeting the diagnostic criteria of DMS-IV-TR; avoid simply giving the label of depression only because of the fatigue, sleep disturbances, and lack of participation in activities due to active arthritis.

Several psychometric scales can be used in the office-based setting to elucidate psychological issues. It is important to understand the severity of confounding treatable factors that can lead to further deterioration of the functional and emotional abilities, such as sleep disturbances, nocturnal pain, and discomfort. The Children's Sleep Habits Questionnaire (CSHQ) is a 33 item questionnaire asking parents to recall sleep behaviors over a typical week. Child-reported Sleep Self-Report (SSR) is a retrospective survey asking children about their sleep pattern over 1 week (60). Quality of life issues can be assessed using the Pediatric Quality of life (PedsQL) rheumatology module.

Psychoeducation of children and parents is a very important step in the treatment plan, although it needs to be provided on an ongoing basis as it cannot achieve its goal if delivered in a one-time informational session. Care should be taken to deliver the message in the context of the child's age as well as his or her ability to acquire and utilize the information. Cognitive behavioral and individual psychotherapy can be used to help the patient understand the state of alexithymia and introverted behaviors (49). Mastery of cognitive behavioral techniques can help a child change his or her view of a chronic debilitating disease such as JRA and to actively engage them in learning how to deal with their illness in an effective way.

Behavioral techniques can all be employed with some degree of success; these include systemic desensitization, breathing exercises, role modeling, behavioral rehearsals, positive reinforcement, distraction strategies, progressive muscle relaxation, hypnosis, and guided imagery (see Chapter 23). Art therapy can be used as a diagnostic and treatment tool. The children with chronic diseases benefit from social skills training, including skill instruction, behavioral training, and problem solving by assessing, negotiating, and developing a plan to deal with a particular social situation.

Family therapy is very important as family members can learn about the disease and learn how to positively affect the disease management. Group therapy provides an excellent platform for the pediatric patients to learn from each other and to receive some guidance from peers (61). Identifying maladaptive patterns of pain perception and pain threshold is important. If needed, focused interventions can be utilized to improve their ability to regulate pain perception by using relaxation, biofeedback, guided imagery, and hypnosis (61).

References

1. Costner MI, Sontheimer RD. Lupus erythematosus. In: Wolff K, Goldsmith LA, Katz SI, Gilchrest BA, Paller AS, Leffell DJ, eds. *Fitzpatrick's dermatology in general medicine*, 7th edn. New York: McGraw Hill Medical, 2008:1515–35.
2. Barnett NK, Weston WL, Krol A, Shishov M, Ede K, Shulman ST, et al. Rheumatic diseases in children, autoinflammatory syndromes in children, and selected systemic diseases with skin manifestations. In: Schachner LA, Hansen RC, eds. *Pediatric dermatology*, 4th edn. Edinburgh: Mosby Elsevier, 2011:1269–1330.
3. Hochberg MC. Updating the American College of Rheumatology revised criteria for the classification of systemic lupus erythematosus. *Arthritis Rheum* 1997;40(9):1725.
4. Lehman TJA. Systemic lupus erythematosus in childhood and adolescence. In: Wallace DJ, Hahn BH, eds. *Dubois lupus erythematosus*, 4th edn. Philadelphia, PA: Lea Febiger, 1993:431.
5. Tucker LB. Caring for the adolescent with systemic lupus erythematosus. *Adolesc Med* 1998;9 (1):59.
6. Lehman TJA, McCurdy D, Spencer C, Silverman E, Harley JB. Prognostic value of antibodies to Ro/SSA, La/SSB, and RNP in children with systemic lupus erythematosus. *Arthritis Rheum* 1990;33:S154.
7. Tan EM, Cohen AS, Fries JF, Masi AT, McShane DJ, Rothfield NF, et al. The 1982 revised criteria for the classification of systemic lupus erythematosus. *Arthritis Rheum* 1982;25(11):1271–7.
8. Hanly JG. Neuropsychiatric lupus. *Curr Rheumatol Rep* 2001;3:205–12.
9. Olfat MO, Al-Mayouf SM. Pattern of neuropsychiatric manifestations and outcome in juvenile systemic lupus erythematosus. *Clin Rheumatol* 2004;23:395–99.
10. Benseler SM, Silverman ED. Review: Neuropsychiatric involvement in pediatric systemic lupus erythematosus. *Lupus* 2007;16:564–71.
11. Sibbitt WL Jr, Brandt JR, Johnson CR, Maldonado ME, Patel SR, Ford CC, et al. The incidence and prevalence of neuropsychiatric syndromes in pediatric onset systemic lupus erythematosus. *J Rheumatol* 2002;29(7):1536–42.
12. The American College of Rheumatology nomenclature and case definitions for neuropsychiatric lupus syndromes. *Arthritis Rheum* 1999;42(4):599–608.
13. Yu HH, Lee JH, Wang LC, Yang YH, Chiang BL. Neuropsychiatric manifestations in pediatric systemic lupus erythematosus: A 20-year study. *Lupus* 2006;15(10):651–7.
14. Muscal E, Nadeem T, Li X, Mian A, Harris TB. Evaluation and treatment of acute psychosis in children with Systemic Lupus Erythematosus (SLE): Consultation-liaison service experiences at a tertiary-care pediatric institution. *Psychosomatics* 2010;51(6):508–14.
15. Devins GM, Edworthy SM, Guthrie NG,Martin L. Illness intrusiveness in rheumatoid arthritis: differential impact on depressive symptoms over the adult lifespan. *J Rheumatol* 1992;19(5): 709–15.
16. Schattner E, Shahar G, Lerman S, Shakra MA. Depression in systemic lupus erythematosus: The key role of illness intrusiveness and concealment of symptoms. *Psychiatry* 2010;73(4):329–40.
17. Fonseca E, Rubio G. Factitious Systemic Lupus Erythematosus. *Lupus* 1993;2:195–7.
18. Bartels CM, Krause RS, Lakdawala VS, et al. Systemic lupus erythematosus (SLE). *Mescape Reference* 2012. http://emedicine.medscape.com/article/332244-overview
19. Schur PH, Wallace DJ. Diagnosis and differential diagnosis of systemic lupus erythematosus in adults. *Wolters Kluwer Health: Up to Date.* http://www.uptodate.com/contents/diagnosis-and-differential-diagnosis-of-systemic-lupus-erythematosus-in-adults
20. Ruiz-Irastorza G, Ramos-Casals M, Brito-Zeron P, Khamashta MA. Clinical efficacy and side effects of antimalarials in systemic lupus erythematosus: A systematic review. *Ann Rheum Dis* 2010;69(1):20.

21. Buratti S, Szer IS, Spencer CH, Bartosh S, Reiff A. Mycophenolate mofetil treatment of severe renal disease in pediatric onset systemic lupus erythematosus. *J Rheumatol* 2001;28(9):2103.
22. Kazyra I, Pilkington C, Marks SD, Tullus K. Mycophenolate mofetil treatment in children and adolescents with lupus. *Arch Dis Child* 2010;95(12):1059.
23. Linden KG, Weinstein GD. Psoriasis: Current perspectives with an emphasis on treatment. *Am J Med* 1999;107(6):595.
24. Lampropoulos CE, Sangle S, Harrison P, Hughes GR, D'Cruz DP. Topical tacrolimus therapy of resistant cutaneous lesions in lupus erythematosus: A possible alternative. *Rheumatology* 2004; 43(11):1383.
25. Muscal E, Bang L, Mian A, Harris TB. Use of aripiprazole in adolescents with a history of lupus-associated psychosis and refractory psychiatric manifestations. *J Psychiatr Pract* 2011;17(3):212–6.
26. Sontheimer RD, Costner MI. Dermatomyositis. In: Wolff K, Goldsmith LA, Katz SI, Gilchrest BA, Paller AS, Leffell DJ, eds. *Fitzpatrick's dermatology in general medicine*, 7th edn. New York: McGraw Hill Medical 2008:1536–83.
27. Miller ML. Clinical manifestations and diagnosis of adult dermatomyositis and polymyositis. *Wolters Kluwer Health: Up to Date.* http://www.uptodate.com/contents/clinical-manifestations-and-diagnosis-of-adult-dermatomyositis-and-polymyositis
28. Paradis CM, Friedman S, Lazar RM,Kula RW. Anxiety disorders in a neuromuscular clinic. *Am J Psychiatry* 1993;150(7):1102–4.
29. Butbul Aviel Y, Stremler R, Benseler SM, Cameron B, Laxer RM, Ota S, et al. Sleep and fatigue and the relationship to pain, disease activity and quality of life in juvenile idiopathic arthritis and juvenile dermatomyositis. *Rheumatology* 2011;50(11):2051–60.
30. Alsanafi S, Werth VP. Evaluating quality of life in dermatomyositis. *Expert Rev Dermatol* 2010;5.6:605.
31. Hundley JL, Carroll CL, Lang W, Snively B, Yosipovitch G, Feldman SR, et al. Cutaneous symptoms of dermatomyositis significantly impact patients' quality of life. *J Am Acad Dermatol* 2006;54(2):217–20.
32. Chalmers A, Sayson R, Walters K. Juvenile dermatomyositis: Medical, social and economic status in adulthood. *Can Med Assoc* J1982;126(1):31–3.
33. Vleugels RA. Management of refractory cutaneous dermatomyositis. *Wolters Kluwer Health: Up to Date.* http://www.uptodate.com/contents/management-of-refractory-cutaneous-dermatomyositis
34. Miller ML, Rudnicki SA. Initial treatment of dermatomyositis and polymyositis in adults. *Wolters Kluwer Health: Up to Date.* http://www.uptodate.com/contents/initial-treatment-of-dermatomyositis-and-polymyositis-in-adults
35. Finlay AY. Quality of life indices. *Indian J Dermatol Venereol Leprol* 2004;70(3):143–8.
36. Finlay AY. Practice Gaps. Dermatologists should better integrate quality-of-life measures to inform and improve clinical decision making: Comment on "The impact of pruritus on quality of life." *Arch Dermatol* 2011;147(10):1157.
37. Alamanos Y, Drosos AA. Epidemiology of adult rheumatoid arthritis. *Autoimmune Rev* 2004; 4:130.
38. Agrawal S, Aggarwal A, Dabadghao S, Naik S,Misra R. Compound heterozygosity of HLA-DR4 and DR1 antigens in Asian Indians increases the risk of extra-articular features in rheumatoid arthritis. *Br J Rheumatol* 1995;34(1):41–4.
39. Firestein GS. Immunologic mechanisms in the pathogenesis of rheumatoid arthritis. *J Clin Rheumatol* 2005;11:S39–S44.
40. Lee DM, Weinblatt ME. Rheumatoid arthritis. *Lancet* 2001;358(9285):903–11.
41. Koskinen E, Hannonen P, Sokka T. Palindromic rheumatism: Longterm outcomes of 60 patients diagnosed in 1967–84. *J Rheumatol* 2009;36(9):1873–5.
42. Schur PH. Overview of the systemic and nonarticular manifestations of rheumatoid arthritis. *Wolters Kluwer Health: Up to Date.* http://www.uptodate.com/contents/overview-of-the-systemic-and-nonarticular-manifestations-of-rheumatoid-arthritis

43. Sayah A, English JC, III. Rheumatoid arthritis: A review of the cutaneous manifestations. *J Am Acad Dermatol* 2005;53(2):191–209.
44. Haverstock CL, Jorizzo JL. Rheumatoid arthritis, rheumatic fever, and gout. In: Wolff K, Goldsmith LA, Katz SI, Gilchrest BA, Paller AS, Leffell DJ, eds. *Fitzpatrick's dermatology in general medicine*, 7th edn. New York: McGraw Hill Medical, 2008:1569–1577.
45. Watts RA, Carruthers DM, Symmons DP, Scott DG. The incidence of rheumatoid vasculitis in the Norwich Health Authority. *Br J Rheumatol* 1994;33(9):832–3.
46. Ackerman, AB, Chongchitnant N, Sanchez J, Guo Y. Histologic Diagnosis of Inflammatory Skin Diseases: An Algorithmic Method Based on Pattern Analysis, 2nd ed, Baltimore: Lippincott Williams & Wilkins; 1997.
47. Erdogdu D, Kasapcopur O, Cimen G, Arisoy N, Kayaalp. Depression, anxiety and pain in juvenile idiopathic arthritis. Poster presentation. 15th Paediatric Rheumatology European Society (PreS) Congress. *Pediatric Rheumatology* 2008;6(Suppl 1):P175.
48. Packham JC, Hall MA. Long-term follow-up of 246 adults with juvenile idiopathic arthritis: functional outcome. *Rheumatology* 2002;41(12):1428–35.
49. Sterling S. *The role of alexithymia and anger in rheumatoid arthritis.* San Francisco, CA: California Institute of Integral Studies, 2008.
50. Rangel L, Garralda ME, Hall A, Woodham S. Psychiatric adjustment in chronic fatigue syndrome of childhood and in juvenile idiopathic arthritis. *Psychol Med* 2003;33(2):289–97.
51. White MM, Chaney JM, Mullins LL, Wagner JL, Hommel KA, Andrews NR, et al. Children's perceived illness uncertainty as a moderator in the parent-child distress relation in juvenile rheumatic diseases. *Rehabil Psychol* 2005;50(3):224–31.
52. Compas BE, Boyer MC, Stanger C, Colletti RB, Thomsen AH, Dufton LM, et al. Latent variable analysis of coping, anxiety/depression, and somatic symptoms in adolescents with chronic pain. *J Consult Clin Psychol* 2006;74(6):1132–42.
53. Margetić B, Aukst-Margetić B, Bilić E, Jelusić M, Tambić Bukovac L. Depression, anxiety and pain in children with juvenile idiopathic arthritis (JIA). *Eur Psychiatry* 2005;20(3):274–6.
54. Labyak SE, Bourguignon C, Docherty S. Sleep quality in children with juvenile rheumatoid arthritis. *Holist Nurs Pract* 2003;17(4):193–200.
55. Tarakci E, Yeldan I, Kaya Mutlu E, Baydogan SN, Kasapcopur O. The relationship between physical activity level, anxiety, depression, and functional ability in children and adolescents with juvenile idiopathic arthritis. *Clin Rheumatol* 2011;30(11):1415–20.
56. Venables PJW, Maini RN. Diagnosis and differential diagnosis of rheumatoid arthritis. *Wolters Kluwer Health: Up to Date.* http://www.uptodate.com/contents/diagnosis-and-differential-diagnosis-of-rheumatoid-arthritis
57. Aletaha D, Neogi T, Silman AJ, Funovits J, Felson DT, Bingham, III CO, et al. Arthritis & rheumatism. 2010 Rheumatoid Arthritis Classification Criteria: An American College of Rheumatology/European League Against Rheumatism Collaborative Initiative. *Arthritis Rheumatism* 2010;62(9):2569–81.
58. Schur PH, Cohen S. Treatment of early, moderately active rheumatoid arthritis in adults. *Wolters Kluwer Health: Up to Date.* http://www.uptodate.com/contents/treatment-of-early-moderately-active-rheumatoid-arthritis-in-adults
59. DiMatteo MR, Lepper HS, Croghan TW. Depression is a risk factor for noncompliance with medical treatment: Meta-analysis of the effects of anxiety and depression on patient adherence. *Arch Intern Med* 2000;160(14):2101–7.
60. Aviel YB, Stremler R, Benseler SM. Sleep and fatigue and the relationship to pain, disease activity and quality of life in juvenile idiopathic arthritis and juvenile dermatomyositis. *Rheumatology* 2011;50:2051–60.
61. Goodman RF. Children with a chronic illness: The interface of medicine and mental health. *NYU Child Study Center Letter* 2001;5:4:1–6.

Manmohan K. Kamboj and Ruqiya Shama Tareen

19 Psychocutaneous manifestations of endocrine disorders

The intricate relationship of cutaneous manifestations of endocrine disorders and their connection with psychosomatic repercussions is quite complex and is being dully recognized. However, more specific interplay of endocrine systems in psychiatric and dermatological disorders is still not very well understood, and our knowledge of this area is still in its early phases. The Neuro-Immuno-Cutaneous-Endocrine (NICE) network is one of the emerging models seeking to understand mind–body relationships and their impact on skin. NICE is a construct of four major organ systems and how they are intertwined and function with regard to the extensive communication systems of neurochemical signals, such as cytokines, neuropeptides, glucocorticoids, and other messenger molecules. This chapter seeks to review endocrine disorders and their cutaneous features, along with psychiatric features and principles of clinical management of these cutaneous and psychiatric issues presenting in the context of major endocrine disorders commonly seen in children and adolescents.

19.1 Introduction

The bidirectional mind and body connection has been acknowledged by the medical professional for a long time; however, when it comes to its implication in our clinical practices, we still are not fully embracing this idea. Skin has been regarded mostly as an encasement protecting our body and internal organs, while most skin conditions are treated in isolation without paying much attention to the underlying mechanisms. More recently we are acknowledging the intricate and multifaceted origins of the cutaneous presentations of various systemic diseases. The Neuro-Immuno-Cutaneous-Endocrine (NICE) network is one of the emerging models seeking to explain mind–body relationships and their impact on skin. NICE is a construct comprising four organ systems and how they are interlinked and communicate with each other utilizing the aid of intricate systems of neurochemical signals involving cytokines, neuropeptides, glucocorticoids, and other messenger molecules (1). This chapter considers some of the endocrine and metabolic disorders that have prominent psychiatric and dermatological presentations (see Table 19.1).

19.2 Diabetes Mellitus

Diabetes mellitus (DM) is an endocrine disorder comprising a heterogeneous group of conditions that result in hyperglycemia either due to insulin deficiency, insulin

Table 19.1: Endocrine disorders and severity of comorbid psychiatric and dermatologic features

Endocrine Disorders	Dermatologic Features	Psychiatric Features
Diabetes Mellitus	++	+++
Disorders of Growth Hormone	+++	+++
Thyroid Hormone Disorders	+++	+++
Adrenal Gland Disorders	++	+++
Disorders of Parathyroid Glands	+++	+++
Disorders of Androgens	++	++
Disorders of Estrogens	+++	++

resistance, or a combination of the two. The common types of DM are listed in Table 19.2.

Diabetes mellitus is one of the most common chronic illnesses. The prevalence of diabetes mellitus is 25.8 million people (18.8 million of these are diagnosed, while 7 million are undiagnosed), which accounts for 8.3% of the population in the United States as of 2011 (2). The prevalence of DM in people younger than 20 years of age is 215,000, which accounts for 0.26% of the population (2).

19.2.1 Clinical features

Patients with DM (Type1DM [T1DM] and Type2DM [T2DM]) may be diagnosed in one of several ways. One is if asymptomatic and diagnosed early with screening tests; another is presentation with classic symptomatology of polyuria, polydipsia, and

Table 19.2: Types of Diabetes Mellitus

Types of Diabetes Mellitus (DM)
Type I Diabetes
Type 2 Diabetes
MODY: Genetic defects of β-cell function
Secondary type of diabetes
• Genetic defects in insulin action
• Diseases of the exocrine pancreas
• Endocrinopathies
• Drug or chemical induced
• Infection
Gestational Diabetes Mellitus

weight loss. Also, there is presentation in a decompensated state with diabetic ketoacidosis (DKA).

19.2.2 Dermatological manifestations

A multitude of dermatologic manifestations may be seen in DM, as listed in Table 19.3 (3). Some of these conditions are caused directly by a state of chronic hyperglycemia and dyslipidemia/hyperlipidemia; others may be caused indirectly by the chronic effects of diabetes on immune function, neuropathy, and macrovascular changes affecting the skin. The underlying pathogenesis of many of these conditions remains unclear. Some of these dermatologic manifestations are now considered.

19.2.2.1 Necrotising fasciitis

This is a specific infection caused by multiple bacterial species including streptococci, *E. coli*, and clostridia (4). The infection starts in the soft tissues and spreads along fascial planes of the trunk, abdomen, and upper arms; it carries a high

Table 19.3: Cutaneous disorders associated with diabetes mellitus

1. Cutaneous disorders seen with higher incidence in patients with DM
Bacterial Infections
• Streptococcal infections
• Staphylococcal infections
• Malignant external otitis
• Necrotizing fasciitis
Fungal Infections
• Candida infections
• Dermatophyte infections
Cutaneous disorders with known underlying etiopathogenesis
• Acanthosis nigricans
• Diabetic limited joint mobility (DLJM) or Scleroderma like syndrome
• Scleroderma diabeticorum
• Eruptive Xanthomas
• Diabetic ulcers
Cutaneous disorders in DM with yet unknown underlying etiopathogenesis
• Diabetic dermatopathy
• Necrobiosis lipoidica diabeticorum

mortality rate up to 40% (4,5). Surgical debridement and appropriate antibiotics are treatments of choice.

19.2.2.2 Necrobiosis lipoidica diabeticorum (NLD)

NLD is seen in patients with DM but may also occur in non-DM patients. It is a chronic granulomatous, cutaneous disorder with characteristic pretibial lesions. The underlying etiology is not clear, but immune pathologic mechanisms as well as some trauma are thought to be important factors of pathogenesis (3,6). Widely ranging prevalence rates have been reported for NLD (7,8). The skin lesions show slow evolution, beginning as dark red, irregular nodules and progressing to atrophic yellowish brown lesions with a reddish border. Ulceration of the overlying skin, sensory neuropathy, and even squamous cell carcinoma has been reported in these lesions (7).

The treatment options available for NLD are unsatisfactory. Multiple agents have been tried with varying results, including topical and intra-lesional glucocorticoids, systemic steroids, aspirin, dipyridamole, topical retinoids, PUVA (psoralen + ultraviolet A), fumaric esters, cyclosporine, anti TNFα (tumor necrosis factor-alpha), and tacrolimus (7,9,10,11,12). Improvement of diabetes control may lead to some improvement in the cutaneous lesions. For ulcerated lesions surgical excision and grafting may be needed (13).

19.2.2.3 Diabetic limited joint mobility syndrome (DLJMS) or Scleroderma-like syndrome

This is characterized by the typical "prayer sign" in which patients are unable to approximate the palmer surfaces of both their hands (as in prayer). When the hands are pressed together with the fingers separated, the palms and interphalangeal (IP) joint spaces are unable to approximate each other. There is accompanying skin thickening as well. Severity of DLJMS correlates with the duration and level of control of the underlying DM; thus, it is not usually seen in the pediatric population. DLJMS may be seen in up to 50% of adult patients (14). Conversely, improvement in diabetes control has shown a decrease in incidence of DLJM and a fourfold lowering of frequency over the last 20 years has been reported (14,15).

19.2.2.4 Scleroderma diabeticorum (SB) /Scleroderma of Buschke

Scleroderma diabeticorum (SB) is a relatively rare cutaneous disorder characterized primarily by non-pitting thickening and hardening of the skin, generally starting in the neck, upper back area, and then progressing to involve the upper chest, shoulders, upper arms, and even the face. SB is not specific to DM but is associated mostly with T2DM (16). Although there is no standard treatment for SB, many therapeutic options have been tried, mostly published in non-controlled reports. Recent publications report success with use of UVA1 and PUVA in combination with other modalities, such as colchicine, physiotherapy, and corticosteroids (17,18). Optimization of diabetes control is encouraged, while physiotherapy may help in joint mobility and respiratory compromise.

19.2.2.5 Acanthosis nigricans (AN)

Acanthosis nigricans (AN) is a condition characterized by velvety, dark appearing, hypertrophic, non-inflamed, exophytic cutaneous lesions. AN initially starts in the axilla and nape of the neck and subsequently has a wide spread distribution to include extensive neck involvement and other flexural surfaces in addition to infra-mammary, lower abdomen, and groin areas. The most common associations of AN are with obesity, hyperinsulinemia, and insulin resistance. It is also noted to be correlated with body mass index regardless of insulin sensitivity (19).

The underlying pathogenesis in DM seems to result from high insulin levels binding and stimulating both the insulin and the IGF1 (insulin like growth factor 1) receptors on keratinocytes and dermal fibroblasts (20). The hyperpigmentation is primarily attributed to hyperkeratosis. The endocrine evaluation should focus on evaluation for hyperinsulinemia, insulin resistance (IR), glycemic status, prediabetes, and T2DM.

There is no effective specific treatment for acanthosis nigricans. Weight loss and improvement in insulin resistance may result in improvement of AN. Cosmetic treatment with topical tretinoin or oral isotretinoin is reported to improve AN (21). Calcipotriol has also been noted to be useful (22). More recent options include long-pulsed alexandrite laser treatment (23).

19.2.3 Psychiatric manifestations

19.2.3.1 Depressive disorders

Psychiatric comorbidity in patients with DM is much more common than is usually acknowledged. In comparison to general populations, depressive symptoms are two to three times more common in patients with DM (24). Non compliance with diabetes care is more frequently seen in young patients with DM, and if so, the presence of an underlying comorbid depressive illness should be investigated. There is a sense of apathy toward their illness in these patients, which leads to chronic poor diabetes control and care. It is difficult to ascertain which of these two conditions come first. A large cohort prospective study evaluated new onset T2DM patients for the new onset of depression, and it was concluded that the rate of new onset depression was not higher than the general population (25). Depression has been proposed as an independent risk factor for developing DM-II (26).

19.2.3.2 Anxiety disorders

There is a higher prevalence of anxiety disorders in patients with DM. This was demonstrated by a study that found that patients with DM had a 17–20% higher lifetime prevalence of an anxiety disorder when compared to their age matched controls without DM (27). Having an anxiety disorder also impacted the child or adolescent's ability to engage fully in diabetes care. The higher levels of anxiety symptoms were associated with less frequent blood glucose monitoring resulting in suboptimal glycemic control, independent of depressive symptoms in adolescents with T1DM (28).

19.2.3.3 Eating disorders

Adolescents with T1DM show a much higher prevalence of eating disorders: 36% versus 4% in the general population (29). Girls with eating disorders typically have a higher basal metabolic index (BMI) than their age matched controls (30). Evidence of eating disorders is not very well established in younger children and adolescents; however, there is evidence for a higher prevalence of body image issues, disturbed eating behavior such as binge eating, dieting, deliberately omitting insulin doses, and excessive exercise in an attempt to lose weight in girls with T1DM as young as 9–13 years of age (30).

Manipulation of insulin doses to attain desired weight has become a major problem in this population. As many as 35.6% of pediatric patients with DM reported misuse of insulin for weight control, and when they were followed up after 8–12 years, they were found to have higher levels of microvascular complications (31). This study concluded that cumulative incidence of eating disorders, if present in childhood or early youth years in DM patients, continues to increase after young adulthood; also, it was strongly associated with long term risks such as higher rates of morbidity and mortality (32).

Quality of life (QoL) is known to be affected in patients with DM, skin diseases, and psychiatric diseases (see Chapter 4). When all three of these are present in one patient, there is no doubt that it can cause significant decline in QoL. Adolescents who have DM with a mean age of 16.1 years and mean duration of illness of 8.2 years were found to have feelings of low self-esteem, disease-related worries, higher levels of depression, and less family support. The levels of QoL were much more reduced in adolescents from low socioeconomic class and minority groups (33).

19.2.4 Management of psychiatric conditions

Early identification is the key in developing a successful treatment plan for DM. It is important for clinicians to know that patients with DM are likely to have other parallel comorbid disease processes, including dermatological (i.e. acanthosis nigricans, others) and psychiatric disorders as well as body image issues, affecting their psychological state. A multidisciplinary approach is necessary in these patients to address these complex concerns, and when behavioral as well as non-behavioral interventions are utilized, the outcomes are significantly improved for not only psychological well-being but also for the systemic disease.

Psychological interventions have shown promise in this regard and include behavior modifications, cognitive behavioral therapy (CBT), biofeedback, distraction techniques, relaxation, and imagery therapy (34). General screening of all DM patients is not necessary, but identifying patients at risk and screening them for psychiatric illness and for QoL issues may help improve the outcome measures for DM while also decreasing the risk of long term complications. A study of 20 patients with T2DM showed improved fasting blood glucose and 2-hour postprandial blood glucose levels when they were treated with progressive relaxation techniques, and biofeedback treatment suggesting that a less anxious state may improve diabetes care (35). In a 4 year follow up of adolescent girls with T1DM and eating disorders, higher incidence of microvascular complications was reported (36). Early recognition of these subjects at risk especially in the first few years of diagnosis for DM may provide opportunities for psychiatric interventions and help prevent these complications in the long term.

19.3 Disorders of growth hormone

Growth hormone (GH) is secreted by the somatotropes in the anterior lobe of the pituitary gland in a pulsatile manner with diurnal variation. The primary regulators of GH are GHRH (growth hormone releasing hormone) for stimulation and somastostatin (GHIF) for inhibition of secretion of GH. The primary function of GH is the stimulation of linear growth, but in addition, GH has multiple metabolic functions. Therefore, growth hormone is important not only in the childhood growing periods but also in adulthood after completion of linear growth.

19.3.1 Acromegaly

Increased GH secretion most commonly results from a pituitary adenoma that leads to an excessive growth in childhood and adolescence. Acromegaly produces increased GH levels after epiphyseal plate closure at puberty. It presents with typical cutaneous and musculoskeletal features along with multiple metabolic disturbances (37). The main clinical features of acromegaly are listed in Table 19.4 (37).

19.3.2 Dermatological manifestations

Most of the cutaneous manifestations seen in acromegaly result from overgrowth of skin, cartilage, and bones giving rise to the characteristic appearance of acromegaly

Table 19.4: Main clinical features of acromegaly

Generalized features
- Fatigue, weakness
- Muscle weakness, bone pains/joint pains
- Arthralgias, parasthesias
- Increased hand, glove, shoe, hat or ring sizes
- Sleep apnea, hypersomnolence
- Galactorrhoea, amenorrhea
- depression
- jaw protrusion, underbite increased space between teeth
- polyuria, polydipsia

Dematological features
- Coarsening of facial features
- Overgrowth of bones and cartilages
- Enlargement of ears, elongation of the nose
- Protrusion of the chin, mandible and zygoma.
- Doughy, thickened skin
- Thickened skin folds and creases
- Thickening of the lips and eyelids
- Thick and hard nails
- Hypertrichosis
- Widely spaced teeth
- Excessive sweating
- Hyperpigmentation – generalized acanthosis nigricans
- Fibromas and skin tags

Acromegaly as part of syndromes
- Carney complex
- McCune Albright syndrome

as mentioned in Table 19.4. The facial, musculoskeletal, and dermatologic features are the physical hallmarks of this condition.

19.3.3 Psychiatric manifestations

Decreased health related quality of life (HRQoL) has been reported with acromegaly, denoting the subjective reduction in physical, emotional, and social well being. Patients complain of low levels of energy, decline in strength, and lack of initiative and spontaneity. Mood lability, irritability, and hostility are also reported (38).

Pantanetti et al reported that psychological symptoms of acromegaly can be divided into three phases: pre-diagnosis, post-diagnosis, and post-surgery. In the *pre-diagnosis* phase, patients experience anxiety, mood lability, and hypochondriasis or fear of having a disease that is not being diagnosed, along with some non-specific symptoms such as sleep disturbances, low self-esteem, and the feeling of losing control over themselves. During the *post-diagnosis/pre-surgery* phase, body image distortions are prominent, giving rise to social withdrawal, helplessness, and depression. Patients feel considerable mixed emotions such as anger, fear, relief, burden, and guilt. In the *post-surgery* phase, body image distortions and social withdrawal persist along with feelings of unmet expectations and fatigue; patients may also experience a decreased interest in life, which gives rise to anger and depression (39).

19.3.4 Diagnostic workup

The laboratory workup reveals elevations of IGF1 and IGFBP3 levels. Oral glucose tolerance testing with GH levels is measured 1 hour after administration of glucose, and this is a very important test. Levels of more than 10 ng/ml make the diagnosis of acromegaly; also, GH levels of less than 5 ng/ml essentially rule out the diagnosis of acromegaly (40). Imaging of the pituitary and peri-pituitary area for anatomical evaluation and localizing of an underlying tumor with magnetic resonance imaging (MRI) is important in making the correct diagnosis.

19.3.5 Clinical management

A multipronged approach is needed for treatment of acromegaly. Surgical therapy is usually the first line of treatment and involves transsphenoidal surgery to remove the underlying GH producing tumor, using stereotactic gamma knife radiosurgery or microsurgery. Medical options to treat acromegaly have improved significantly and are often now used as options of first choice (41). Two options of medications that are used aim to negate the effect of GH; one is by inhibiting GH secretion by using agents such as octreotide and lanreotide (42,40) and the other is by using a GH receptor blocking agent such as pegvisomant (43). Cabergoline and bromocriptine may also be helpful in reducing prolactin and GH levels by acting on the central dopamine receptors; these are more effective in tumors that secrete prolactin as well (44). Long term follow-up is required in all these patients. IGF1 levels, revaluation of GH production by dynamic studies, and imaging to follow tumor size may be needed as indicated (45).

19.3.6 Management of dermatological manifestations

No specific treatment is recommended for the cutaneous manifestation per se. Treatment of the inhibition of GH results in partial improvement of acromegalic facial features; also, hand swelling is reduced and the skin becomes softer as well as thinner following appropriate treatment (46).

19.3.7 Management of psychiatric manifestations

Depression, irritability, and hostility usually improve after the successful treatment of acromegaly. Treatment with lanreotide was found to significantly improve psychological distress, sense of psychological well-being, and social anxiety as well as fears (39). At times depression and anxiety, especially related to social situations, persist and may require treatment with psychotherapy, such as cognitive behavior therapy, and psychotropic medications, such as selective serotonin reuptake inhibitors.

19.4 Thyroid hormone disorders

Thyroid hormone plays a very important role in normal growth, development, and in the metabolic functioning of the body at the cellular level. An intact hypothalamo-pituitary-thyroid axis is needed to maintain normal thyroid function. The two main categories of thyroid dysfunction are *hypothyroidism*, characterized by low thyroid hormone levels, and *hyperthyroidism*, which features high thyroid hormone levels.

19.4.1 Hypothyroidism

Hypothyroidism may be congenital or acquired. Congenital hypothyroidism (CH) has an incidence of about 1:3,000 to 4,000; it is commonly due to thyroid dysgenesis with an anatomical defect in thyroid gland or dyshormogenesis with an enzymatic defect in thyroid hormone formation or even iodine deficiency in endemic iodine deficiency areas (47). Babies born with congenital hypothyroidism are at risk for developing severe mental retardation. It is extremely important to start them on thyroid hormone replacement at the earliest, preferably within the first 2 weeks of life. All newborns in the United States and many developed countries are screened for CH on the newborn screen.

Acquired hypothyroidism is acquired later in life and may be due to multiple underlying causes. Autoimmune hypothyroidism, also referred to as Hashimoto's thyroiditis is most common in the teen years and is also more common in girls with a male to female ratio of 1:5. There may also be a positive family history of Hashimoto's thyroiditis or Graves disease in patients with autoimmune thyroid disease.

19.4.2 Hyperthyroidism

Excessive thyroid hormone levels (T4 and T3) result in hyperthyroidism. The most common cause of hyperthyroidism is also autoimmune, with thyroid stimulating immunoglobulins responsible for increased thyroid hormone formation. Other causes include a toxic nodule, thyroid adenoma, sub-acute thyroiditis, or a TSH secreting pituitary tumor.

19.4.3 Clinical features of thyroid disorders

Early clinical features of thyroid dysfunction are very non-specific, varied, and may be quite subtle. The clinical presenting signs and symptoms for hypothyroidism and hyperthyroidism are listed in Tables 19.5 and 19.6.

Table 19.5: Main clinical features of hypothyroidism

General features
• Lethargy, easy fatigability
• Constipation
• Cold intolerance
Growth
• Growth failure
• Delayed puberty
• Precocious puberty (rarely in severe hypothyroidism)
Dermatologic features
• Dry, cool skin
• Pallor
• Carotenemia
• Myxedema
• Coarse brittle hair
• Excessive hair loss
Menstrual disturbances – Meno-metorrhagia
Pseudo-hypertrophy of calf muscles
Hung-up deep tendon reflexes
Thyrotrope hyperplasia and pituitary enlargement
• Headaches, vomiting, visual disturbances

Table 19.6: Clinical features of hyperthyroidism

General features
- Weight loss
- Increased appetite
- Loose stools

Dermatologic features
- Dermopathy

Ophthalmologic features
- Exophthalmos
- Lid lag
- Ophthalmoplegia
- Conjunctival inflammation

Cardiovascular features
- Palpitations
- Poor exercise tolerance
- Tachycardia
- Cardiac murmurs
- Hypertension
- Widened pulse pressure

Emotional/Behavioral features
- Hyperactivity
- Poor concentration
- Nervousness
- Poor school performance

Irregular periods: Oligomenorrhea

Features associated with coexisting autoimmune conditions

19.4.4 Dermatological manifestations of hypothyroidism

Cutaneous features seen in hypothyroidism include discoloration that is pale, dry, cool, sallow, and yellowish orange (48). This is likely due to relative peripheral vasoconstriction and lowered body temperature; also, cutaneous deposits of beta carotene contribute to the discoloration. This is believed to be due to the sluggish metabolism of beta carotene to vitamin A in the liver. These skin changes are noted to be generalized in distribution all over the body without any specific localization.

Myxedema is the most characteristic cutaneous finding in hypothyroidism. Hypothyroidism needs to be severe enough and of long term duration for myxedema to be seen in its characteristic description. Myxedema is also generalized but may be noted to be more prominent in the face, hands, and feet. The skin is swollen, doughy, and waxy but non-pitting; wound healing may be impaired as well (48). Facial features in myxedema include broadened thickened nose, puffy eyelids, macroglossia, and thickened lips. Histologically there is accumulation of mucopolysaccharides such as chondroitin sulfate and hyaluronic acid. Treatment of hypothyroidism results in improvement or resolution of the myxedema (48).

Nail changes in hypothyroidism include brittle thickened nails with striations. Hair changes include scalp hair loss, which may be patchy or generalized; the hair is noted to be dry, brittle, and exhibiting slow growth. Loss of eyebrows characteristically involves the outer one third. Also, there are case reports of association of hypothyroidism with muco-cutaneous candidiasis (49), bullous pemphigoid (50), alopecia areata (51), and autoimmune connective tissue disorders (52).

19.4.5 Dermatological manifestations of hyperthyroidism

In contrast to changes seen in hypothyroidism, the skin in hyperthyroidism is noted to be soft, velvety, moist, and warm; the skin may be tender while sweatiness and pruritus may be increased. This is due to peripheral vasodilation and increased blood flow in the skin. The nails may be normal, shining and brittle, or they may be concave with onycholysis, also referred to as "plumber's nails" (48). The hair is soft and thin with evidence of hair loss. Vitiligo is also noted to be more common in hyperthyroidism, especially Graves disease. Most of these skin features are noted to resolve on treatment of hyperthyroidism; however, the vitiligo does not show any improvement even after treatment of the hyperthyroidism as it may share the common underlying auto-immune etiology.

Thyroid dermopathy is mostly seen with hyperthyroidism as a late manifestation, and generally occurs in conjunction with ophthalmopathy (53). The typical dermopathy lesions are bilateral and may be diffuse or well circumscribed; it is most commonly found on the anterior lower legs and is described as painless, non-pitting nodules or plaques. The skin lesions may be variably pigmented and indurated or waxy in texture (48). Histologically there is thickening of the dermis, deposition of mucin as well as hyaluronic acid in the interstitium, and there is separation of the collagen fibrils (53,54). Biopsy of these lesions should be avoided as there is poor wound healing. The lesions may be seen in other areas of the body as well. There is a correlation between thyroid disease and chronic urticaria, although an underlying etiology has not been clearly defined (55).

19.4.6 Psychiatric manifestations

Multiple psychiatric features are noted in thyroid disorders and include Hashimoto's encephalopathy, depressive disorders, bipolar disorder, anxiety disorders, psychotic disorders, and attention deficit hyperactivity disorder (ADHD).

19.4.6.1 Hashimoto's encephalopathy

This is commonly seen in the 9 to 17 year age group and is an acute condition presenting with features such as decreased levels of alertness, dysphoric mood, cognitive decline, anxiety, restlessness, and hallucinations. Focal neurological symptoms may be present as well (56).

19.4.6.2 Depressive disorders

This is commonly seen in hypothyroidism. The depression often remains undiagnosed and untreated in the pediatric population. Generally its onset is insidious with vague symptoms such as easy fatigability, slow cognitive processing, impaired memory, and decline in school performance. The symptomatology of hypothyroidism and depression overlaps significantly, thereby making it difficult at times to notice coexisting depression in these patients (57,58).

19.4.6.3 Bipolar disorder

Although generally associated with hyperthyroidism, acute mania and hypomania have been reported in cases of severe hypothyroidism; however, evidence for such presentation is not robust in the pediatric population. Pediatric bipolar disorder, when treated with lithium on a long term basis, can cause hypothyroidism. Hyperthyroidism is also associated with depression, mania, and hypomania. A prospective cohort study showed increased rates of re-admission with depressive disorder or bipolar disorder in patients with hyperthyroidism versus controls; the risk was greatest in the first 6 months after index hospitalization (59).

19.4.6.4 Anxiety disorders

Hyperthyroidism may present with symptoms of anxiety, dysphoric mood, restlessness, irritability, and hyperactivity – all of which can be part of an anxiety state. These symptoms may be present for 6–12 months prior to the onset of a true thyrotoxicosis state. Anxiety was the most frequent psychiatric symptom seen in as many as 72% of patients with thyrotoxicosis, along with shakiness and irritability in 77% and 78%, respectively (60). Specific phobia (61) and panic disorder with agoraphobia has also been reported with hyperthyroidism (59).

19.4.6.5 Psychotic disorders

Myxedema madness is now extremely rare, but it was commonly seen prior to the availability of exogenous thyroxine as an effective treatment. Patients presented with severe depression and psychotic features such as paranoia, hallucinations, and delusions. If left untreated it can lead to myxedema coma, which can be potentially fatal (58).

19.4.6.6 Attention deficit hyperactivity disorder (ADHD)

This is a highly controversial topic among pediatric providers from different disciplines. There is a high familial incidence of ADHD and generalized resistance to thyroid hormone (GRTH). About 5.4% of children with ADHD were noted to have a thyroid abnormality compared to 1% of controls (62). Weiss et al reported that although ADHD is characterized by hyperactivity, the most common association in children with ADHD was found to be hypothyroidism; in addition, hyperthyroidism, which is commonly considered in the differential diagnosis of ADHD, was not prominent in their sample of 277 children (62).

19.4.7 Diagnostic workup

A definitive diagnosis of thyroid dysfunction is made by evaluation of thyroid function tests (TFTs) preferably with free thyroxine (FT4), total thyroxine (total T4) level, and thyroid stimulating hormone (TSH) level; in certain specific situations a triiodothyronine (T3) level may be needed as in T3 toxicosis. In order to determine the underlying autoimmune status, a number of tests can be done to measure antithyroglobulin (ATG), antithyroperoxidase (TPO) antibodies, TSH receptor autoantibodies (TRAbs), and thyroid stimulating immunoglobulins (TSI). Serial FT4 and TSH levels are used to titrate for adequacy of the dose of thyroid hormone. Imaging with a thyroid or thyroid/neck ultrasound should be performed if there is a concern about thyroid enlargement with any irregularity (including nodules) or if there are palpable neck lymph nodes. If the functional status needs to be evaluated, as in the case of an autonomous thyroid nodule or toxic nodule, radioactive iodine (RAI) uptake and scan may be done.

19.4.8 Management of hypothyroidism

The treatment for hypothyroidism is by replacement therapy with thyroid hormone, namely levothyroxine (LT4), which is available commercially under different brand names. Relative dose requirements vary with age from 10–15 mcg/kg/day in newborns to 1–2 mcg/kg/day in older children/adolescents.

19.4.9 Management of hyperthyroidism

There are three main treatment options available for the treatment of hyperthyroidism: medications, radioactive iodine ablation therapy, and surgery.

Table 19.7: Comparison of anti-thyroid medications

	PTU	MMI
Dosing	Q8h initially, then twice or thrice a day	Q8h initially then once or twice a day
Compliance	Metallic taste, poor compliance	Better compliance
Potency	Less potent	More potent
Dose	5–10 mg/kg/day	0.5–1.0 mg/kg/day
Risk of hepatitis	Higher risk of hepatitis	Lower risk
Use in pregnancy	Relatively preferred	Higher teratogenicity

19.4.9.1 Medication

The main groups of medications are propylthiouracil (PTU) and methimazoles (e.g. Tapazole). The doses and scheduling of these medications and their main side effects are outlined in Tables 19.7 and 19.8.

19.4.9.2 Radioactive iodine ablation therapy (RAI)

In adults RAI is the first treatment of choice, whereas in the pediatric population (especially in the preteen period and even in adolescents), a trial of medical therapy for 1–2 years may be given before giving RAI; this is based on the possibility of spontaneous disease remission. However, there is a current move toward increased use of RAI in the adolescent population as well. RAI completely ablates the thyroid gland; therefore post-ablation, the patient becomes hypothyroid needing lifelong thyroid hormone replacement.

Table 19.8: Side effects of antithyroid medications

Major complications – may be seen in up to 1% of patients
Agranulocytosis
Hepatitis
Minor complications – may be seen in up to 25% of patients
Elevated liver enzymes
Leukopenia
Skin rash
Granulocytopenia
Arthritis
Lymphadenopathy

19.4.9.3 Surgical therapy

Depending on the underlying cause, surgery for focal nodule excision or total thyroidectomy may be the surgical options available. This is the preferred mode of treatment in cases of large glands and in younger children. There are concerns about risks of excessive bleeding, permanent hypoparathyroidism, and vocal cord paralysis as potential side-effects.

19.4.10 Management of psychiatric disorders

19.4.10.1 Depression and anxiety

First line treatment of depression associated with hypothyroidism is to optimize thyroid hormone replacement and normalize thyroid function tests. Treatment of depressive disorder that persists after euthyroid status is achieved depends on the severity of the depression. Mild to moderate adjustment disorder with depressed and anxious mood as well as dysthymic disorder with low-grade depression may respond well to psychotherapeutic approaches such as supportive psychotherapy, individual psychotherapy, and cognitive behavioral therapy (see Chapter 23).

In cases of depression of moderate to severe degree and moderate to severe anxiety states (including generalized anxiety, panic disorder with or without agoraphobia, and social phobia) that are impacting the patient's functional abilities to a significant degree, a trial of psychotropic medications at optimal dose and for adequate duration is indicated. Selective serotonin reuptake inhibitors (SSRIs) are the first line medication for depression and severe anxiety states (63). The risk of suicidal ideation should be taken in account but should not deter a clinician from treating these pediatric patients. Emergence of suicidal ideation with SSRIs is most common in the first few weeks of starting the treatment, and during this period, the patient should be closely monitored by the physician (63).

19.4.10.2 Bipolar disorders

Lithium is the gold standard for treatment of bipolar disorders. Lithium is indicated for the treatment of acute manic and depressive episodes as well as the maintenance of bipolar disorder. Lithium can be used in children under 12 years of age at dose of 10–30 mg/kg/day. Adolescents are more likely to respond to a dose of 1200–1800 mg/day in divided doses with an aim to reach steady lithium serum levels in the range of 0.8–1.2 mmol/liter (64). Acne and weight gain are the side effects that can severely impact self-esteem and body image concerns in adolescents.

Conditions leading to lithium toxicity include those leading to dehydration and drug interactions with many medications (including non-steroidal anti-inflammatory drugs [NSAIDs] and tetracyclines). Lithium toxicity can present with altered mental status, diarrhea, nausea with or without vomiting, slurred speech, drooling, muscle twitching, blurred vision, irregular heart rate, and peripheral edema. Lithium toxicity is a potentially fatal condition and should be considered as a medical emergency, which requires immediate hospitalization and possible hemodialysis if the lithium level is critical. Close monitoring of thyroid function and renal function is recommended (65).

19.5 Adrenal gland disorders

The adrenal gland disorders may present with either hypofunction resulting in hypocortisolemia or hyperfunction resulting in hypercortisolemia. Both these conditions may be associated with significant cutaneous manifestations irrespective of the underlying cause. The HPA (hypothalamic-pituitary-adrenal) axis comprises the hypothalamus secreting CRH (corticotropin releasing hormone), which stimulates the corticotrophs in the anterior pituitary to secrete ACTH (adrenocorticotropin hormone); this in turn stimulates the secretion of glucocorticoids and sex steroids. Mineralocorticoids are predominantly under the control of the renin-angiotensin system.

19.5.1 Hypoadrenocorticism (adrenal insufficiency [AI] or Addison disease [AD])

The adrenal dysfunction results in deficiency of one or all of the adrenal hormones, namely glucocorticoids, mineralocorticoids, and adrenal androgens. The underlying disorder leading to adrenal insufficiency may be acquired or congenital. The most common form of acquired adrenal insufficiency (AI) in the United States is due to autoimmune disorders. However, the most common worldwide cause of AI is infection with tuberculosis causing damage to the adrenal gland. AI may be isolated or may be a component of the autoimmune polyglandular syndromes 1 and 2 (APS1 and APS2). Another common and important cause of adrenal insufficiency is also iatrogenic in which there may be suppression of the HPA axis noted with as little as about 2 weeks of pharmacologic treatment with glucocorticoids. Various kinds of enzymatic defects of the adrenal biosynthetic hormone pathway (as noted in congenital adrenal hyperplasia) are also an important cause of adrenal insufficiency.

19.5.1.1 Clinical presentation

Most of the systemic features of acute insufficiency are non-specific. Clinical features of AI are listed in Table 19.9 (66).

19.5.1.2 Dermatologic manifestations

The most pathognomic cutaneous feature of adrenal insufficiency is hyperpigmentation. Generalized hyperpigmentation of the skin is noted that may have been present

Table 19.9: Clinical features of adrenal insufficiency

Systemic features
• Anorexia
• Weight loss
• Easy fatigability
• Abdominal pain
• Sparse pubic and axillary hair
• Postural hypotension
• Shock, coma, and even death
Cutaneous features
• Hyperpigmentation
–Skin
–Mucous membrane
–Nails
• Vitiligo- in association with underlying autoimmune etiology

for many years prior to seeking medical attention. Although there is a generalized tan-like hyperpigmentation, the darkening is more pronounced in the skin folds, creases of the hands, nipples, genitalia, and linea alba; it may also present as freckling. The mucous membrane, more specifically the oral mucosa, may reveal hyperpigmentation including darkening of the gum lines (67). The nails reveal hyperpigmented horizontal bands.

19.5.1.3 Psychiatric manifestations

Adrenal insufficiency (AI) may present with depression, anxiety, symptoms of asthenia-like fatigue, lack of energy, decline in strength, loss of appetite leading to weight loss, and in younger children, failure to thrive. Women may present with decreased libido. When QoL issues of these patients were studied, about 50% of patients with primary AI considered themselves unfit to work, and 30% needed help for their household chores (68). Affective disturbance, cognitive impairment, and behavioral problems have also been reported with AI. Addisonian crisis may present with disturbances of consciousness as well as hallucinations and delusions.

19.5.1.4 Treament

Glucocorticoid replacement is essential, and failure to do so is life threatening. Patients with adrenal insufficiency also cannot mount an adequate cortisol response during stress situations; therefore, "stress dosing" is needed for adequate physiologic function during these times. This broadly includes giving 2 to 5 times the routine physiologic dose depending on the degree of stress. Patients are also educated about the use of injectable hydrocortisone for use in emergency situations when oral dosing may not be feasible. Mineralocorticoid replacement if indicated is done by the use of fludrocortisone. Additional salt supplementation may be accomplished with added salt in the diet.

The replacement of DHEA (dehydroepiandrosterone) in primary adrenal insufficiency is not routinely recommended (69,70). The two main concerns in acute AI are hypovolemia and hypoglycemia. The patients may be hypotensive as well as dehydrated and may be in shock. There may be associated hyponatremia and hyperkalemia. Therefore, appropriate fluid resuscitation with normal saline to restore intravascular volume is needed. The fluids should contain adequate dextrose concentration (5–10%) as needed to prevent ongoing hypoglycemia after initial correction of hypoglycemia using concentrated dextrose.

19.5.1.5 Management of psychiatric conditions

Acute delirium in the setting of adrenal insufficiency requires intensive treatment in the inpatient setting. Delirium in children may remain undiagnosed. There are no clear guidelines available to treat delirium in the pediatric population, and treatment measures are extrapolated from adult treatment guidelines. Haloperidol presents risk of extrapyramidal symptoms, and one should be prudent in its use in the pediatric population with the smallest effective dose possible for the shortest duration required. Atypical antipsychotics such as risperidone, olanzapine, and quetiapine may also be used for shorter periods of time. Most of the symptoms of neurasthenia respond well to the initiation of glucocorticoid therapy. However, it may take time for symptoms of anxiety and depression to improve completely.

19.5.2 Hyperadrenocorticism (Cushing syndrome)

Excessive cortisol production may cause Cushing syndrome (CS) because of central (pituitary or hypothalamic lesions), adrenal, or extra adrenal lesions. Exogenous glucocorticoid administration may also result in the same clinical picture as well. In fact, the most common cause of Cushing syndrome is exogenous glucocorticoid administration. The main causes of CS are listed in Table 19.10 (66,71).

19.5.2.1 Clinical features

Patients with Cushing syndrome may have chronic nonspecific symptoms. There is history of weight gain, which is described as centripetal obesity characterized by truncal obesity and thinning of the limbs; in addition, there is progressive proximal muscle weakness, symptoms of sexual dysfunction, menstrual irregularities, poor

Table 19.10: Causes of Cushing Syndrome

Exogenous steroids (treatment with oral and parenteral steroids)
Endogenous steroid overproduction
• ACTH producing pituitary adenoma
• Nelson syndrome
Adrenal lesions
• Adrenal adenoma, carcinoma
• Adrenal hyperplasia (micronodular or macronodular)
• Carney complex
• McCune Albright syndrome
Ectopic ACTH production
• Extra adrenal lesions
• Oat cell or small cell lung tumors
• Carcinoid tumors

wound healing, pathologic fractures, increased infections, and psychological manifestations, including depression and emotional lability. The pressure effect of pituitary tumors may present with visual disturbances and headaches; also, there can be features of deficiency of other anterior pituitary hormones. There may be new onset hypertension or worsening of pre-existing hypertension (66).

19.5.2.2 Dermatological manifestations

The main dermatological features of CS are thinning and atrophy of the skin. There is easy bruisability because of this thinning and ecchymosis; also, there can be bruising that is out of proportion to the degree of trauma. Wide, purplish striae are seen because of stretching of the skin and the skin becoming translucent due to thinning, through which the underlying vasculature can be seen (72,73,74). These striae are different from the ones seen in obesity and pregnancy. Dilated skin capillaries also appear as telangiectasias, especially on the face; therefore, the face not only looks round but also plethoric, giving the appearance of the typical "moon facies." There may be generalized increased hair growth or hypertrichosis. The concomitant finding of significant hirsutism and acne may alert the clinician to the probability of co-secretion of excessive amounts of adrenal androgens as well.

19.5.2.3 Psychiatric manifestations

Psychiatric features of Cushing disease are difficult to distinguish from the neurovegetative symptoms of a major depressive episode. Starkman et al found a statistically significant correlation between the severity of psychiatric symptoms and levels of cortisol and ACTH (75). The level of psychiatric disability was reported to be very severe in 11% and mild in 34% of these patients (75). Almost all of these patients complained of lassitude and lack of energy, while as many as 86% stated that they felt very irritable; in fact, anger and irritability were the first symptoms to emerge in most patients (75). The irritability in combination with verbal dyscontrol, sensitivity to stimuli, and an urge to express their frustration may result in anger outbursts (75).

About 77% of patients with Cushing syndrome complain of having depressed mood with frequent crying spells. The depression was intermittent, lasting for 1–3 days, and lack of anhedonia differentiates it from a major depressive episode (75). When standardized psychometric scales were used to delineate between the transient depressive symptoms and a major depressive episode, about 58% of patients fulfilled the diagnostic criteria of the American Psychiatric Association's (APA's) *Diagnostic and Statistical Manual of Mental Disorder* (DSM-IV-TR) for major depression (76).

Although manic and hypomanic episodes have been reported in association with hypercortisolism, the frequency of these episodes is much lower (30%) during the course of Cushing's syndrome (76). Anxiety appeared to be quite significant whether it is present with or without depression. Loosen et al reported 79% of the patients in their study developed generalized anxiety disorder, while panic disorder was seen in 53% (77). Cognitive difficulties were frequently reported, including difficulty in concentrating reported by 66%, memory problems in 83%, and speeding thoughts as well as thought blocking in one third (75,78). Psychotic symptoms were less common, seen in about 10% of patients, and included paranoia, perceptual distortions, and depersonalization usually as part of a depressive or bipolar episode (75). Body image issues leading to social withdrawal were reported by 46%; these patients felt ashamed due to the physical and dermatological stigmata of Cushing's syndrome and did not like to be seen in public (75,78).

19.5.2.4 Clinical diagnosis

The diagnosis of Cushing syndrome can be difficult, especially in the early stages. A high index of suspicion is needed when a combination of suggestive features is noted. An endocrinology expert consultation is recommended to pursue further workup and treatment. Multiple testing methods and repeated testing may be needed before a definitive diagnosis is made. Testing may include 24 hour urinary free cortisol, late night serum and/or salivary cortisol levels, low dose dexamethasone suppression test, and a combination of 48 hour low dose dexamethasone suppression test along with CRH stimulation.

Once the hypercortisolemia and a diagnosis of Cushing syndrome are established, it is important to identify the underlying etiology. It is important to define whether the high cortisol is ACTH dependent or ACTH independent; also, it should be determined whether the pathology of excessive ACTH production is in the pituitary gland or there is ectopic ACTH production. High dose dexamethasone suppression test and CRH testing are used for defining these issues. Further delineation of anatomic defects can be accomplished by an adrenal gland/abdominal computed tomography (CT) scan to look for adrenal tumors. Also, a magnetic resonance imaging (MRI) of the pituitary can be done for localization of pituitary adenomas. Other tests can include inferior petrosal sinus venous sampling for lateralization of ACTH production as well as abdominal and chest CT scans to rule out ectopic ACTH production. Also, octerotide scintigraphy may be useful in localizing ACTH producing ectopic tumors (D1).

19.5.2.5 Treatment

Surgical, medical, and/or radiation therapy or a combination of these measures may be needed to cure the underlying cause. Considerations for long term follow up include surveillance for recurrence of the underlying process and for evaluation and replacement of any concomitant hormone deficits. The treatment of the underlying disease processes is now addressed.

Cushing syndrome (exogenous)

The exogenous glucocorticoid treatment/source should be evaluated, and dosing is minimized if possible; also, early discontinuation of exogenous glucocorticoids as indicated should be encouraged. Steroid treatment for more than 10–14 days may result in adrenal insufficiency. A gradual and careful steroid taper needs to be given, and physiologic doses of steroids may be given until the patient is evaluated for adrenal insufficiency. If the Cushing syndrome is due to an adrenal source, unilateral or bilateral adrenalectomy may be needed depending on the underlying histopathology.

Cushing disease (endogenous)

The underlying cause of hypercortisolemia in Cushing disease is in the pituitary gland. The treatment options are based on further delineation of the underlying lesion. Treatment of choice for pituitary adenoma is transphenoidel removal of the adenoma. If surgery is not possible or not indicated, various methodologies may be used to irradiate the gland. There is ongoing risk of developing panhypopituitarism. If none of these options are feasible, bilateral adrenalectomy may have to be done to negate the effects of excessive ACTH. These patients will become dependent on glucocorticoid and mineralocorticoid replacement for the rest of their lives.

Some medical treatment options include ketoconazole, mitotane, metyrapone, aminoglutethimide, etomidate, and trilostane. These agents inhibit steroidogenesis. Mifepristone (RU486), octreotide, bromocriptine, valproic acid, and cyproheptadine are other medical options that are still under investigation but may be useful (66,71). Adrenal insufficiency may develop secondary to any of these treatment modalities.

Careful monitoring, evaluation, and replacement for glucocorticoids as well as mineralocorticoids is mandatory and best done under the care of an endocrinologist.

19.5.2.6 Management of psychiatric conditions

Treatment of any psychiatric condition, when presenting during the course of Cushing's disease, is to first focus on treating the underlying cause of the hypercortisolism. However, the psychiatric symptoms may persist after the successful treatment of the Cushing syndrome, or they may be of such severe intensity that they are impacting a child's ability to function at the age appropriate level. Then a thorough evaluation is indicated to see if these symptoms are meeting the diagnostic criteria of a formal psychiatric disorder, with subsequent development of a multidisciplinary treatment plan or referral to a psychiatrist.

Non-medication alternatives such as individual and family psychotherapy should be discussed (especially cognitive behavioral therapy [CBT] and interpersonal therapy [IPT]) as a first option if the disease is of mild to moderate severity. SSRIs are now considered first line treatment for depression and anxiety, and several of them are approved for the use on the pediatric population (79). Please see Fig 19.1 for the illustration of Texas algorithm for treatment of depression in children & adolescents. Emergence of suicidal ideation in this population reported with use of SSRIs should be taken in consideration at the onset of the treatment with a thorough evaluation of suicide assessment before initiation of treatment; also, a close follow up is needed, especially during the first few weeks after starting the medication. A thorough assessment of suicide risk during the course of treatment is important, especially in the earlier phase and whenever doses are adjusted; this can be achieved during a clinical session with the patient by asking appropriate questions to assess the risk of suicide and can be aided by using a standardized suicide assessment scale, such as the Columbia Suicide Severity Rating Scale.

19.6 Disorders of parathyroid glands

The metabolism of calcium, vitamin D, and parathyroid hormone is closely interrelated. The physiologic role of the parathyroid (PTH) at multiple levels is to maintain normocalcemia. The main causes of parathyroid gland disorders are listed in Table 19.11 and Table 19.12 (80,81).

19.6.1 Hypoparathyroidism

Signs and symptoms of hypocalcemia are generally related to those of increased neuromuscular irritability because of hypocalcemia. The generalized clinical features

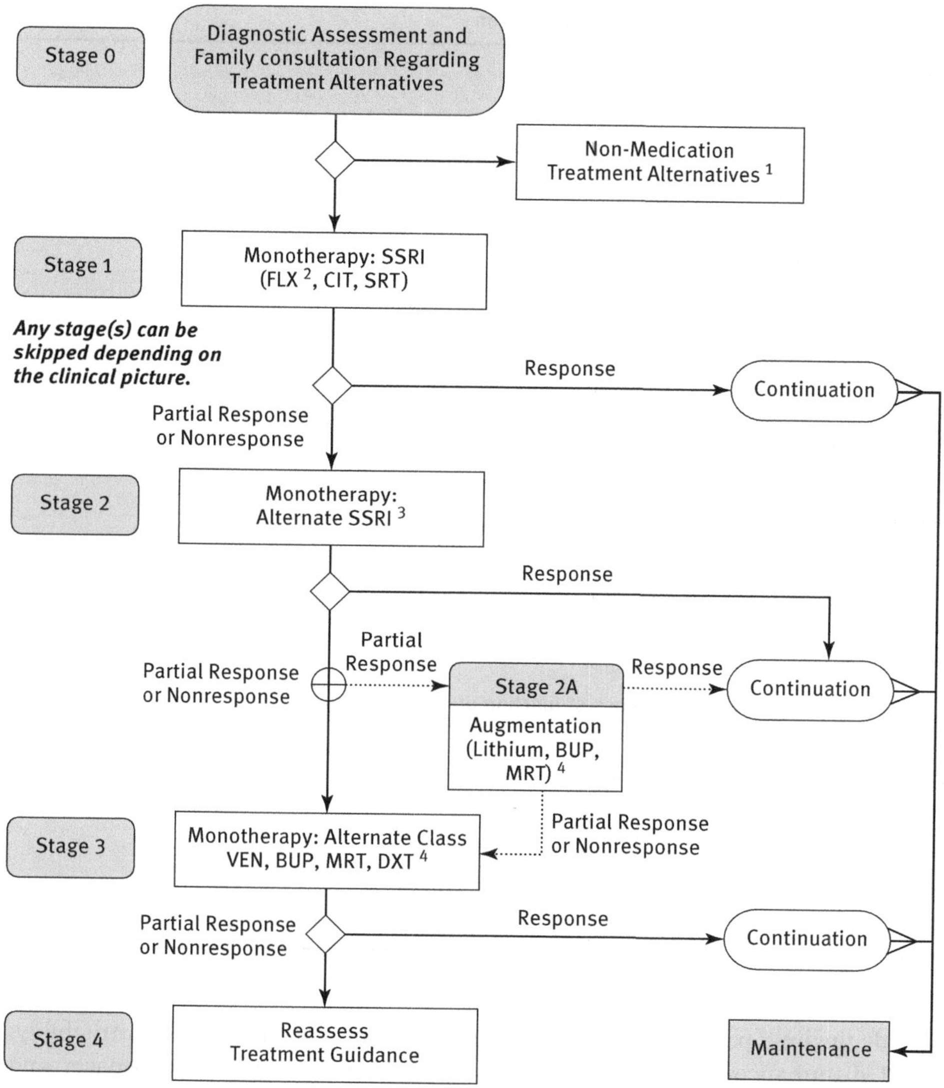

[1] Evidence-based psychotherapy can be used at any stage in the algorithm.
[2] FLX (fluoxetine) is the only antidepressant with and FDA-approved indication for depression in youth.
[3] SSRI - Selective serotonin reuptake inhibitor (including: citalopram [CIT], escitalopram, fluxetine [FLX], paroxetine [not recommended for preadolescents], sertraline [SRT])
[4] VEN = venlafaxine: BUP = bupropion: MRT = mirtazapine: DXT = duloxetine

Figure 19.1: Texas Algorithm for Treatment of Depression in Children & Adolescents. Medication algorithm for treating children and adolescents who meet DSM-IV criteria for major depressive disorder. FDA = U.S. Food and Drug Administration. Revised based on Hughes et al. (1999) (79).

Table 19.11: Common causes of hypoparathyroidim

Transient neonatal hypoparathyroidism
Congenital hypoparathyroidism
• Autosomal recessive:
–Familial isolated
–Sajad-Sakati syndrome
• Autosomal dominant:
–Gain of function mutation of CASR
–Barakat syndrome
–Isolated familial
• X-linked recessive
DiGeorge syndrome
Kenny-Caffey syndrome
Mitochondrial disorders-Kearns-Sayre Syndrome
Pseudohypoparathyroidism
• Type I
• Type I
• Pseudo-Pseudohypoparathyroidism
• Blomstrand Chrondrodysplasia-loss of function of PTHR1
Acquired hypoparathyroidism
• Autoimmune polyglandular syndrome 1
• Post-surgical hypoparathyroidism
• Post-radiation hypoparathyridism
• Infilterative-hemachromatosis, Wilsons disease, Sarcoidosis
• Idiopathic

include tingling, parasthesias, muscle cramps, fatigue, seizures, anxiety, irritability, mood disturbances, and personality changes; also seen are laryngospasm and bronchospasm giving dyspnea, wheezing, and hoarseness. The neuromuscular irritability can be demonstrated by the Chvostek's sign and Trousseau's sign. Parkinsonism, extrapyramidal choreo-athetoid movements, ataxia, dysphagia, and dysarthria may also be seen.

19.6.1.1 Dermatologic manifestations

Cutaneous findings generally include dry, coarse skin as well as skin puffiness. Abnormal dentition and ocular cataracts may also be seen. There are case reports of congenital primary Albright's hereditary osteodystrophy with osteoma cutis or subcutaneous calcifications (82,83,84). Mucocutaneous candidiasis (involving the

Table 19.12: Common causes of hyperparathyroidism

Primary Hyperparathyroidism
• Single benign adenoma: after radiation exposure
Parathyroid hyperplasia-involving all 4 glands
• Familial isolated hyperparathyroidism
• MEN 1
• MEN 2
• Familial hypocalciuric hypercalcemia
• Hyperparathyroidism + jaw tumor syndrome
Secondary hyperparathyroidism
• Chronic renal failure
• Post-renal transplantation
• Chronic hyperphosphatemia
• Resistance to parathyroid hormone
• Rickets and Vitamin D deficiency
Tertiary hyperparathyroidism
• Autonomous parathyroid function
Parathyroid cancer (rare)

oral cavity, skin, nails, and vagina) occurs, which is often intractable and in conjunction with adrenal insufficiency; it can occur as a part of the triad with hypoparathyroidism in APS1. Multiple case reports about the coexistence of impetigo herpetiformis with hypoparathyroidism also exist, especially in relation to generally the last trimester of pregnancy. The exact etiology of this entity remains unclear (85,86). These lesions are described as polycyclic, edematous, red patches bordered by tiny pustules in a herpetiform distribution; the old lesions dry and become scaly (87,88).

19.6.1.2 Psychiatric manifestations

Hypocalcaemia is the main reason for the development of depression, irritability, and anxiety. Hypocalcemia can result in seizures and multiple psychiatric manifestations (including depression and other psychiatric conditions), which can occur in up to 60% of patients with DiGeorge syndrome (89).

19.6.1.3 Diagnostic workup

Serum calcium and ionized calcium are usually low, and serum phosphorous is usually elevated. Serum parathyroid hormone (PTH) is low in primary hypoparathyroidism but high in pseudohypoparathyroidism. In secondary hypoparathyroidism, however, the PTH is low but serum calcium is elevated. Serum magnesium and 25 hydroxy vitamin D (25 OHD) levels should be measured to rule out hypomagnesemia and vitamin D deficiency. Also, 24 hour urinary calcium excretion measurements for measuring hypercalciuria (as in familial hypercalciuric hypocalcemia [FHH]) should be done. Imaging is not useful per se for making the diagnosis of hypercalcemia or hyperparathyroidism. However, imaging studies such as ultrasonography, sestamibi nuclear scan, CT scan and MRI are useful to guide surgical therapy and to look for distant disease or recurrence.

19.6.1.4 Treatment of hypoparathyroidism

These patients need consultation and follow-up with an endocrinologist. The identification and treatment of underlying etiology is helpful. PTH is now commercially available; however, it is probably one of the only hormones not approved for hormone replacement therapy as yet by the U.S. Food and Drug Administration. The mainstay of medical therapy is calcium and vitamin D replacement. Vitamin D replacement is with the bioactive form of vitamin D, which is 1,25 dihydroxy vitamin D (1,25 diOHD) (E10).

In the absence of PTH, the 1 alpha hydroxylation of vitamin D, converting 25OHD to the active 1,25diOHD, does not occur. Therefore, these patients need to be treated directly with 1,25 diOHD, which helps maintaining normocalcemia by promoting calcium absorption in the intestines and in the renal tubules, while decreasing serum phosphorous. In patients who undergo total parathyroidectomy (of all 4 glands) auto transplant of parathyroid gland in the forearm prevents permanent hypoparathyroidism. Close monitoring and follow-up of these patients is necessary with monitoring of serum calcium and phosphorous levels. Renal calcium excretion is monitored by serial urine calcium/creatinine ratios and renal ultrasounds to monitor for nephrocalcinosis.

19.6.1.5 Management of psychiatric conditions

Correction of hypocalcemia in hypoparathyroidism results in significant improvement in psychiatric symptomatology. Psychotropic medications are indicated in the interim while hypoparathyroid state is being corrected (90).

19.6.2 Hyperparathyroidism

Hyperparathyroidism results from overproduction of parathyroid hormone, resulting in severe metabolic disturbances primarily due to hypercalcemia. It is less common in children and adolescents than in adults.

19.6.2.1 Clinical features

Hyperparathyroidism presents in a widely ranging spectrum varying from being asymptomatic, having minimal nonspecific generalized vague symptomatology, to severe complications; the severe state occurs from severe hypercalcemia and results in essentially a hypercalcemic parathyroid crisis with dehydration, alteration of sensorium, and coma (80). Nephrocalcinosis, renal stones, and renal failure may occur. Other features less commonly seen in the pediatric population include peptic ulcers disease, low bone density, osteopenia, and osteoporosis (80).

19.6.2.2 Dermatological manifestations

Various cutaneous manifestations seen include generalized pruritis, calciphylaxis, and calcinosis cutis. *Calcinosis cutis* is characterized by deposition of calcium salts (mainly hydroxyapatite) in the skin, usually involving all layers of skin. The lesions of calcinosis cutis appear as yellowish-white deposits of varying sizes in the skin presenting as small milia-like lesions or as lesions of tumorous calcinosis (3,91,92). These lesions are otherwise generally benign. Various treatment modalities are available, such as sodium sulphate or cellulose phosphate, injections of triamcinolone in the lesions, or surgical removal (92).

General pruritis is observed in patients with hyperparathyroidism, which is believed to be related to hypercalcemia rather than levels of parathyroid hormone (91). Calciphylaxis is generally seen in the setting of secondary hyperparathyroidism mostly in patients with chronic renal insufficiency. The skin lesions are described as livid, reddish, and necrotic; also, they are noted to be painful, may advance to necrosis, and cause scarring. These lesions are generally found widespread all over the body including finger tips, thighs, ankles, and buttocks (92). Parathyroidectomy induces improvement of the calciphylaxis lesions.

19.6.2.3 Psychiatric manifestations

Neuropsychiatric changes can present in about 39% to 50% of patients suffering from primary hyperparathyroidism according to different studies (90,93). One prospective review of 405 patients suggested that psychiatric presentation in hyperparathyroidism can be divided into three different categories: (a) a confusional state, which can progress to stupor and coma; (b) depression and psychosis especially paranoid delusions; and (c) a pseudo-neurotic state with lethargy, fatigue, anorexia, mood lability, and weakness.

Patients with hyperparathyroidism present with significant depression and anxiety symptoms. Women with hyperthyroidism tend to have significantly higher scores on depression scales than controls. They also demonstrated a more significant deficit when tested for verbal memory and verbal abstraction. Hypomagnesemia is also known to cause visual-spatial disturbances, visual hallucinations, and paranoid delusion (90,93).

19.6.2.4 Treatment of hyperparathyroidism

The principles of treatment include treatment of hypercalcemia and its complications, concerns related to high PTH levels, and treatment of the underlying cause. Therapeutic options are further grouped into non-surgical and surgical. There is ongoing controversy about the decision and timing to pursue surgical options (94). Recommendations for non-surgical candidates include close clinical follow up and periodic laboratory testing that includes serum calcium and creatinine levels every 6 months as well as bone density evaluation every year. Other measures include maintaining moderate calcium and vitamin D intake as per guidelines, maintaining adequate hydration, regular physical activity, and avoiding immobilization.

Intravenous hydrations and loop diuretics are mainstays of management for acute hypercalcemia. Calcimimetic agents such as cinacalcet are very useful in reducing serum PTH levels and leading to decrease in serum calcium levels (95). The main indications for medication include symptomatic hypercalcemia in primary hyperparathyroidism when surgery is not an option, secondary hyperparathyroidism in chronic renal failure, and hypercalcemia in parathyroid malignancy (95).

19.6.2.5 Management of psychiatric conditions

Psychiatric presentation of primary hyperparathyroidism responds very well to the correction of metabolic and hormonal disturbances. Short term management of acute confusional and psychotic symptoms may require inpatient hospitalization and management with antipsychotic medications as well.

19.7 Disorders of hormones of the reproductive system

Both androgens and estrogens are present in males and females, although the relative amounts of each of these are different. A dysbalance of these hormone levels in males and females therefore causes different clinical presentations. Hypo/hyperestrogenemia and hypo/hyperandrogenemia are the main biochemical scenarios that need to be considered in males and females.

19.8 Androgen disorders

19.8.1 Hypogonadism in males

During *in utero* and early neonatal periods congenital malformation of the testis may result from different underlying etiologies, including chromosomal disorders or defects in androgen synthesis or action; this results in physical maldevelopment of the external male genitalia. In the pubertal period hypogonadism may develop with low androgen levels due to hypogonadotropic hypogonadism with inadequate gonadotropin production leading to complete or partial failure of pubertal development. There can also be hypergonadotropic hypogonadism, which results from primary testicular failure. Both these types of hypogonadism result in low androgen levels and delayed onset and/or progression of puberty; at times this can result in no or minimal pubertal development. The cutaneous features of low androgen levels in males at this stage include minimal or inadequate growth of the male external genitalia, minimal development or absence of pubic/axillary/facial terminal hair, absence of male voice changes, and no acne.

19.8.1.1 Treatment

The underlying cause will need to be addressed if possible. Symptomatic and specific treatment involves replacement of androgen (testosterone) in these patients, irrespective of the underlying cause. Testosterone replacement results in normal pubertal development. Treatment with GnRH or with gonadotropins in the case of hypogonadotropic hypogonadism will also offer the same therapeutic results and may also be able to address fertility concerns. In puberty, testosterone injections are generally provided every 3 to 4 weeks, in progressively increasing doses, until the adult doses are achieved (96).

19.8.1.2 Hypergonadism in males

Excessive androgen levels in males may cause early pubertal features in childhood and precocious puberty. The underlying pathology, such as androgen producing tumors or congenital adrenal hyperplasia, needs to be diagnosed and treated.

19.8.2 Androgen disorders in Females

Androgens in females are produced in adrenal glands and ovaries, with some conversion of weak to more potent androgens in the periphery (i.e. skin and adipose tissue). Hyperandrogenemia in the form of polycystic ovarian syndrome (PCOS) is the most common hormonal disorder in females with a prevalence of about 8% in women in the reproductive age group in the United States. The common causes of hyperandrogenemia in females are listed in Table 19.13 (97).

19.8.2.1 Clinical features

Excess androgen exposure *in utero* causes virilization of the external genitalia. This is generally noted at birth initiating further diagnostic evaluation. In infancy and the pre-pubertal period, girls may present with evidence of virilization in the form of

Table 19.13: The common causes of hyperandrogenemia in females

Exogenous androgen exposure:
–Direct exposure to the female herself
–Indirect exposure from mother to fetus
Congenital adrenal hyperplasia
Polycystic ovarian syndrome
Androgen secreting tumors
Cushing syndrome
Pregnancy
Hyperprolactinemia
Hyperthecosis

premature adrenarche; there can be early onset of pubic hair, axillary odor, axillary hair, seborrhea, and acne. In adolescents and adult females, the presentation of hyperandrogenemia generally presents with menstrual irregularities, including oligomenorrhea and amenorrhea; dermatologic findings are discussed in the following sections (*vida infra*).

19.8.2.2 Dermatological manifestations

Dermatological conditions include hirsutism, acne, acneform lesions, and seborrhea. Acanthosis nigricans can be seen if there is associated obesity. Other clinical features include evidence of virilization generally depending on the level of underlying hyperandrogenemia; these include clitoromegaly, laryngeal hypertrophy causing hoarseness of voice, and androgenetic alopecia.

19.8.2.3 Diagnostic workup

Based on the history and clinical findings as discussed previously (*vida supra*), hormone work up is obtained to confirm hyperandrogenemia and to evaluate for underlying causes. The main laboratory workup is listed in Table 19.14 (98,99).

19.8.2.4 Treatment of androgen disorders in females

Treatment options are aimed at addressing the underlying cause as well the particular manifestation of hyperandrogenemia.

Obesity, hyperinsulinemia, insulin resistance, prediabetes

If associated with hyperandrogenemia, these will need treatment. Lifestyle modifications for weight control and weight loss are recommended while metformin therapy for improving the insulin sensitivity may be needed as well.

Table 19.14: Laboratory workup for hyperandrogenemia

Initial hormone work up
Androgen work up:
• Testosterone, Free Testosterone, SHBG*
• 17- Hydroxy progesterone
• DHEAS**
Non-Androgen hormone work up:
• FT4, TSH
• FSH, LH
• Estradiol
• Prolactin
• Pregnancy test
Further Testing (as indicated)
• ACTH Stimulation test
• 24 hour urinary free cortisol
• 2 hour glucose tolerance test
• Dexamethasone suppression test
• GnRH/Leuprolide stimulation test
Imaging
• Pelvic ultrasonography
• MRI/CT scan of the adrenal gland

*SHBG – Sex Hormone Binding Globulin; **DHEA

Hyperandrogenemia

Oral contraceptive pills (OCPs) are the treatment of choice. OCPs work by decreasing the androgen levels (both adrenal and ovarian) and increasing the sex hormone-binding globulin (SHBG) levels. Some OCPs, such as the ones with drospirenone, also block androgen function at the receptor level. OCPs can regulate the menstrual cycle and also improve acne as well as hirsutism. Cardiovascular risk factors for estrogen use need to be considered.

Hirsutism

Improvement in regrowth of hair is noted on OCPs. However, the existing hair growth needs to be addressed. Various temporary hair removal options are available and include hair removal creams, waxing, and threading. Eflornithine is an anticancer drug that blocks ornithine carboxylase in the hair follicle, thus reducing hair growth. Topical eflornithine has been shown to be an effective treatment for hirsutism and has few side effects (100). However, its effects rapidly reverse after discontinuing treatment. Permanent/semi-permanent methods of hair removal, including electrolysis and laser hair removal, are becoming popular as well, although they still remain expensive. Oral anti-androgens are available, including spironolactone, finasteride, and flutamide, but as of yet, they are approved by the U.S. FDA for this purpose.

19.8.2.5 Acne vulgaris

Topical acne preparations include appropriate cleansing agents, topical creams and lotions with salicylic acid, antibiotics, benzoyl peroxide, and retinoids (see Chapter 7). Other adjunctive therapies such as laser treatments or chemical peels may be needed in some cases, which are best addressed by a dermatologist. In addition to topical skin care, oral agents are generally required for severe acne. These may include oral antibiotics and oral isotretinoin; acne may improve dramatically on OCPs.

19.8.2.6 Congenital adrenal hyperplasia (CAH)

These patients need glucocorticoid replacement and mineralocorticoid replacement (if salt wasting type). Surgical treatment of genital ambiguity may be needed as appropriate.

19.9 Estrogen disorders

19.9.1 Estrogen disorders in males

Estrogen excess can lead to gynecomastia. It is important to differentiate physiologic, pubertal gynecomastia from pathologic gynecomastia, including the rare breast cancer in males. Medical treatment using anti-estrogens or estrogen receptor blockers may be used; however, these are noted not to offer consistent benefits nor response for improvement in gynecomastia (101). Surgical removal may be undertaken if desired.

19.9.2 Estrogen disorders in females

Estrogen deficiency can result from the normal physiologic menopause. There is hypogonadotropic hypogonadism resulting from inadequate gonadotropin production because of a hypothalamic or pituitary concern; there can also be hypergonadotropic hypogonadism resulting from primary ovarian damage/dysfunction.

19.9.2.1 Clinical features

Estrogen deficiency in the pubertal period can lead to delayed or absent puberty. In post menopausal woman, the skin reveals atrophy, dryness, and wrinkling. Estrogens are also thought to inhibit hair growth and suppress function of the sebaceous glands.

19.9.2.2 Treatment

Estrogen replacement therapy reverses the cutaneous changes caused by estrogen deficiency. The need for estrogen replacement should be assessed on an individual basis (102).

19.9.3 Psychiatric manifestations of disorders of androgen and estrogens

Hyperandrogenic states have been associated with aggressive behavior in animals and humans. Some research studies have focused on finding an association of higher levels of androgen to the socially maladaptive and aggressive behaviors in children and adolescents. Van Goozen et al studied 24 school age children with a diagnosis of oppositional defiant disorder (ODD). The plasma concentration of dehydroepiandrosterone sulfate (DHEAS) was measured in these children and compared with controls without any psychiatric illness and controls with other psychiatric conditions. In children with ODD, DHEAS level was significantly higher in comparison to the control groups (103).

Another study showed that 47 adolescent girls with high levels of aggression diagnosed with conduct disorder had higher levels of plasma free testosterone, lower levels of sex hormone binding globulin, and lower cortisol to DHEA ratios than the girls who had conduct disorder but did not display much aggression (104). One third of the adolescents diagnosed with bipolar disorder complained of irregular menstrual periods and were found to be more susceptible to develop polycystic ovarian syndrome (PCOS) when treated with certain mood stabilizers like valproic acid. There is an indication that these girls may have premorbid higher levels of androgens (105).

Autistic spectrum disorders (ASD) are characterized by deficits in reciprocal social interactions, difficulties in verbal and non-verbal expression, and stereotypic behavior. There is a strong male predilection, with autism four times and Asperger's syndrome 10 times more common in boys than in girls, indicating a possible role of testosterone. The theory of extreme male brain (EMB) proposes that the developing brain has two different dimensions: systematizing or male dimension and empathizing or female dimension. It is hypothesized that children with ASD have EMB, which causes the systematizing domain to be overdeveloped at the expense of empathizing, thus depriving them of having an innate ability to negotiate novel social situations (106). In female children with ASD the androgen receptor gene encoding is found to be defective, possibly predisposing them to develop ASD (107).

19.9.3.1 Management of psychiatric conditions in disorders of androgen and estrogens

Opposition defiance disorder (ODD) seldom exists as the only psychiatric problem; for example, about 60% of children with ODD will develop conduct disorder, and more than half of these children also have attention deficit hyperactivity disorder (ADHD). Mood disorders, especially bipolar disorder, are also highly comorbid with ODD. In cases where ODD is the only diagnosis, beneficial management includes psychosocial intervention, especially individual and family interventions, behavior modifications, and behavior therapy utilizing a contingency reward system (see Chapter 23).

If psychosocial therapies do not show any significant improvement in 2–3 months, then a trial of psychotropic may be indicated. There is some evidence that medications used to treat ADHD, such as atomoxetine and stimulants, can also be beneficial in treating ODD. When mood disorders coexist with ODD, the treatment should involve appropriate treatment of the mood disorder, which may also result in improvement in symptoms of ODD (108). Conduct disorders, when not amenable to psychosocial interventions, may respond to psychopharmacological interventions such as mood stabilizers, especially lithium, carbamazepine, and valproate. Stimulant medications, such as methylphenidate, may also be helpful even in the absence of comorbid ADHD. Typical neuroleptics, such as haloperidol and pimozide, have shown benefits, but the concern about extrapyramidal side effects limits the use of haloperidol on an ongoing basis. Atypical neuroleptics such as risperidone have also been shown to be effective in decreasing aggressive and disruptive behaviors (109).

19.10 Conclusion

This chapter reviews endocrine disorders and their cutaneous features, along with psychiatric features and principles of clinical management of these cutaneous and psychiatric issues presenting in the context of major endocrine disorders commonly seen in children and adolescents. The relationship between these various paradigms are complex, and much is yet to be learned. A multidisciplinary team is needed to help pediatric patients with endocrine disorders complicated by dermatological features. Fortunately, there is much that can be done to help these children and adolescents lead a productive life during their pediatric years as well as in adulthood.

References

1. O'Sullivan RL, Lipper G, Lerner EA. The neuro-immuno-cutaneous-endocrine network: Relationship of mind and skin. *Arch Dermatol* 1998;134(11):1431–5.
2. Centers for Disease Control and Prevention. 2011 National Diabetes Facts Sheet. http://www.cdc.gov/diabetes//pubs/factsheet11.htm
3. Kalus AA, Chien AJ, Olerud JE. Diabetes mellitus and other endocrine diseases. In: Wolff K, Goldsmith LA, Katz SI, Gilchrest BA, Paller AS, Leffell DJ, eds. *Fitzpatrick's dermatology in general medicine*, 7th edn. New York: McGraw Hill, 2008:1461–84.
4. Joshi N, Caputo GM, Weitekamp MR, Karchmer, AW. Infections in patients with diabetes mellitus. *N Engl J Med* 1999;341:1906–12.
5. Olerud JE. Diabetes and the skin. In: Porte D Jr, Sherwin RS, Baron A, eds. *Ellenburg and Rifkin's diabetes mellitus*, 6th edn. New York: McGraw-Hill, 2003:895.
6. Krause WKH. Cutaneous manifestations of endocrine diseases. *Diabetes mellitus and glucagonoma*, ch. 10. Berlin: Springer, 2010:121–41.
7. Muller SA, Winkelmann. Necrobiosis lipoidica diabeticorum. A clinical and pathological investigation of 171 cases. *Arch Dermatol* 1966;93(3):272–81.
8. O'Toole ET, Kennedy U, Nolan JJ, Young MM, Rogers S, Barnes L. Necrobiosis lipoidica: Only a minority of patients have diabetes mellitus. *Br J Dermatol* 1999;140(2): 283–6.
9. Petzelbauer P, Wolff K, Tappeiner G. Necrobiosis lipoidica: Treatment with systemic corticosteroids. *Br J Dermatol* 1992;126(6):542–5.
10. Kreuter A, Knierim C, Stucker M, Pawlak F, Rotterdam S, Altmeyer P, et al. Fumaric acid esters in necrobiosis lipoidica: Results of a prospective, non-controlled study. *Br J Dermatol* 2005;153 (4):802–7.
11. Alexis AF, Strober BE. Off-label dermatologic uses of anti-TNF-a therapies. *J Cutan Med Surg* 2005;9(6):296–302.
12. Rallis E, Korfitis C, Gregoriou S, Rigopoulos D. Assigning new roles to topical tacrolimus. *Expert Opin Investig Drugs* 2007;16(8):1267–76.
13. Dubin BJ, Kaplan EN. The surgical treatment of necrobiosis lipoidica diabeticorum. *Plast Reconstr Surg* 1977;60(3):421–8.
14. Silverstein JH, Gordon G, Pollock BH, Rosenbloom AL. Long-term glycemic control influences the onset of limited joint mobility in type 1 diabetes. *J Pediatr* 1998;132(6):944–7.
15. Infante JR, Rosenbloom AL, Silverstein JH, et al. Changes in frequency and severity of limited joint mobility in children type with type 1 diabetes mellitus between 1976–78 and 1998. J *Pediatr* 2001;138(1):33–7.
16. Meguerditchian C, Jacquet P, Béliard S, Benderitter T, Valéro R, Carsuzza F, et al. Scleredema adultorum of Buschke: An under recognized skin complication of diabetes. *Diabetes Metab* 2006;32(5):481–4.
17. Thumpimukvatana N, Wongopraparut C, Lim HW. Sclerederma diabeticorum successfully treated with ultraviolet A1 phototherapy. *J Dermatol* 2010;37(12):1036–9.
18. Yuksek J, Sezer E, Koseoglu D, Markoc F, Yildiz H. Sclerederma treated with broad-band ultraviolet A phototherapy plus colchicine. *Photodermatol Photoimmunol Photomed* 2010;26(5): 257–60.
19. Schwartz RA, Janniger CK. Childhood acanthosis nigricans. *Cutis* 1995;55(6):337–41.
20. Kahn CR, Flier JS, Bar RS, Archer JA, Gorden P, Martin MM, et al. The syndromes of insulin resistance and acanthosis nigricans: Insulin-receptor disorders in man. *N Engl J Med* 1976; 294(14):739–45.
21. Bohm M, Luger TA, Metz D. treatment of mixed-type acanthosis nigricans with topical calcipotriol. *Br J Dermatol* 1998;139(5):932–4.

22. Blobstein SH. Topical therapy with tretinoin and ammonium lactate for acanthosis nigricans by substitution of an analogue (acipimox) in a patient with type V hyperlipidemia. *Br J Dermatol* 1992;126(4):412–4.
23. Rosenbach A, Ram R. Treatment of Acanthosis nigricans of the axillae using a long-pulsed (5-msec) alexandrite laser. *Dermatol Surg* 2004;30(8):1158–60.
24. Levenson JL. Psychiatric issues in endocrinology: Updates in psychosomatic medicine and consultation-liaison psychiatry. *Prim Psychiatry* 2006;13(4):27–30.
25. Brown LC, Majumdar SR, Newman SC, Johnson JA. History of depression increases risk of type 2 diabetes in younger adults. *Diabetes Care* 2005;28(5):1063–7.
26. Anderson RJ, Freeeland KE, Clouse RE. The prevalence of comorbid depression in adults with diabetes. *Diabetes Care* 2001;24(6):1069–78.
27. Li C, Barker L, Ford ES, Zhang X, Strine TW, Mokdad AH. Diabetes and anxiety in US adults: Findings from the 2006 behavioral risk factor surveillance system. *Diabet Med* 2008;25(7): 878–81.
28. Herzer M, Hood KK. Anxiety symptoms in adolescents with type 1 diabetes: Association with blood glucose monitoring and glycemic control. *J Pediatr Psychol* 2010;35(4):415–25.
29. Jones JM, Lawson ML, Daneman D. Eating disorders in adolescent females with and without type 1 diabetes: Cross sectional study. *BMJ* 2000;320(7249):1563–6.
30. Nielsen S. Eating disorders in females with type 1 diabetes: An update of a meta-analysis. *Eur Eat Disord Rev* 2002;10:241–54.
31. Daneman D, Rodin G, Jones J. Eating disorders in adolescent girls and young adult women with type 1 diabetes. *Diabetes Spectrum* 2002;15(2):83–105.
32. Peveler RC, Bryden KS, Neil HAW. The relationship of disordered eating habits and attitudes to clinical outcomes in young adult females with type 1 diabetes. *Diabetes Care* 2005;28(1):84–8.
33. Delamater AM. Quality of life in youths with diabetes. *Diabetes Spectrum* 2000;13:42.
34. Kibby MY, Tyce VL, Mulhern RK. Effectiveness of psychological intervention for children and adolescents with chronic medical illness: A meta-analysis. *Clin Psychol Rev* 1998;18(1):103–17.
35. Jablon SL, Nalibof BD, Gilmore SL. Effects of relaxation training on glucose tolerance and diabetic control in type II diabetes. *Appl Psychophysiol Biofeedback* 1997;22(3): 155–69.
36. Rydall AC, Rodin GM, Olmsted MP, Devenyi RG, Daneman D. Disordered eating behavior and micro-vascular complications in young women with insulin-dependent diabetes mellitus. *N Engl J Med* 1997;336(26):1849–54.
37. Ezzat S. Acromegaly. *Endocrinol Metab Clin North Am* 1997;26(4):703–23.
38. Trepp R, Everst R, Stettler C. Assessment of quality of life in patients with uncontrolled vs. controlled acromegaly using the Acromegaly Quality of Life Questionnaire (AcroQoL). *Clin Endocrinol* 2005;63(1):103–10.
39. Pantanetti P, Sonino N, Arnaldi G. Self image and quality of life in acromegaly. *Pituitary* 2002;5 (1):17–9.
40. Ezzat S, Serri O, Chik CL, Johnson MD, Beauregard H, Marcovitz S, et al. Canadian consensus guidelines for the diagnosis and management of acromegaly. *Clin Invest Med* 2006;29:29–39.
41. Melmed S, Casanueva F, Cavagnini F, Chanson P, Frohman LA, Gaillard R, et al. Consensus statement: Medical management of acromegaly. *Eur J Endocrinol* 2005;153(6):737–40.
42. Newman CB. Medical therapy for acromegaly. *Endocrinol Metab Clin North Am* 1999;28(1): 171–90.
43. Trainer PJ, Drake WM, Katznelson L, Freda PU, Herman-Bonert V, van der Lely AJ, et al. Treatment of acromegaly with the growth hormone-receptor antagonist pegvisomant. *N Engl J Med* 2000;342(16):1171–7.
44. Sandret L, Maison P, Chanson P. Place of cabergoline in acromegaly: A meta-analysis. *J Clin Endocrinol Metab* 2011;96(5):1327–35.

45. GiustinaA, Chanson P, Bronstein MD, Klibanski A, Lamberts S, Casanueva FF, et al. A consensus on criteria for cure of acromegaly. *J Clin Endocrinol Metab* 2010;95(7):3141–8.
46. Krause WKH. Cutaneous manifestations of endocrine diseases. *Anterior pituitary hormones*, ch. 2. Berlin: Springer, 2009:9–20.
47. Büyükgebiz A. Congenital hypothyroidism clinical aspects and late consequences. *Pediatr Endocrinol Rev* 2003;1(2):185–90.
48. Kalus AA, Chien AJ, Olerud JE. Diabetes mellitus and other endocrine diseases. In: Wolff K, Goldsmith LA, Katz SI, Gilchrest BA, Paller AS, Leffell DJ, eds. *Fitzpatrick's dermatology in general medicine*. New York: McGraw-Hill, 2008:1461–84.
49. Coleman R, Hay RJ. Chronic mucocutaneous candidiasis associated with hypothyroidism: A distinct syndrome? *Br J Dermatol* 1997;136:24.
50. Callen JP, McCall MW. Bullous pemphigold and Hashimoto's thyroiditis. *J Am Acad Dermatol* 1981;5(5):558–60.
51. Puavilai S, Puavilai G, Charuwichitratana S, Sakuntabhai A, Sriprachya-Anunt S. Prevalence of thyroid diseases in patients with alopecia areata. *Int J Dermatol* 1994;33(9):632–3.
52. BiroE, Szekanecz Z, Czirjak L, Danko K, Kiss E, Szabo NA, et al. Association of systemic and thyroid autoimmune diseases. *Clin Rheumatol* 2006;25(2):240–5.
53. Fatourechi V, Pajouhi M, Fransway AF. Dermopathy of Graves disease (pretibial myxedema). Review of 150 cases. *Medicine* (Baltimore) 1994;73(1):1–7.
54. Ai J, Leonhardt JM, Heymann WR. Autoimmune thyroid diseases: Etiology, pathogenesis, and dermatologic manifestations. *J Am Acad Dermatol* 2003;48(5):641–59.
55. Dreskin SC, Andrews KY. The thyroid and urticaria. *Curr Opin Allergy Clin Immunol* 2005;5 (5):408–12.
56. Mahmud FH, Lteif AN, Renaud DL, Reed AM, Brands CK. Steroid-responsive encephalopathy associated with Hashimoto's thyroiditis in an adolescent with chronic hallucinations and depression: Case report and review. *Pediatrics* 2003;112(3):686–90.
57. O'Brien RF, Kifuji K, Summergrad P. Medical conditions with psychiatric manifestations. *Adolesc Med Clin* 2006;17(1):49–77.
58. Roberts CG, Landenson PW. Hypothyroidism. *Lancet* 2004;363(9411):793–03.
59. Thomsen AF, Kvist TK, Andersen PK, Kessing LV. Increased risk of affective disorder following hospitalisation with hyperthyroidism – a register-based study. *Eur J Endocrinol* 2005;152(4): 535–43.
60. Stern RA, Robinson B, Thorner AR, Arruda JE, Prohaska ML, Prange AL Jr. A survey study of neuropsychiatric complaints in patients with Graves' disease. *J Neuropsychiatry Clin Neurosci* 1996;8(2):181–5.
61. Ficarra BJ, Nelson RA. Phobia as a symptom in hyperthyroidism. *Am J Psychiatry* 1947;103 (5):831.
62. WeissRE, Stein MA, Trommer B, Refetoff S. Attention deficit hyperactivity disorder and thyroid function. *J Pediatr* 1993;123(4):539–45.
63. Kamboj MK, Tareen RS. Management of nonpsychiatric medical conditions presenting with psychiatric manifestations. *Pediatr Clin North Am* 2011;58(1):219–41.
64. Kowatch RA, DelBello MP. Pharmacotherapy of children and adolescents with bipolar disorder. *Psychiatr Clin North Am* 2005;28(2):385–97.
65. National Institute of Mental Health. Bipolar disorder in children and teens: A parent's guide. http://www.nimh.nih.gov/health/publications/bipolar-disorder-in-children-and-teens-a-parents-guide/what-treatments-are-available-for-children-and-teens-with-bipolar-disorder.shtml
66. Miller WL, Achermann JC, Fluck CE. The adrenal cortex and its disorders. In: Sperling MA, ed. *Pediatric endocrinology*. Philadelphia, PA: Saunders Elsevier, 2008:444–511.

67. Shah SS, Oh CH, Coffin SE, Yan AC. Addisonian pigmentation of the oral mucosa. *Cutis* 2005; 76(2):97–9.
68. Arit W, Allollo B. Adrenal Insufficiency. *Lancet* 2003;361(9372):1881–93.
69. Libè R, Barbetta L, Dall'Asta C, Salvaggio F, Gala C, Beck-Peccoz P, et al. Effects of dehydroepiandrosterone (DHEA) supplementation on hormonal, metabolic and behavioral status in patients with hypoadrenalism. *J Endocrinol Invest* 2004;27(8):736–41.
70. van Thiel SW, Romijn JA, Pereira AM, Biermasz NR, Roelfsema F, van Hemert A, et al. Effects of dehydroepiandrostenedione, superimposed on growth hormone substitution, on quality of life and insulin-like growth factor I in patients with secondary adrenal insufficiency: A randomized, placebo-controlled, cross-over trial. *J Clin Endocrinol Metab* 2005;90(6):3295–303.
71. Adler GK. Cushing Syndrome. http://emedicine.medscape.com/article/117365
72. Krause WKH. Cutaneous manifestations of endocrine diseases. *Adrenocortical Hormones*, ch. 5. Berlin: Springer, 2010:45–56.
73. Shibli-Rahhal A, Van Beek M, Sclechte JA. Cushing's syndrome. *Clin Dermatol* 2006;24(4): 260–5.
74. Feingold KR, Elias PM. Endocrine-skin interactions. Cutaneous manifestations of adrenal disease, pheochromocytomas, carcinoid syndrome, sex hormone excess and deficiency, polyglandular autoimmune syndromes, multiple endocrine neoplasia syndromes, and other miscellaneous disorders. *J Am Acad Dermatol* 1988;19(1):1–20.
75. Starkman MN, Schteingar DE, Schork MA. Depressed mood and other psychiatric manifestations of Cushing's syndrome: Relationship to hormone levels. *Psychosom Med* 1981;43(1):3–18.
76. Sonino N, Fallo F, Fava GA. Psychosomatic aspects of Cushing's syndrome. *Rev Endocr Metab Disord* 2010;11(2):95–104.
77. Loosen PT, Chambliss B, de Bold CR, Shelton R, Orth DN. Psychiatric phenomenology in Cushing's disease. *Pharmacopsychiatry* 1992;25(4):192–8.
78. Starkman MN, Schteingar DE. Neuropsychiatric manifestations of patients with Cushing's syndrome. *Arch Int Med* 1981;141(2):215–19.
79. Hughes CW, Emslie GJ, Crismon ML, Posner K, Birmaher B, Ryan N, et al. Texas children's medication algorithm project: Update from Texas consensus conference panel on medication treatment of childhood major depressive disorder. *J Am Acad Child Adolesc Psychiatry* 2007;46(6): 667–86.
80. Root AW, Diamond FB Jr. Disorders of mineral homeostasis in the newborn, infant, child, and adolescent. In: Sperling MA, ed. *Pediatric endocrinology*. Philadelphia, PA: Saunders Elsevier, 2008:686–769.
81. Salen PN. Hyperparathyroidism in emergency medicine. http://emedicine.medscape.com/article/766906
82. Aslan Y, Gedik Y, Okten A, Aksoy A, Cimşit G, Ari N. Congenital primary hypoparathyroidism presented with extensive cutaneous and subcutaneous calcifications. *Turk J Pediatr* 1999;41 (2):253–7.
83. Jeong KH, Lew BL, Sim WY. Osteoma cutis as the presenting feature of albright hereditary osteodystrophy associated with pseudopseudohypoparathyroidism. *Ann Dermatol* 2009;21(2): 154–8.
84. Trüeb RM, Panizzon RG, Burg G. Cutaneous ossification in Albright's hereditary osteodystrophy. *Dermatology* 1993;186(3):205–9.
85. Gueydan M, Folchetti G, Christofilis MA, Valéro R, Grob JJ, Vialettes B. Impetigo herpetiformis, a rare manifestation of severe hypocalcemia. *Ann Endocrinol* 2002;63(6):502–4.
86. Sárdy M, Preisz K, Berecz M, Horváth C, Kárpáti S, Horváth A. Methotrexate treatment of recurrent impetigo herpetiformis with hypoparathyroidism. J Eur Acad Dermatol Venereol2006; 20(6):742–3.

87. Wolf R, Tartler U, Stege H, Megahed M, Ruzicka T. Impetigo herpetiformis with hyperparathyroidism. J Eur Acad Dermatol Venereol2005;19(6):743–6.
88. Lotem M, Katzenelson V, Rotem A, Hod M, Sandbank M. Impetigo herpetiformis: A variant of pustular psoriasis or a separate entity? J Am Acad Dermatol1989;20(2):338–41.
89. Phillip N, Bassett A. Cognitive, behavioural and psychiatric phenotype in 22q11.2 deletion syndrome. *Behav Genet* 2011;41(3):403–12.
90. Velasco PJ, Manshadi M, Breen K, Lippmann S. Psychiatric aspects of parathyroid disease. *Psychosomatics* 1999;40(6):486–90.
91. Ståhle-Bäckdahl M, Hägermark O, Lins LE, Törring O, Hilliges M, Johansson O. Experimental and immunohistochemical studies on the possible role of parathyroid hormone in uraemic pruritus. *J Intern Med* 1989;225(6):411–5.
92. Krause WKH. *Cutaneous manifestations of endocrine diseases*. Berlin: Springer,2010:35–44.
93. Walker MD, Mcmohan DJ, Inabnet WB. Neuropsychological features in primary hyperparathyroidism: A prospective study. *J Clin Endocrinol Metab* 2009;94(6):1951–8.
94. Bilezikian JP, Potts JT Jr, Fuleihan Gel-H, Kleerekoper M, Neer R, Peacock M, et al. Summary statement from a workshop on asymptomatic primary hyperparathyroidism: A perspective for the 21st century. National Institutes of Health Consensus Development Conference Panel. NIH conference. Diagnosis and management of asymptomatic primary hyperparathyroidism: consensus development conference statement. *Ann Intern Med* 1991;114(7):593–7.
95. Khan A, Grey A, Shoback D. Medical management of asymptomatic primary hyperparathyroidism: Proceedings of the third international workshop. *J Clin Endocrinol Metab* 2009;94(2): 373–81.
96. Witchel SF, Lee PA. Ambiguous genitalia. In: Sperling MA, ed. *Pediatric Endocrinology*. Philadelphia, PA: Saunders Elsevier, 2008:127–64.
97. Rosenfield RL. Definition, pathogenesis and etiology of polycystic ovary syndrome in adolescents. In: Rose BD, ed. *Up to Date*. Wellesley, MA: Up to Date, 2009.
98. Kamboj MK, Patel DR. Polycystic ovarian syndrome: A diagnostic and therapeutic challenge. *J Pediatr Sci* 2010;2:e4.
99. Rosenfield RL. Clinical features and diagnosis of polycystic ovary syndrome in adolescents. In: Rose BD, ed. *Up to Date*. Wellesley, MA: Up to Date, 2009.
100. Hickman JG, Huber F, Palmisano M. Human dermal safety studies with eflornithine HCl 13.9% cream (Vaniqa), a novel treatment for excessive facial hair. *Curr Med Res Opin* 2001;16(4): 235–44.
101. Plourde PV, Reiter EO, Jou HC, Desrochers PE, Rubin SD, Bercu BB, et al. Safety and efficacy of anastrozole for the treatment of pubertal gynecomastia: A randomized, double-blind, placebo-controlled trial. J Clin Endocrinol Metab2004;89(9):4428–33.
102. Santen RJ, Allred DC, Ardoin SP, Archer DF, Boyd N, Braunstein GD, et al. Postmenopausal hormone therapy: An Endocrine Society scientific statement. *J Clin Endocrinol Metab* 2010;95(7 Suppl 1):s1–s66.
103. van Goozen SH, van den Ban E, Matthys W, Cohen-Kettenis PT, Thijssen JH, van Engeland H. Increased adrenal androgen functioning in children with oppositional defiant disorder: A comparison with psychiatric and normal controls. *J Am Acad Child Adolesc Psychiatry* 2000;39(11): 1446–51.
104. Pajer K, Tabbah R, Gardner W. Adrenal androgen and gonadal hormone levels in adolescent girls with conduct disorder. *Psychoneuroendocrinology* 2006;31(10):1245–56.
105. Joffe H, Hayes FJ. Menstrual cycle dysfunction associated with neurologic and psychiatric disorders: Their treatment in Adolescents. *Ann NY Acad Sci* 2008; 1135:219–29.
106. Baron-Cohen S. The extreme male brain theory of autism. *Trends Cogn Sci* 2002; 6(6):248–54.

107. Henningsson S, Jonsson L, Ljunggren E, Westberg L, Gillberg C, Råstam M, et al. Possible association between the androgen receptor gene and autism spectrum disorder. *Psychoneuroendocrinology* 2009;34(5):752–61.
108. Turgay A. Psychopharmacological treatment of oppositional defiant disorder. *CNS Drugs* 2009;23(1):1–17.
109. Gérardin P, Cohen D, Mazet P. Drug treatment of conduct disorder in young people. *Eur Neuropsychopharmacol* 2002;12(6):361–70.

Manmohan K. Kamboj and Ruqiya Shama Tareen

20 Inborn errors of metabolism with psychiatric and dermatologic features

Inborn errors of metabolism (IEMs) may involve any of the physiologic, biochemical, and metabolic pathways characterized by developmental delays, neuropsychiatric manifestations, and characteristic dermatological features. Psychiatric conditions may manifest much earlier and often may be the only type of symptoms presents, predating the presentation of symptoms related to other systems sometimes by many years. The psychiatric and cognitive symptoms seen in IEM are of wide variety and range from vague, nonspecific symptoms to severe psychosis and delirium. Some of these disorders are considered in this chapter with respect to their psychodermatologic aspects.

20.1 Introduction

Inborn errors of metabolism (IEMs) comprise a wide range of heritable disorders, most of which are autosomal recessive. Many of these have a high rate of morbidity and mortality if undiagnosed or diagnosed late. However, early diagnosis and timely institution of appropriate interventions may result in significant clinical improvement. Many of these defects are therefore screened for on newborn screening programs (NBS).

IEMs may involve any of the physiologic, biochemical, and metabolic pathways characterized by developmental delays, neuropsychiatric manifestations, and typical cutaneous features. IEMs are relatively rare but often overlooked underlying causes of psychiatric presentations in children and adolescents.

Psychiatric conditions may manifest much earlier and often may be the only type of presenting symptoms, predating the presentation of symptoms related to other systems sometimes by many years (). The psychiatric and cognitive symptoms seen in IEM are of wide variety and range from vague nonspecific symptoms to severe psychosis and delirium. Some of these disorders are discussed in more detail with respect to their psychodermatologic aspects in this chapter. See Table 20.1 as well as Figures 20.1 and 20.2.

20.2 Phenylketonuria [PKU]

Phenylketonuria (PKU) is also called Følling disease, phenylalanine hydroxylase deficiency, hyperphenylalaninemia, and OMIM # 261600. PKU was the first clearly

Table 20.1: Frequency of dermatologic and psychiatric features in some of IEM in pediatric population

Metabolic Disorders	Dermatologic Features	Psychiatric Features	Mental Retardation
Phenylketonuria	++	+++	+
Hartnup Disease	++	++	+
Alkaptonuria	+	+	+
Homocystinuria	++	++	+
Homocystinuria	++	++	+
Porphyria	++	+++	
Wilson's Disease	++	++	+/−

delineated inborn error of metabolism and has been on the newborn screen (NBS) program in the United States since the 1960s. In fact the NBS has been referred to as the "PKU screen." The diagnostic testing was first implemented by Guthrie (3). The incidence of PKU varies greatly in different countries and ethnicities; overall, the incidence in the Caucasian population is about 1:11,000 and 1:50,000 in the African Americans. Males and females are affected equally (4).

20.2.1 Genetics and pathophysiology

PKU is an autosomal recessive metabolic disorder of the metabolism of the amino acid phenylalanine. The defect is a mutation in the phenylalanine hydroxylase gene resulting in accumulation of phenylalanine.

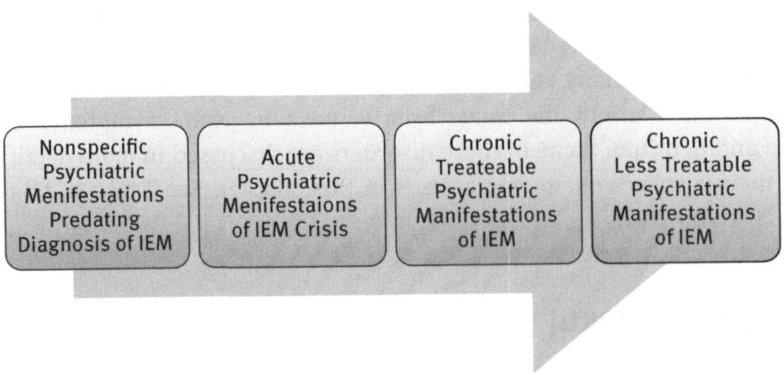

Figure 20.1: Psychiatric Manifestations of Inborn Errors of Metabolism [IEM] Adapted from Sedel F et al (1).

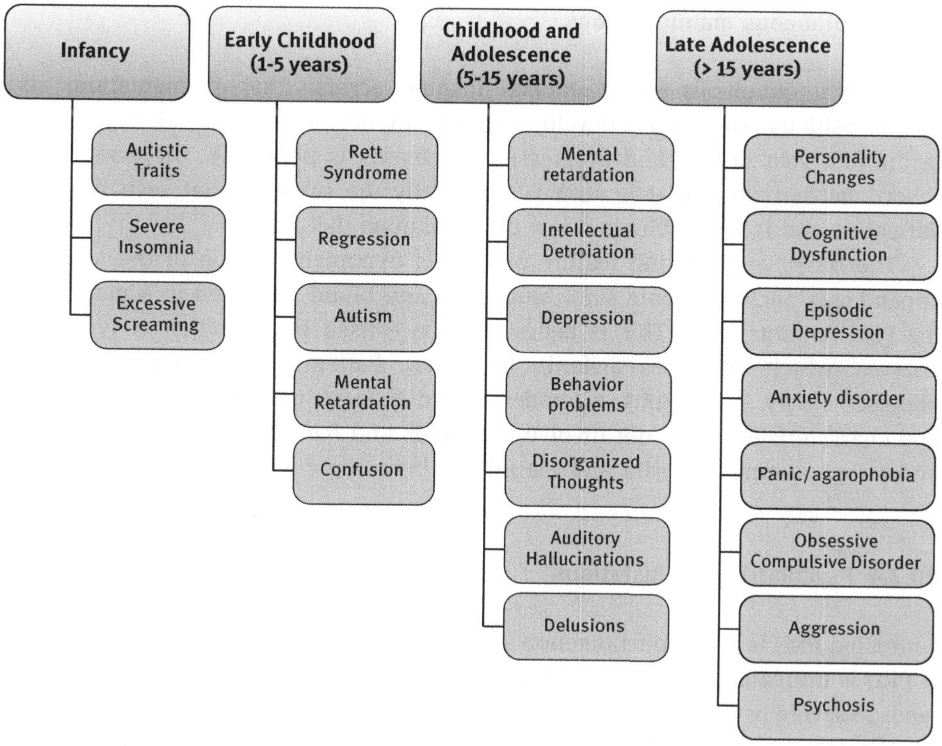

Figure 20.2: Psychiatric manifestations in disorders of inborn error of metabolisms in pediatric population. (2)

20.2.2 Clinical features

The clinical features seen in PKU are the result of accumulation of phenylalanine. Neonates are born normal, and as the levels of phenylalanine start accumulating, the clinical features are noted progressively after the first few weeks/months of life. Newborns may present with typical symptomatology if the mother herself has PKU and was poorly controlled during pregnancy. Clinical hallmarks of the disease include the following (4,5):

- Neurological features consisting of mental retardation, seizures, and microcephaly are significant. There may be irritability, hyperactivity, and self-destructive behavior as well.
- Features include excessive heavy vomiting, growth failure, and failure to thrive. A mousy odor is noted in the sweat and urine secondary to the accumulation of phenylacetic acid.

20.2.3 Cutaneous manifestations

The typical cutaneous manifestations include eczema, hypopigmentation, and photosensitivity. The eczema develops early in infancy, is seen in 20–50% of infants in the first year of life, and progressive worsening is noted (4). The eczema and seborrheic dermatitis that is seen is essentially the same as that seen in atopic dermatitis and is reversible on a low phenylalanine diet.

The other very striking feature of PKU is hypopigmentation of the skin and appendages, including pale skin, blue eyes, and blond hair seen in a majority of the PKU patients (4,6). This is believed to be caused by inhibition of tyrosinase enzyme, which decreases melanin formation. Patients also exhibit significant photosensitivity. Edematous, scleroderma-like changes develop in the extremities and characteristically do not involve the hands and feet (7,8). Segmental sclerosis and atrophoderma of Pasini and Pierini has been reported in PKU (9).

20.2.4 Psychiatric manifestations

Untreated PKU is a rare phenomenon since the advent of NBS prompting treatment. If PKU is untreated, the structural brain damage caused by elevated phenylalanine leads to severe psychiatric symptoms and mental retardation. Autistic disorders have been associated with PKU, especially when it is not diagnosed and treated early on, with a reported prevalence rate of about 5.7%. However, other studies have reported a much higher rate of up to 20% (10). Even when treated early, PKU can have substantial psychiatric and psychological comorbidity.

Many children and adolescents may present with non-specific psychological difficulties to their providers, at times vague enough to make the distinction difficult between problematic behavior versus underlying psychiatric illness. In this group the psychiatric illness is at times attributed to discontinuation of the special PKU diet, leading to cognitive, emotional, and behavioral symptoms (11). However, there are reports that strict adherence to dietary restrictions may not guarantee that these children will not develop psychiatric problems later in life (12).

Children with PKU who are treated early tend to have intelligence quotient (IQ) in normal range, albeit decline in IQ over time is seen at a rate of 1.8 to 3.8 points for each corresponding increase of 100 µmol/l in phenylalanine level (12). These behavioral problems, especially in boys, were not in correlation with their IQ levels, which was different from the observation in girls with early treated PKU who tended to have behavioral problems if their IQ was lower than the 75th percentile (13). The executive function difficulties include a slow processing speed (14).

The role of keeping the serum phenylalanine levels under good control by a low phenylalanine diet has been studied in several other studies. In this research children with early-treated PKU who were not on a strict phenylalanine diet regime were compared to children who followed such regimes. There were significant differences between these groups in terms of attention deficits, emotional development, deviant behavior, social isolation, introversion, low self-esteem, less autonomy, low threshold for frustration tolerance, and low motivation, which is reflected in low academic achievement and impulsiveness (12). Thus, compliance with the low phenylalanine diet is recommended.

Some of the American Psychiatric Association's (APA's) *Diagnostic and Statistical Manual of Mental Disease* (DSM-IV) diagnoses that are seen more frequently in children who do not have good metabolic control are attention deficit hyperactivity disorder (ADHD), depressive disorders of various degrees, oppositional defiance disorder, encopresis, and various types of phobias (11). Children who were treated and continued on a good diet regime with good metabolic control when evaluated for their quality of life were found to be better adjusted psychologically but still demonstrated some negative emotions and were described as less happy and less confident (11).

Research has looked at children with PKU who were either treated late or who stopped following the dietary regimen after the first few years; they tend to have many more psychological disturbances as adults than their counterparts who were treated early and stayed on a life-long dietary regimen. The group with limited treatment tend to have serious mood and thought anomalies, social alienation, and difficulties interpreting social cues in interpersonal relations; they also had impaired executive functioning leading to lesser degree of adjustment in life (11).

Depressive disorders are the most commonly found disorders in adolescents and young adults with PKU and are more frequently noted in females versus males. Anxiety spectrum disorders are the second leading diagnosis seen in PKU patients, especially panic attacks with or without agoraphobia and specific phobia. Psychosis including hallucinations and delusions are the most dramatic but an infrequent presentation of PKU and are mostly seen in untreated or metabolically compromised individuals.

20.2.5 Laboratory diagnosis

The laboratory diagnosis of PKU essentially involves the demonstration of increased phenylalanine or its end products and demonstration of phenylpyruvic hydroxylase deficiency as well as genetic testing for the gene mutation. This is summarized in Figure 20.3 (4,5,15,16).

20.2.6 Management

The foundation of PKU treatment is strict dietary restrictions to implement a low phenylalanine diet; this diet results in the reduction of serum phenylalanine levels.

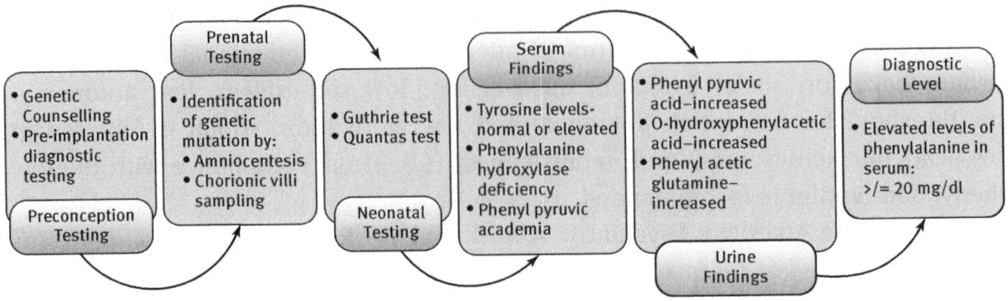

Figure 20.3: Diagnostic testing for phenylketonuria.

The dietary restrictions need to continue lifelong (17,18,19). The cutaneous findings as well as the neurologic and psychologic manifestations are all noted to be reversible with strict dietary control. The same restrictions in diet apply to pregnant women with PKU starting in the preconception period and continued through pregnancy; this plan can minimize fetal effects of PKU (20,21). Phenylalanine-free formulas are now available as well.

Tetrahydrobiopterin-responsive PKU has been shown to respond well to treatment with tetrahydrobiopterin (22). Other options that have been studied include the use of large neutral amino acid substitution and recombinant or pegylated phenylalanine-ammonia lyase. Gene therapy offers promise for PKU management in the future as well (23,24).

Psychoeducation of the child and family is especially aimed at enhancing compliance with the low phenylalanine diet and its impact on the long term prognosis for metabolic and cognitive aspects of disease. Psychosocial support is very important for improving compliance and outcomes. Summer camps for children and adolescents with PKU can be very effective when trying to teach them adherence to special diets and other aspects of this disease while engaging them in fun activities. In recent years, with the advent of the social media, peer to peer information and expertise can be exchanged easily via social network groups and websites (25).

Patients with PKU have inherent cognitive difficulties, which can cause problems for them when planning and executing the low protein regimens and may result in frustration, poor compliance, and non-adherence with dietary restrictions. Individual and family counseling aiming at enhanced understanding about the special food restriction and change in lifestyle may help patients who struggle with this difficult task (12). Specific treatment of psychiatric disorders with psychotropic medications has not been studied in the PKU population. General measures of treating such disorders may be employed under care of a multidisciplinary team including a psychiatrist.

20.3 Hartnup disease

Hartnup disease [HD] is also known as Hartnup disorder or OMIM# 234500. It was initially described in 1956 and is the second most common aminoaciduria with an overall incidence of 1:30,000.

20.3.1 Genetics and pathophysiology

Hartnup disease (HD) is caused by an impairment of the neutral amino acid transport system B0AT1 in the kidneys and small intestines. The genetic lesion is a mutation of the SLC6A9 gene on chromosome 5p15.33 that is inherited in an autosomal recessive manner (26,27,28).

20.3.2 Cutaneous manifestations

Patients may be asymptomatic, though the typical cutaneous features are that of a photosensitive pellagra-like skin rash with lesions that may be painful. Blistering may occur in severe presentations. The skin lesions may leave a depigmented area after a phase of yellowish brown hyperpigmentation (5).

20.3.3 Psychiatric manifestations

Children with HD can present with a variety of symptoms, which may be mild and nonspecific, or they may be significant and serious and significantly impact the patient's daily functioning. Most of the children with Hartnup disease have IQs in normal ranges, though earlier studies reported declining IQs over time. Hersov et al suggested that this finding may be attributed to multiple factors, especially detrimental effects of multiple hospitalizations due to severe disease states, poor school performance because of missed days, and possibly having difficulty in adjusting to daily life routines after each hospitalization (5).

Such factors along with the burden of a lifelong illness with repeated attacks could also explain the behavioral problems reported in some of the children with HD who develop aggressive personalities and bullying attitudes with peers as well as defiance toward adults. Children with HD can be apathetic or very labile, with high levels of irritability and depressive mood; at times, they can develop more severe symptoms, including confusion, depersonalization, hallucinations, and delusions (29). Other reported neuropsychological features include mental retardation, emotional lability, cerebellar ataxia, headaches, seizures, and hypertonia (5,30).

20.3.4 Laboratory findings

Aminoaciduria of all neutral amino acids (except proline) is diagnostic, while serum amino acid levels are usually normal (5).

20.3.5 Management

The treatment is basically centered on a protein-rich diet. Supplementation with about 200–400 mg/day of nicotinic acid is therapeutic for the cutaneous manifestations and even ataxia (5). The use of effective topical sunscreen is essential. Nonspecific psychiatric symptoms respond rapidly to the correction of the underlying metabolic abnormality. Patel et al reviewed a case of a 10 year old who presented with confusion, agitation, flailing of limbs, abnormal tone of speech for 15 days duration, and all psychiatric symptoms along with cutaneous symptoms that responded well to treatment with niacin (31).

20.4 Homocystinuria

Homocystinuria is also called hyperhomocystinuria, CBS deficiency, cystathionine beta synthase deficiency, and OMIM# 236200. It is an IEM of the amino acid methionine, which results in multisystemic pathology. Homocystinuria is a rare IEM worldwide, and in the United States there is an incidence of about 1:300,000. The incidence varies greatly geographically with prevalence for northern European countries reported to be 1:64,000. It is noted to be more common in males than females (5).

20.4.1 Genetics and pathophysiology

Homocystinuria is an autosomal recessive disorder caused by deficiency of cystathionine synthase. The results of the enzymatic deficiency is the elevation of serum and urine levels of both methionine and homocystine, and the deposition of homocystine in multiple organ systems giving rise to its multiple clinical manifestations (5). The genetic mutation maps to chromosome 21q22.3.

20.4.2 Clinical features

The main clinical features of homocystinuria include developmental delay and the involvement of the central nervous system as well as ophthalmologic and vascular complications. These are briefly summarized in Figure 20.4 (5,32).

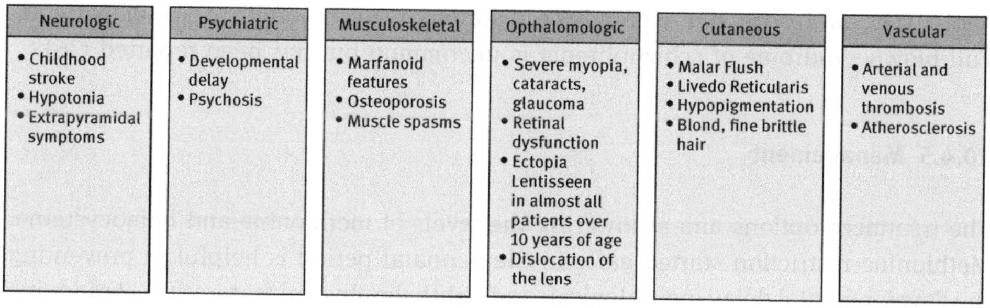

Figure 20.4: Clinical features of homocystinuria.

20.4.3 Cutaneous manifestations

The cutaneous manifestations include changes in the skin and hair. The skin is noted to be pale with large pores; malar flush and livedoreticularis may be noted on the face. Pigmentary dilution resulting from the inhibition of the metabolism of tyrosine causes hypo-pigmentation of the skin and hair (33). The hair is noted to be fine, thin, brittle, and blonde.

20.4.4 Psychiatric Manifestations

Mental retardation with IQs in range of 60 or below is reported in about half of children who have homocystinuria. Mental retardation predisposes these children to other neuropsychiatric symptoms at times when the metabolic disorder is not compensated or due to any other type of stress. Surgery under general anesthesia may unmask the cystathione β-synthase deficiency for the first time; the post-surgical course can be complicated with encephalopathy marked by confusion, disorientation, cognitive deficit, psychosis presenting with persecutory delusion, auditory as well as visual hallucination, and paranoia (34). Visual hallucinations have also been reported in isolation in patients who underwent removal of dislocated lenses resulting in acute postoperative visual deprivation.

Neuropsychiatric symptoms may be the first and only symptoms in about 2.8% of patients, leading to initial presentation for treatment. Ryan et al presented a case of a 17-year-old male with no previous medical or psychiatric history except some difficulties in attention span but no established diagnosis of ADHD; he presented with florid psychosis, tearfulness, agitation, tremulousness along with extreme anxiety, and feeling of impending danger (35).

About 51% of adults with homocystinuria have some level of neuropsychiatric symptoms. Mood disorders, especially episodic depression, are reported in about 10% of patients, personality disorders in about 19%, behavioral dysregulation in about 17%, and obsessive compulsive disorders were reported in 5% of patients. Full-blown syndrome of schizophrenia is uncommon but has been reported (36).

20.4.5 Management

The treatment options aim at lowering the levels of methionine and homocysteine. Methionine restriction started early in the neonatal period is helpful in preventing the developmental delay, neurological, and ophthalmological features (5). Pyridoxine treatment with 250–500 mg/day of vitamin B6 is useful in the pyridoxine-sensitive homocystinuria patients in preventing the thromboembolic events and in the treatment of cutaneous manifestations (37). The use of betaine and folic acid are also very effective in reducing the methionine levels (38). Vitamin B12 supplementation is also noted to be useful.

Patients with homocystinuria who have mental retardation are highly susceptible to develop acute psychotic symptoms and should be monitored closely in cases of physical stress, especially if undergoing surgery. Pre-surgical evaluation should include an emphasis on correction of any cysteine deficiency and efforts to normalize the levels before surgery, especially if long acting NMDA receptors antagonist like thiopental and ketamine are going to be used as an anesthetic; an NMDA receptor is a specific type of ionotropic glutamate receptor.

When treating psychotic symptoms one should avoid high potency dopaminergic 2 (D2) blockers such as haloperidol or other typical neuroleptics, which can cause serious extrapyramidal side effects, such as acute muscle dystonia or catatonia and mutism. Newer atypical neuroleptics with lowest D2 blocking properties are preferred in such cases. Benzodiazepines, such as clonazepam and baclofen, have been used effectively in patients with homocystinuria who develop extrapyramidal symptoms (39).

20.5 Porphyrias

Porphyrias are inborn errors of heme metabolism. Porphyrins are precursors of the heme molecules, which is a part of the hemoglobin molecule. Porphyria results from enzymatic defects at the multiple steps of heme synthesis. Therefore, depending on the enzymatic defect, there are different kinds of porphyrias, all of which result in increased accumulation and excretion of precursors and varying clinical manifestations.

20.5.1 Genetics and prevalence

Congenital erythropoietic porphyria (CEP) is inherited in an autosomal recessive manner; all other types of porphyrias are inherited in an autosomal dominant pattern. Overall, prevalence of all kinds of porphyrias is about 5 per 100,000 (40). Porphyria cutaneatarda (PCT) is the most common, and CEP is rare (41,42).

20.5.2 Clinical features

The porphyrias may be acute or chronic depending on the presenting signs and symptoms; these are summarized in Table 20.2 (43). Episodes of acute intermittent abdominal pain with discrepancy between the severity of pain and actual clinical findings are characteristic; muscular weakness, focal neurological deficits, and seizures may be seen (44).

20.5.3 Cutaneous manifestations

The cutaneous manifestations are typically seen in variegate porphyria, hereditary coproporphyrias, and porphyria cutaneatarda. Sub-epidermal bullous lesions,

Table 20.2: Main types of porphyrias

Acute porphyrias

Types:

- Acute intermittent porphyria [AIP]
- Hereditary Corpropophyria
- Variegate porphyria
- ALA-D deficiency porphyria

Main features:

- Acute abdominal pain attacks
- Neurological deficits
- Psychiatric symptoms
- Red colored urine

Chronic porphyrias

Types:

- Congenital erythropoietic porphyria [CEP]
- Erythropoieticprotoporphyria [EP]
- Porphyria cutaneatarda [PCT]
- Hepato- erythropoietic porphyria [HEP]

Main features:

- Cutaneous manifestations
- No acute attacks
- May or may not have any neurologic and/or hepatic involvement

epidermal atrophy, and scleroderma-like changes, followed by hyperpigmented and then hypopigmented lesions on healing, are seen and represent the spectrum of cutaneous lesions in this condition (43). The photosensitive skin lesions are observed to improve when sun exposure is decreased. Petechiae and purpura may be noted in erythropoieticprotoporphyria. Hypertrichosis and loss of eyelashes as well as eyebrows may occur. The face may reveal severe mutilation of the cartilaginous structures (43).

20.5.4 Psychiatric manifestations

Acute intermittent porphyria, variegate porphyria, and coproporphyria all present with many neuropsychiatric symptoms. Prevalence of acute porphyria in hospitalized psychiatric patients has been reported to be between 0.21% to 1.6%; most of these patients were admitted due to a psychotic episode and had diagnoses of schizophrenia, schizoaffective disorder, or atypical psychosis. Alcohol intake, especially red wine and whiskey, can precipitate an acute porphyria attack with acute psychotic symptoms. Adolescents and young adults with eating disorders or maladaptive eating behaviors are at high risk for porphyria with neuropsychiatric manifestations precipitated by restricting food intake and following a strict dietary regimen with low carbohydrate intake to lose weight.

Post-pubertal adolescents can also develop cyclical psychiatric episodes associated with luteal phase porphyria attacks, which, if mild to moderate in nature, can be confused with premenstrual dysphoric syndrome. Children exposed to any medications that can deplete intracellular heme (due to induction of hepatic cytochrome *P*-450 enzyme pathways) can experience acute porphyria attacks with severe psychiatric symptoms (45, 46). Psychotic episodes with auditory hallucinations, persecutory delusion, ideas of references, social isolation, and catatonia can be mistaken as schizophrenia. Bipolar disorder has also been reported, including mood lability, hypomania, elated mood, distractibility, social disinhibition, decreased sleep, and grandiosity.

In children and adolescents behavioral problems can be due to an acute porphyria attack and include oppositional defiance disorder, conduct disorders, social disruption, hyperactivity, and encopresis. It is not surprising that patients are diagnosed with somatoform disorders (i.e., conversion disorder and somatization disorder) due to the episodic nature and varied combinations of the physical, neurologic, and psychiatric symptoms.

Patients with repeated attacks of porphyria also develop persistent depressive and anxiety spectrum disorders. When those with porphyria were asked to rate their subjective sense of depression and anxiety, about 15% reported feeling depressed, while about 22% reported a moderate to severe degree of anxiety (47). Anxiety disorder usually presents as generalized anxiety, although panic disorder with or without agoraphobia and obsessive compulsive disorder also have been reported.

Having an episodic illness with serious physical and psychiatric symptoms impacts this patient's general sense of well-being, which was reflected in patients with porphyria who rated their quality of life not only lower than healthy controls but also lower than the patients with diabetes mellitus (see Chapters 4 and 19). They were also found to have much lower levels of achievements in different areas of life such as employments, relationships, and family structure (48).

20.5.5 Laboratory diagnosis

The measurements of porphyrins and precursors of porphyrins in urine and stool are the most important initial studies to establish the diagnosis. Once the initial diagnosis is made, further specific specialized testing offered in specialty laboratories can be undertaken. This includes genetic studies for mutation analysis, prenatal diagnosis, and genetics screening of the family when feasible (43). Details of further testing are not discussed in this writing.

20.5.6 Management

An acute porphyria attack may be life-threatening and needs emergent, intensive management. Prevention of porphyria attacks should be at the forefront of any treatment plan. It is also very important to avoid exposure to any of the offending medications and agents. Most symptoms and findings need symptomatic treatment, close intensive monitoring, and management of pain, dehydration, and electrolyte disturbances; precipitating agents should be withdrawn (43). Details of treatment can also be found at the EPIs (The European Porphyria initiative) website: www.Porphyria_Europe.org.

The use of hemearginate has been found to be the most useful specific therapeutic agent. Avoidance of sun exposure as well as a use of effective mechanical and biochemical sunscreen is mandatory (49). Acute psychiatric symptoms usually respond to reversal of metabolic derangement, although chronic depression and anxiety disorders may require specific psychopharmacologic treatment. Many antidepressants can cause a porphyria attack such as tricyclic antidepressants (TCAs) and monoamine oxidase inhibitors (MAOIs); thus, TCAs and MAOIs should be avoided as they can induce a porphyria attack (Table 20.3) (45).

There is no clear data available for more commonly used psychotropics, such as selective serotonin reuptake inhibitors (SSRIs) or other such agents for use in porphyrias. Data about the use of SSRIs even in adult patients with porphyria is at best conflicting. A clinician should carefully weigh the risk of the interaction at hepatic cytochrome *P*-450 enzyme pathway inducing a porphyria attack versus letting patients suffer from depression and anxiety, which have shown to impact the

Table 20.3: Porphyria-inducing medications and other substances

Some Psychotropic Agents Causing Porphyria
Sedatives: Barbiturate, Chloral hydrate
Benzodiazepines: Alprazolam, Chlorodiazepoxide, Diazepam, Midazolam
Antidepressants: Amitriptyline
Mood Stabilizers: Valproate Acid, Carbamazepine
Neuroleptics: Haloperidol
Substance of Abuse: Nicotine, Alcohol, Cocaine, Amphetamines

quality of life significantly (47). When selecting a SSRI or other related medications, care should be taken to choose one that has the least possibility to interact at hepatic cytochrome *P*-450 enzyme pathways. Most of the medications are predominantly metabolized through four of the major pathways: Cyp2D6, Cyp3A4, Cyp1A2, and Cyp2C enzymes (2C9, 2C10, 2C19); also, one or more of these pathways can be utilized by the same medication.

SSRIs are potent inhibitors of Cyp2D6. Fluoxetine and paroxetine are the most potent inhibitors among this group, while citalopram and escitalopram are the least potent inhibitors; sertraline is somewhere in the middle. Fluvoxamine is an SSRI that is commonly used to treat obsessive compulsive disorder and is the only one in this group that is a very potent inhibitor of CYP1A2 (50). One case report has presented successful treatment of a first acute porphyria attack with the use of fluoxetine 20 mg daily; it was continued for 6 months and further attacks during this time were not reported (51). Another case report also noted successful treatment of a woman with porphyria and learning disabilities utilizing fluoxetine (52).

Education regarding abstinence from smoking, alcohol, amphetamines, and cocaine is very important, and patients may need referral to appropriate resources for individual and group therapy focused on developing coping skills in order to overcome impulses to abuse such substances. Young adults can be referred to Alcoholics Anonymous and other such programs to continue abstinence from substances of abuse.

20.6 Conclusion

Inborn errors of metabolism (IEMs) comprise a wide range of heritable disorders, most of which are autosomal recessive. They may involve any of the physiologic, biochemical, and metabolic pathways characterized by developmental delays, neuropsychiatric manifestations, and characteristic dermatological features. Psychiatric conditions may manifest much earlier and often may be the only type of symptoms seen, predating the presentation of symptoms related to other systems sometimes by many years. The psychiatric and cognitive symptoms seen in IEM are of wide variety and range from vague, nonspecific symptoms to severe psychosis and delirium. Many of these have a high rate of morbidity and mortality if undiagnosed or diagnosed late. However, early diagnosis and timely institution of appropriate interventions may result in significant clinical improvement. IEMs reviewed in this discussion are phenylketonuria, hartnup disease, homocystinuria, and the porphyrias.

References

1. Sedel F, Baumann N, Turpin JC. Psychiatric manifestations revealing inborn errors of metabolism in adolescents and adults. *J Inherit Metab Dis* 2007;30(5):631–41.
2. Mayatepek E. Psychiatric disease. In: Hoffmann GF, Zschocke J, Nyhan WL, eds. *Inherited metabolic diseases: A clinical approach.* New York: Springer, 2010:177–80.
3. Guthrie R, Susi A. A simple phenylalanine method for phenylketonuria in large populations of newborn infants. *Pediatrics* 1963;32:338–43.
4. Itin PH, Goldsmith LA. Cutaneous changes in errors of amino acid metabolism. In: Wolff K, Goldsmith LA, Katz SI, Gilchrest BA, Paller AS, Leffell DJ, eds. *Fitzpatric's dermatology in general medicine,* 7th edn. New York: McGraw-Hill, 2007:1219–28.
5. Izakovic J. Hereditary metabolic disorders. In: Schachner LA, Hansen RC, eds. *Pediatric dermatology,* 4th edn. Edinburgh: Mosby-Elsevier, 2011:503–24.
6. Scriver CR, Kaufman S. Hyperphenylalaninemia: Phenylalanine hydroxylase deficiency In: Scriver CR, Sly WS, Childs B, Beaudet AL, Valle D, Kinzler KW, et al, eds. *Metabolic and molecular basis of inherited disease,* 8th edn. New York: McGraw-Hill, 2001;1667.
7. Al-Mayouf SM, Al-Owain MA. Progressive sclerodermatous skin changes in a child with phenylketonuria. *Pediatr Dermatol* 2006;23(2):136–8.
8. Nova MP, Kaufman M, Halperin A. Scleroderma-like skin indurations in a child with phenylketonuria: A clinicopathologic correlation and review of the literature. *J Am Acad Dermatol* 1992;26 (2):329–33.
9. Lasser AE, Schultz BC, Beaff D, Bielinski S, Kirschenbaum B. Phenylketonuria and scleroderma. *Arch Dermatol* 1978;114(8):1215–7.
10. Baieli S, Pavone L, Meli C, Fiumara A, Coleman M. Autism and phenylketonuria. *J Autism Dev Disord* 2003;33(2):201–4.
11. Brumm VL, Bilder D, Waisbern SE. Psychiatric symptoms and disorders in phenylketonuria. *Mol Genet Metab* 2010;99(Suppl 1):S59–63.
12. Stevenson JE, Hawcroft J, Lobascher M. Behavioral deviance in children with early treated phenylketonuria. *Arch Dis Child* 1979;54(1):14–8.
13. Channon S, Mockler C, Lee P. Executive functioning and speed of processing in phenylketonuria. *Neuropsychology* 2005;19(5):679–86.
14. Gentile JK, Ten Hoedt AE, Bosch AM. Psychosocial aspects of PKU: Hidden disabilities – A review. *Mol Genet Metab* 2010;99(Suppl 1):S64–7.
15. Abadie V, Berthelot J, Feillet F, Maurin N, Mercier A, de Baulny HO, et al. Neonatal screening and long-term follow-up of phenylketonuria: The French database. *Early Hum Dev* 2001;65(2):149–58.
16. Verlinsky Y, Rechitsky S, Verlinsky O, Strom C, Kuliev A. Preimplantation testing for phenylketonuria. *Fertil Steril* 2001;76(2):346–9.
17. Holtzman NA, Kronmal RA, van Doorninck W, Azen C, Koch R. Effect of age at loss of dietary control on intellectual performance and behavior of children with phenylketonuria. *N Engl J Med* 1986;314(10):593–8.

18. Weglage J, Pietsch M, Denecke J, Sprinz A, Feldmann R, Grenzebach M, et al. Regression of neuropsychological deficits in early-treated phenylketonurics during adolescence. *J Inherit Metab Dis* 1999;22(6):693–705.
19. Waisbren SE, Noel K, Fahrbach K, Cella C, Frame D, Dorenbaum A, et al. Phenylalanine blood levels and clinical outcomes in phenylketonuria: A systematic literature review and meta-analysis. *Mol Genet Metab* 2007;92(1,2):63–70.
20. Rohr FJ, Doherty LB, Waisbren SE, Bailey IV, Ampola MG, Benacerraf B, et al. New England Maternal PKU Project: Prospective study of untreated and treated pregnancies and their outcomes. *J Pediatr* 1987;110(3):391–8.
21. Cipcic-Schmidt S, Trefz FK, Fünders B, Seidlitz G, Ullrich K. German maternal phenylketonuria study. *Eur J Pediatr* 1996;155 (Suppl 1):S173–6.
22. Muntau AC, Röschinger W, Habich M, Demme lmair H, Hoffmann B, Sommerhoff CP, et al. Tetrahydrobiopterin as an alternative treatment for mild phenylketonuria. *N Engl J Med* 2002; 347(26):2122–32.
23. Scriver CR. The PAH gene, phenylketonuria, and a paradigm shift. *Hum Mutat* 2007;28(9):831–45.
24. Harding CO. Progress towards a cell-directed therapy for phenylketonuria. *Clin Genet* 2008; 74:97–104.
25. Gentile J, Fickie MR, Waisbren S. Phenylketonuria: Outcomes and treatment. *Pediatric Health* 2008:2(2):225–34.
26. Bröer S. Apical transporters for neutral amino acids: Physiology and pathophysiology. *Physiology* 2008;23:95–103.
27. Seow HF, Bröer S, Bröer A, Bailey CG, Potter SJ, Cavanaugh JA, et al. Hartnup disorder is caused by mutations in the gene encoding the neutral amino acid transporter SLC6A19. *Nat Genet* 2004;36(9):1003–7.
28. Broer S, Cavanaugh JA, Rasko JE. Neutral amino acid transport in epithelial cells and its malfunction in Hartnup disorder. *Biochem Soc Trans* 2005;33(1):233–6.
29. Hersov LA, Rodnight R. Hartnup disease in psychiatric practice: Clinical and biochemical features of three cases. *J Neurol Neurosurg Psychiatry* 1960;23:40–5.
30. Levy H. Hartnup Disorder. In: Scriver CR, Sly WS, Childs B, Beaudet AL, Valle D, Kinzler KW, et al, eds. *Metabolic and molecular basis of inherited disease*, 8th edn. New York: McGraw Hill, 2001.
31. Patel AB, Prabhu AS. Hartnup Disease. *Indian J Dermatol* 2008;53(1):31–2.
32. Baloghova J. Dermatologic manifestations of homocystinuria. http://emedicine.medscape.com/article/1115062
33. Reish O, Townsend D, Berry SA, Tsai MY, King RA. Tyrosinase inhibition due to interaction of homocyst[e]ine with copper: The mechanism for reversible hypopigmentation in homocystinuria due to cystathionine beta-synthase deficiency. *Am J Hum Genet* 1995; 57(1):127–32.
34. Eschweiler G, Rosin R, Their P, Giedke H. Postoperative psychosis in homocystinuria. *Eur Psychiatry* 1997;12(2):98–101.
35. Ryan MM, Sidhu RK, Alexander J, Megerian JT. Homocystinuria presenting as psychosis in an adolescent. *J Child Neurol* 2002;17(11):859–60.
36. Abbott MH, Folstein SE, Abbey H, Pyeritz RE. Psychiatric manifestations of homocystinuria due to cystathionine beta-synthase deficiency: Prevalence, natural history, and relationship to neurologic impairment and vitamin B6-responsiveness. *Am J Med Genet* 1987;26(4):959–69.
37. Reish O, Townsend D, Berry SA, Tsai MY, King RA. Tyrosinase inhibition due to interaction of homocyst[e]ine with copper: The mechanism for reversible hypopigmentation in homocystinuria due to cystathionine beta-synthase deficiency. *Am J Hum Genet* 1995;57(1):127–32.
38. Ueland PM, Holm PI, Hustad S. Betaine: A key modulator of one-carbon metabolism and homocysteine status. *Clin Chem Lab Med* 2005;43(10):1069–75.

39. Burlina AP, Edini C, Burlina AB. Treatment of extrapyramidal symptoms in a patient with homozygous homocystinuria. *J Inherit Metab Dis* 2002;25(2):135–6.
40. Anderson KE, Sassa S, Bishop DF, Desnick RJ. Disorders of heme biosynthesis: X-linked sideroblastic anemia and the porphyrias. In: Scriver CR, Sly WS, Childs B, Beaudet AL, Valle D, Kinzler KW, et al, eds. *Metabolic and molecular basis of inherited disease,* 8th edn. New York: McGraw Hill, 2001:2991–3062.
41. Bulat V, Lugović L, Situm M, Buljan M, Bradić L. Porphyria cutaneatarda as the most common porphyria. *Acta Dermatovenerol Croat* 2007;15(4):254–63.
42. Maniangatt SC, Panicker JN, Thomas M, Pavithran K. A rare case of porphyria. *Ann Acad Med Singapore* 2004;33(3):359–61.
43. Poblete-Gutiérrez P, Wiederholt T, Merk HF, Frank J. The porphyrias: Clinical presentation, diagnosis and treatment. *Eur J Dermatol* 2006;16(3):230–40.
44. Foran SE, Abel G. Guide to porphyrias. A historical and clinical perspective. *Am J Clin Pathol* 2003;119(Suppl):S86–93.
45. European Porphyria Network. Drugs that should be avoided in the acute porphyrias. http://www.porphyria-europe.com/03-drugs/selecting-drug-unsafe.asp
46. Crimlisk HL. The little imitator-porphyria: A neuropsychiatric disorder. *J Neurol Neurosurg Psychiatry* 1997;62(4):319–28.
47. Millward LM, Kelly P, King A. Anxiety and depression in the acute porphyrias. *J Inherit Metab Dis* 2005;28(6):1099–107.
48. Millward LM, Kelly P, Deacon A, Senior V, Peters TJ. Self-rated psychosocial consequences and quality of life in the acute porphyrias. *J Inherit Metab Dis* 2001;24(7):733–47.
49. Harper P, Wahlin S. Treatment options in acute porphyria, porphyria cutaneatarda, and erythropoieticprotoporphyria. *Curr Treat Options Gastroenterol* 2007;10(6):444–55.
50. Wroblewski B, Glenn MB. The cytochrome P-450 drug metabolizing enzyme system: an overview of potential clinically important drug interactions. *J Head Trauma Rehabil* 2002;17(6):571–4.
51. Mercan S, Karamustafalioglu O, Tanriverdi N, Oba S. Safety of fluoxetine treatment in a case of acute intermittent porphyria. *Int J Psychiatr Clin Pract* 2003;7(4):281–3.
52. Beber E, Cooper SA. Depression and porphyria: Safe use of fluoxetine in a woman with learning disabilities. *Int J Psychiatr Clin Pract* 1998;2(4): 303–5.

Part VI: SPECIAL ISSUES IN MANAGEMENT OF PSYCHOCUTANEOUS DISORDERS

Joseph L. Calles

21 Psychiatric complications of dermatological treatments

It has been observed for quite some time that patients who suffer from dermatologic diseases also often struggle with emotional symptoms. As more therapeutic agents have been discovered for the treatment of dermatologic disorders, so too has it been appreciated that some of those treatments can produce their own emotional symptoms. The aim of this discussion is to familiarize clinicians who treat cutaneous diseases with (a) the psychiatric symptoms that can derive from dermatologic treatments, (b) the psychopathology that can be comorbid with dermatologic diseases, and (c) the potential drug–drug interactions that can arise during the concurrent treatment of dermatologic and psychiatric pathology.

21.1 Introduction

The therapeutic options for the treatment of dermatologic disorders have expanded over time and are a combination of specific dermatological agents as well as drugs that have been borrowed from other areas of medicine. Along with the increasing availability and use of medications has come the increased risk of potential adverse drug reactions (ADRs). Physicians who treat skin disorders are familiar with the most common ADRs to the most common agents that they prescribe, e.g. gastrointestinal upset from antibiotics. What may not be as familiar to physicians are the possible central nervous system (CNS) effects of dermatological treatments, especially those that present as psychopathology. This chapter reviews the medications used in dermatologic practice that are most commonly associated with the development of psychiatric symptoms. There will also be a brief overview of some of the potential problems that can arise when concurrently treating dermatologic and psychiatric disorders.

21.2 Epidemiology

A Danish literature review on ADRs in children found that the largest share of ADRs (in 9–83% of studies) was reported for systemic anti-infective agents (1). That same review also found that 5–46% patients reported experiencing “nervous system and psychiatric disorders” as side effects to medications from all classes (1). The Danish group subsequently reviewed the ADRs associated with off-label (i.e. outside the approved age group) prescribing in children and adolescents (2). Off-label vs. approved prescribing was more likely to lead to a serious ADR (60% vs. 35%). The medication group that included "dermatologicals" was one of three groups with the highest share of serious off-label ADRs (2). This study did not categorize ADRs by organ system affected.

The accurate measurement of incidence and prevalence of psychiatric symptoms as ADRs in dermatologic practice has been limited by the under-recognition and under-documentation of this association. This becomes apparent when reviewing the literature, as most ADRs are published as either single case reports or as small case series. Given these limitations, what follows are descriptions of the medications used in dermatology that are most likely to produce psychiatric symptomatology.

21.3 Clinical features by medication category

21.3.1 Antibacterial agents

The fluoroquinolones are used to treat abscesses, cellulitis, and skin ulcers, as well as uncomplicated cutaneous infections in patients who are allergic to the penicillins. Of all the different types of antibiotics used in dermatologic practice, the fluoroquinolones are the most likely to be associated with psychiatric ADRs. In France, between 1985 and 2002, there were a reported 590 psychiatric ADRs to the fluoroquinolones (3). Among the highest reported symptoms were confusion (51%), hallucinations (27%), agitation (13%), and delirium (12%). There were also less frequent reports of anxiety, mania, and depression. All agents from this medication class were implicated, and most had been administered orally.

An Italian study compared the rates of ADRs among the different fluoroquinolones and between them and other types of antibacterial agents (4). Although the fluoroquinolones produced fewer cutaneous ADRs, they were associated with significantly higher rates of CNS (12.2% vs. 3.6%) and psychiatric (9.3% vs. 1.8%) ADRs. The most frequently reported serious psychiatric reaction was hallucinations. Abouesh and colleagues reviewed published and unpublished reports of mania induced by antimicrobial agents (5). The unpublished reports were obtained from the World Health Organization (WHO) and the U.S. Food and Drug Administration (FDA). WHO reported 82 cases (mostly adults) of antimicrobial-related mania, of which 14.4% were associated with ciprofloxacin, 12% with ofloxacin, and 3.6% with norfloxacin. The FDA similarly provided data on 61 adult cases, 23% of which were associated with fluoroquinolones, and of those, all but 3 cases were related to ciprofloxacin.

The macrolide antibiotics are also used to treat abscesses, ulcers, and numerous other cutaneous infections; erythromycin is also commonly used to treat acne vulgaris. In the previously cited review (5), in the data provided by the WHO, clarithromycin-related mania accounted for 27.6% of cases and erythromycin-related mania for 6%. In that same review, of the FDA-reported cases of antimicrobial-related mania, 31 of 61 (50.8%) were associated with clarithromycin; 3 cases were related to erythromycin (5).

A report from Turkey described a 12-year-old boy with pneumonia that developed symptoms of mania after just one dose of clarithromycin (6). An older case report describes a 4-year-old boy who was prescribed erythromycin for an upper respiratory infection (7). He developed uncontrollable, alternating crying and laughing, which abated upon discontinuation of the drug. A subsequent, inadvertent re-treatment with erythromycin produced identical symptoms, which once again went away when the drug was stopped. The authors made the point that the child did not experience similar symptoms with other antibiotics.

There are scattered reports in the literature of other antimicrobial agents producing psychiatric symptomatology, including depersonalization related to minocycline (8), delirium related to cephalexin (9), and psychosis related to cotrimoxazole (10).

21.3.2 Antiviral agents

Some of the most common cutaneous virus-related eruptions are due to the herpes simplex virus (HSV) and the related varicella-zoster virus (VZV). In the United States there are currently five FDA-approved oral agents to treat herpes infections. What is interesting – but not necessarily surprising – is that the neuropsychiatric ADRs associated with these agents are usually reported in patients with renal failure or who are on other medications with the potential for causing their own neuropsychiatric ADRs (11).

Not all patients, however, have had those risk factors. For example, a 63-year-old male developed depression, paranoid delusions, and suicidal ideation 5 days after starting intravenous acyclovir (for widespread HSV dermatitis) (12). Treatment with haloperidol for 2 days and discontinuation of the acyclovir (in that order) led to a rapid resolution of the psychosis, but the persistent depression was ultimately treated with an antidepressant. The patient had normal renal functioning; however, he had previously been treated for chronic lymphocytic leukemia with chlorambucil and prednisone, which were discontinued prior to the use of acyclovir. After discussing the complexities of the case, the authors conclude that the most likely explanation for the symptoms is acyclovir-related neurotoxicity.

A brief conference abstract describes a 22-year-old, previously healthy female who was started on acyclovir for VZV infection (13). She developed irritable mood and grandiose delusions 72 hours after the medication was initiated, and she was psychiatrically hospitalized for persistent symptoms 2 weeks after discontinuing the acyclovir. Her symptoms resolved with haloperidol after only modest improvement when treated with olanzapine.

21.3.3 Corticosteroids

The synthetic glucocorticoids are commonly used to treat inflammatory dermatoses and are administered systemically when the conditions are severe, widespread, or non-responsive to topical steroid treatments. The long term use of these agents can have profound adverse physiologic effects, including effects on the CNS (14). Neuropsychiatric ADRs from corticosteroids vary depending on patient age, the dosage, and duration of steroid use. For example, the young and the elderly are more sensitive to the adverse cognitive effects, such as inattention, poor concentration, and memory difficulties.

Regarding mood disturbances, short term, high-dose pulse treatment with corticosteroids is more likely to precipitate mania, whereas longer term treatment is more likely to be associated with depression (14). Data from a French database demonstrated that glucocorticoid-related neuropsychiatric ADRs in children and adolescents were more likely to occur in cases of overdosage or high dosage (combined 44.2% of the total) (15). In that study, the most common ADRs were agitation/excitation in 43.4% and sleep disturbances in 18.4% of the patients. Although “steroid psychosis” is often mentioned as a possible ADR, it was only identified in 8.1% of the patients. Adults treated with corticosteroids are twice as likely as controls to develop psychosis (16).

21.3.4 Dapsone

The sulfone drug dapsone is FDA-approved for the treatment of dermatitis herpetiformis and leprosy and is used off-label for several other dermatoses. The earliest reports of dapsone-related psychiatric ADRs were of psychosis in African patients being treated for leprosy (17). There have been two reports of non-psychotic psychiatric disturbances related to dapsone treatment of non-leprosy dermatologic conditions. The first report was of a 37-year-old female with erythema multiforme who rapidly developed hypomania, followed by depression, after starting dapsone (18). The second was of a 35-year-old male with dermatitis herpetiformis who had been treated for 6 months with dapsone before experiencing depression and anger after each dose of the medication (19).

21.3.5 Antimalarial agents

The antimalarial drugs chloroquine and hydroxychloroquine are approved for the treatment of the variable cutaneous manifestations of systemic lupus erythematosus (SLE). These agents are also used off-label for several other dermatoses. The better-tolerated hydroxychloroquine is preferred over chloroquine as the latter is associated with many more ADRs, including the neuropsychiatric variety. Chloroquine has been implicated in producing symptoms of mania. A 33-year-old male was prescribed chloroquine (along with proquanil) for malaria prophylaxis (20). After each dose of chloroquine he experienced arousal, and with continued use he became irritable, overly active, and talkative, with racing thoughts as well as grandiose delusions; he also maintained a clear sensorium. A series of six patients, ages 17–38 years of age, were started on chloroquine for the presumptive diagnosis of malaria (21). All of the patients developed symptoms of mania, which included irritable/labile mood, increased or "irrelevant" speech, decreased sleep, and grandiosity.

Chloroquine can also produce a clinical picture of psychosis, and younger patients may be at particular risk for that reaction. A series of 10 Indian children, ages 5–12 years of age, developed psychotic symptoms (not detailed) when exposed to initial and subsequent doses of chloroquine, with resolution of symptoms upon drug discontinuation (22). A 15-year-old female with SLE developed a psychotic, confusional state that was presumed to be secondary to phencyclidine, until it was discovered that she had been taking chloroquine (purchased from India) instead of the prescribed hydroxychloroquine (23).

21.3.6 Retinoids

A variety of dermatologic disorders have been treated using the retinoid drugs, especially acitretin for psoriasis and isotretinoin for acne vulgaris, as they are FDA-approved for those indications. Isotretinoin is the most commonly prescribed retinoid as acne is prevalent in the adolescent population (see Chapter 7). There has been some controversy surrounding use of isotretinoin as there had been reports of it causing depression and even suicide. Subsequent studies have not found a correlation between use of this drug and those particular adverse outcomes (24,25); also, some reports have documented improvements in depression and quality of life with this medication (26,27).

The aforementioned data do not mean that the retinoids are devoid of psychiatric ADRs. A male with acne vulgaris, and without a prior history of psychiatric illness, developed symptoms of obsessive compulsive disorder (OCD) at age 23, about 7 years after treatment with isotretinoin was initiated (28). The OCD was treated with fluvoxamine, which precipitated a mixed manic-depressive state, which in turn was unsuccessfully treated with carbamazepine. The patient was finally free of OCD and bipolar symptoms with a combination of fluvoxamine and olanzapine. In individuals with pre-existing bipolar disorder and acne, treatment with isotretinoin destabilizes mood in the majority, and mood is generally restabilized upon discontinuation of the drug (29).

21.3.7 Interferons

This family of secretory glycoproteins comprises two main types and several classes. They are used primarily in the treatment of viral and neoplastic disorders but have also been used in other dermatoses. Interferons are known for their neurotoxic effects, which can manifest as delirium, depression, and – rarely – mania and psychosis (30). The major depressive disorder (MDD) that is secondary to the effects of interferon-alpha is virtually indistinguishable from primary MDD (31). The risk of developing mood instability and mania associated with interferon-alpha-2b may be increased when interferon doses fluctuate, are reduced, or are halted (32). The risk may persist for up to 6 months after discontinuation of the interferon.

21.3.8 Other agents

Cyclosporine is a non-cytotoxic immunosuppressive agent that is FDA-approved for the treatment of psoriasis (see Chapter 6) and is used off-label for numerous other dermatoses. A 44-year-old man with a known history of paranoid schizophrenia had an exacerbation of his psychiatric symptoms when his psoriasis was treated with cyclosporine A (33). The symptoms resolved, and the psoriasis was successfully treated when the cyclosporine was replaced with etanercept.

21.4 Differential diagnosis

An important distinction needs to be made between the psychiatric symptoms that are ADRs to dermatologic treatments and the symptoms of psychiatric disorders that are comorbid with dermatologic disorders. This is important, as psychiatric symptoms and disorders are fairly common in individuals with skin diseases, a topic that is discussed in Chapter 24 in this book.

21.5 Management

The clinical management of the psychiatric symptoms produced by dermatologic treatments can be facilitated by following some basic principles. First, stop the offending agent, if possible. This may involve a risk-benefit decision, especially if the medication is effective and there are no suitable alternatives. Second, if the dermatologic treatment is efficacious enough to warrant continued use, treat the psychiatric symptoms or syndrome.

The clinician should be aware of important aspects of the use of psychotropic medications in that scenario. Some of the drugs used to treat psychiatric disorders may cause cutaneous ADRs. Also, depending on how the drugs are metabolized, concurrent use of certain dermatologic agents and psychotropic agents could make one or the other less effective or could lead to untoward results, such as toxicity. Finally, at any point in the process, consider initiating non-pharmacologic therapies, especially if the psychiatric symptoms (e.g. depression or anxiety) are thought to be psychological responses to the dermatologic condition (see Chapter 23).

21.5.1 Drug–drug interactions

As previously noted, committing to continued treatment with a dermatologic agent concurrent with the use of a psychotropic agent can either (a) make the agents used less effective, and/or (b) raise the level of those agents and increase the risk for an adverse, possibly dangerous outcome. It is important for clinicians to be familiar with some of the more common drug interactions. Table 21.1 lists the drug–drug interactions between carbamazepine and the related oxcarbazepine and various dermatologic agents; the other mood stabilizers are much less likely to interact with dermatologic medications. Table 21.2 lists the antipsychotics and the dermatologic agents that can affect antipsychotic blood levels. Table 21.3 describes some notable interactions between selected antidepressants and dermatologic medications.

21.5.2 Non-pharmacologic interventions

Whether psychiatric symptoms are a psychological reaction to the dermatologic condition, an adverse medication effect, or a comorbid psychiatric disorder, all patients can benefit from more than strict medical treatments. Educating patients and their families about the dermatologic disease, the connection to psychosocial changes, and the effects of medications can alleviate anxiety and despondency. If available in the community, referral to a patient support group can be immensely helpful.

Table 21.1: Drug–drug interactions: dermatologic and mood stabilizer medications

Mood stabilizer	Dermatologic	Effect
Carbamazepine (CBZ)	Erythromycin, troleandomycin, clarithromycin, ketaconazole, itraconazole, fluconazole, and voriconazole	Can increase CBZ levels
	Cyclosporine, corticosteroids, doxycycline, itraconazole	CBZ can decrease the levels of these medications
Oxcarbazepine (OXC)	Cyclosporine	OXC can decrease the levels of this medication

Table 21.2: Drug–drug interactions: dermatologic and antipsychotic medications

Antipsychotic	Cytochrome P450 Inhibitors*	Cytochrome P450 Inducers**
Risperidone	Erythromycin, clarithromycin, telithromycin, fluconazole, ketoconazole, itraconazole, voriconazole, ciprofloxacin, norfloxacin	Glucocorticoids
Olanzapine	Fluoroquinolones, ciprofloxacin, interferon	Nafcillin
Quetiapine	(see Risperidone)	(see Risperidone)
Aripiprazole	(see Risperidone)	(see Risperidone)
Ziprasidone	(see Risperidone)	(see Risperidone)
Clozapine	(see Olanzapine)	(see Olanzapine)

*Can increase antipsychotic blood levels; ** Can decrease the antipsychotic blood levels

Early and comprehensive psychological supports can sometimes obviate the need for psychotropic medications, avoiding the potential adverse reactions that were previously noted. If psychiatric treatment is initiated, psychosocial interventions can improve compliance and response (see Chapter 23).

21.6 Conclusion

The clinical management of dermatologic diseases is complicated by high rates of psychiatric symptomatology. It can be further complicated when the decision is made to treat the emotional symptoms with psychotropic medications. This chapter provides an overview of the psychopathology associated with the treatments for dermatologic disorders and the complexities of the concurrent use of dermatologic and psychiatric medications. It is hoped that this information will stimulate further study in this interesting and challenging area of pediatrics.

Table 21.3: Drug–drug interactions: dermatologic and antidepressant medications

Antidepressant	Dermatologic	Effect
Fluoxetine	Fluconazole	Increased risk of cardiotoxicity, including prolonged QTc interval
Citalopram	Fluconazole	Increased risk of serotonin syndrome
Fluvoxamine	Cyclosporine	Increased risk of cyclosporine toxicity
Duloxetine	Ciprofloxacin	Increased duloxetine levels

References

1. Aagaard L, Christensen A, Hansen EH. Information about adverse drug reactions reported in children: a qualitative review of empirical studies. *Br J Clin Pharmacol* 2010;70(4):481–91.
2. Aagaard L, Hansen EH. Prescribing of medicines in the Danish paediatric population outwith the licensed age group: Characteristics of adverse drug reactions. *Br J Clin Pharmacol* 2011; 71(5):751–7.
3. Fluoroquinolones: Psychiatric adverse effects. *Prescrire Int* 2008;17(93):20.
4. Leone R, Venegoni M, Motola D, Moretti U, Piazzetta V, Cocci A, et al. Adverse drug reactions related to the use of fluoroquinolone antimicrobials: An analysis of spontaneous reports and fluoroquinolone consumption data from three Italian regions. *Drug Saf* 2003;26(2):109–20.
5. Abouesh A, Stone C, Hobbs WR. Antimicrobial-induced mania (antibiomania): A review of spontaneous reports. *J Clin Psychopharmacol* 2002;22(1):71–81.
6. Fidan T, Fidan V. Clarithromycin-induced mania in a child. *Int J Clin Pharmacol Ther* 2009;47 (6):402–4.
7. Cohen IJ, Weitz R. Psychiatric complications with erythromycin. *Drug Intell Clin Pharm* 1981;15 (5):388.
8. Cohen PR. Medication-associated depersonalization symptoms: Report of transient depersonalization symptoms induced by minocycline. *S Med J* 2004;97:70–3.
9. Penttilä J, Pasila K, Tiisala A, Sipiläinen P. Delirium in an adolescent patient during treatment with cephalexin. *J Adolesc Health* 2006;39(5):782–3.
10. Weis S, Karagülle D, Kornhuber J, Bayerlein K. Cotrimoxazole-induced psychosis: A case report and review of literature. *Pharmacopsychiatry* 2006;39(6):236–7.
11. Rashiq S, Briewa L, Mooney M, Giancarlo T, Khatib R, Wilson FM. Distinguishing acyclovir neurotoxicity from encephalomyelitis. *J Int Med* 1993;234(5):507–11.
12. Sirota P, Stoler M, Meshulam B. Major depression with psychotic features associated with acyclovir therapy. *Drug Intell Clin Pharm* 1988;22(4):306–8.
13. Vâzquez Caubet JC, Bautista Garrido O, Marín Mayor M, Sanz Fuentenebro J. P02–298 – Acyclovir-induced psychosis with manic symptoms after treating adult chickenpox. *Eur Psychiatry* 2011;26 (suppl 1):894.
14. Fietta P, Fietta P, Delsante G. Central nervous system effects of natural and synthetic glucocorticoids. *Psychiatry Clin Neurosci* 2009;63(5):613–22.
15. Tavassoli N, Montastruc-Fournier J, Montastruc JL; French Association of Regional Pharmacovigilance Centres. Psychiatric adverse drug reactions to glucocorticoids in children and adolescents: A much higher risk with elevated doses. *Br J Clin Pharmacol* 2008;66(4):566–7.
16. Fardet L, Kassar A, Cabane J, Flahault A. Corticosteroid-induced adverse events in adults: Frequency, screening and prevention. *Drug Saf* 2007;30(10):861–81.
17. Daneshmend TK. The neurotoxicity of dapsone. *Adverse Drug React Acute Poisoning Rev* 1984;3 (1):43–58.
18. Carmichael AJ, Paul CJ. Idiosyncratic dapsone induced manic depression. *BMJ* 1989;298 (6686):1524.
19. Gawkrodger D. Manic depression induced by dapsone in patient with dermatitis herpetiformis. *BMJ* 1989;299(6703):860.
20. Lovestone S. Chloroquine-induced mania. *Br J Psychiatry* 1991;159(1):164–5.
21. Akhtar S, Mukherjee S. Chloroquine induced mania. *Int J Psychiatry Med* 1993;23(4):349–56.
22. Bhatia MS. Chloroquine-induced recurrent psychosis (brief report). *Indian J Med Sci* 1996;50 (11):302–4.
23. Collins GB, McAllister MS. Chloroquine psychosis masquerading as PCP: A case report. *J Psychoactive Drugs* 2008;40(2):211–4.

24. Cohen J, Adams S, Patten S. No association found between patients receiving isotretinoin for acne and the development of depression in a Canadian prospective cohort. *Can J Clin Pharmacol* 2007;14(2):e227–33.
25. Marqueling AL, Zane LT. Depression and suicidal behavior in acne patients treated with isotretinoin: A systematic review. *Semin Cutan Med Surg* 2007;26(4):210–20.
26. Hahm BJ, Min SU, Yoon MY, Shin YW, Kim JS, Jung JY, et al. Changes of psychiatric parameters and their relationships by oral isotretinoin in acne patients. *J Dermatol* 2009;36(5):255–61.
27. Kaymak Y, Taner E, Taner Y. Comparison of depression, anxiety and life quality in acne vulgaris patients who were treated with either isotretinoin or topical agents. *Int J Dermatol* 2009;48(1): 41–6.
28. Fornaro M. Obsessive-compulsive disorder with bipolar diathesis following isotretinoin therapy remitting upon treatment with olanzapine and fluvoxamine. *Neuropsychiatr Dis Treat* 2010;6: 719–22.
29. Schaffer LC, Schaffer CB, Hunter S, Miller A. Psychiatric reactions to isotretinoin in patients with bipolar disorder. *J Affect Disord* 2010;122(3):306–8.
30. Patten SB. Psychiatric side effects of interferon treatment. *Curr Drug Saf* 2006;1(2):143–50.
31. Lotrich FE. Major depression during interferon-alpha treatment: Vulnerability and prevention. *Dialogues Clin Neurosci* 2009;11(4):417–25.
32. Greenberg DB, Jonasch E, Gadd MA, Ryan BF, Everett JR, Sober AJ, et al. Adjuvant therapy of melanoma with interferon-alpha-2b is associated with mania and bipolar syndromes. *Cancer* 2000;89(2):356–62.
33. Di Nuzzo S, Zanni M, De Panfilis G. Exacerbation of paranoid schizophrenia in a psoriatic patient after treatment with cyclosporine A, but not with etanercept. *J Drugs Dermatol* 2007;6(10):1046–7.

Misha M. Heller, Meagan Barrett, Stefani Takahashi,
Jenny Murase, and Josephine L. Howard

22 Dermatologic manifestations of psychotropic medications

Psychotropic medications including mood stabilizers, antidepressants, anxiolytics, antipsychotics, and stimulants are increasingly being prescribed to pediatric and adolescent patients. These medications are known to cause adverse cutaneous reactions. Although most dermatologic manifestations of psychotropic medications are benign, some may require immediate medical attention. This chapter reviews the clinical features of common adverse cutaneous reactions, serious and life-threatening cutaneous reactions, and general dermatologic conditions frequently associated with psychotropic medications. Ultimately, with the knowledge of how to recognize the cutaneous patterns of these adverse drug reactions, the clinician should be better able to identify the offending agents and offer appropriate therapeutic management.

22.1 Introduction

In the past two decades, there has been a considerable increase in the pediatric and adolescent use of psychotropic medications (1). Dermatologic side effects associated with psychotropic medications are common, and the majority of these adverse reactions are benign and easily treated (2,3). However, rare, serious, and life-threatening events do occur. Understanding the types of common and potentially life-threatening dermatologic side effects is critically important as it helps the clinician to identify the offending agent. The purpose of this chapter is to discuss the presentation and management of various types of adverse cutaneous drug reactions (ACDRs) seen with psychotropic medications; this includes those seen with mood stabilizing agents, antidepressants, anxiolytics, antipsychotics, and stimulants. Table 22.1 provides a complete list of the psychotropic medications described here.

22.1.1 Epidemiology

In a hospital setting, ACDRs to any medication are estimated to occur in approximately 2% of patients (4,5,6). The prevalence of ACDRs to psychotropic medications are thought to be significantly higher. Studies have reported that as many as 5% of patients experience ACDRs while taking psychotropic medications. However, it is difficult to assess the true prevalence of ACDRs since many cases are not reported in the literature (7,8).

Table 22.1: List of psychotropic medications

Mood Stabilizing Agents	Antidepressants			
	SSRIs	**TCAs**	**MAOIs**	**Other Antidepressants**
Lithium*	Fluoxetine**	Desipramine	Phenelzine	Bupropriont
Carbamazepine	Fluvoxamine**	Nortriptyline**	Tranylcypromine	Venlafaxine
Valproic acid	Paroxetine**	Protriptyline	Isocarboxazid	Mirtazapine
Lamotrigine	Sertraline**	Amitriptyline**		Trazodone**
Oxcarbazepine	Citalopram	Doxepin		
Gabapentin	Escitalopram**	Clomipramine**		
Topiramate		Imipramine**		

Anxiolytics		Antipsychotics		Stimulants
Benzodiazepines	**Non-Benzodiazepine**	**Atypicals**	**Typicals**	
Alprazolam	Buspirone††	Risperidone*‡	Haloperidol	Dextroamphetamine†
Diazepam††		Aripiprazole*‡	Pimozide	Methylphenidate†
Clonazepam		Ziprasidone	Chlorpromazine	Lisdexamfetamine†
Lorazepam††		Quetiapine*‡	Perphenazine	
		Olanzapine*‡	Thioridazine	
		Clozapine	Trifluoperazine	
			Fluphenazine	
			Prochlorperazine	

Abbreviations: SSRIs = selective serotonin reuptake inhibitors, TCAs = tricyclic antidepressants, and MAOIs = monoamine oxidase inhibitors.
*This medication is approved for pediatric use for the treatment of bipolar disorder.
**This medication is approved for pediatric use for the treatment of major depressive disorder and/or obsessive compulsive disorder.
†This medication is approved for pediatric use for the treatment of ADHD.
††This medication is approved for pediatric use for the treatment of anxiety.
‡This medication is approved for pediatric use for the treatment of schizophrenia.
This table indicates all the psychotropic medications discussed in this chapter that can cause dermatologic side effects.

22.2 Diagnosis

In order to diagnose a drug eruption, it is essential to collect a complete history of all the medications, both prescription and non-prescription, that the patient has taken.

A timeline can be helpful in assessing the timing of exposure to the medication relative to the cutaneous eruption. Determine how the medication in question was administered (i.e. topical, oral, intramuscular, or intravenous). One should assess whether the patient has any associated symptoms (i.e. fevers, chills, diarrhea, etc.). Determine if the patient has any known drug allergies and if other family members have had unusual drug reactions. Evaluate for other medical problems that may predispose the patient to drug reactions. Also, one should perform a thorough physical examination with a detailed account of primary skin lesions, secondary skin changes, as well as the distribution and configuration of these lesions.

The suspected medication should be withdrawn as soon as possible. This is especially crucial in life-threatening drug eruptions, such as Stevens-Johnson syndrome (SJS) and toxic epidermolysis necrolysis (TEN). All medications that are not essential should be discontinued. These medications can later be reintroduced slowly, one by one. The patient can also be rechallenged with the medication in question. Although this is the most definitive diagnostic approach of determining the offending agent, it can be potentially dangerous and should never be performed if the medication in question can cause a serious drug eruption (9).

22.3 Pathogenesis

Most drug reactions are due to a hypersensitivity reaction with an underlying immunologic response. The offending drug and its metabolites act as haptens covalently binding to peptides, thereby eliciting a specific cell-mediated or humoral immune response. In contrast, drug reactions resulting from a non-immunologic response can be attributed to many factors, such as cumulative dose toxicity, drug overdose, and drug–drug interactions (9).

Immunologically mediated drug reactions are classified as Type I (Immunoglobulin-E mediated reactions), Type II (cytotoxic reactions), Type III (Immunoglobulin-G or -M mediated reactions), or Type IV (delayed-type hypersensitivity reactions). Examples of drug-induced type I reactions of the skin include urticaria and angioedema. If the medication is given orally, there can be a 1–2 hour delay before symptoms occur. However, with intravenous administration, symptoms can occur almost immediately. Regardless of the route of administration, anaphylaxis may develop.

Classic examples of type II reactions are antibiotic-induced hemolytic anemia and thrombocytopenic purpura. However, an alternative type II reaction can be autoimmune bullous diseases (e.g. drug-induced pemphigus). Type III reactions include serum sickness and leukocytoclastic vasculitis. Serum-sickness usually takes place about 1 to 3 weeks following the drug administration. Drug-induced type IV reactions of the skin include exanthematous reactions, fixed drug eruptions, lichenoid reactions, SJS, and TEN (9).

22.4 Categories

A useful method of simplifying the many dermatologic manifestations of psychotropic medications is to group them into three broad categories: common adverse cutaneous reactions, serious and life-threatening cutaneous reactions, and general dermatologic conditions. The first category represents the common adverse cutaneous reactions (e.g. pruritus, exanthematous drug eruptions, urticaria and angioedema, fixed drug eruption, photosensitivity, pigmentation, diaphoresis, and alopecia) (see Table 22.2).

The second category consists of serious and life-threatening cutaneous reactions (e.g. erythema multiforme, SJS, TEN, drug hypersensitivity syndrome, vasculitis, exfoliative dermatitis, and anaphylaxis) (see Table 22.3). The third category includes cutaneous reactions that can cause an exacerbation or initiation of a general dermatologic condition (e.g. acne, psoriasis, seborrhea, and lichenoid eruptions) (see Table 22.4) (10,11,12,13). Please see Tables 22.5 to 22.13, which identify the ACDRs observed with each class of psychotropic medications.

22.5 Common adverse cutaneous reactions

22.5.1 Pruritus

Pruritus (or itching) can occur secondary to other ACDRs, or as a primary adverse drug effect. Pruritus has been reported in almost all psychotropic medications (10). Pruritus may be localized or generalized. Patients often report more intense itching at nighttime. On physical examination, patients may demonstrate a range of findings, from normal skin to severe areas of excoriation. Other possible etiologies of pruritus can include metabolic and endocrine diseases, malignancy, hematologic diseases, hepatic diseases, infections, infestation, and underlying dermatologic conditions.

If, however, the pruritus is a result of the psychotropic medication, discontinuation of the offending agent generally resolves symptoms, but it is not always necessary to do. When the patient is responding well to the medication, the clinician may consider continuing the psychotropic medication and providing the patient with symptomatic treatment. Emollients and anti-itch lotions can be helpful in alleviating pruritus. Oral therapies such as antihistamines, tranquilizers, and opiate antagonists can also provide significant relief (9,10,11,12,13,14,15,16,17).

22.5.2 Exanthematous eruptions

Exanthematous (or morbilliform) eruptions are the most common form of ACDRs and can occur with nearly all psychotropic medications (10). The cutaneous reaction

Table 22.2: Cutaneous adverse reactions of psychotropic medications

Cutaneous Adverse Reactions	Mood Stabilizers	SSRI	TCAs	MAOIs	Other Anti-depressants	Benzodi-azepines	Non-Benzodi-azepines	Atypical Antipsy-chotics	Typical Antipsychotic	Stimulants
Pruritus	Lithium (<1%) Carbamazepine (<1%) Valproic acid (>5%) Lamotrigine (3%) Gabapentin (1%) Topiramate (2%)	Fluoxetine (2%) Fluvoxamine Paroxetine (<1%) Sertraline (<1%) Citalopram (<10%) Escitalopram (<1%)	Desipramine Nortriptyline Protriptyline Amitriptyline Doxepin Clomipramine (6%) Imipramine (3%)	Phenelzine (13%) Tranylcypromine	Bupropion (4%) Venlafaxine (1–10%) Trazodone (<1%)	Alprazolam Diazepam Clonazepam Lorazepam	Buspirone (1%)	Risperidone (<1%) Aripiprazole Olanzapine (>1%) Clozapine (<1%)	Haloperidol (<1%) Pimozide Chlorpromazine (1–10%) Perphenazine Trifluoperazine Fluphenazine (<1%) Prochlorperazine (1–10%)	Methylphenidate
Exanthems	Lithium Valproic acid Lamotrigine (1–10%)	Fluoxetine (4%) Fluvoxamine Paroxetine (<1%) Sertraline (<1%) Citalopram	Desipramine Nortriptyline Protriptyline Amitriptyline Doxepin Clomipramine Imipramine (1–6%)	Phenelzine Tranylcypromine Isocarboxazide (7%)	Bupropion (<1%) Venlafaxine (<1%) Trazodone	Alprazolam Diazepam Clonazepam Lorazepam	Buspirone	Aripiprazole Olanzapine (<1%) Clozapine	Haloperidol Pimozide Chlorpromazine (>5%) Perphenazine Trifluoperazine Fluphenazine Prochlorperazine	Methylphenidate
Urticaria	Lithium Carbamazepine Valproic acid Lamotrigine (<1%)	Fluoxetine (4%) Fluvoxamine (<1%) Paroxetine (<1%)	Desipramine Nortriptyline Protriptyline Amitriptyline Doxepin	Phenelzine Tranylcypromine	Bupropion Venlafaxine (<1%) Trazodone	Alprazolam Diazepam Clonazepam Lorazepam	Buspirone (<1%)	Risperidone Aripiprazole Ziprasidone (5%) Olanzapine (<1%)	Haloperidol Pimozide Chlorpromazine Perphenazine Thioridazine Trifluoperazine	Dextroamphetamine (<1%) Methylphenidate

(Continued)

Table 22.2: Cutaneous adverse reactions of psychotropic medications (*Continued*)

Cutaneous Adverse Reactions	Mood Stabilizers	SSRI	TCAs	MAOIs	Other Anti-depressants	Benzodi-azepines	Non-Benzodi-azepines	Atypical Antipsy-chotics	Typical Antipsychotic	Stimulants
	Gabapentin Topiramate	Sertraline (<1%) Citalopram	Clomipramine (1%) Imipramine					Clozapine (<1%)	Fluphenazine Prochlorperazine	
Pigmentation	Lithium (<1%) Carbamazepine Gabapentin Topiramate (<1%)	Fluoxetine (<1%) Fluvoxamine (<1%) Paroxetine (<1%) Sertraline (<1%) Citalopram	Desipramine (blue-gray) Amitriptyline Clomipramine Imipramine		Venlafaxine (<1%)	Diazepam		Risperidone (1%) Olanzapine (<1%)	Haloperidol (<1%) Pimozide Chlorpromazine (<1%) Perphenazine (<1%) (blue-gray) Thioridazine (<1%) (blue-gray) Trifluoperazine (<1%) (blue-gray) Fluphenazine (<1%) (blue-gray) Prochlorperazine (<1%)	
Diaphoresis	Carbamazepine (1–10%) Valproic acid Lamotrigine (<1%) Oxcarbazepine (3%) Topiramate (2%)	Fluoxetine (8%) Fluvoxamine (<7%) Paroxetine (11%) Sertraline (8%)	Desipramine (1–10%) Nortriptyline (1–10%) Protriptyline (1–10%) Amitriptyline (1–10%)	Bupropion (5%) Venlafaxine Mirtazapine Trazodone (>1%)		Alprazolam Diazepam Clonazepam (>10%) Lorazepam (>10%)	Buspirone	Risperidone Aripiprazole Ziprasidone Quetiapine (1–10%) Olanzapine (>1%) Clozapine (6%)	Haloperidol Pimozide Perphenazine Trifluoperazine Fluphenazine Prochlorperazine	Dextroamphetamine (1–10%) Methylphenidate

		Citalopram (11%) Escitalopram (5%)	Doxepin (1–10%) Clomipramine (29%) Imipramine (1–25%)							
Alopecia	Lithium (10–19%) Carbamazepine Valproic Acid (7%) Lamotrigine (1%) Oxcarbazepine Gabapentin Topiramate (>1%)	Fluoxetine (<1%) Fluvoxamine (<1%) Paroxetine (<1%) Sertraline (<1%) Citalopram Escitalopram (<1%)	Desipramine (<1%) Nortriptyline (<1%) Protriptyline (<1%) Amitriptyline (<1%) Doxepin (<1%) Clomipramine (<1%) Imipramine (<1%)	Bupropion (<1%) Venlafaxine (<1%) Trazodone		Clonazepam Lorazepam	Buspirone (<1%)	Risperidone (<1%) Aripiprazole Ziprasidone (<1%) Quetiapine Olanzapine (<1%)	Haloperidol (<1%) Thioridazine	Methylphenidate

Table 22.3: Serious and Life-Threatening Cutaneous Reaction of Psychiatric Medications

Serious Cutaneous Reactions	Mood Stabilizers	SSRI	TCAs	Other Antidepressants	Benzodiazepines	Antipsychotics	Stimulants
Erythema Multiforme	Lithium Carbamazepine Valproic acid (<1%) Lamotrigine Oxcarbazepine	Fluoxetine Paroxetine Sertraline (<1%) Citalopram	Desipramine Nortriptyline Protriptyline Amitriptyline Doxepin Clomipramine (6%) Imipramine (3%)	Bupropion	Clonazepam Lorazepam	Quetiapine Clozapine (<1%)	Methylphenidate
Stevens-Johnson syndrome	Carbamazepine (1–10%) Valproic acid Lamotrigine (1–10%) Oxcarbazepine Gabapentin	Fluoxetine Fluvoxamine Paroxetine Sertraline		Bupropion Venlafaxine	Alprazolam Lorazepam		Lisdexamfetamine
Toxic Epidermolysis Necrosis	Carbamazepine (1–10%) Valproic acid Lamotrigine Oxcarbazepine	Fluoxetine Fluvoxamine (<1%) Paroxetine		Venlafaxine		Thioridazine Fluphenazine Prochlorperazine Clozapine (<1%)	Dextroamphetamine Lisdexamfetamine
Hypersensitivity Syndrome	Carbamazepine Valproic acid Lamotrigine (1–10%)	Fluoxetine	Desipramine Amitriptyline Clomipramine	Bupropion Trazodone	Diazepam	Thioridazine	Methylphenidate (1–10%) Lisdexamfetamine

	Oxcarbazepine Gabapentin						
Vasculitis	Lithium Carbamazepine Valproic Acid Gabapentin	Fluoxetine Paroxetine Citalopram	Desipramine Nortriptyline Protriptyline Amitriptyline Doxepin Clomipramine Imipramine	Trazodone	Diazepam	Olanzapine (<1%) Clozapine (<1%) Chlorpromazine Thioridazine	Methylphenidate
Exfoliative Dermatitis	Lithium (1%) Carbamazepine	Fluoxetine Fluvoxamine (<1%) Paroxetine	Desipramine Amitriptyline Doxepin Imipramine	Bupropion Venlafaxine (<1%) Mirtazapine	Diazepam	Risperidone Aripiprazole Ziprasidone Haloperidol Chlorpromazine Perphenazine Trifluoperazine	Methylphenidate
Anaphylactoid Reactions	Lamotrigine	Fluoxetine (<1%) Fluvoxamine Escitalopram (<1%)	Amitriptyline	Bupropion Venlafaxine	Diazepam	Risperidone Quetiapine Chlorpromazine (<1%) Perphenazine Thioridazine Trifluoperazine Fluphenazine Prochlorperazine (1–10%)	Lisdexamfetamine

Abbreviations: SSRIs = selective serotonin reuptake inhibitors, TCAs = tricylic antidepressants, and MAOIs = monoamine oxidase inhibitors.
This table represents the serious and life-threatening cutaneous reactions as a result of psychotropic medications.
If indicated, the incidence of the specific adverse cutaneous reactions is given (1).

Table 22.4: Psychotropic medication–induced dermatologic conditions

Dermatologic Condition	Mood Stabilizers	SSRI	TCAs	Other Antidepressants	Anxiolytics	Atypical Antipsychotics	Typical Antipsychotic
Lichenoid Reaction	Lithium Carbamazepine	Fluoxetine	Amitriptyline Imipramine	Venlafaxine (<1%)		Risperidone Olanzapine	Chlorpromazine Thioridazine
Acneform Eruption	Lithium Carbamazepine Valproic acid Lamotrigine (1%) Oxcarbazepine Gabapentin (>1%) Topiramate (>1%)	Fluoxetine (<1%) Fluvoxamine (<1%) Paroxetine (<1%) Sertraline (<1%) Escitalopram (<1%)	Desipramine Nortriptyline Protriptyline Amitriptyline Clomipramine (2%) Imipramine	Bupropion (1–10%) Venlafaxine (<1%) Mirtazapine	Alprazolam Diazepam Buspirone (<1%)	Risperidone Aripiprazole Quetiapine	Haloperidol
Psoriasis	Lithium (2%) Carbamazepine Valproic acid Gabapentin	Fluoxetine (<1%) Paroxetine Citalopram		Venlafaxine (<1%) Mirtazapine		Risperidone (<1%) Aripiprazole Olanzapine	
Seborrhea	Lithium Valproic acid Gabapentin Topiramate (<1%)	Fluoxetine (<1%) Fluvoxamine (<1%) Paroxetine	Clomipramine		Buspirone	Risperidone Aripiprazole Olanzapine (<1%)	Haloperidol Chlorpromazine Perphenazine Thioridazine Trifluoperazine Fluphenazine Prochlorperazine

Abbreviations: SSRIs = selective serotonin reuptake inhibitors, TCAs = tricylic antidepressants, and MAOIs = monoamine oxidase inhibitors. This table represents general dermatologic conditions that are initiated or exacerbated by psychotropic medications. If indicated, the incidence of the specific adverse cutaneous reactions is given (10).

Table 22.5: Mood stabilizer–induced dermatologic conditions

Lithium	Carbamazepine	Valproic Acid	Lamotrigine	Oxcarbazepine	Gabapentin	Topiramate
Acneform eruption	Alopecia	Alopecia (7%)	Alopecia (1%)	Alopecia	Alopecia	Alopecia (>1%)
Alopecia (10–19%)	Acneform eruption	Acneform eruption	Acneform eruption (1%)	Acneform eruption	Acneform eruption (>1%)	Acneform eruption (>1%)
Angioedema	Angioedema (<1%)	Diaphoresis	Anaphylactoid reactions	Angioedema	Diaphoresis	Diaphoresis (2%)
Erythema multiforme	Erythema multiforme	Erythema multiforme (<1%)	Angioedema (1–10%)	Diaphoresis (3%)	Exanthems	Exanthems (<1%)
Exanthems	Erythroderma	Exanthems (5%)	Diaphoresis (<1%)	Erythema multiforme	Hypersensitivity	Photosensitivity (<1%)
Exfoliative dermatitis (1%)	Exanthems (>5%)	Fixed eruption	Erythema multiforme	Exanthems	Photosensitivity	Pigmentation (<1%)
Pigmentation (<1%)	Exfoliative dermatitis	Hypersensitivity	Exanthems (1–10%)	Hypersensitivity	Pigmentation	Pruritus (2%)
Pruritus (<1%)	Fixed eruption (<1%)	Photosensitivity	Fixed eruption	Photosensitivity	Pruritus (1%)	Seborrhea (<1%)
Psoriasis (2%)	Hypersensitivity	Pruritus (>5%)	Hypersensitivity (1–10%)	SJS	Psoriasis	Urticaria (<15)
Seborrheic dermatitis	Lichenoid eruption	Psoriasis	Photosensitivity	TEN	Seborrhea	
Urticaria	Photosensitivity	Seborrhea	Pruritus (3%)		SJS	
Vasculitis	Pigmentation	SJS	SJS (1–10%)		Urticaria	
	Pruritus (<1%)	TEN	TEN		Vasculitis	
	Psoriasis	Urticaria	Urticaria (<1%)			
	SJS (1–10%)	Vasculitis				
	TEN (1–10%)					
	Urticaria					
	Vasculitis					

Abbreviations: SJS = Stevens-Johnson Syndrome, TEN = toxic epidermolysis necrosis.
This table specifies the adverse cutaneous drug reactions observed among the mood stabilizing agents. If indicated, the incidence of the specific adverse cutaneous reactions is given (10)

Table 22.6: Dermatologic side effects of selective serotonin reuptake inhibitors

Fluoxetine	Fluvoxamine	Paroxetine	Sertraline	Citalopram	Escitalopram
Alopecia (<1%)	Alopecia (<1%)	Alopecia (<1%)	Alopecia (<1%)	Alopecia	Alopecia (<1%)
Acneform eruption (<1%)	Anaphylactoid reactions	Acneform eruption (<1%)	Acneform eruption (<1%)	Angioedema	Acneform eruption (<1%)
Anaphylactoid reactions (<1%)	Angioedema	Angioedema (<1%)	Angioedema	Diaphoresis (11%)	Anaphylactoid reactions
Angioedema	Diaphoresis (<7%)	Diaphoresis (11%)	Diaphoresis (8%)	Erythema multiforme	Diaphoresis (5%)
Diaphoresis (8%)	Exanthems	Erythema multiforme	Erythema multiforme (<1%)	Exanthems	Pruritus (<1%)
Erythema multiforme	Exfoliative dermatitis (<1%)	Exanthems (<1%)	Exanthems (<1%)	Photopigmentation	
Exanthems (4%)	Photosensitivity (<1%)	Exfoliative dermatitis	Fixed eruption	Photosensitivity	
Exfoliative dermatitis	Pigmentation (<1%)	Photosensitivity (<1%)	Photosensitivity (<1%)	Pruritus (<10%)	
Hypersensitivity	Pruritus	Pigmenation (<1%)	Pigmentation (<1%)	Psoriasis	
Lichenoid eruption	Seborrhea (<1%)	Pruritus (<1%)	Pruritus (<1%)	Urticaria	
Photosensitivity	SJS	Psoriasis	SJS	Vasculitis	
Phototoxicity (<1%)	TEN (<1%)	Seborrhea	Urticaria (<1%)		
Pigmentation (<1%)	Urticaria (<1%)	SJS			
Pruritus (2%)		TEN			
Psoriasis (<1%)		Urticaria (<1%)			
Seborrhea (<1%)		Vasculitis			
Serum sickness					
SJS					
TEN					
Urticaria (4%)					
Vasculitis					

Abbreviations: SJS = Stevens-Johnson Syndrome, TEN = toxic epidermolysis necrosis.
This table specifies the adverse cutaneous drug reactions observed with the selective serotonin reuptake inhibitors. If indicated, the incidence of the specific adverse cutaneous reactions is given (10)

Table 22.7: Cutaneous side effects of tricyclic antidepressants

Desipramine	Nortriptyline	Protriptyline	Amitriptyline	Doxepin	Clomipramine	Imipramine
Alopecia (<1%)	Alopecia (<1%)	Alopecia (<1%)	Alopecia (<1%)	Alopecia (<1%)	Alopecia (<1%)	Alopecia (<1%)
Acneform eruption	Acneform eruption	Acneform eruption	Acneform eruption	Diaphoresis (1–10%)	Acneform eruption (2%)	Acneform eruption
Angioedema	Diaphoresis (1–10%)	Angioedema	Anaphylactoid reactions	Erythroderma	Diaphoresis (29%)	Angioedema (<1%)
Diaphoresis (1–10%)	Exanthems	Diaphoresis (1–10%)	Angioedema	Exanthems	Exanthems	Diaphoresis (1–25%)
Exanthems	Photosensitivity (<1%)	Exanthems	Diaphoresis (1–10%)	Photosensitivity (<1%)	Hypersensitivity	Exanthems (1–6%)
Exfoliative dermatitis	Phototoxicity	Photosensitivity (<1%)	Erythroderma	Pruritus	Photosensitivity (<1%)	Exfoliative dermatitis
Hypersensitivity	Pruritus	Phototoxicity	Exanthems	Urticaria	Pigmentation	Fixed eruptions (<1%)
Photosensitivity (1%)	Urticaria	Pruritus (1–5%)	Exfoliative dermatitis	Vasculitis	Pruritus (6%)	Lichenoid eruption
Pigmentation (blue-gray)	Vasculitis	Urticaria	Fixed eruption		Psoriasis	Photosensitivity (<1%)
Pruritus		Vasculitis	Hypersensitivity		Seborrhea	Pigmentation
Urticaria			Lichenoid eruption		Urticaria (1%)	Pruritus (3%)
Vasculitis			Photosensitivity (<1%)		Vasculitis	Urticaria
			Pigmentation			Vasculitis
			Pruritus			
			Urticaria			
			Vasculitis			

This table specifies the adverse cutaneous drug reactions observed with the tricyclic antidepressants. If indicated, the incidence of the specific adverse cutaneous reactions is given (10)

Table 22.8: Dermatologic side effects of monoamine oxidase inhibitors

Phenelzine	**Tranylcypromine**	**Isocarboxazid**
Angioedema	Diaphoresis	Diaphoresis
Diaphoresis	Exanthems	Exanthems (7%)
Exanthems	Photosensitivity (<1%)	Photosensitivity (4%)
Photosensitivity	Pruritus	Pruritus (4%)
Pruritus (13%)	Urticaria	
Urticaria		

This table specifies the adverse cutaneous drug reactions observed with the monoamine oxidase inhibitors. If indicated, the incidence of the specific adverse cutaneous reactions is given (10)

Table 22.9: Cutaneous side effects of other antidepressants

Bupropion	**Venlafaxine**	**Mirtazapine**	**Trazodone**
Alopecia (<1%)	Alopecia (<1%)	Acneform eruption	Alopecia
Acneform eruption (1–10%)	Acneform eruption (<1%)	Angioedema	Angioedema
Anaphylactoid reactions	Anaphylactoid reactions	Diaphoresis	Diaphoresis (>1%)
Angioedema	Angioedema	Exfoliative dermatitis	Erythema multiforme
Diaphoresis (5%)	Diaphoresis	Exfoliative dermatitis	Exanthems
Edema (>1%)	Erythema multiforme	Photosensitivity	Exfoliative dermatitis
Erythema multiforme	Exanthems (<1%)	Seborrhea	Hypersensitivity
Exanthems (<1%)	Exfoliative dermatitis (<1%)		Photosensitivity
Exfoliative dermatitis	Lichenoid eruption (<1%)		Pruritus (<1%)
Hypersensitivity	Photosensitivity (<1%)		Psoriasis
Photosensitivity (<1%)	Pigmentaton		Urticaria
Pruritus (4%)	Pruritus (1–10%)		Vasculitis
Psoriasis	Psoriasis (<1%)		
SJS	Seborrhea		
Urticaria	SJS		
	TEN		
	Urticaria (<1%)		

Abbreviations: SJS = Stevens-Johnson Syndrome, TEN = toxic epidermolysis necrosis.
This table specifies the adverse cutaneous drug reactions observed with the other antidepressants. If indicated, the incidence of the specific adverse cutaneous reactions is given (10)

Table 22.10: Dermatologic side effects of anxiolytics

Alprazolam	Diazepam	Clonazepam	Lorazepam	Buspirone
Acneform eruption	Acneform eruption	Alopecia	Alopecia	Alopecia (1%)
Angioedema	Anaphylactoid reactions	Angioedema	Diaphoresis (>10%)	Acneform eruption (<1%)
Diaphoresis (16%)	Angioedema	Diaphoresis (>10%)	Erythema multiforme	Diaphoresis
Exanthems	Diaphoresis (>10%)	Erythema multiforme	Exanthems	Exanthems
Photosensitivity	Exanthems	Exanthems	Fixed eruption	Pruritus (1%)
Phototoxicity	Exfoliative dermatitis	Pruritus	Pruritus	Rash(<1%)
Pruritus	Fixed eruption (<1%)	Urticaria	SJS	Seborrheic dermatitis
SJS	Hypersensitivity		Urticaria	Urticaria (<1%)
Urticaria	Pigmentation			
	Pruritus			
	Urticaria			
	Vasculitis			

Abbreviations: SJS = Stevens-Johnson Syndrome
This table specifies the adverse cutaneous drug reactions observed with anxiolytics. If indicated, the incidence of the specific adverse cutaneous reactions is given (10)

generally occurs 1–2 weeks following the start of new medication. If the medication is rechallenged, it can occur within just a few days. The lesions are often described as maculopapular in pattern. They tend to appear as erythematous macules, evolve to papules, and then progress into confluent plaques. The eruption begins on the upper trunk and then spreads outward to extremities in a bilateral and symmetric distribution. The patient may complain of intense pruritus. A low-grade fever may also be present. The eruption typically resolves in 1–2 weeks without complications.

Many drugs can induce exanthemous eruptions. However, anticonvulsants, along with antibiotics (e.g. aminopenicillins, sulfonamides, and cephalosporines), are known to cause the highest incidences of drug-induced exanthems. The differential diagnosis is primarily viral exanthems, particularly in pediatric populations. The clinician should always rule out more severe drug-induced reactions. High temperature, mucous membrane involvement, or painful lesions may suggest SJS or TEN. In drug-induced exanthems, withdrawal of the offending agent is of utmost importance. Therapy is largely supportive; oral antihistamines and topical corticosteroids are generally sufficient, but severe reactions may require systemic steroids (9,10,11,12,13,14,15,16,17).

Table 22.11: Cutaneous adverse effects of atypical antipsychotic medications

Risperidone	Aripiprazole	Ziprasidone	Quetiapine	Olanzapine	Clozapine
Alopecia (<1%)	Alopecia	Alopecia (<1%)	Alopecia	Alopecia (<1%)	Angioedema
Acneform eruption (<1%)	Acneform eruption	Angioedema	Acneform eruption	Angioedema	Diaphoresis (6%)
Anaphlactoid reactions	Angioedema	Diaphoresis	Anaphlactoid reactions	Diaphoresis (>1%)	Erythema multiforme (<1%)
Angioedema	Diaphoresis	Exfoliative dermatitis (<1%)	Angioedema	Exanthems (<1%)	Exanthems
Diaphoresis (<1%)	Exanthems	Photosensitivity	Diaphoresis (1–10%)	Hypersensitivity	Photosensitivity
Exfoliative dermatitis (<1%)	Exfoliative dermatitis	Urticaria (5%)	Erythema multiforme	Lichenoid eruption	Pruritus (<1%)
Hypersensitivity	Pruritus		Hypersensitivity	Photosensitivity (<1%)	SJS (<1%)
Lichenoid eruptions (<1%)	Psoriasis		Photosensitivity (<1%)	Pigmentation (<1%)	Urticaria (<1%)
Photosensitivity (1–10%)	Seborrhea			Pruritus (>1%)	Vasculitis (<1%)
Pigmentation (1%)	SJS			Psoriasis	
Pruritus (<1%)	Urticaria			Seborrhea (<1%)	
Psoriasis (<1%)				Urticaria (<1%)	
Seborrhea				Vasculitis	
Urticaria					

Abbreviations: SJS = Stevens-Johnson Syndrome
This table specifies the adverse cutaneous drug reactions observed with the atypical antipsychotics. If indicated, the incidence of the specific adverse cutaneous reactions is given (10)

Table 22.12: Cutaneous adverse effects of typical antipsychotics

Haloperidol	Pimozide	Chlorpromazine	Perphenazine	Thioridazine	Trifluoperazine	Fluphenazine	Prochlorperazine
Alopecia (<1%)	Diaphoresis	Anaphlactoid reactions (<1%)	Anaphylactoid reactions	Alopecia	Anaphylactoid reactions	Anaphylactoid reactions	Anaphylactoid reactions (1–10%)
Acneform eruption	Exanthems	Angioedema (<1%)	Angioedema	Anaphylactoid reactions	Angioedema	Angioedema (<1%)	Diaphoresis
Diaphoresis	Photosensitivity	Erythema multiforme (<1%)	Diaphoresis	Angioedema (<1%)	Diaphoresis	Diaphoresis	Exanthems
Exanthems	Pigmentation	Exanthems (>5%)	Exanthems		Erythema	Exanthems	Exfoliative dermatitis
Exfoliative dermatitis	Pruritus	Exfoliative dermatitis	Exfoliative dermatitis	Erythema multiforme	Exanthems	Exfoliative dermatitis	Fixed eruption (<1%)
Photosensitivity (<1%)	Urticaria	Fixed eruption (<1%)	Photosensitivity	Exanthems	Exfoliative dermatitis	Photosensitivity	Photosensitivity (1–10%)
Pigmentation (<1%)		Lichenoid eruption	Pigmentation (<1%) (blue-gray)	Exfoliative dermatitis	Fixed eruption	Pigmentation (<1%) (blue-gray)	Phototoxicity
Pruritus (<1%)		Photosensitivity (1–10%)	Pruritus	Hypersensitivity	Photosensitivity (1–10%)	Pruritus (<1%)	Pigmentation (<1%)
Seborrheic dermatitis		Phototoxicity	Seborrhea	Lichenoid eruption	Pigmentation (<1%) (blue-gray)	Seborrhea	Pruritus (1–10%)
Urticaria		Pigmentation (<1%)	Urticaria	Photosensitivity (1–10%)	Pruritus	TEN	Seborrhea
		Pruritus (1–10%)		Phototoxicity	Seborrhea	Urticaria	TEN
		Seborrheic dermatitis		Pigmentation (<1%) (blue-gray)	Urticaria		Urticaria
		TEN (<1%)		Seborrhea			
		Urticaria		TEN			
		Vasculitis		Urticaria			
				Vasculitis			

Abbreviations: SJS = Stevens-Johnson Syndrome
This table specifies the adverse cutaneous drug reactions observed with the typical antipsychotics. If indicated, the incidence of the specific adverse cutaneous reactions is given (10)

Table 22.13: Cutaneous side effects of stimulant medications

Dextroamphetamine	Methylphenidate	Lisdexamfetamine
Diaphoresis (1–10%)	Alopecia	Anaphylactoid reactions
Rash (<1%)	Angioedema	Angioedema
TEN	Diaphoresis	Hypersensitivity
Urticaria (<1%)	Erythema multiforme	SJS
	Exanthems	TEN
	Exfoliative dermatitis	Urticaria
	Fixed eruption	
	Hypersensitivity (1–10%)	
	Photosensitivity	
	Pruritus	
	Urticaria	
	Vasculitis	

Abbreviations: SJS = Stevens-Johnson Syndrome, TEN = toxic epidermolysis necrosis.
This table specifies the adverse cutaneous drug reactions observed with the stimulant medications. If indicated, the incidence of the specific adverse cutaneous reactions is given (10)

22.5.3 Urticaria and angioedema

Urticaria, the second most common form of ACDRs, can occur with any of the psychotropic medications (10). Urticaria is characterized as a transient, often pruritic eruption of papules and plaques that are edematous and erythematous. Large wheals can appear anywhere on the body, including the palms, soles, and scalp. Lesions can vary in size and morphology. Depending on prior sensitization, lesions can present within minutes to several days after drug exposure. They generally last a few hours, but less than 24 hours. If, however, the lesions persist for more than 24 hours and demonstrate residual petechiae, the clinician should suspect a possible urticarial vasculitis.

Angioedema represents transient edema of the deep dermal, subcutaneous, and submucousal tissue. Patients typically present with swelling of the face and, less frequently, of the extremities. If the larynx, epiglottis, or surrounding tissues are affected, the patient may be at risk of impaired swallowing and upper airway obstruction. Angioedema is associated with urticaria in about half of all cases, and it can progress to anaphylaxis, a medical emergency (see Section 22.6.6).

Other drugs implicated in urticaria include penicillins, cephalosporines, sulfonamides, and NSAIDs. Other drugs responsible for angioedema are penicillins, NSAIDs, ACE inhibitors, and monoclonal antibodies. Treatment of drug-induced urticaria and angioedema involves discontinuing the offending agent. For uncomplicated cases, oral antihistamine H1 and H2 are often prescribed. However, patients presenting with laryngeal angioedema require immediate medical attention. These patients should be given epinephrine and corticosteroids, and if necessary, their upper airway should be secured (9,10,11,12,13,14,15,16,17).

22.5.4 Fixed drug eruptions

Fixed drug eruptions have been observed with mood stabilizers (i.e. carbamazepine, valproic acid, and lamotrigine), SSRIs (i.e. sertraline), TCAs (i.e. amitriptyline and imipramine), benzodiazepines (i.e. diazepam and lorazepam), typical antipsychotics (i.e. chlorpromazine, trifluoperazine, and prochloperazine), and stimulants (i.e. methylphenidate) (10). This cutaneous reaction is characterized by well-circumscribed lesions (solitary or multiple) that recur in exactly the same site with repeated exposure to the offending drug. The color varies from red, red-brown, dusky red, to violaceous; the size often ranges from just a few millimeters to more than 10 cm. Patches or plaques are most typical, but bullae can develop. Lesions are often found on the genitalia, palms, soles, and mucosa.

Tetracyclines, sulfonamides, acetaminophen, and NSAIDs are several other drugs capable of causing a fixed drug eruption. Removal of the offending drug is the primary treatment. Topical corticosteroids may be helpful; however, post-inflammatory hyperpigmentation frequently persists for weeks to months (9,10,11,12,13,14,15,16,17).

22.5.5 Photosensitivity

The majority of the antipsychotic agents can lead to a photosensitive drug reaction (10). Typical antipsychotics (containing phenothiazine-structure) and tricyclic antidepressants are frequently implicated in causing photosensitivity. There are two types of photosensitivity: phototoxicity and photoallergy. Phototoxic reactions are more common and develop within days of beginning a new medication. Phototoxic reactions depend both on the drug dosage and the duration of sun exposure. Clinically, patients present with an exaggerated sunburn, yet they report shorter than expected sun exposure time. The cutaneous reaction is limited to sun-exposed areas. Patients will demonstrate erythema and edema, followed by desequamation and hyperpigmentation. Besides typical antipsychotics, the drugs frequently associated with phototoxic reactions include tetracyclines, NSAIDs, fluoroquinolones, amiodarone, and psoralens. Rather than discontinuing the offending agent, it may be possible to decrease the dosage of the medication, limit sun exposure, or both.

Photoallergic reactions are less common. They are a cell-mediated hypersensitivity response in which ultraviolet irradiation converts the drug into a photoallergen that can induce an immune response. They tend to occur 1–2 weeks after initiation of the offending agent. Clinical manifestations are eruptions that can be eczematous, maculapopalar, vesicular, lichenoid, urticarial, or bullous. The reaction begins in sun-exposed areas but often extends beyond these sun-exposed areas. Chronic exposure to photoallergic medications can lead to continued photosensitivity months to years after the offending drug is discontinued. Additional photoallergic drugs include thiazide diuretics, sulfonamides, sulfonylureas, quinine, quinidine, antimalarials, and NSAIDs. Patients should be advised to avoid sun exposure, wear sun protective clothing, and apply broad-spectrum sunscreen (9,10,11,12,13,14,15,16,17).

22.5.6 Pigmentation

Pigmentary changes can result from the drug itself, or the drug can disrupt melanin formation, or both mechanisms can be involved. Drug-induced pigmentation is associated with the mood stabilizers lithium, carbamazepine, gabapentin, and topiramate. Prolonged exposure to these mood stabilizers can produce a patchy brown pigmentation, especially on the face, neck, and arms. With removal of the offending agent, the discoloration slowly fades.

Of the antidepressants, TCAs are most often described to cause drug-induced pigmentation. Reported cases of discoloration with all of the SSRIs (except escitalopram) can be found, but they are rare. Drug-induced pigmentation is also associated with typical antipsychotics, but it is less common with atypical antipsychotics. Pigmentation is usually slate-gray or blue-gray in color. Besides the skin, the cornea and lens can be affected. Drug-induced pigmentation occurs with long term drug exposure but generally improves with time after discontinuation of the offending drug. Exposure to minocycline, amiodarone, chloroquine, and heavy metals are other drugs that incite pigmentary changes (9,10,11,12,13,14,15,16,17).

22.5.7 Diaphoresis

Diaphoresis (an increase in perspiration) has been noted in patients treated with all classes of psychotropic mediations. It is especially common with many of the SSRIs, TCAs, and benzodiazepines (10). Symptomatic treatment using aluminum chloride-containing antiperspirants may be helpful (9,10,11,12,13,14,15,16,17).

22.5.8 Alopecia

With respect to psychotropic medications, mood-stabilizing agents and antidepressants are most often implicated in causing drug-induced alopecia (hair loss).

Though less frequent, many of the other classes of psychiatric medications are known to cause this side effect as well (10). Drug-induced hair loss can be localized or generalized. It usually affects the scalp and is a non-scarring alopecia that is reversible when the drug is discontinued. Other etiologies of non-scarring alopecia should be ruled out. These include alopecia areata, androgenic alopecia, telogen effluvium, trichotillomania, thyroid disease, and iron deficiency (see Chapters 1 and 14).

Drug-induced alopecia secondary to psychotropic mediations can cause a tremendous emotional burden on patients and can interfere with medication compliance. Withdrawal of the offending agent is the most definitive treatment. An alterative therapy is to recommend zinc and selenium supplementation. Topical minoxidil is sometimes prescribed to speed hair regrowth (9,10,11,12,13,14,15,16,17).

22.6 Serious and life-threatening cutaneous reactions

22.6.1 Erythema multiforme

There are many possible etiologies for erythema multiforme, though about 90% of cases are precipitated by infections (e.g. herpes simplex virus and mycoplasma pneumonia). In contrast, drug-induced erythema multiforme represents less than 10% of all cases. Primarily, the offending drugs are anticonvulsants, along with NSAIDs, sulfonamides, and other antibiotics. Albeit less frequent, reports of drug-induced erythema multiforme have been observed with antidepressants, anxiolytics, antipsychotics, and stimulants (10).

Erythema multiforme is an acute, self-limited, but potentially recurrent condition. There are two forms of erythema multiforme: erythema multiforme major and erythema multiforme minor. Both feature the characteristic erythematous "target" (or iris-shaped) papules. Lesions generally favor distal extremities and the face. They tend to appear within 24–72 hours but remain fixed for at least 1 week. In contrast to erythema multiforme minor, erythema multiforme major is distinct in that patients develop severe mucosal involvement and systemic symptoms. Occasionally, vesiculobullous lesions are present. Treatment should involve prompt withdrawal of the offending agent, and a dermatologist should be urgently consulted (9,10,11,12,13,14,15,16,17).

22.6.2 Stevens-Johnson Syndrome and Toxic Epidermolysis Necrolysis

Stevens-Johnson syndrome (SJS) and toxic epidermal necrolysis (TEN) are rare but potentially fatal, adverse mucocutaneous reactions. These conditions are almost always drug-induced. Anticonvulsants (i.e. carbamazepine, valproic acid, lamotrigine, oxcarbazepine, gabapentin), penicillins, sulfonamide antibiotics, and NSAIDs are among the medications most frequently associated with SJS and TEN. Though less common, specific antidepressants (i.e. fluoxetine, fluvoxamine, paroxetine, sertraline, bupropion, venlafaxine), benzodiazepines (i.e. alprazolam, lorazepam), antipsychotics (i.e. aripiprazole, clozapine, chlorpromazine, thioridazine, fluphenazine, prochlorperazine), and stimulants (i.e. dextroamphetamine, lisdexamfetamine) have also been reported to precipitate these conditions (10).

SJS and TEN present as extensive areas of exfoliation as a result of keratinocyte cell death and consequent separation of skin at the dermal-epidermal junction. SJS and TEN vary in disease severity. SJS, SJS-TEN overlap, and TEN are defined as epidermal detachment of less than 10%, 10–30%, and more than 30% body surface areas, respectively. Patients usually experience a prodrome with fever, malaise, and arthralgia. Mucosal membrane involvement and significant systemic symptoms occur in nearly all cases; erosions, hemorrhage, and crusting of the oral mucosa are characteristic. Lesions tend to be most severe on the trunk and face, but they can appear on any part of the body.

Both TEN and SJS typically occur 1–3 weeks after starting the offending drug. Mortality rates approach 5% for SJS and 35% for TEN. Thus, early diagnosis and immediate discontinuation of the responsible drug are crucial. Patients should be monitored in the intensive care facility or burn unit. Fluid correction, nutritional support, pain control, and other supportive care should be promptly initiated. Intravenous immunoglobulin may also prove to be beneficial. The offending drug should never be rechallenged, as symptoms can quickly return upon re-exposure (9,10,11,12,13,14,15,16,17).

22.6.3 Drug hypersensitivity syndrome

Mood stabilizing agents are frequently associated with drug hypersensitivity syndrome, though certain psychotropic agents (i.e. desipramine, amitriptyline, clomipramine, bupropion, trazodone, diazepam, risperidone, quetiapine, olanzapine, thioridazine, methylphenidate, lisdexamfetamine) have also been implicated (10). Drug hypersensitivity syndrome consists of the following triad: fevers, rash, and internal organ involvement. The cutaneous eruption generally begins 1 to 8 weeks following the first prolonged course of drug therapy. Symptoms can begin with fever, malaise, and pharyngitis. This is followed by a cutaneous eruption in about 85% of cases. Cutaneous involvement varies from an exanthematous eruption to erythroderma, SJS, and TEN. Generalized lymphadenopathy, hepatitis, nephritis, and pneumonitis are serious internal organ manifestations. Immediate discontinuation of the offending drug is essential as this syndrome has a high risk of morbidity and mortality. Systemic steroids may be necessary. In all cases, patients should be evaluated by appropriate specialists experienced in treating this life-threatening condition (9,10,11,12,13,14,15,16,17).

22.6.4 Vasculitis

Vasculitis has been observed with mood stabilizers (i.e. lithium, carbamazepine, valproic acid, and gabapentin), SSRIs (i.e. fluoxetine, paroxetine, citalopram), TCAs (all of them), other antidepressants (i.e. trazodone), benzodiazepines (i.e. diazepam), atypical antipsychotics (i.e. olanzapine and clonzapine), the typical antipsychotics (i.e. chlorpromazine and thioridazine), and stimulants (i.e. methylphenidate) (10). Drug-induced vasculitis is an inflammation of small dermal venules that is believed to be triggered by the deposition of immune complexes. This activates the complement cascade leading to an inflammatory response that damages the vessel walls. The vasculitis can occur 1–3 weeks following drug initiation.

Clinically, vasculitis appears as purpura primarily on the lower extremities. As the disease progresses, the lesions may become palpable. Less common clinical findings include papules, ulcers, pustules, urticaria, subcutaneous nodules, and digital necrosis. Patients may complain of fever, myalgia, arthralgias, and headaches. On physical examination, peripheral neuropathy, peripheral edema, and tachypnea may be noted. Biopsy should be performed to confirm the diagnosis.

Vasculitis can be idiopathic in nature, or secondary to infections (e.g. streptococcus, tuberculosis, and hepatitis B or C), autoimmune connective tissue disease (e.g. systemic lupus erythematous, Sjögren syndrome), or other drugs (e.g. penicillins, ACE inhibitors, sulfonamides). In drug-induced vasculitis, discontinuation of the offending agent often resolves symptoms rapidly. Often, no additional treatment is needed. Systemic corticosteroids may be helpful in cases of significant systemic involvement (9,10,11,12,13,14,15,16,17).

22.6.5 Exfoliative dermatitis

Exfoliative dermatitis (also known as erythroderma or red man syndrome) has multiple etiologies, the most common being psoriasis, atopic dermatitis, cutaneous T-cell lymphoma, and drug reactions. Carbamazepines rank among the common drug-related causes of exfoliative dermatitis. Other responsible drugs can include allopurinol, beta-lactam antibiotics, gold, sulfasalazine, and sulfonamides. Less frequently, exfoliative dermatitis has been associated with several of the medications found within each class of antipsychotics, with the exception of MAOIs (10).

Clinically, exfoliative dermatitis appears as generalized erythema and scaling. It is a serious medical problem. Patients often require hospitalization as they frequently develop impaired thermoregulation, tachycardia, loss of fluid as well as proteins, and peripheral edema. The suspected drug should be discontinued immediately, while optimal supportive care should be given. Topical corticosteroids, oral antihistamines, systemic corticosteroids, or intravenous immunoglobulins are all possible therapeutic options. In refractory cases, cyclosporine may be prescribed (9,10,11,12,13,14,15,16,17).

22.6.6 Anaphylactoid reactions

Anaphylaxis is an acute life-threatening emergency. It has been associated with many psychotropic agents. Specifically, anaphylaxis has been described with mood stabilizers (i.e. lamotrigrine), SSRIs (i.e. fluoxetine, fluvoxamine, escitalopramine), TCAs (i.e. amitripytiline), other antidepressants (i.e. bupropion, venlafaxine), atypical antipsychotics (i.e. risperidone, quetiapine), typical antipsychotics (nearly all of them), and stimulants (i.e. lisdexamfetamine) (10). Anaphylaxis develops rapidly, just minutes following drug exposure. It presents with skin manifestations of urticaria or angioedema, as well as systemic findings such as hypotension, tachycardia, or shock (i.e. hemodynamic instability). Prompt discontinuation of the offending medication is crucial. Patients should be hospitalized for observation, and upper airway management may be necessary. Systemic corticosteroids, oral antihistamines, and subcutaneous epinephrine are often required (9,10,11,12,13,14,15,16,17).

22.7 General dermatologic conditions

22.7.1 Acneiform eruptions

Among the psychotropic medications, lithium is perhaps the most notorious drug for inducing acne-like eruptions. Other drugs suspected of inciting or aggravating acne include other mood stabilizers, as well as the SSRIs, TCAs, other antidepressants, anxiolytics, atypical antipsychotics (i.e. risperidone, aripiprazole, and quetiapine), and typical antipsychotics (i.e. haloperidol) (10). Acneiform drug eruptions consist of papulopustular eruptions, usually without comedones. It is clinically distinct from acne vulgaris because of its rapid onset and monomorphous pattern. Use of anabolic steroids, corticosteroid, isoniazide, iodides, bromides, and inhibitors of the epidermal growth factor receptor are known to cause drug-induced acneiform eruptions. Depending on the disease severity, therapies include benzoyl peroxide, topical antibiotics, oral tetracyclines, oral contraceptives, and systemic isotretinoin (see Chapter 7) (9,10,11,12,13,14,15,16,17).

22.7.2 Psoriasiform eruption

Similar to ACE inhibitors, beta-blockers, antimalarials, gold, and interferons, *lithium* ranks as one of the leading causes of drug-induced psoriasiform eruptions. Other mood stabilizers (i.e. carbamazepine, valproic acid, and gabapentin), SSRIs (i.e. fluoxetine, paroxetine, and citalopram), TCAs (i.e. clomipramine), other antidepressants (i.e. bupropion, venlafaxine, trazadone), and atypical antidepressants (i.e. risperidone, aripiprazole, and olanzapine) have also been reported in cases of psoriasiform eruption, though less frequently (10). This cutaneous reaction presents as well-demarcated, erythematous papules and plaques with micaceous scaling. Lesions may be localized or generalized. They tend to be symmetrically distributed, with a predilection for the elbows, knees, and scalp. Discontinuation of the offending agent is usually advised. Treatment largely depends on disease severity. Therapeutic options range from high-potency topical corticosteroids to phototherapy, methotrexate, cyclosporine, and biologics (9,10,11,12,13,14,15,16,17).

22.7.3 Seborrheic eruption

Reported cases of seborrheic eruptions are noted with typical antipsychotics (nearly all of them), atypical antipsychotics (i.e. risperidone, aripiprazole, and olanzapine), mood stabilizers (i.e. lithium, valproic acid, gabapentin, topiramate), SSRIs (i.e. fluoxetine, fluvoxamine, paroxetine), TCAs (i.e. clomipramine), other antidepressants (i.e. venlafaxine and mirtazapine), and non-benzodiazepines (i.e. buspirone) (10). Seborrheic eruptions appear as poorly circumscribed erythematous, red-yellow plaques with fine scaling. Eruptions occur in areas rich in sebaceous glands such as the scalp, nasolabial region, eyebrows, ears, anterior chest, and intertriginous areas. Discontinuation of the medication can be helpful but not always indicated. Medicated shampoos (containing ketoconazole, zinc pyrithone, selenium sulfide, or tar), low-potency corticosteroids, or antifungal creams may be recommended (9,10,11,12,13,14,15,16,17).

22.7.4 Lichenoid eruption

Anticonvulsants (i.e. lithium and carbamazepine), SSRIs (i.e. fluoxetine), TCAs (i.e. amitriptyline and imipramine), other antidepressants (i.e. venlafaxine), atypical antipsychotics (i.e. risperidone and olanzapine), and typical antipsychotics (i.e. chlorpromazine and thioridazine) have been identified as causing drug-induced lichenoid eruptions (10).

Clinically, these eruptions mimic lichen planus. However, there are several features that can help distinguish lichen planus and lichenoid drug eruption. Lesions seen with lichen planus are flattened-topped, polygonal, violaceous papules that coalesce into plaques. They are found on wrists, flexor forearms, lower legs, and genitalia. In contrast, lesions of lichenoid drug eruptions are more eczematous, psoriasiform, or pityriasis rosea-like. They are more generalized, often sparing the classic sites of lichen planus. The mucosa is usually not involved. In addition, unlike in lichen planus, hyperpigmentation often occurs and may persist. Other associated drugs include antibiotics, gold salts, ACE inhibitors, beta-blockers, lipid-lowering agents, and NSAIDs.

It is difficult to estimate the efficacy of various therapies for drug-induced lichenoid eruption. In general, high-potency topical corticosteroids are first-line therapy, while systemic corticosteroids may be needed for widespread involvement. Other possible treatments include topical calcineurin inhibitors, phototherapy, oral metronidazole, antimalarials, and systemic retinoids (9,10,11,12,13,14,15,16,17).

22.8 Conclusion

Adverse cutaneous reactions to psychotropic medications are common. In a small, yet significant proportion of these reactions, the dermatologic manifestations can be life threatening. It is, therefore, imperative that a clinician can recognize these clinical presentations and identify all probable offending agents. Whenever possible, the offending psychotropic medication should be discontinued. If, however, the patient requires long term therapy for a psychiatric condition, the patient should be placed on the lowest effective dosage of that medication or switched to another psychotropic medication that is less prone to such adverse effects. Ultimately, the clinician must weigh the therapeutic benefits of continuing therapy against the risks of the cutaneous symptoms.

References

1. Vitiello B. Research in child and adolescent psychopharmacology: rRecent accomplishments and new challenges. *Psychopharmacology* (Berl) 2007;191:5–13.
2. MacMorran WS, Krahn LE. Adverse cutaneous reactions to psychotropic drugs. *Psychosomatics* 1997;38:413–22.
3. Garnis-Jones S. Dermatologic side effects of psychopharmacologic agents. *Dermatol Clin* 1996;14:503–8.
4. Bigby M, Jick S, Jick H, Arndt K. Drug-induced cutaneous reactions. A report from the Boston Collaborative Drug Surveillance Program on 15,438 consecutive inpatients, 1975 to 1982. *JAMA* 1986;256:3358–63.
5. Drake LA, Dinehart SM, Farmer ER, et al. Guidelines of care for cutaneous adverse drug reactions. *J Am Acad Dermatol* 1996;35:458–61.
6. Arndt KA, Jick H. Rates of cutaneous reactions to drugs. A report from the Boston Collaborative Drug Surveillance Program. *JAMA* 1976;235:918–23.

7. Litvak R, Kaelbling R. Dermatological side effects with psychotropics. *Dis Nerv Syst* 1972;33: 309–11.
8. Srebrnik A, Hes JP, Brenner S. Adverse cutaneous reactions to psychotropic drugs. *Acta Derm Venereol Suppl* (Stockh) 1991;158:1–12.
9. McKenna JK, Leiferman KM. Dermatologic drug reactions. *Immunol Allergy Clin North Am* 2004;24:399–423, vi.
10. Litt's D.E.R.M. (Drug Eruption & Reactions Manual) Database. http://www.drugeruptiondata.com/info/index/type/contact.
11. Warnock JK, Morris DW. Adverse cutaneous reactions to mood stabilizers. *Am J Clin Dermatol* 2003;4:21–30.
12. Warnock JK, Morris DW. Adverse cutaneous reactions to antidepressants. *Am J Clin Dermatol* 2002;3:329–39.
13. Warnock JK, Morris DW. Adverse cutaneous reactions to antipsychotics. *Am J Clin Dermatol* 2002;3:629–36.
14. Sterry W, Paus R, Burgdorf WHC. *Dermatology*. New York: Thieme, 2006.
15. James WD, Berger TG, Elston DM, Odom RB. *Andrews' diseases of the skin: Clinical dermatology*, 10th edn. Philadelphia, PA: Saunders Elsevier, 2006.
16. Marks JG, Miller JJ, Lookingbill DP. *Lookingbill and Marks' principles of dermatology*, 4th edn. Philadelphia, PA: Saunders Elsevier, 2006.
17. Bolognia J, Jorizzo JL, Rapini RP. *Dermatology*. London: Mosby, 2003.

Philip D. Shenefelt

23 Non-pharmacological approaches to treat psychocutaneous disorders

Children and adolescents can often benefit from nonpharmacological interventions for psychocutaneous disorders with minimal if any side effects. Interventions include acupuncture, aromatherapy, biofeedback, brief dynamic psychotherapy, cognitive behavioral therapy (CBT) methods, energy acupressure techniques such as emotional freedom techniques (EFT), eye movement desensitization and reprocessing (EMDR), hypnosis, music, placebo, and suggestion. Age-appropriate modifications permit tailoring the interventions to individual patients. Adding elements of age-appropriate fun and storytelling often will motivate the patient to cooperate. Biofeedback can often incorporate a video or audio game-like, age-appropriate approach to engage the patient. CBT must also be age-appropriate, starting at about age 8, and can incorporate storytelling as well as straight talk. EFT can be done for the pediatric patient as infants, toddlers, and preschoolers, while EFT can be taught to elementary school age and adolescent patients. EMDR can be used with older preschoolers, elementary school age, and adolescent patients. Hypnoidal techniques such as rocking can be used with infants and toddlers. Older preschoolers and elementary school age patients generally shift into imaginative trance quite easily, with a peak of hypnotizability between ages 8 and 12. Elementary school age and adolescent patients can be taught self-hypnosis as well. For low hypnotizables, distraction will likely be the key element, while for moderate hypnotizables sensory or time distortion will be key; dissociation or fantasy will predominate for high hypnotizables. Music can calm anxious children. Placebo can be used when age and ethically appropriate. Appropriately phrased suggestions can benefit older preschoolers, elementary school age, and adolescent patients.

23.1 Introduction

The skin and the nervous system form next to each other in the ectoderm of the fetus. They remain interconnected physically as well as biochemically and interact in childhood and throughout life. The various touch receptors in the skin comprise the body's largest sense organ. The skin–nervous system interactions result in significant psychosomatic or behavioral influences on many dermatologic conditions. Psychoneuroimmunology elucidates the biological basis of how the brain and nerves alter immune responses in common skin disorders such as atopic dermatitis, psoriasis, and urticaria (1). These interactions and influences allow non-pharmacologic psychotherapeutic interventions such as acupressure or tapping on meridian points, aromatherapy, biofeedback, cognitive behavioral therapy, hypnosis, music, placebo, and suggestion to produce positive effects on many dermatologic diseases.

23.2 Non-pharmacological modalities

23.2.1 Acupuncture

Needle acupuncture with focal stimulation of cutaneous nerves at specified sites has been reported to be helpful in the treatment of acne, atopic dermatitis, postherpetic neuralgia, psoriasis, and urticaria (2). Generally these have been single case reports or case series in the Chinese literature. The treatment sites correspond to specific numbered acupuncture points on the 12 lateral and 2 midline meridians. A complex system relating the meridians to specific hollow and solid organs is described in traditional Chinese medicine. Nonsterile acupuncture needles carry a risk of blood-borne pathogen infection. Use in some children may be limited by aversion to needles. Non-needle acupuncture methods include moxibustion, cupping, acupressure, and more recently laser acupuncture. Tapping at acupuncture sites is discussed in Section 23.2.6.

23.2.2 Aromatherapy

Direct skin contact aromatherapy with application of a fragrant essential oil diluted in a carrier oil has been used for atopic dermatitis, contact dermatitis, psoriasis, and seborrheic dermatitis. While some topical pharmacological effect cannot be excluded, the olfactory stimulation activates nerves that extend directly adjacent to the limbic system in the brain. According to reports, oil of Bergamont (caution – photosensitizer) has been reported to have antiseptic and antidepressant properties.

Geranium oil is reported to be antiseptic, antidepressant, and a stimulator of granulation tissue. Jasmine oil is said to have antidepressant, sedative, and relaxant properties. Lavender oil reportedly has analgesic, antiseptic, bactericidal, anti-inflammatory, and sedative effects. Lemon balm (*Melissa officinalis*) is said to have antidepressant effects, while sandalwood oil is reported to have antiseptic and antidepressant qualities.

Other essential oils that have been used include benzoin, chamomile, frankincense, myrrh, sweet marjoram, and thyme. The carrier oils such as avocado oil, coconut oil, evening primrose oil, sweet almond oil, and wheat germ oil also may have some topical pharmacologic activities (3). These are based on case reports and case series. Massage with carrier oil with or without essential oil added resulted in significant improvement in children aged 3–7 years with atopic dermatitis resistant to other treatments in a case series (4). As an adverse effect, allergic contact dermatitis has been reported from direct contact aromatherapy (5).

Noncontact aromatherapy coupled with relaxation can link a specific fragrance with the relaxation response. That specific fragrance can then be used as a conditioned stimulus to induce the relaxation response. In a study of 6- to 12-year-old children who smelled fragrances of essential oils (i.e. of ginger, lavender, lemon, peppermint, spearmint, and sweet orange), positive effects on mood and energy were reported (6). Preference ranking by non-Latino Caucasian males of which one oil to take home in descending order were lemon, sweet orange, peppermint, spearmint, lavender, and ginger. Non-Latino Caucasian females preferred the same order. Latino males noted as preferences in descending order spearmint, sweet orange, lemon, and lavender. Latino females preferred sweet orange, spearmint, and lemon. Some of the fragrances evoked memories in some of the participants (6).

23.2.3 Biofeedback

Biofeedback involves the use of instruments to provide real time visual or auditory feedback about specifically measureable biological activities. Biofeedback training can improve skin problems that have an autonomic nervous system component such as biofeedback of galvanic skin resistance (GSR) for hyperhidrosis and biofeedback of skin temperature for dyshidrosis and Raynaud's syndrome (7). Children 7 to 16 years old have proven to be especially adept at skin temperature biofeedback (8). Incorporating a game or some play aspect into the biofeedback can help to maintain the child's interest and motivation.

Biofeedback may result in some improvement in atopic dermatitis (9). Hypnosis may enhance the effects obtained by biofeedback (10,11). Heart rate variability biofeedback with handheld electronic devices such as the emWave Personal Stress Reliever or StressEraser can promote relaxation and improve skin conditions worsened by stress.

An inexpensive and simple biofeedback device for finger temperature is a temperature-sensitive color changing card that Barrios used to promote relaxation in school children (12). He is the inventor of the Stress Control Card that has a heat sensitive color changing biofeedback thermometer placed on a credit card sized card having color indications from colder black through red and green to warmer blue; this is similar in function to the well known mood ring. It measures ranges of finger temperatures, giving biofeedback of vasoconstriction versus vasodilatation associated with autonomic activity. Colder finger temperatures are a result of sympathetic nervous system vasoconstriction, which, when the person is in an environment of normal room temperature, often reflects stress. The higher finger temperature is associated with relaxation. Relaxation can benefit most inflammatory skin disorders, including atopic dermatitis and psoriasis.

23.2.4 Brief dynamic psychotherapy

Individual brief dynamic psychotherapy in children as young as 5 years old was found to significantly benefit children with atopic dermatitis in a randomized control trial (13). A total of 11–18 sessions were required over a 6 month period.

23.2.5 Cognitive behavioral therapy methods

Cognitive behavioral therapy (CBT) methods help to alter dysfunctional thought patterns (cognitive) or actions (behavioral) that damage the skin through scratching or picking and interference with dermatologic therapy (14). These methods include habit reversal therapy. Skin diseases in children 8 years old and older that are responsive include acne excoriée (Chapter 7), atopic dermatitis (Chapter 5), factitious cheilitis, hyperhidrosis, lichen simplex chronicus, needle phobia, neurodermatitis, onychotillomania, prurigo nodularis, trichotillomania (Chapter 12), and urticaria (see Chapter 1).

Adding hypnosis to CBT can facilitate virtual aversive therapy and enhance desensitization and other cognitive behavioral methods (11). A randomized controlled trial using CBT for atopic dermatitis aimed to reduce scratching frequency and stress (15). The subjects maintained scratching diaries and were instructed in habit reversal techniques, relaxation techniques, distraction techniques, positive self talk, and application of ice to itchy skin. Assessments at 1 year for CBT showed significantly improved atopic skin conditions with significantly decreased topical corticosteroid use compared with standard dermatological treatment or education groups (15).

23.2.6 Emotional freedom techniques (EFT)

Emotional freedom techniques (EFT) are related to acupressure (16). EFT starts with selecting a negatively emotionally charged memory or problem area and then focusing intently on that thought or memory or condition, pressing on the subclavicular "sore spot," and repeating an affirmation such as "Even though I have this problem with _______, I deeply and completely accept myself," while progressively tapping with the finger on a series of up to 14 specific acupuncture sites on the head, chest, and hand.

For infants, toddlers, and preschoolers, this tapping process can be done for them, either directly on them or on a surrogate. Older children and adolescents can be taught to use the technique themselves. EFT can neutralize negative emotional charged memories or problem areas, reducing anxiety, and enhancing performance (16). Anecdotally reported improvements or resolution of skin conditions in children on www.EFTuniverse.com include acne, allergic contact dermatitis, atopic dermatitis, lupus erythematosus, needle phobia, procedure anxiety, psoriasis, and warts.

A controlled comparison of EFT with EMDR (see Section 23.2.7) in a study that included older adolescents showed that for post traumatic stress disorder (PTSD), both produced significant therapeutic gains (17). Some children do develop PTSD as a result of life events that were overwhelmingly traumatic to them, including hospitalizations and medical procedures. Reducing emotional distress often results in improvement of inflammatory skin conditions such as acne, atopic dermatitis, and psoriasis.

23.2.7 Eye Movement Desensitizing and Reprocessing (EMDR)

Eye movement desensitizing and reprocessing (EMDR) also involves selecting a negatively emotionally charged memory or problem area and focusing on that thought; then, the person does an alternating bilateral activity such as following a finger from side to side with the eyes (18), hearing alternating left and right tones through headphones, feeling alternating left and right vibrations in handheld paddles, or alternately tapping left and right distal thighs or upper arms. It is slightly more effective than EFT in producing positive benefits in PTSD (17). The efficacy of EMDR in children has been evaluated in a meta-analysis. The post-treatment effect size was medium and significant (19). When combined with the EFT affirmations it becomes a hybrid known as Wholistic Hybrid derived from EMDR and EFT (WHEE), reducing anxiety and enhancing performance (20). EMDR has been reported effective for improving atopic dermatitis and psoriasis (21).

23.2.8 Hypnosis

Hypnosis consists of guiding the patient into a trance state of narrowed awareness, focused attention, selective wakefulness, and heightened suggestibility for a specific purpose such as relaxation, pain or pruritus reduction, or habit modification. Autogenic training and guided imagery are considered to be forms of hypnosis. Autogenic training has a specific method of trance induction. Guided imagery intentionally involves trance induction, while storytelling often induces spontaneous trance. Meditation is a close cousin to hypnosis. Both hypnosis and meditation involve the use of trance phenomena.

Hypnosis is a Western concept and focuses more on fixing something, while meditation is more of an Eastern concept and focuses more on centering and balance. Both can reduce psychological roadblocks to healing. The hypnotic trance has objectively documented differences in regional cerebral blood flow (22) and electroencephalographic (EEG) patterns compared with the usual waking state (23). The use of hypnosis may improve or clear numerous skin disorders, including acne excoriée, alopecia areata, atopic dermatitis, congenital ichthyosiform erythroderma, dyshidrotic dermatitis, erythromelalgia, furuncles, glossodynia, herpes simplex, hyperhidrosis, ichthyosis vulgaris, lichen planus, neurodermatitis, nummular dermatitis, post-herpetic neuralgia, pruritus, psoriasis, rosacea, trichotillomania, urticaria, verruca vulgaris, and vitiligo (24) (see Chapter 1).

Most children ages 4 and older are good hypnotic subjects, with hypnotic ability reaching a peak at around age 8 to 12 (25). Thereafter, there is some mild decline in hypnotizability into adulthood. A randomized controlled trial showed hypnosis to result in significantly greater resolution of verrucae than controls (26). A small pilot study that was a randomized controlled trial with psoriasis demonstrated significant improvement in high hypnotizables (27). A randomized controlled trial using autogenic training, a form of hypnosis, revealed after 1 year that atopic dermatitis patients had significantly improved skin and significant reduction in corticosteroid use compared with standard dermatological treatment or education groups (15). Similarly a non-randomized controlled trial utilizing hypnotic suggestions demonstrated that atopic patients had significant improvement and significantly less use of topical corticosteroids by 6 weeks and maintained this pattern for up to 2 years compared with controls (28).

Hypnosis is most useful in high and medium hypnotizables, and should generally not be used with those having schizophrenia or mental retardation. Relaxation with hypnosis can reduce anxiety and pain associated with dermatologic procedures. Hypnoanalysis has been successful in reducing erythema nodosum, herpes simplex reactivation, neurodermatitis, neurotic excoriations, rosacea, urticaria, and verrucae (29,30). Hypnoanalysis of 41 consecutive cases of verrucae resistant to prior hypnotic suggestion, including 11 prepubertal children and 5 adolescents, resulted in the warts resolving in 31 cases (31).

23.2.9 Music

Slow calming music, such as classical music with a tempo of 60 to 70 beats per minute, has been demonstrated to reduce anxiety in children in a waiting room in an emergency department setting (32). This technique can also be used for relaxation of children prior to and during skin procedures. The slower tempo helps to shift the child out of sympathetic into parasympathetic dominance with its ensuing relaxation. Another approach has been to loan an MP3 player (iPod Nano) to individual children while in the pediatric emergency department. The MP3 players were color coded with different kinds of music for infants/toddlers, preschoolers, school-aged children, and adolescents (33). This method is more expensive but allows provision of age-appropriate music. A systemic review of randomized control trials using music therapy for children listed and assessed the various studies and their results (34).

23.2.10 Placebo

Positive expectations and a positive doctor–patient relationship can affect the child's experience of treatment, can reduce pain, and may influence outcome. Negative expectations can produce negative nocebo results (35). Care must be taken in selecting language that will have a positive rather than negative effect on the child. Research on the placebo effect illustrates that the natural healing capacities of individuals can be enhanced and nurtured (36). The placebo effect for some common dermatologic conditions, such as acne and urticaria, is about 30% (37). The Griesemer index (38) rates dermatologic disorders on a percentage scale from 100% to 0% based on emotional triggering of the condition. Those disorders higher on the Griesemer scale are more likely to have a significant placebo effect. Younger children are often easily influenced, while adolescents may resist influence by physicians and parents. Ethical considerations often limit the application of the placebo in clinical practice.

23.2.11 Suggestion

Suggestion in the usual alert conscious state can be used to change subjective perceptions, to reduce pain, and may influence outcome. Reports of the efficacy of suggestion in treating verruca vulgaris have since been confirmed numerous times to a greater or lesser degree (39). Younger children often are in a hypnoidal state of consciousness as they play imaginatively and often readily accept suggestions. Resistant toddlers can sometimes be directed to do the opposite to get the desired effect, while resistant adolescents are more difficult to reach except through peers.

23.3 Conclusion

Skin disorders in children can have a significant effect on the psyche, and the psyche can have a significant effect on skin disorders through psychoneuroimmunoendocrine and behavioral mechanisms. Since many inflammatory skin disorders are triggered or aggravated by stress, it is important to teach children and adolescents to practice safe stress using non-pharmacological methods. Psychocutaneous treatments are safe non-pharmacological methods for improving skin disorders that have a significant psychological component; these treatments include acupuncture, biofeedback, brief psychodynamic therapy, CBT methods, EFT, EMDR, hypnosis, music, placebo, or suggestion. Further robust research is needed to reappraise and clarify the utility of some of these techniques in children and adolescents.

References

1. Tausk F, Elenkov I, Moynihan J. Psychoneuroimmunology. *Dermatol Ther* 2008;21:22–31.
2. Chen CJ. Acupuncture, electrostimulation, and reflex therapy in dermatology. *Dermatol Ther* 2003;16(2):87–92.
3. Walsh D. Using aromatherapy in the management of psoriasis. *Nurs Stand* 1996;11:53–6.
4. Anderson C, Lis-Balchin M, Kirk-Smith M. Evaluation of massage with essential oils on childhood atopic eczema. *Phytother Res* 2000;14:452–5.
5. Weiss RR, James WD. Allergic contact dermatitis from aromatherapy. *Am J Contact Derm* 1997;8:250–1.
6. Fitzgerald M, Culbert T, Finkelstein M, Green M, Johnson A, Chen S. The effect of gender and ethnicity on children's attitudes and preferences for essential oils, a pilot study. *Explore* 2007;3:378–85.
7. Sarti MG. Biofeedback in dermatology. *Clin Dermatol* 1998;16:711–4.
8. Delaney DC, Olson K, Labbe EE. Skin temperature biofeedback: Evaluation of non-clinical children's responses. *J Behav Ther Exp Psychiat* 1992;23:37–42.
9. Haynes SN, Wilson CC, Jaffe PG, Britton BT. Biofeedback treatment of atopic dermatitis: Controlled case studies of eight cases. *Biofeedback Self Regulation* 1979;4:195–209.
10. Dikel W, Olness K. Self-hypnosis, biofeedback, and voluntary peripheral temperature control in children. *Pediatrics* 1980;66:335–40.
11. Shenefelt PD. Biofeedback, cognitive-behavioral methods, and hypnosis in dermatology: Is it all in your mind? *Dermatol Ther* 2003;16:114–22.
12. Barrios AA. *Towards greater freedom and happiness*. Los Angeles, CA: SPC Press, 1985.
13. Linnet J, Jemec GBE. Anxiety level and severity of skin condition predicts outcome of psychotherapy in atopic dermatitis patients. *Int J Dermatol* 2001;40:632–6.
14. Levenson H, Persons JB, Pope KS. Behavior therapy and cognitive therapy. In: Goldman HH, ed. *Review of general psychiatry*, 5th edn. New York; McGraw-Hill, 2000;472.
15. Ehlers A, Stangier U, Gieler U. Treatment of atopic dermatitis: A comparison of psychological and dermatological approaches to relapse prevention. *J Consult Clin Psychol* 1995;63:624–35.
16. Craig G. *The EFT Manual*. Santa Rosa, CA: Energy Psychology Press, 2008.
17. Karatzias T, Power K, Brown K, McGoldrick T, Begum M, Young J, Loughran P, Chouliara Z, Adams S. A controlled comparison of the effectiveness and efficiency of two psychological therapies for posttraumatic stress disorder: Eye movement desensitization and reprocessing vs. emotional freedom techniques. *J Nerv Ment Dis* 2011;199:372–8.
18. Shapiro F. *Eye movement desensitization and reprocessing (EMDR): Basic principles, protocols, and procedures*, 2nd ed. New York: Guilford, 2001.
19. Rodenburg R, Benjamin A, de Roos C, Meijer AM, Starns GJ. Efficacy of EMDR in children: A meta-analysis. *Clin Psychol Rev* 2009:29:599–606.
20. Benor DJ, Ledger K, Toussaint L, Hett G, Zaccaro D. Pilot study of emotional freedom techniques, wholistic hybrid derived from eye movement desensitization and reprocessing and emotional freedom technique, and cognitive behavioral therapy for treatment of test anxiety in university students. *Explore* 2009;5:338–40.
21. Gupta MA, Gupta AK. Use of eye movement desensitization and reprocessing (EMDR) in the treatment of dermatologic disorders. *J Cutan Med Surg* 2002;6:415–21.
22. Rainville P, Hofbauer RK, Bushnell MC, et al. Hypnosis modulates activity in brain structures involved in the regulation of consciousness. *J Cognit Neurosci* 2002;14(6):887–901.
23. Freeman R, Barabasz A, Barabasz M, Warner D. Hypnosis and distraction differ in their effects on cold pressor pain. *Am J Clin Hypn* 2000;43:137–48.
24. Shenefelt PD. Hypnosis in dermatology. *Arch Dermatol* 2000;136:393–9.

25. Morgan AH, Hilgard ER. Age differences in susceptibility to hypnosis. *Internat J Clin Exper Hypn* 1973;21:78–85.
26. Spanos NP, Stenstrom RJ, Johnston JC. Hypnosis, placebo, and suggestion in the treatment of warts. *Psychosom Med* 1988;50:245–60.
27. Tausk F, Whitmore SE. A pilot study of hypnosis in the treatment of patients with psoriasis. *Psychother Psychosom* 1999;495:1–9.
28. Stewart AC, Thomas SE. Hypnotherapy as a treatment for atopic dermatitis in adults and children. *Br J Dermatol* 1995;132:778–83.
29. Shenefelt PD. Psychocutaneous hypnoanalysis: Detection and deactivation of emotional and mental root factors in psychosomatic skin disorders. *Am J Clin Hypn* 2007;50:131–6.
30. Shenefelt PD. Hypnoanalysis for dermatologic disorders. *J Altern Med Res* 2010;2(4):439–45.
31. Ewin DM. Hypnotherapy for warts (verruca vulgaris): 41 consecutive cases with 33 cures. *Am J Clin Hypn* 1992;35:1–10.
32. Holm L, Fitzmaurice L. Emergency department waiting room stress: Can music or aromatherapy improve anxiety scores? *Ped Emerg Care* 2008;24(12):836–8.
33. Young T, Griffin E, Phillips E, Stanley E. Music as distraction in a pediatric emergency department. *J Emergency Nurs* 2010;33:472–3.
34. Mrazova M, Celec P. A systemic review of randomized control trials using music therapy for children. *J Alt Compl Med* 2010;16:1089–95.
35. Speigel D. Placebos in practice (editorial). *BMJ* 2004;329:927–8.
36. Di Blasi Z, Reilly D. Placebos in medicine: Medical paradoxes need disentangling. (letter). *BMJ* 2005;330:45.
37. Gupta MA, Gupta AK. Psychodermatology: An update. *J Am Acad Dermatol* 1996;34:1030–46.
38. Griesemer RD. Emotionally triggered disease in a dermatological practice. *Psychiatr Ann* 1978;8:49–56.
39. Ullman M. On the psyche and warts: I. Suggestion and warts: A review and comment. *Psychosom Med* 1959;21:473–88.

Ruqiya Shama Tareen and Anam Nisar Tareen

24 Psychiatric disorders frequently encountered in dermatology practices

Dermatology and primary care offices appear to be unlikely settings to encounter psychiatric disorders; however, many psychiatric conditions are frequently encountered in dermatologic clinics, primary care offices, and inpatient settings. The association between skin disorders and psychiatric illnesses has been recognized for several decades, but the level of our understanding is still at the initial stages. The presence of comorbid psychiatric conditions in dermatology patients often complicates the treatment plan and creates a viscous cycle where both disease processes keep perpetuating each other. The estimates about the prevalence of psychiatric conditions in pediatric and adult patients with skin diseases have been wide ranging and intriguing. There are indications that this awareness is growing, but further appreciation and understanding are needed to help our pediatric and adult patients with psychodermatologic conditions. In this chapter, many common psychiatric conditions are discussed with major emphasis on their clinical management in outpatient settings. Disorders considered include major affective disorders (such as major depression and bipolar disorders), common anxiety spectrum disorders (such as social phobia and obsessive compulsive disorder), and some commonly encountered personality disorders in patients with skin conditions.

24.1 Introduction

This chapter focuses on primary psychiatric conditions commonly seen in dermatologic and primary care practices, whether they are a consequence of psychophysiologic dermatologic disease (such as psoriasis or atopic dermatitis) or resulting from self consciousness, stigmas, and low self-esteem due to a disfiguring skin disease (such as acne, vitiligo, alopecia, others). Primary psychiatric conditions presenting with dermatological findings are discussed elsewhere in this publication, such as body dysmorphic disorders (Chapter 9), delusional infestations (Chapter 10), trichotillomania (Chapter 12), and many others. Many times dermatologists and primary care clinicians are the only physicians with whom these patients will have a trusting relationship in context of their skin disease; also, this therapeutic relationship may be the only place where a window of opportunity exists to evaluate, investigate, and possibly treat these psychiatric conditions. This review seeks to provide a synopsis of some of the commonly encountered psychiatric disorders for any clinician who is treating children and adolescents for their dermatological condition, whether one is a dermatologist, pediatrician, or other primary care clinician.

24.1.1 Epidemiology

There is a wide variation in estimates about how many of the patients presenting to dermatologic and primary care practices have comorbid psychiatric illnesses. For example, studies have reported that about 30% of patients attending outpatient dermatology practices and 60% of patients who were hospitalized due to their dermatologic disease are found to have comorbid psychiatric illnesses (1). Other research has also reported similar prevalence ranging from 33% to 71% in different countries and in different treatment settings (2). Some skin diseases were found to have much higher prevalence of psychiatric disorders, and these include urticaria, pruritus, acne, herpes virus infections, and alopecia areata. Psychiatric comorbidity was found to be associated with having more than one skin disease, a past history of skin disease, and complaints of dermatologic symptoms with no evidence of any skin disease (2).

24.2 Mood disorders

24.2.1 Epidemiology

A child has a 10% to 25% risk of developing depression if one of the parents is diagnosed with a mood disorder, and this risk is doubled when both parents have such an illness (3). Adoption studies are limited but have shown that if children had genetic predisposition, but were raised by adoptive parents, they still had a two-fold risk of developing depression. Twin studies have provided the most significant evidence by showing that monozygotic twins had a concordance rate for any mood disorder of up to 70% to 90%, in comparison to dizygotic twins who have a much lower concordance rate of 16% to 35% (3). Figure 24.1 provides a simplified description of various types of mood disorders. Box 24.1 provides diagnostic criteria (SIG E CAPS mnemonic) for major depressive disorders (MDD).

24.2.1.1 Major depressive disorder (MDD)

MDD is a common disorder affecting about 2% to 5% of the pediatric and adolescent population. Prevalence rate of depression in young children under 13 years of age is 2.8%. In adolescents ages 13–18 years it affects 4.6% of boys versus 5.9% of girls (4). Costello et al conducted a meta-analysis of 26 epidemiological studies with the total of 60,000 children born between 1965 and 1995 (4). This study concluded that there is no evidence of increased prevalence of depression over the last 30 years; also, there were no gender differences in prevalence of depression in young and prepubescent children (4). After attaining puberty girls have double the risk of developing depression than boys. MDD is seen much more frequently in children and adolescents with chronic physical illness and disabilities. MDD is also prevalent is many chronic dermatologic conditions, especially in chronic disfiguring conditions (4).

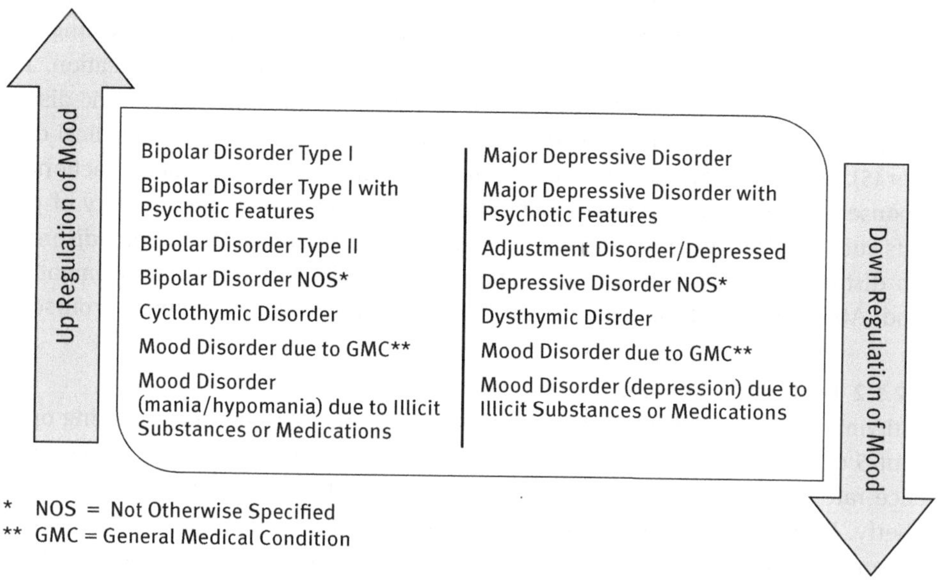

Figure 24.1: Spectrum of mood disorders.

Box 24.1 SIG E CAPS Mnemonic for Evaluation of MDD from *Diagnostic Statistical Manual of Mental Disorders*. 4th edn, text rev. Washington, DC: American Psychiatric Association, 2000

Depressed mood most of the day, nearly every day or irritable mood in children and adolescent along with any four of the following;

S Sleep disturbances: Early, middle (maintaining sleep), and late insomnia (early morning awakenings) or hypersomnia

I Interest*: Anhedonia, markedly diminished interest in almost all activities most of the day, nearly every day

G Guilt: Excessive or inappropriate guilt, rumination, feelings of worthlessness, nearly every day

E Energy: Decline in energy level, feeling tired, sluggish, excessive fatigue, nearly every day

C Concentration: Inability to focus and concentrate, nearly every day (may reflect in significant decline in academic performance)

A Appetite: More then 5% change in weight in 1 month in either direction; in children failure to make expected weight gain

P Psychomotor Activity: Amotivation, decline in activity level, lying around, versus restlessness, inability to sit down or relax

S Suicidal Ideation: Recurrent suicidal thoughts, hopelessness and helplessness with or without intent or a plan, or a suicide attempt

*In absence of depressed or irritable mood anhedonia or loss of interest must be present with other (≥ 4) symptoms in order to make a diagnosis of MDD.

A major depressive episode is described as a pervasive sense of depression that lasts for at least 2 weeks; it is characterized by neurovegetative symptoms including sleep disturbances, anhedonia or loss of interest in pleasurable activities, cognitive difficulties, decline in appetite and energy, change in psychomotor activity level, feelings of worthlessness, hopelessness with tendency to ruminate, and suicidal ideation. In order to make a diagnosis of MDD, it is necessary to exclude other psychiatric disorders, substance-induced mood disorder, and mood disorder caused by a medical disorder (5). Depressive symptoms as part of bereavement and in adjustment reaction in response to a major life event stressor should also be excluded. The majority of patients suffering from depression for at least 6–9 months will have a recurring disorder with distinct episodes of depression separated by periods of some improvement in mood. About 20% of these patients will have a chronic – almost lifetime – course.

24.2.1.2 Dysthymic disorder

Dysthymic disorder or dysthymia is relatively uncommon in children, affecting only about 5 children in 100,000; however, as the children approach puberty, the incidence rate steadily increases until it reaches a prevalence rate of 5 in 1,000 after puberty. Dysthymia is a low intensity depression of chronic nature usually starting with an early life event. Most cases start around 6–13 years of age (6). The child presenting with dysthymia commonly responds to a query about time of onset with "as long as I can remember." About 73% of patients reported suffering from this illness for ≥ 5 years, and 42% reported ≥ 10 years of duration (6).

The American Psychiatric Association's (APA's) *Diagnostic and Statistical Manual of Mental Disorders*, Fourth Edition (DSM-IV-TR) defines dysthymic disorder as a depressive state that lasts at least for 1 year in children and adolescents (5). Box 24.2 provides diagnostic criteria for dysthymia in children and adolescents. Longstanding depression gives rise to a characteristic personality with dependence on others, clinginess, demanding nature, interpersonal sensitivity, self doubt, low self-esteem, passivity, and a pessimistic outlook about life. About 50% to 70% of patients with dysthymia have a comorbid personality disorder. Substance abuse is also very frequently encountered in this disorder along with anxiety disorder (6).

Box 24.2 Diagnostic Criteria for Evaluation of Dysthymia in Children and Adolescents, from *Diagnostic Statistical Manual of Mental Disorders*, 4th edn, text rev. Washington, DC: American Psychiatric Association, 2000

Depressed mood for most of the day, for more days than not, for at least 1 year (never without symptoms for more than 2 months at a time during this year) along with two or more of the following symptoms:

Insomnia (early, middle, or late) or hypersomnia
Low energy level, excessive fatigue
Poor focus and concentration or indecisiveness
Increase or decrease in appetite
Feelings of hopelessness

24.2.1.3 Adjustment disorder

Adjustment disorder is a psychological response to an identifiable psychosocial stressor with a prevalence of 2–8% in the community; however, it increases up to 12% in patients who are hospitalized due to a medical condition (5). Adjustment disorder is classified as (a) with depressed mood, (b) with anxiety, (c) mixed with depression and anxiety, and (d) with disturbances of emotion and conduct. The symptoms appear within 3 months of a stressful event and usually resolve within 6 months of resolution of the index event. If symptoms are severe enough to impact functioning, then they can be more quickly resolved by such management as short term supportive therapy, interpersonal therapy, or cognitive behavioral therapy. In some cases symptoms continue to persist after 6 months, at which point adjustment disorder is labeled as chronic and may require more long term psychotherapy.

24.2.1.4 Depressive disorder not otherwise specified (NOS)

This is a category that can be used to label any depressive disorder that does not meet the full criteria of MDD, dysthymia, or adjustment disorder (with depressed mood or mixed with depression and anxiety). At present proposed research criteria of minor depression also reside in this category. Minor depression is a depressive state that meets the duration criteria of 2 weeks and presents with at least two but less than five symptoms required for MDD diagnosis (5).

24.2.2 Diagnosis of depressive disorders

A thorough history is important to obtain, paying special attention to the child or adolescent's developmental history, patient and family's psychiatric, alcohol/substance abuse, and medical history; also, obtain a thorough review of current or recently used medications, immunization status, family dynamic, psychosocial trauma and stressors, school performance and peer relationships, and any significant functional decline. Any medical conditions contributing to the depressive state should be ruled out. A diagnosis of depression in children younger than 6 years can be very difficult as developmentally they cannot identify their emotional state and express it in a meaningful way. Play therapy and parallel parental interviews are helpful in such cases. In school-aged children direct interviews with short simple questions can be useful.

A semi structured or guided interview-based instrument can be used to clarify the diagnosis. Commonly used measures are the Schedule for Affective Disorders and Schizophrenia in School-age Children-Present and the Lifetime Version (K-SADS-PL) and Child and Adolescent Psychiatric Assessment (CAPA); however, these instruments also depend on the expertise of the interviewer to utilize the questions in the most meaningful way and to follow up on the answers (7).

24.2.3 Differential diagnosis of depressive disorders

Table 24.1 provides a differential diagnosis of depressive disorders.

24.2.4 Management of depressive disorders

Developing a treatment plan depends on the severity of the episode (i.e. mild, moderate or severe), and if the episode is severe, is it with or without psychosis? The mild to moderate depressive episodes, especially the first episode, should always be treated with psychosocial support and psychotherapy. Supportive psychotherapy, interpersonal therapy (IPT), cognitive behavioral therapy (CBT), group therapy, and family therapy have all been shown to be effective in mild cases of depression (8). CBT was shown to be superior in the treatment of depression in comparison to supportive and family therapy (9). More serious episodes and recurrent episodes that fail

Table 24.1: Differential diagnosis of depressive disorders

Disorder	Duration	Functional Decline	Associated Findings
Major Depressive Disorder	2 weeks or more	Significant	Prominent neurovegetative symptoms
Dysthymic Disorder	1 year or more	Moderate	Able to function albeit at lower level
Adjustment Disorder with Depression	3–6 months	Initial decline with return to normal level	Depression within 3 months of an event, resolves within 6 months
Bipolar Disorder, Depressed	Variable	Significant	History of mania or hypomania in past
Schizoaffective Disorder, Depressed	Variable	Significant	History of psychosis in past in absence of depression
Substance Induced Depression	Variable	Significant	History of current substance abuse or dependence
Depressive Disorder due to GMC*	Related to the course of GMC	Dependent on course of GMC	GMC is etiologically related to depression via a pathophysiologic mechanism, i.e. hypothyroidism
Depressive Disorder NOS**	Variable	Not significant	Not meeting criteria of any of above
Grief and Bereavement	2 months (highly variable)	Initial decline with return to normal level	Reaction to death of loved one. Guilt, yearning for and hearing voice of loved one

*GMC = General Medical Condition
**NOS = Not Otherwise Specified

to respond to psychosocial support and psychotherapy should be assessed carefully for a trial of psychotropic medications.

The TADS (Treatment for Adolescents with Depression Study) compared the treatment outcomes in adolescents 12–17 years of age in 13 academic centers and clinics in the United States. The subjects were divided into four treatment groups: (a) only cognitive behavioral therapy, (b) fluoxetine 10–40 mg/day, (c) combination of fluoxetine 10–40 mg /day and CBT, and (d) placebo group. After 12 weeks the fluoxetine and fluoxetine with CBT groups showed robust response rates of 60.6% and 71% respectively. A naturalistic study over the next 1 year showed that almost 60% stayed in remission (10).

The TORDIA trial (Treatment of SSRI-Resistant Depression in Adolescents) was also a multicenter study in adolescents 12–18 years of age who failed to respond to an adequate trail of selective serotonin reuptake inhibitors (SSRI) with an optimal dose for 2 months duration (9). The subjects were randomized to switch to (a) a different SSRI including fluoxetine, paroxetine, sertraline, and citalopram; (b) switch to a serotonin-norepinephrine reuptake inhibitor (SNRI) venlafaxine; (c) switch to a second SSRI plus CBT; and (d) switch to SNRI plus CBT. Both combination groups (SNRI+CBT) and (SSRI+CBT) were found to be superior to the medication switch alone (9).

The Texas children medication algorithm (TCMA) was released in 1999 after a consensus conference of national experts (11).The TCMA agreed that results from experiments about treatment of mental illness in adults can be extrapolated and applied to treatment in children and adolescents. It also emphasized the importance of psychoeducation of children and parents about illness and treatment options being offered (11). Recommendations of the panel are illustrated in Figure 24.2.

24.3 Bipolar spectrum disorders

Pediatric bipolar disorder (PBD) has created a robust debate in the field of psychiatry in the last few years. One side argues that PBD is almost non-existent in young children, while the other side of the debate point out the findings that about 16% of children presenting for a psychiatric evaluation do in fact have PBD (12). Lifetime prevalence of bipolar disease (BD) in general is around 0.4% to 1.6% (5). Approximately 10–15% of adolescents who were diagnosed with MDD (recurrent) developed BD later on in life (5). Wozniak et al reported that of children diagnosed with PBD, 70% developed this disorder very early in life (5 years old or younger) (13). It was also reported that 23% of these children with early onset pediatric bipolar disorder (EOPBD) reported having manic symptoms on almost a continuous basis (13).

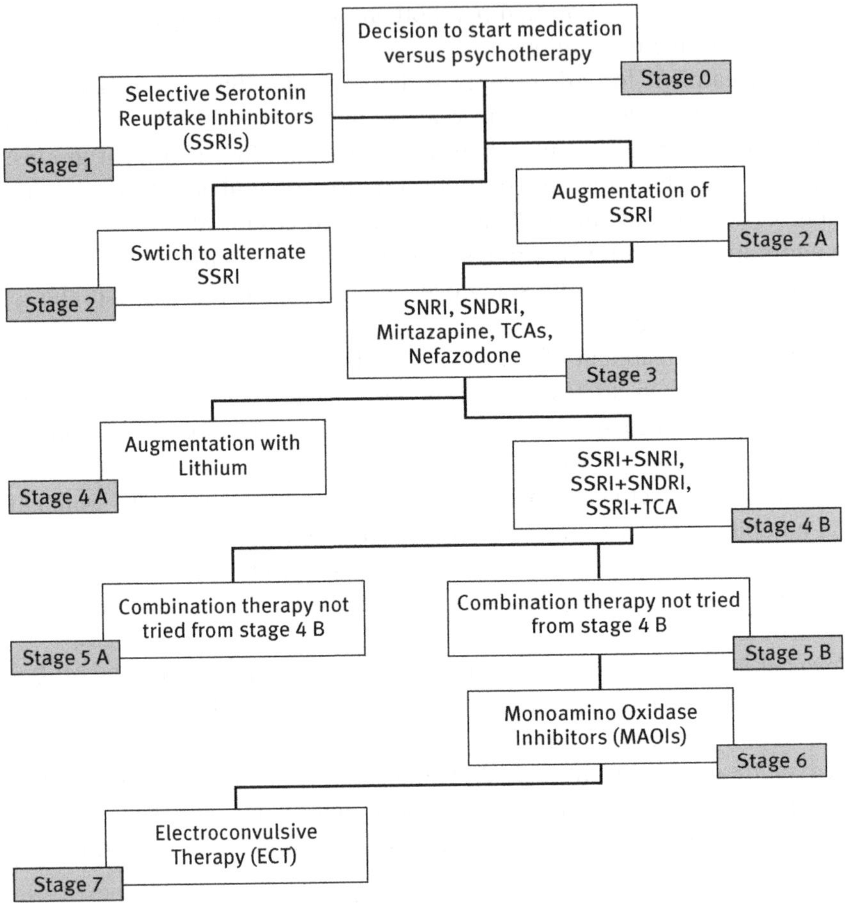

Figure 24.2: The Texas Children Medication Algorithm 1999.

24.3.1 Types of bipolar disorders

24.3.1.1 Bipolar disorder type I

The main difficulty in diagnosing PBD is that children, especially very young children, do not present with typical manic episodes lasting for a full week. They present with affective instability of very rapid type known as ultradian cycling of mood symptoms. Ultradian cycling is an ultra-rapid cycling of mood happening on a daily basis. Children usually do not present with euphoria or grandiosity (a criteria required by the DSM-IV-TR for the diagnosis of a PBD); also, they have not accumulated mountains of debts, legal problems, and relationship problems as is commonly seen in adults as a consequences of their bipolar disorder (PD).

Many researchers have argued that irritable mood, which is almost synonymous with PBD and EOPBD, should be considered as the cardinal symptom of mania in children instead of euphoria and grandiosity (13). The proponents for this change argue that the irritability, which is considered a non-specific symptom when seen in PBD and EOPBD, has a quite distinct flavor and is much more severe and qualitatively different from the irritability seen in other disorders. Typical episodes of EOPBP are not discrete as in adolescents and adults but tend to be prolonged, sometimes for years. Prepubertal children tend to have more mixed episodes, with or without psychosis, ultra rapid cycling, and hyperactivity (13).

This creates diagnostic confusion with attention deficit hyperactivity disorder (ADHD) and, at times, leads to misdiagnosis of the child with ADHD; indeed, the two disorders are highly comorbid, making the diagnosis more difficult. One must rule out any other psychiatric disorders, medications, or substance-induced euphoria and hyperthermia, and any mania-induced by a general medical condition. See Box 24.3 that lists the DIG FAST mnemonic for evaluation of mania and hypomania.

Box 24.3 DIG FAST Mnemonic for Evaluation of Mania and Hypomania based on criteria from *Diagnostic Statistical Manual of Mental Disorders*, 4th edn, text rev. Washington, DC: American Psychiatric Association, 2000

Presence of only one manic episode characterized by a distinct period of abnormally and persistently elevated, expansive, or irritable mood, lasting at least *1 week for mania* and *≥ 4 days for hypomania* with *≥ 3 (4 if the mood is only irritable)* of the following symptoms have persisted throughout this period

D Distractibility (i.e. attention too easily drawn to unimportant or irrelevant external stimuli)
I Increase in goal-directed activity (socially, at work or school, or sexually) or psychomotor agitation
G Grandiosity or inflated self-esteem (not usually seen in children)
F Flight of ideas or subjective experience that thoughts are racing
A Activity, excessive involvement in activities that have a high potential for painful consequences
S Sleep disturbances, decreased need for sleep (e.g., feels rested after only 3 hours of sleep)
T Talkative, more than usual or pressure to keep talking

A mixed episode of BD-I is characterized by the presence of some manic and some depressive symptoms that are present together nearly every day in the same 1 week period. The episode should be severe enough to cause marked decline in occupational functioning or in interpersonal relationships and social activities, or it is so disturbing that it necessitates hospitalization to prevent harm to the patient or others. Mixed episodes of severe degree occur when the symptoms present with psychotic features (5).

24.3.1.8 Bipolar disorder II (BD-II)

BD-II is a syndrome with many depressive episodes interspersed with hypomanic episodes. A hypomanic episode is defined by the DSM-IV-TR as "a distinct period of persistently elevated, expansive, or irritable mood, lasting at least 4 days, that is clearly different from the usual non-depressed mood to a significant degree." BD-II is not diagnosed if the hypomanic episode caused marked impairment in social or occupational functioning resulted in psychiatric hospitalization or caused legal consequences; if such things happened, it was most likely due to an overt manic episode. Another distinguishing feature is psychosis, which, if present, rules out BD-II (5).

24.3.1.9 Cyclothymia

A disorder of exclusion, cyclothymia requires establishing the duration criteria of 1 year during which period the child or adolescent has experienced numerous periods of hypomania alternating with numerous periods of low intensity depressive episodes. During this period the patient must not be symptom-free for more than 2 months. Cyclothymia appears to develop early on in life with some cases as early as 6 years of age. Van Meter et al found an 83% rate of comorbid ADHD (14). The same study also pointed out that most children with cyclothymia had a positive family history of mood disorders and many other psychiatric disorders, suggesting a different type of genetic predisposition (14). As in dysthymia due to the early onset and chronic course, these children tend to develop a pattern of being emotionally overactive, characterized by hypersensitivity, impulsivity, and aggressiveness comprising a personality style known as the cyclothymic-hypersensitivity temperament.

24.3.1.10 Bipolar disorder not otherwise specified (BD-NOS)

BD-NOS is considered as a diagnosis when the child or adolescent presents with clinical features of a bipolar disorder but either the severity of the symptoms or the duration of the illness does not meet the criteria of BD-I, BD-II, or cyclothymic disorder. The American Academy of Child and Adolescent Psychiatry Practice Parameter guidelines of 2007 suggest that BD-NOS should be used in children in whom the manic symptoms are of shorter duration to meet the requirement of mania, or hypomania, or in children who continue to have chronic manic symptoms that constitute their baseline functioning (15).

24.3.2 Diagnosis of bipolar disorders

The WASH-U-KSADS is a modified version of KSADS (Kiddie Schedule for Affective Disorders and Schizophrenia) to better assess EOPBD and PBD (16). WASH-U-KSADS is a screening tool that has shown excellent reliability and should be used when reaching a definitive diagnosis of PBD or EOPBD based on clinical presentation is difficult (16). The Childhood Behavior Checklist (CBCL) is another good psychometric scale that assesses for psychopathology and behavior problems in those 4–18 years of age; it is a screening tool with proven reliability. The Young Mania Rating Scale (YMRS) is another widely used scale that has high validity and reliability in the diagnosis of pediatric bipolar disorder (14).

24.3.3 Differential diagnosis of bipolar disorders

Table 24.2 lists a differential diagnosis for bipolar disorders.

24.3.3.1 Psychotherapeutic Management

Psychoeducation of the child, adolescent, and parents develops a better understanding of the illness, its course, and the importance of adhering to the treatment plan. Time-limited cognitive behavioral therapy (CBT) can also help to create an understanding of the disease and develop some healthy attitudes and coping skills. The irritability, hyperthymia, anger, and at times aggression toward others can be very disturbing for the parents and siblings; thus, family therapy can be very beneficial

Table 24.2: Differential diagnosis of bipolar disorder

Disorder	Duration	Functional Decline	Associated Features
Bipolar Disorder I	1 week long manic episode	Significant	Significant irritability,
Bipolar Disorder II	≥4 days of hypomania	Variable	Irritability, depressive episodes
Bipolar Disorder NOS	Not meeting duration or symptom intensity of mania or hypomania	Not significant	Nonspecific symptoms, some irritability
Cyclothymic Disorder	≥4 days of hypomania/ depression	Not significant	Rapid cycling hypomania/ mild depressive episodes
ADHD*	Continuous symptoms	Variable	Hyperactivity, inattention, restlessness
Substance induced	Variable	Variable	Evidence of recent or continuous substance abuse
Borderline Personality Disorder	Continuous symptoms	Variable	Affective instability, impulsivity, erratic behavior Frequent suicidal and parasuicidal behavior

in these cases. In situations where behavioral problems are the main concern, structured behavioral therapy with contingencies and reward systems may prove effective. Ideally the treatment providers should pay close attention to developing and implementing coping skills, teaching patients about symptom management, identifying signs and symptoms of relapse to prevent relapse, and bolstering academic as well as social functioning.

24.3.3.2 Psychotropic Management

The International Society for Bipolar Disorders (ISBD) has released guidelines for the monitoring of patients who are undergoing long term pharmacotherapy for bipolar disorders (17). Physicians are asked to thoroughly analyze the medical history, paying close attention to personal and family history of diabetes mellitus, coronary artery disease, thyroid or renal disease, and substance abuse. Baseline weight/waist circumference should be collected to calculate body mass index (BMI). Baseline assessments should be obtained before embarking on any medication trial; these include assessments of blood pressure, renal function, complete blood count, liver function, fasting blood sugar, and lipid profile (17).

There are no clear guidelines for the pharmacotherapy of PBD and EOPBD at present. Clinicians have to extrapolate from the various consensus guidelines and algorithms in existence for the management of bipolar disorder in adults. The inherent risk in this approach is that there are no data to support that the medications that are effective in adults are going to be effective and safe in children and adolescents. Recommendations for the treatment of adult BD, based on the four leading consensus guidelines (18), are summarized in Figures 24.3 and 24.4 for easy reference.

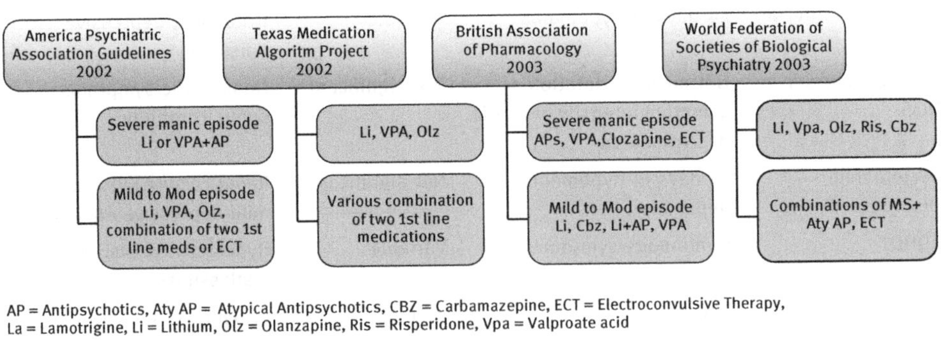

Figure 24.3: Comparison of consensus guidelines for treatment of a manic episode of bipolar disorder (adult) adopted from Fountoulakis KN et al. Treatment guidelines for bipolar disorder: a critical review. *J Aff Dis* 2005; 86:1–10.
AP=Antipsychotics, Aty AP= Atypical Antipsychotics, CBZ=Carbamazepine, ECT= Electroconvulsive Therapy, La= Lamotrigine, Li = Lithium, Olz=Olanzapine, Ris=Risperidone, Vpa= Valproate acid

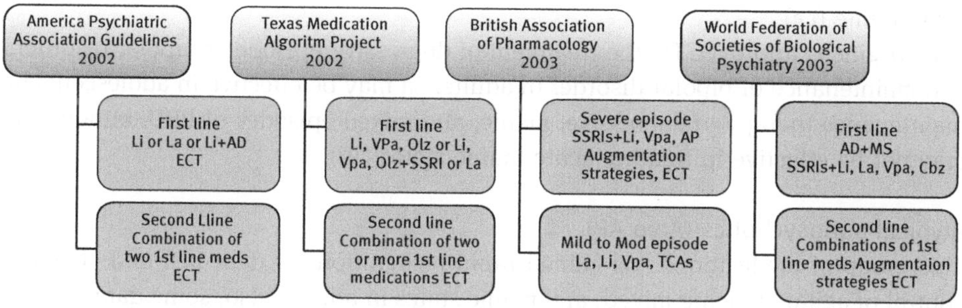

Figure 24.4: Comparison of consensus guidelines for treatment of a depressive episode of bipolar disorder (adult) adopted from Fountoulakis KN et al. Treatment guidelines for bipolar disorder: a critical review. *J Aff Dis* 2005; 86:1–10.

Mood stabilizers

A mild to moderate manic or mixed episode and depressive phase of PBD can be treated with mood stabilizer monotherapy, which is considered the first line treatment by most guidelines. In case of severe, agitated manic or mixed episode, augmentation with an antipsychotic may be necessary, at least for the short term.

Lithium (Li)

This is the medication treatment of choice and was the first mood stabilizer to be approved by the U.S. Food and Drug Administration (FDA) for the treatment of mania in patients ≥ 12 years of age. Lithium, although very effective in controlling manic episodes in adolescents, may not be able to control symptoms in very young children or in children and adolescents with mixed episodes. It is also not recommended in those who have a rapid cycling pattern, who abuse substances, or who have comorbid ADHD, conduct disorder, or a personality disorder (19). A therapeutic level for acute phase, between 0.8–1.2 mEq/l, is optimal in adults. This level should be checked every 3–6 months to achieve a therapeutic level of 0.6 to 1.0 mEq/l during the maintenance phase (19).

Valproic acid (Vpa)

Valproic acid (Vpa) has been shown to be effective in treating a mixed or manic episode in adolescents. Caution should be taken in the treatment selection of pediatric patients with Vpa, especially young girls, because of the risk of developing hirsutism and polycystic ovarian disease (PCOD). Another major side effect is the risk of fulminant hepatitis in very young children and hematological side effects in general.

Carbamazepine (Cbz)

An effective agent in adults, Cbz has shown mixed results in children and adolescents (19). Hematological side effects (especially agranulocytosis) and drug interactions at the P-450 isoenzyme hepatic pathway further limits its use in pediatric patients.

Lamotrigine (La)

Lamotrigine is approved for the treatment of depressive episode of bipolar disorder, and maintenance of bipolar disorder in adults. La may be effective in adolescents in maintenance therapy of depressive, manic, and mixed episodes of PBD, although it may not be effective in treating acute manic states (19).

Atypical antipsychotics (Atyp AP)

This group of medications has gained rapid recognition for their fast and effective control of agitated, acute mixed, and manic states in adults; also, some data is present to support efficacy in children and adolescents. The American Academy of Child and Adolescent Psychiatry (AACAP) recommends use of atypical antipsychotics (such as olanzapine, risperidone, or quetiapine) as a first-line agent in treatment of manic or mixed episodes of PBD (15). The US FDA has since approved other Atyp AP such as aripiprazole for use in the children. The long term use of these medications in children may lead to excessive weight gain as well as the associated risk of developing metabolic syndrome, hyperglycemia, and, in some cases, diabetes mellitus. Table 24.3 provides a comparison of various atypical antipsychotics.

Risperidone (Ris)

The first Atyp AP to be approved by the FDA for the treatment of mania missed episode of PBD in children, risperidone has shown a 59% response rate in controlling acute manic and mixed states in one randomized placebo control trial (RPCT) (19,20). Hyperprolactinemia is seen in more than 80% of patients; thus, it is recommended to obtain a base line prolactin level and then recheck this level every 6 months (19,20).

Olanzapine (Olz)

Approved by FDA for the treatment of mixed and manic episodes of PBD, olanzapine has shown a 48% response rate and a remission rate of 35% in PBD (19). Side effects

Table 24.3: Comparison of atypical antipsychotic medications

Atypical AP	Age	Mg/day	WtG*	Other Side Effects
Risperidone	10–17 y	0.5–2.5		Somnolence, Hyperprolactinaemia
Olanzapine	13–17 y	2.5–10	3.7 kg	Somnolence, Hyperprolactinaemia, increase BG, lipids, uric acid, possibility of DM/DKA**
Quetiapine	10–17 y	50–600	1.7 kg	Somnolence, sedation and dizziness
Ziprasidone†	10–17 y	80–160		Sedation, nausea, headache, fatigue dizziness
Aripiprazole	10–17 y	2–30	0.7kg	Akathisia, somnolence, fatigue, blurred vision, drooling, and dizziness

*= Mean Weight Gain.

**= Diabetes Mellitus and Diabetic Ketoacidosis.

†= Not approved by FDA for use in children.

include somnolence, elevation of prolactin level that was more pronounced in boys, and elevation of fasting glucose, total cholesterol, and uric acid; also, there was a transient increase in hepatic alanine and aspartate transaminase levels (19,20).

Quetiapine (Que)

The FDA has approved quetiapine for treatment of acute manic episodes in children and adolescents as a monotherapy agent, or as an adjunct for mood stabilizers. In a 3 week trial it has shown a 61% response rate versus 37% for placebo (19,20).

Ziprasidone (Zip)

Although not currently approved for treatment of PBD, a 4 week multicenter, double blind, randomized control trial in children with acute manic and mixed symptoms showed a 62% response rate (19,20). Careful selection of patients is important; this includes inquiring about family history of any sudden cardiac arrests and paying attention to any comorbid medical illness or concurrent medications, which can cause prolongation of QT interval. This is a concern associated with all atypical antipsychotics but which was first reported with ziprasidone (19,20).

Aripiprazole (Arp)

This medication was recently approved for the treatment of manic and mixed episodes PBD in children and adolescents as well as maintenance therapy of PBD (19,20). In a 4 week randomized control trial, it has shown a response rate of 54%.; about 19% of these subjects reported akathisia or inability to relax, which usually responds to decreasing the dose or stopping medication (19,20).

24.4 Anxiety spectrum disorders

Anxiety disorders are the most common psychiatric disorders among children and adolescents (21). Girls are more likely than boys to develop anxiety disorder once they are 6 years or older. Figure 24.5 provides a list of the incidence of anxiety spectrum disorders in childhood and adolescence.

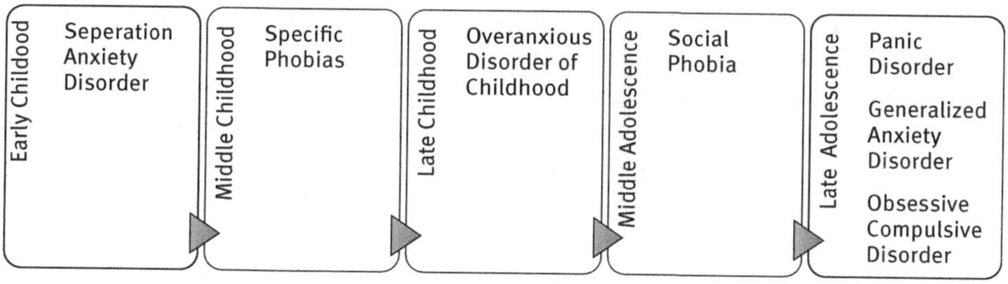

Figure 24.5: Usual incidence of anxiety spectrum disorders across childhood and adolescence.

24.4.1 Obsessive compulsive disorder

Obsessive compulsive disorder (OCD) is more frequently seen in children and adolescents who present to dermatologic practices with the cutaneous manifestation being the primary and, at times the only, presenting symptom. Most commonly pediatric OCD manifests itself in dermatology clinics as acne excoriée, trichotillomania, onychotillomania, and onychophagia (22). The DSM-IV-TR defines OCD as the presence of either recurrent obsessions or compulsions; symptoms are present for 1 hour or more per day, while obsessions and compulsions are not due to the presence of another mental disorder. In adults an additional criteria is that these symptoms are recognized as a product of one's own mind ("ego-dystonic"), but in the case of children, this criteria is waived. OCD can occur in very young children but is more commonly seen in late adolescence.

The prevalence increases from 0.17% in school age children to 0.3% in mid adolescence and finally reaching 0.53% to 4% in late adolescence (21). OCD is slightly more common in young boys than girls, but the gender difference disappears around puberty. Children with this disorder have a 4-fold prevalence of OCD in the parents and first-degree relatives. Familial association is most commonly seen with early onset of OCD in childhood (21).

Children with OCD have shown some specific anomalies on neuroimaging studies, most noticeably smaller volume of basal ganglia and larger size of thalamus as compared to children without OCD. There is evidence that the frontal cortical-striatal-thalamo-cortical neuronal network in OCD is very hyperactive, suggesting a lack of usual inhibitory control. Neuroimmunological links have been proposed in childhood-onset OCD. Pediatric autoimmune neuropsychiatric disorder-associated with streptococcus (PANDAS) is an autoimmune sequelae of group β-hemolytic streptococcus infection; similar to Sydenham's chorea and rheumatic fever, PANDAS is highly associated with OCD. Children with strong genetic predisposition to OCD tend to have a high risk of developing comorbid tic disorders (23).

24.4.1.1 Clinical features

Obsessive compulsive disorder (OCD) can be diagnosed with the presence of only obsession(s) or only compulsion(s), but in most cases of OCD they coexist. Obsessions are intrusive, unwanted, recurrent thoughts or images that are disturbing and create a sense of tension in the child or adolescent. In order to release the anxiety and tension created by the intrusive obsessive thoughts, the child attempts to create a reaction pattern called "compulsions." Obsessions can be of different types such as fear of contamination, fear of disease, need for symmetry and organization, fear of causing harm to others or self, or extreme religious and moral values. Some of the common compulsions include excessive washing, cleaning, cleansing, and purifying rituals, checking and rechecking, counting, organizing, arranging, need for touching, and rubbing. Preoccupation with numbers, colors, and shapes and assigning them a special significance is also common. OCD is highly comorbid with other anxiety disorders, mood disorders, ADHD, and childhood disruptive disorders.

OCD is seen quite often in dermatology practices, and thus, the dermatologist may be the first, and at times the only, physician who would come across these patients and diagnose the underlying OCD. Koblenzer et al has proposed the term "dermo-OCD"(DOCD) to describe the presentation of OCD in dermatology. DOCD comprises obsessions related to the appearance of fear of infestations as well as infections and resulting compulsions attempting to neutralize the anxiety and fear affecting skin and appendages (24). See Box 24.4.

Box 24.4 Dermato-Obsessive Compulsive Phenomenon Proposed by Koblenzer et al.

Obsessional worries about skin disorders
- Loosing or thinning of hair
- Skin anomalies (perceived)
- Skin contamination
- Infestations and infection
- HIV phobia
- Moles transforming in skin cancer
- Scarring from acne
- Emanating bad body odor

Compulsive dermatologic expressions
- Trichotillomania
- Chronic pruritus
- Neurotic excoriations
- Onychotillomania
- Onychphagia/dermatophagia
- Cheilitis facticia
- Localized neurodermatitis
- Irritant dermatitis
- Dermatological lesions caused by repeated mechanical trauma of touching, rubbing, picking, etc.

24.4.1.2 Clinical diagnosis

The Childhood Behavior Checklist (CBCL) contains an obsessive compulsive scale (OCS) that was validated to be used individually to screen for OCD and demonstrated good validity and reliability (25). The Leyton Obsessive Inventory – Children's Version (LOI-CV) short form is also a good screening tool in clinic settings. In adolescents some of the screening tools used for adults can be employed, such as the Yale Brown Obsessive Compulsive Scale (YBOCS). Please also see Appendix II for a more comprehensive list of psychometric scales that can be used in primary care or dermatologic practices (26).

24.4.1.3 Psychiatric management

Establishing a therapeutic alliance and reassurance benefits the child most and enhances the chance of success of any treatment plan. Delineating goals of treatment is important, including decreasing the time spent in OCD behavior, developing coping skills, and encouraging compliance by the child or adolescent and family with the treatment regimen. There are no guidelines for the treatment of OCD in children and adolescents; however, the general principles used in adults can serve as guidelines to devise a pediatric treatment plan. The APA treatment guidelines recommend using CBT, especially utilizing exposure and relapse prevention (ERP) or SSRIs as first line of treatment. OCD can be difficult to treat due to its waxing and waning course as well as high propensity of being comorbid with other psychiatric disorders (27). Several optimizing, alternate, adjunct, and augmentative strategies have been proposed for adults; these are illustrated in Figure 24.6.

24.4.2 Social anxiety disorder (SAD)

Social anxiety disorder (SAD), also known as social phobia, has a prevalence of 0.6% to 3.5% with equal gender distribution and a peak incidence in middle adolescence (28). The DSM-IV-TR defines SAD as a marked or persistent fear of being scrutinized in one or more social or performance situations. In children and adolescents SAD must occur in peer situations and not only when having an encounter with adults. Children also may not recognize that this fear is irrational, which is one of the criteria for diagnosis of SAD in adults.

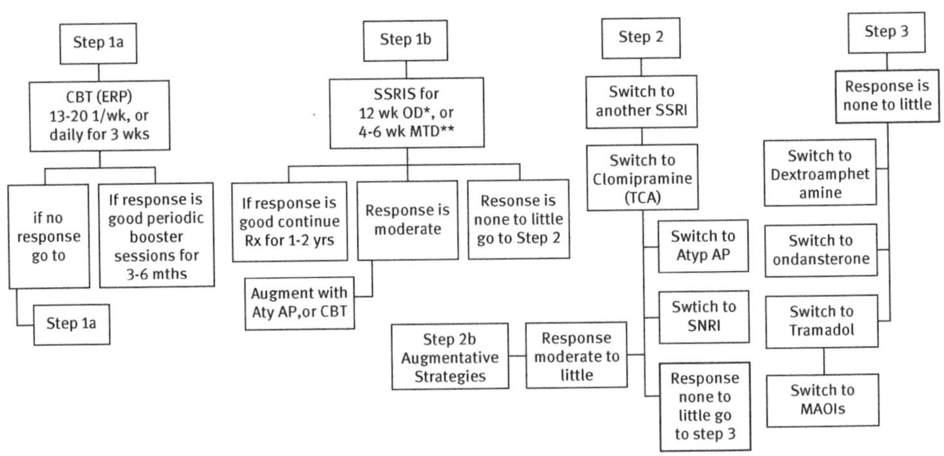

Figure 24.6: APA guidelines for treatment of OCD in adults.

SAD is considered generalized when almost all social situations are feared. In children and adolescents the SAD can be incapacitating and may involve a variety of situations, including performance anxiety related to participating in class, taking part in extracurricular activities, public speaking, and social situations involving interpersonal interactions experienced in dating, carrying out a casual conversation with peers, and attending social events. Children with SAD isolate themselves and have less academic achievement than their peers. Social stigma of altered appearance resulting from various skin diseases is highly associated with SAD in children and adolescents (29); these skin disorders include acne, atopic dermatitis, psoriasis, vitligo, alopecia areata, and other skin conditions producing actual or perceived "ugliness." Diagnostic criteria for social phobia are listed in Box 24.5.

Box 24.5 DSM-IV-TR Diagnostic Criteria for Social Phobia in Children and Adolescents

A marked and persistent fear of one or more social or performance situations in which the person is exposed to unfamiliar people or to possible scrutiny by others

Evidence of capacity for age-appropriate social relationships with familiar people and the anxiety must occur in peer settings, not just in interactions with adults

The anxiety may be expressed by crying, tantrums, freezing, or shrinking from social situations with unfamiliar people.

Avoidance of social or performance situations, or else endured with intense anxiety or distress. The duration of the condition must be at least 6 months

SP is not due to the direct physiological effects of a substance or a general medical condition and is not better accounted for by another mental disorder.

24.4.2.1 Clinical diagnosis

The Liebowitz Social Anxiety Scale (LSAS) is a 24-item test that is an effective aid in reaching a diagnosis of social anxiety disorder (30). Fear of Negative Evaluation Scale (FNE) is a 30-item self-report and the Social Avoidance and Distress Scale (SADS) is a 28-item self-report scale encompassing different aspects of social anxiety, including fear, anxiety, discomfort, distress, and avoidance of social situations (30).

24.4.2.2 Psychotherapeutic management

Mainstay of treatment is psychotherapy, including individual and group therapy; these management tools have demonstrated effectiveness, although most patients with avoidant personality are very reluctant to disclose personal information in group settings. CBT is also very effective, especially involving gradual desensitization to intrapersonal and social situations. CBT provided to anxious child was found to be superior to the CBT provided to family of anxious child (31).

24.4.2.3 Psychotropic management

Selective serotonin reuptake inhibitors (SSRIs) are the first line of treatment for all anxiety disorders. At present there are no large prospective studies in the pediatric population regarding psychotropic use for the treatment of anxiety disorder. The RUPP (Research Units on Pediatric Psychopharmacology) Anxiety Study Group have studied SSRIs in children and adolescents with anxiety spectrum disorders and presented their findings in 2001 (32).

Fluvoxamine (Flx)

The 128 participants aged 6–17 years were randomized to receive treatment either with fluvoxamine or placebo for 8 weeks with and without supportive psychotherapy (SPT). The Flx + SPT group showed far superior response of 76% versus the 29% response rate in the placebo +SPT group.

Fluoxetine

Fluoxetine was studied in 15 children age 6–11 years in selective mutism, a subtype of social phobia. Fluoxetine was found superior to placebo, but its effect was not statistically different (33). Another open label trial of 21 children and adolescents with selective mutism ages 5–14 years showed a 76% improvement in social anxiety and facilitation of speech in school and public settings (34). Youth 7–17 years of age diagnosed with generalized anxiety disorder, separation anxiety disorder, and social phobia showed improvement in anxiety scores as well as in functional abilities with fluoxetine (35). Children who continued to take fluoxetine 20 mg daily showed much greater outcomes on most measures at their 1 year follow up.

Paroxetine

Paroxetine has shown to be effective in SAD in a double blind randomized control trial (RCT) of 319 children and adolescents 8–17 years of age; the group treated with paroxetine had a 77% positive response versus the 38% seen with placebo (36). Decreased appetite, insomnia, and mild gastrointestinal upset were common side effects reported in the paroxetine-treated group.

Sertraline

Pediatric patients 5 to 17 years of age with generalized anxiety disorder (GAD) were treated with 50 mg a day of sertraline in a 9 week double-blind, RCT (37). Those prescribed the sertraline demonstrated significant improvement in psychic and somatic anxiety as well as significant improvement on all five domains of the Hamilton anxiety scale and on clinical global impression (37).

24.4.3 Eating disorders

Eating disorders were previously considered as conditions that affected primarily adolescents and those in early adulthood; however, they are now being diagnosed in more and more young children. Any activities that require pursuit of a thin habitus (e.g. ballet, figure skating, gymnastics, swimming, and others) place a greater focus on how a child or adolescent perceives his or her body and how it should appear to others; this is also true for those with future aspiration to be in professions such as modeling, acting, dancing, and various sports. Girls are more frequently affected by eating disorders, but young males with a homosexual orientation or those taking part in weight conscious sports (such as wrestling) are associated with increased risks of eating disorders (38). There is a greater male preponderance and a much more dramatic weight loss when children develop eating disorders under 13 years of age (38). Eating disorders are divided into four distinct groups: anorexia nervosa (AN), bulimia nervosa (BN), binge eating disorder (BED), and eating disorders not otherwise specified (EDNOS).

24.4.3.1 Anorexia nervosa (AN)

Anorexia nervosa (AN) has a strong genetic predisposition with a 7% likelihood of having a first degree relative with AN; twin studies have shown a 33% to 84% heritability pattern (38). Although AN predominantly affects 20–30 per 100,000 predominantly young girls, boys are also at risk, although they make up only 10% of these patients (38,39). The DSM-IV-TR describes AN as refusal to maintain body weight at or above the minimal normal weight for age and height, or failure to make expected weight gain during a period of growth, leading to a body weight that is less than 85% of that expected. In postmenarcheal girls absence of three consecutive menstrual cycles is one of the diagnostic criteria (40). These persons are also preoccupied with a fear of gaining any weight despite being overly thin, and they have a disturbance in the way they perceive and experience their bodies. They also place undue influence on body weight or shape. They are highly critical of themselves and are in denial of the seriousness of their current lower than expected body weight. AN is subdivided into two types: restricting and purging types.

24.4.3.2 Bulimia nervosa (BN)

Bulimia nervosa (BN) affects about 3.2% of young females and about 1.1% of young males with a high heritability rate of 28% to 83% (38).The DSM-IV-TR defines BN as recurrent episodes of binge eating in a discrete period of time associated with a sense of lack of control over eating during the episodes; this is followed by inappropriate compensatory behavior in order to prevent weight gain, such as self-induced vomiting, fasting, excessive exercise, or misuse of laxatives, diuretics, enemas, or other medications (40). These young people are excessively preoccupied with their body image, and self-evaluation is unduly influenced by body shape and weight (40).

In order to diagnose a patient with BN one must make sure that these maladaptive behaviors have occurred at least twice a week for 3 months of time, as episodic eating-related behavior not meeting the duration criteria occur much more often. Eaton DK et al conducted the Youth Risk Behavior Surveillance (YRBS) of American teenagers, which showed that 46% of females and 30% of males admitted at least one binge episode during their lifetime; also, 60% of females and 30% of males had attempted to lose weight by different means during the preceding 30 days (41). About 12% had restricted food and fasted for more than 24 hours to lose weight. About 6.4% of females and 2.2% of males reported self-induced vomiting or laxative use, while 7.5% of girls and 4.2% of boys reported using other medications in an effort to lose weight (41).

24.4.3.3 Binge eating disorder (BED)

Binge eating disorder (BED) affects about 2% to 4% of the population starting in adolescence. The diagnostic criteria of BED includes recurrent binge eating episodes, as defined in BN, accompanied with at least three of the maladaptive behaviors; these include eating much more rapidly than normal, eating until feeling uncomfortably full, eating large amounts of food when not feeling physically hungry, eating alone, and feeling disgusted, depressed, or very guilty after overeating. The binge eating occurs, on average, at least 2 days a week for a continuous 6 month duration (40).

24.4.3.4 Eating disorder not otherwise specified (EDNOS)

Eating disorder not otherwise specified (EDNOS) is a category that is used when the eating disorder does not meet the criteria of any of the other mentioned disorders but exhibits some features of these eating disorders. It is much more commonly diagnosed than other eating disorders with a prevalence of 0.5% to 14% of the population (38). EDNOS is diagnosed when the criteria for anorexia nervosa are met but the patient has normal weight with regular menses; it can also be diagnosed if a patient meets all the criteria for bulimia nervosa but has less than two binging episodes per week in the last 3 months. A person who maintains normal body weight but displays inappropriate compensatory behavior after ingestion of small amounts of food is also diagnosed with EDNOS. These inappropriate behaviors include chewing and spitting repeatedly, without swallowing significant amounts of food. EDNOS is also seen when recurrent episodes of binging are present in the absence of inappropriate compensatory behavior.

24.4.3.5 Clinical features

Eating disorders present with many prominent dermatologic signs and symptoms; indeed, some may be seen by a dermatologist for their skin problems before they present to, or are noticed by, any other physician, including a psychiatrist. Gupta et al has described four different ways in which an eating disorder patient develops skin manifestations: (a) due to the impact of dietary alterations or starvation, (b) due to self-induced vomiting, (c) due to the abuse of laxative or diuretics, and (d) because of highly comorbid self-induced dermatitis (42).

The most common reported dermatological symptom was xerosis or generalized dryness of the skin, which was seen in 84% of those with BN and 96% with AN, followed by acne in 59% with AN and 70% with BN. Alopecia (mostly of diffuse frontal type) was reported in 61% to 67% of patients with eating disorders. Hypertrichosis lanuginosa was present in 77% of AN patients. In another study, acne was seen in 70% of BN and 60% of AN patients (39). Dental caries were seen in 40% to 47% of patients with eating disorders.

Other cutaneous signs found in approximately 10% to 30% of these patients were nail fragility, onychophagia, Russell's sign, seborrheic dermatitis, interdigital intertrigo, hand dermatitis, onychoschizia, depapillated tongue, angular cheilitis, and dental enamel erosion. Opaque fragile hair was seen in almost 41% of patients with BN. About 12% to 21% of patients had comorbid factitious dermatitis in the form of acne excoriée and erythema abigne due to intentional exposure to low intensity heat, cigarette burns, and other forms of self-induced cutaneous trauma (39).

24.4.3.6 Differential diagnosis

Differential diagnosis of eating disorders is displayed in Table 24.4.

24.4.3.7 Clinical diagnosis

Electrolyte abnormalities are common, including hypomagnesemia, hypophosphatemia, and hypokalemia; others include hypochloremic metabolic alkalosis,

Table 24.4: Differential diagnosis of eating disorders

Disorder	Restricting	Purging	Binging	Others
Anorexia Nervosa	Positive	Positive	Negative	Type I restricting Type II purging type
Bulimia Nervosa	Negative	Positive	Positive	Binging & purging at least twice a week for 3 months
Binge Eating Disorder	Negative	Positive	Positive	Binging at least 2 days a week for 6 months
Eating Disorder NOS	Positive/ Negative	Positive/Negative	Positive/ Negative	Not meeting full criteria any ED

hyperamylasemia, and hypercarotinemia. Leukopenia with relative lymphocytosis and anemia are also common findings. Electrocardiography shows low voltage, bradycardia, S-T segment depression, and Q-T and T wave changes that may result in cardiac arrhythmias (43).

Several psychometric scales can be used to evaluate eating disorders, including self-reports such as the Eating Disorder Inventory-2 (EDI-2), Body Shape Questionnaire (BSQ), and Three Factor Eating Questionnaire (TFEQ). Semi-structured interviews can also be helpful in confirming the diagnosis once clinical suspicion of a eating disorder arises; these include the Eating Disorder Examination (EDE) and the Child Eating Disorder Examination Questionnaire (ChEDE-Q), which is derived from the adult EDE (43,44,45,46).

24.4.3.8 Psychotherapeutic management

Cognitive behavioral therapy (CBT)has proven to be effective in treatment of eating disorders, but weight loss after the end of treatment can occur. CBT in bulimia nervosa is shown to be more effective, resulting in abstinence from binging and purging along with sustaining the improvement even after 1 year.

24.4.3.9 Psychotropic management

Psychotropic medications are indicated in cases where psychotherapy has not been beneficial or in some cases where medications can be used as adjunct to psychotherapy. Cyproheptadine is an H2 blocker that has been shown to be marginally effective in anorexia nervosa but can have a negative effect in bulimia nervosa patients. SSRIs have shown little impact on weight gain in anorexia nervosa patients, but they can impact positively on other aspects of eating disorders, including depression, anxiety, OCD symptoms, and relapse prevention. Fluoxetine in high doses of 60 mg per day was effective in patients with bulimia nervosa when compared to placebo. Antipsychotics and mood stabilizers have been used in those with eating disorders, especially if there is comorbid condition requiring such treatment; however, no large studies are available at this time (47).

24.5 Personality disorders (PDs)

24.5.1 Introduction

Personality disorders (PDs) are defined in the DSM-IV-TR as enduring, inflexible, and pervasive patterns of inner experience and behavior that deviate markedly from the expectations of these individuals' cultures. PDs are manifested in any of two of four domains, including one's way of perceiving self and others, inappropriate emotional response and affective expression, deficit in interpersonal functioning, and a problem in impulse control. One of the qualifying criteria that must be met is that the personality traits are stable and its onset can be traced back at least to adolescence or early adulthood (48). It is estimated that about 10% to 20% of the general population meet criteria for some kind of personality disorder; however, this number rises to almost 50% among psychiatric inpatients and those presenting to emergency departments with psychiatric emergencies. PDs commonly encountered in medical settings, especially in dermatology clinics, are now considered.

24.5.2 Clinical diagnosis

There are several very well developed and highly valid tests to assess personality disorders. The Millon Clinical Multiaxial Inventory (MCMI) and the Minnesota Multiphasic Personality Inventory (MMPI) are the two most widely used tests in this regard. The MCMI consists of 344 true and false questions and was developed to uncover specific personality traits, styles of coping, and clinical personality syndromes. The Personality Assessment Inventory (PAI) is a 344 items inventory that comprises 22 scales. The MMPI is a much broader assessment of psychiatric disorders, including personality disorders, and it has more than 500 questions assessing 9 different domains of psychological functioning.

24.5.2.1 Borderline personality disorder (BPD)

The prevalence of borderline personality disorder (BPD) in the general population is estimated to be around 1% to 2%; however, the prevalence is almost 10 to 15 times higher in medical settings such as emergency rooms and inpatient psychiatric hospitals. BPD accounts for almost one third of all the diagnosed personality disorders (49). Several theories have been proposed about the origin and development of BPD without any definitive evidence supporting any one of them. The disease usually manifests itself in adolescence and early adulthood, although some of the features can be seen at an early age. It appears that early difficulties in differentiation–individuation, abuse (especially of a sexual nature), and neglect predispose these children to develop a sense of real or perceived rejection and abandonment, which is the hallmark of BPD (49).

The main feature of BPD is affective instability or mood labiality that leads to many misinterpretations and misjudgments of interpersonal relationships, highly impulsive and self-destructive behavior leading to lifelong patterns of painful consequences, and a chronic sense of loneliness and inner emptiness, which they try to fill with whatever they consider will bring them companionship and happiness. Box 24.6 lists DSM-IV-TR diagnostic criteria for the borderline personality disorder.

Box 24.6 Diagnostic Criteria for Borderline Personality Disorder, *Diagnostic and Statistical Manual of Mental Disorders*, 4th edn, text rev. Washington, DC: American Psychiatric Association, 2000

Pervasive pattern of instable mood, self image, in a variety of settings indicated by 5 or more of the following:

Efforts to avoid real or imagined abandonment
Intense and unstable interpersonal relationships
Identity disturbance reflected in unstable self image
Impulsive reckless behavior; overspending, overindulgence in sex, drugs, food, etc.
Recurrent suicidal and parasuicidal behavior like cutting and other self-mutilation
Affective instability: short intense mood swings, lasting for hours or few days
Chronic sense of emptiness
Uncontrollable rage, usually inappropriate to the situation
Transient paranoia and dissociative symptoms usually in response to stress related

Management

Patients with borderline personality disorders can present as a dilemma for clinicians because of their presentation with a plethora of symptoms and high levels of comorbidity with Axis I disorders. The treatment plan should reflect a full assessment and management of these comorbid disorders. BPD is a highly heterogeneous disorder both at inter- and intraindividual levels. The treatment plan should be individualized and developed collaboratively with the patient and family; also, it needs to be flexible in order to adapt to the changes in symptoms at different times in the same individual over the course of the illness (50). BPD patients tend to use splitting by idealizing and devaluing team members, which can fracture the team effort and derail the success of the treatment plan. If multiple team members are involved, they should be aware of this inherent risk and make efforts for open lines of communication and collaboration within this team on each level (50).

Psychodynamic/psychoanalytic psychotherapy and group therapy have shown some effectiveness and can be used with each other. Dialectical behavior therapy (DBT) is a manual-based therapy that consists of 1 hour long weekly sessions of individual therapy along with 2.5 hours of group therapy for specific skill development for 6 months to 1 year. DBT has shown success in decreasing rates of admissions to psychiatric units with self-destructive behaviors. Suicidal and parasuicidal behaviors are very common, and about 8% to 10% of patients with BPD commit suicide (48). DBT promotes an understanding of the origin of these destructive impulses and encourages self-reflection to avoid acting upon these dangerous impulses. The second step is to work on behaviors interfering with therapy, such as not respecting personal boundaries, splitting, and non-compliance; then, the therapy focuses on behaviors interfering with the patient's quality of life (50).

Most patients with BPD require some form of pharmacotherapy along with psychological therapy due to following reasons: (a) affective instability, (b) impulse dyscontrol, (c) dissociative symptoms, and (d) comorbid disorders on Axis I. Paton et al conducted a review of the treatment of BPD and found 19 randomized placebo controlled trials with a total of 609 patients treated with either placebo or one of 20 drugs belonging to different psychotropic groups (51). This study concluded that the evidence for the efficacy of antipsychotics is weak, even though they are commonly prescribed in patients with borderline personality disorder because of the high frequency of transient psychotic symptoms (51).

Affective instability and impulse control issues are the main indications for use of antidepressants in this population. SSRIs are shown to be effective in stabilizing mood and decreasing the impulsive destructive behavior by some open studies, although evidence provided by RCTs is not robust (51). Due to the high comorbidity of bipolar disorder with BPD, mood stabilizers are often used for patients with borderline personality disorders. Lithium and divalproex have shown some efficacy that was not replicated in RCTs (51). In terms of anxiolytics, benzodiazepines are best to avoid as they are disinhibiting and may aggravate impulse dyscontrol and aggression toward others as well as increase self-destructive behaviors (51).

24.5.2.2 Avoidant personality disorder

It is estimated that avoidant personality disorder affects 0.5% to 2.4% of the general population, and overall is more prevalent in women than in men. The disorder is characterized by a pattern of avoidance based on anxiety, which, over time, works to hinder the patient from forming both healthy social and interpersonal relationships. Individuals who develop this disorder are often described as being introverted, socially awkward, anxious in social settings, and having a low self-esteem. Sensitive to rejection, they are cautious of situations that may cause them embarrassment or cause people to judge and/or criticize them. It is difficult to distinguish avoidant personality disorder from other Axis I anxiety disorders (such as social phobia) as many of the symptoms are easily interchangeable. The one defining feature of the disorder is that sufferers avoid social situations because of a fear of rejection, despite the fact that they desperately desire social interactions and interpersonal relationships (49).

24.5.2.3 Obsessive compulsive personality disorder (OCPD)

Obsessive compulsive personality disorder (OCPD) is prevalent in approximately 1% of the general population and is seen more often in men than in women. Those who develop this disorder are known for being strict, parsimonious, stubborn, and perfectionist. They are often inflexible and spend large portions of their time fixating on small, often inconsequential details, which over time prevents them from completing their larger goals. This fixation on perfection marks them workaholics and deters them from delegating tasks or working well with others. Over time their rigidity makes it difficult for them to form close and lasting interpersonal relationships. OCPD and OCD differ mainly because OCPD is ego-syntonic, while OCD patients consider their preoccupation, compulsions, and obsessions as detrimental to their quality of life; people with OCPD view their "quirks" as positive characteristics that make them superior to others (49).

Medications such as clomipramine and SSRIs that are effective in OCD may not be useful in OCPD; however, sometimes they are used to treat comorbid OCD and other anxiety as well as depression symptoms. Psychotherapeutic interventions are useful as patients with OCPD want to perform well in therapy as they want to do well in other areas of life, although their desire for perfectionism may become a hurdle in therapy. The aim of therapy is to explore the roots of such rigid and overbearing standards set forth by the patients for themselves and how to change that to a healthier pattern of living. CBT has shown the most efficacy in this regard especially by addressing the rigid schema of these patients about self and the world around them (49).

24.6 Conclusion

The delicate interplay of psychiatry and dermatology is multifactorial. Many patients who are categorized as a dermatology patient or a psychiatric patient may have a disease process with symptomatology of both. Patients presenting with primary dermatologic disease not responding to optimal dermatological care may have an underlying psychiatric disease complicating the index illness, and the treating physician should be mindful about this possibility.

References

1. Hughes JE, Barraclough BM, Hamblin LG. Psychiatric symptoms in dermatology patients. *Br J Psychiatry* 1983;143:51–4.
2. Picardi A, Abeni D, Melchi CF. Psychiatric morbidity in dermatological outpatient: An issue to be recognized. *Br J Dermatol* 2000;143:983–91.
3. Kaplan HI, Sadock BJ, Sadock VA. *Kaplan and Sadock's synopsis of psychiatry 2007*. Philadelphia, PA: Wolter Kluwer/Lippincott Williams Wilkins, 2007:532.
4. Costello EJ, Erkanli A, Angold A. Is there an epidemic of child or adolescent depression? *J Child Psychol Psychiatry* 2006;47:12:1263–71.
5. American Psychiatric Association. *Diagnostic and statistical manual of mental disorders*, 4th edn, text rev (DSM-IV-TR). Washington, DC: APA, 2000.
6. Invernizzi G, Mauri MC, Waintraub L. Antidepressant efficacy in the treatment of dysthymia. *European Neuropsychopharmacology* 1997;7:329–36.

7. Ryan ND. Diagnosing pediatric depression. *Biol Psychiatr* 2001;49:1050–4.
8. Ryan ND. Treatment of depression in children and adolescents. *Lancet* 2005;366:933–40.
9. TADS Team. The Treatment for Adolescents with Depression Study (TADS): Outcomes over 1 year of naturalistic follow-up. *Am J Psychiatry* 2009;166:10:1141–9.
10. Brent D, Emslie G, Clarke G. Switching to another SSRI or to venlafaxine with or without cognitive behavioral therapy for adolescents with SSRI-resistant depression: The TORDIA randomized controlled trial. *JAMA* 2008;299;8:901–13.
11. Hughes CW, Emsile GJ, Crismon ML. The Texas Children's Medication Algorithm Project: Report of the Texas Consensus Conference Panel on Medication Treatment of Childhood Major Depressive Disorder. *J Am Acad Child Adolesc Psychiatr* 1999;38(11):1442–54.
12. Danielyn A, Pathak S, Kowatch RA. Clinical characteristics of bipolar disorder in very young children. *J Affect Disord* 2007;97:51–9.
13. Wozniak J, Biederman J, Kwon A, Mick,E. How cardinal are cardinal symptoms in pediatric bipolar disorder? An examination of clinical correlates. *Biol Psychiatr* 2005;58: 583–8.
14. VanMeter A, Youngstrom EA, Youngstrom JK. Examining the validity of cyclothymic disorder in a youth sample. *J Affect Disord* 2011;132(1,2):55–63.
15. McClellan J, Kowatch R, Findling RL. Practice parameter for the assessment and treatment of children and adolescents with bipolar disorder. AACAP Official Action. *J Am Acad* 2007;46 (1): 107–25.
16. Geller B, Warner K, Williams M. Prepubertal and young adolescent bipolarity versus ADHD: Assessment and validity using the WASH-U-KSADS, CBCL and TRF. *J Affect Disord* 1998;51 (2):93–100.
17. Ng F, Mammen OK, Wilting I. The International Society for Bipolar Disorders (ISBD) consensus guidelines for the safety monitoring of bipolar disorder treatments. *Bipolar Disord* 2009;11(6): 559–595.
18. Fountoulakis KN, Vieta E, Sanchez-Moreno J. Consensus treatment Guidelines for bipolar disorder; a critical review. *J Affect Disord* 2005;86(1):1–10.
19. Thomas T, Stansifer L, Findling RL. Psychopharmacology of Pediatric Bipolar Disorders in Children and Adolescents. *Pediatr Clin North Am* 2011;58(1):173–87.
20. Singh MK, Ketter TA, Chang KD. Atypical antipsychotics for acute manic and mixed episodes in children and adolescents with bipolar disorder: Efficacy and tolerability. *Drugs* 2010;70(4): 433–42.
21. Kaplan HI, Sadock BJ, Sadock VA. *Kaplan and Sadock's synopsis of psychiatry*. Philadelphia: Wolter Kluwer/Lippincott Williams Wilkins, 2007.
22. Koo JY, Smith LL. Obsessive-compulsive disorders in the pediatric dermatology practice. *Pediatr Dermatol* 1991;8(2):107–13.
23. Murphy TK, Sajid M, Soto O. Detecting pediatric autoimmune neuropsychiatric with streptococcus children with obsessive-compulsive disorder and tic. *Biol Psychiatry* 2004;55(1):61–8.
24. Koblenzer C. Psychiatric syndromes of interest to dermatologists. *Int J Dermatol* 1993;32 (2):82–8.
25. Fineberg NA, Bangalore KR, Moberg J. Clinical Screening for Obsessive-Compulsive and Related Disorders. *Isr J Psychiatry Relat Sci* 2008;45(3);151–63.
26. Bamber D, Tamplin A, Park RJ. Development of a Short Leyton Obsessional Inventory for Children and Adolescents 2002. *J Am Acad Child Adolesc Psychiatry* 2002; 41(10):1246–52.
27. Lambert M. APA releases guidelines on treating obsessive-compulsive disorder. *Am Fam Physician* 2008;78(1):131–35.
28. Heimberg RG, Stein MB, Hiripi E. Trends in the prevalence of social phobia in the United States: A synthetic cohort analysis of changes over four decades. *Eur Psychiatry* 2000;15(1):29–37.
29. Kent G. Social anxiety and disfigurement: The moderating effects of fear of negative evaluation and past experience. *Br J Clin Psychol* 2001;40(1):23–34.

30. Evren B, Evren C. Relationship Between Alexithymia and Social Anxiety in Female Outpatients with Dermatological Disorder Presenting for Psychiatric Consultation. *J Clin Psychol Med Sett* 2007;14(3):258–65.
31. Bodden DHM, Bögels SM, Nauta MH. Child Versus Family Cognitive-Behavioral Therapy in Clinically Anxious Youth: An Efficacy and Partial Effectiveness Study. *J Am Acad Child Ado Psychiatry* 2008;47(12):1384–1394.
32. Walkup J, Labellarte M, Riddle MA, Pine DS, Greenhill L, Fairbanks J, et al. An open-label extension of the research units on pediatric psychopharmacology anxiety study. *J Child Adolesc Psychopharmacol* 2002;12(3):175–88.
33. Black B., Uhde T.W. Treatment of elective mutism with fluoxetine: A double-blind, placebo-controlled study. *J Am Acad Child Adolesc Psychiatry* 1995;34(6):701–03.
34. Dummit SE, Klein RG, Trancer NK. Fluoxetine treatment of children with selective mutism: An open trial. *J Am Acad Child Adolesc Psychiatry* 1996;35(5):615–21.
35. Clark DB, Birmher B, Axelson DA, Monk K. Fluoxetine for the treatment of childhood anxiety disorders. *J Am Acad Child Adolesc Psychiatry* 2003;42(4):415–23.
36. Wagner KD, Berard R, Stein R. A multicenter, randomized, double-blind, placebo-controlled trial of paroxetine in children and adolescents with social anxiety disorder. *Arch Gen Psychiatry* 2004;61(11):1153–62.
37. Rynn MA, Siqueland L, Rickels K. Placebo-controlled trial of sertraline in the treatment of children with generalized anxiety disorder. *Am J Psychiatry* 2001;158(12):2008–14.
38. Sigel EJ. Eating disorders. In: Hay WW Jr, Levin MJ, Sondheimer JM, Deterding RR, eds. *Current pediatric diagnosis and treatment,* 19th edn. New York: McGraw Hill, 2009.
39. Glorio R, Allevato M, Pablo AD. Prevalence of cutaneous manifestations in 200 patients with eating disorders. *Int J Dermatology* 2000;39(5):348–53.
40. American Psychiatric Association. *Diagnostic and statistical manual of mental disorders*, 4th edn, text revision (DSM-IV-TR). Washington, DC: APA, 2000:589–94.
41. Eaton DK, Kann L, Kinchen S, Shanklin S. Youth Risk Behavior Surveillance: United States 2007. *MMWR Surveil Summ* 2008;57(4):1–131.
42. Gupta MA, Gupta AK, Haberman HF. Dermatologic signs in anorexia nervosa and bulimia nervosa. *Arch Dermatol* 1987;123(10):1386–90.
43. Wiseman CV, Harris WA, Halmi KA. Eating Disorders. *Med Clin North Am* 1998;82(1): 145–59.
44. Jansen E, Mulkens S, Hamers H, Jansen A. Assessing eating disordered behavior in overweight children and adolescents: Bridging the gap between a self-report questionnaire and a gold standard interview. *Netherland J Psychol* 2007;63(3):93–7.
45. Lavoisy G, Guefi JD, Vera L, Dardennes R, Rouillon. Evaluation of perturbed body image in eating disorders using the Body Shape Questionnaire. *Encephale* 2008;34(6):570–76.
46. Mazzeo ES, Aggen SH, Anderson C, Tozzi F, Bulk CM. Investigating the structure of the eating inventory (three-factor eating questionnaire): A confirmatory approach. *Int J Eat Disord* 2003: 34(2):255–64.
47. Mitchell JE, DeZawan M, Roerig JL. Drug therapy for patients with eating disorders. *Curr Drug Targets CNS Neurol Disord* 2003;2(1):17–29.
48. American Psychiatric Association. *Diagnostic and statistical manual of mental sisorders*, 4th edn, text revision (DSM-IV-TR). Washington, DC: APA, 2000:685–729.
49. Janowsky D. Chapter 30. Personality Disorders. In: Ebert MH, Loosen PT, Nurcombe B, Leckman JF, eds. *Current diagnosis and treatment: Psychiatry,* 2nd edn. New York: McGraw-Hill, 2011.
50. *Practice guidelines* for the treatment of patients with borderline personality disorder. American Psychiatric Association. *Am J Psychiatry* 2001;158(10):1–52.
51. Paton C, Okocha C. Pharmacological treatment of borderline personality disorder. *J Psychol Intensive Care* 2005;1(2):105–16.

APPENDIX

25 About the editors

Ruqiya Shama Tareen, MD, MBBS, DDSc, is an Associate Professor of Psychiatry at Michigan State University College of Human Medicine (East Lansing, Michigan, USA). She serves as full time teaching faculty and as the Director of Women's Behavioral Health program at the Psychiatry Residency Program at Western Michigan University School of Medicine (Kalamazoo, Michigan, USA). She trained as a dermatologist at the University of Wales, Cardiff in the United Kingdom and worked as a dermatologist for several years; later, she completed residency training in psychiatry at Michigan State University/Kalamazoo Center for Medical Studies (Kalamazoo, Michigan, USA). She also acquired subspecialty training in psychosomatic medicine and works as a consultation liaison faculty in two large area hospitals affiliated with the psychiatry residency program. Pursuing her passion of psychiatric issues prevalent with women, Dr. Tareen also founded and supervises a resident based Women's Behavioral Health Clinic and an elective for senior residents, namely Women's Behavioral Health Track at the Psychiatry Residency Program at Michigan State University/Kalamazoo Center for Medical Studies. With her strong background in dermatology, psychiatry, and psychosomatic medicine, it is only natural that psychodermatology is her area of interest. Dr. Tareen has a strong background in both teaching and research and has received several awards, as well as had several of her works published in these various areas of interest. E-mail: tareen@kcms.msu.edu

Donald E. Greydanus, MD, Dr. HC (ATHENS), FAAP, FSAM (Emeritus), FIAP (HON), is Professor of Pediatrics and Human Development at Michigan State University College of Human Medicine (East Lansing, Michigan, USA) and Professor and Chair of the Department of Pediatrics, Western Michigan University School of Medicine (Kalamazoo, Michigan, USA). He received the 1995 American Academy of Pediatrics' Adele D. Hofmann Award for "Distinguished Contributions in Adolescent Health," the 2000 Mayo Clinic Pediatrics Honored Alumnus Award for "National Contributions to the field of Pediatrics," and the 2003 William B Weil, Jr., MD Endowed Distinguished Pediatric Faculty Award from Michigan State University College of Medicine for "National and international recognition as well as exemplary scholarship in pediatrics." He also received the 2004 Charles R Drew School of Medicine (Los Angeles, CA) Stellar Award for contributions to pediatric resident education and was awarded an honorary membership in the Indian Academy of Pediatrics – an honor granted to only a few pediatricians outside of India. He was the 2007–2010 Visiting Professor of Pediatrics at Athens University, Athens, Greece, and received the Michigan State University College of Human Medicine Outstanding Community Faculty Award in 2008. In 2010 he received the title of Doctor Honoris Causa from the University of Athens (Greece) as a "distinguished scientist who through outstanding work has bestowed praise and credit on the field of adolescent medicine (Ephebiatrics)." In 2010 he received the Outstanding Achievement in Adolescent Medicine Award from the Society for Adolescent Medicine "as a leading force in the field of adolescent medicine and health." He is a past Chair of the National Conference and Exhibition Planning Group (Committee on Scientific Meetings) of the American Academy of Pediatrics and member of the Pediatric Academic Societies' (SPR/PAS) Planning Committee (1998 to Present). In 2011 he was elected to The Alpha Omega Alpha Honor Society (Faculty member) at Michigan State University College of Human Medicine, East Lansing, Michigan. He is a member of the Appeals Committee for the Pediatrics' Residency Review Committee (RRC) of the Accreditation Council for Graduate Medical Education (Chicago, IL) in both adolescent medicine and general pediatrics and has numerous publications in adolescent health and lectureships in many countries on adolescent health. E-mail: Greydanus@kcms.msu.edu

Mohammad Jafferany, MD, is Clinical Assistant Professor in the Department of Psychiatry, College of Human Medicine and Osteopathic Medicine, Michigan State University, East Lansing, Michigan, United States and Director of the Psychodermatology Clinic, Jafferany Psychiatric Services, PLC Saginaw, Michigan. He is also Staff Psychiatrist at Tuscola Behavioral Health Systems in Caro, Michigan and a consultant Psychodermatologist in private practice. He completed adult psychiatry residency at Hennepin County Medical center in Minneapolis, Minnesota and did his fellowship training in child and adolescent psychiatry at University of Washington in Seattle, Washington State. He also trained as a dermatologist and practiced for more than 10 years before his psychiatry training. He has authored more than a dozen publications in the field of psychodermatology, and he specializes in psychocutaneous disorders and cutaneous self injurious behavior. He is on the peer review board of various scientific journals in psychiatry and dermatology. His work has been quoted in several textbooks of dermatology. He is a regular speaker on the topics in psychodermatology and has presented his work in national and international conferences. He is also one of the organizers of annual meetings of the Association of Psychocutaneous Medicine of North America. E-mail: mjafferany@yahoo.com

Dilip R Patel, MD, FAAP, FSAM, FAACPDM, FACSM, is professor in the Department of Pediatrics and Human Development at the Michigan State University College of Human Medicine, East Lansing, Michigan, USA. He is a full time teaching faculty member in the Department of Pediatrics at the Western Michigan University School of Medicine (Kalamazoo, Michigan, USA). Dr Patel has subspecialty training and interests in neurodevelopmental disabilities, developmental-behavioral pediatrics, adolescent medicine and sports medicine. He has published numerous papers on wide ranging topics in these areas and has edited several special symposia and books. E-mail: patel@kcms.msu.edu

Joav Merrick, MD, MMedSci, DMSc, is professor of pediatrics, child health and human development affiliated with Kentucky Children's Hospital, University of Kentucky, Lexington, United States and the Division of Pediatrics, Hadassah Hebrew University Medical Centers, Mt Scopus Campus, Jerusalem, Israel; the medical director of the Health Services, Division for Intellectual and Developmental Disabilities; Ministry of Social Affairs and Social Services, Jerusalem, and the founder and director of the National Institute of Child Health and Human Development in Israel. Dr Merrick has numerous publications in the field of pediatrics, child health and human development, rehabilitation, intellectual disability, disability, health, welfare, abuse, advocacy, quality of life and prevention and received the Peter Sabroe Child Award for outstanding work on behalf of Danish Children in 1985 and the International LEGO-Prize ("The Children's Nobel Prize") for an extraordinary contribution towards improvement in child welfare and well-being in 1987. E-mail: jmerrick@zahav.net.il

26 FDA approved psychotropic medication indications for children and adolescents

Class	Medication	FDA Indication for Children
Antidepressants	Fluoxetine	7 years and older, for depression, OCD
Sertraline		6 years and older, for OCD
Paroxetine		No
Citalopram		No
Escitalopram		12 years and older, for depression
Fluvoxamine		8 years and older, for OCD
Venlafaxine		No
Mirtazapine		No
Bupropion		No
Trazodone		No
Amitriptyline		12 years and older, for depression
Desipramine		No
Nortriptyline		6 years and older, for depression
Doxepin		12 years and older, for mixed anxiety and depression
Duloxetine		No
Anxiolytics	Clonazepam	Up to 10 years or 30 kg, for seizures
Alprazolam		No
Lorazepam		12 years and older, for anxiety insomnia (oral)
Mood Stabilizers	Lithium	12 years and older, for bipolar disorder
Valproate		10 years and older, for epilepsy
Carbamazepine		Pediatric, for epilepsy
Oxcarbazepine		2 years and older, for partial seizures, adjunct
Lamotrigine		2 years and older, for partial seizures, Lennox-Gastaut syndrome, adjunct

(Continued)

Class	Medication	FDA Indication for Children
Gabapentin		3–12 years, for partial seizures, adjunct
Antipsychotics	Haloperidol	3 years and older, for Tourette syndrome, severe problematic or hyperactive behavior (after stimulant failure), schizophrenia
Risperidone		5 years and older, for irritability in autism; 13 years and older, for schizophrenia; 10 years and older, for bipolar I
Olanzapine		13–17 years, for acute bipolar I, mixed or manic; 13–17 years, for schizophrenia
Quetiapine		13–17 years, for schizophrenia; 10–17 years, for acute bipolar I, mania and maintenance
Ziprasidone		No
Aripiprazole		6–17 years, for autistic disorder; 13–17 years, for schizophrenia; 10 years and older, for acute bipolar I
Droperidol		2 years and older, for postoperative nausea and vomiting prophylaxis
Chlorpromazine		6 months – 12 years, for behavioral syndrome; pediatric
Stimulants		Methylphenidate
6 years and older, for ADHD and Narcolepsy		
Dextroamphetamine		6 years and older, for ADHD and Narcolepsy
Others		Atomoxetine
6 years and older, for ADHD		
Guanfacine		12 years and older
Intuniv		6–17 years for ADHD

27 Common psychiatric terms

Affective disorders Disorders of mood include Major Depressive Disorder, Dysthymic disorder, Depressive Disorder, NOS, Adjustment Disorder, Bipolar Disorder type I and II, and NOS.

Agoraphobia An unrealistic fear of being in public places or open spaces from which escape may be difficult or embarrassing like a grocery store, being in a line, or in a crowd.

Akathisia Motor restlessness ranging from a feeling of inner disquiet, often localized in the muscles, to inability to sit still or lie quietly, a side effect of some antipsychotic drugs.

Akinesia A side effect of the antipsychotic drugs characterized by a general lack of motor movement in the patient, as well as a slowing down of speech and responsiveness.

Alexithymia A state of deficiency in understanding, processing, or describing emotions.

Amnesia Complete or transient loss of memory.

Anhedonia Loss of interest and/or pleasure in usual activities associated with depression.

Anorexia nervosa An eating disorder in which an individual restricts food intake or uses other means like purging, diuretics, laxatives, and excessive exercise to keep their weight at what they think is their body weight. Diagnosis is made when they weigh less than 85% the expected weight but still control eating because of a self-perception of being overweight.

Anxiety Apprehension, tension, or uneasiness that stems from the anticipation of a danger, whose source is largely unknown.

Apathy Lack of any kind of feeling, emotion, interest, or concern.

Attachment Emotional relationship between a child and the "regular" caregiver.

Ataxia Disturbance of coordination of voluntary muscular movement.

Attitude The learned construct of like and dislike, which affect how to respond to people, concepts, and events in an evaluative way.

Body image How one perceives the self and one's body.

Bipolar Disorder Also known in the past as manic depressive disorder; characterized by mood swings that range from the episodes of depression to mania.

Biofeedback A self-regulatory technique by which an individual acquires voluntary control over biological processes by using signals from their own bodies.

Biopsychosocial model A modern model of health and illness that suggests links among the nervous system, the immune system, cognitive processing, environmental factors, and behavioral styles can put people at risk for illness.

Bulimia nervosa An eating disorder characterized by episodes of binge eating followed by purging in an effort to maintain a certain body weight.

Catatonia Immobility with muscular rigidity or inflexibility and at times excitability, most often seen in schizophrenia.

Cognitive Refers to the mental process of comprehension, judgment, memory, and reasoning, as contrasted with emotional and volitional processes.

Comorbidity The experience of more than one physical or psychiatric disorder at the same time.

Compulsion An insistent, repetitive, intrusive, and unwanted urge to perform and act that is contrary to one's ordinary wishes and standard.

Consciousness A state of awareness of internal events and of the external environment.

Confabulation Fabrication of facts or events in response to questions about events that are not recalled because of memory impairment, commonly seen in alcoholic dementia.

Confusion Disturbed orientation in respect to time, place, or person.

Coping The process of dealing with internal or external demands that are perceived to be threatening or overwhelming.

Countertransference The therapist's partly unconscious or conscious emotional reactions to the patient.

Decompensation The failure of defense mechanisms, leading to an exacerbation of pathological process.

Delusion A firm, fixed idea not amenable to rational explanation and maintained despite objective evidence to the contrary.

Depersonalization An alteration in the perception or experience of the self so that the feelings of one's own reality is temporarily lost; a sense of unreality.

DSM-IV-TR The current diagnostic and statistical manual of the American Psychiatric Association that classifies, defines, and describes mental disorders.

Dysphemia A state of depression, restlessness, anxiety, discontent, irritability, or feeling unwell or unhappy.

Dysphoria An unpleasant emotion such as sadness, sorrow, and anguish.

Dysthymia A less severe form of depression. When a person may experience chronic depression nearly most of the day more often than not for at least 2 years. At least two of the following must be present: poor appetite or overeating, insomnia or hypersomnia, low energy or fatigue, low self-esteem, poor concentration, or feelings of hopelessness.

Dystonia Acute tonic muscular spasms, often of the tongue, jaw, eyes, and neck but sometimes of the whole body. Reactions may come on quickly and dramatically. A treatable side effect of antipsychotic drugs.

Ecolalia Repetition (echoing) of words or phrases of others.

Echopraxia The pathological repetition by imitation of the movements of another person.

Ego The part of personality that operates on the base of reality in order to bring a balance between instinctual drives and urges and social and moral values.

Hallucinations A sensory impression in the absence of any external stimuli; can arise in respect to any sensory modality – visual, auditory, olfactory, tactile, or gustatory.

Homeostasis A state of constancy or equilibrium of the internal conditions of the body.

Ideas of influence The conviction that one's behavior, including one's thoughts, is being influenced in some way by an external agency, when in fact it is not.

Insight oriented therapy A technique by which the therapist guides a patient toward gaining understanding between present symptoms and their origin in the past.

Intelligence quotient (IQ) An index derived from standardized tests of intelligence: computed as an IQ test score.

Major depressive disorder A mood disorder characterized by persistent feelings of depression over a 2 week period, with neurovegetative symptoms like sleep and appetite disturbances, anhedonia, lack of motivation, cognitive impairment, and feelings of guilt with or without suicidal thoughts.

Manic episode A sustained period of 4 days to a week of abnormally elevated or irritable mood, euphoria, grandiosity, and increased arousal and energy.

Mood A pervasive and sustained emotion that in the extreme markedly colors one's perception of the world. Examples of mood include depression, elation, and anger.

Object Freudian term meaning an object (usually mother) an infant drives toward for satiation.

Object relations theory A modern adaptation of Freud's psychoanalytic theory proposed by Melanie Klein view that the objects can be people (mother, father, others) or things, such as transitional objects with which we form attachments. These initial attachments are incorporated into a self and become the building blocks of the self-system and the way in which to make future relationships.

Obsession A persistent, unwanted idea or impulse that cannot be eliminated by logic or reasoning.

Obsessive compulsive disorder (OCD) A psychiatric disorder characterized by unreasonable thoughts and fears (obsessions) that lead one to do repetitive behaviors (compulsions).

Panic attacks Sudden onset of intense apprehension, fearfulness, or terror accompanied by physiological changes.

Paranoid Ideation Suspiciousness or non-delusional belief that one is being harassed, persecuted, or unfairly treated.

Morality A system of beliefs and values that ensures that individuals will keep their obligations to others in society and will behave in ways that do not interfere with the rights and interests of others.

Phobia An obsessive, persistent, unrealistic, intense fear of an object or situation.

Posturing Maintaining an unusual or awkward posture for a considerable amount of time.

Posttraumatic stress disorder (PTSD) An anxiety disorder characterized by the persistent reexperience of traumatic events through distressing recollections, dreams, hallucinations, or dissociative flashbacks; develops in response to a event where a person's life is threatened or they witness somebody else's life in danger.
Pseudodementia Clinical features resembling a dementia that are not due to organic brain dysfunction or disease.
Psyche Sense of self or the totality of the human mind, conscious and unconscious.
Psychomotor Agitation Excessive motor activity associated with a feeling of inner tension; the activity is usually nonproductive and repetitious.
Psychomotor Retardation Visible generalized slowing down of physical reactions, movements, and speech.
Psychodynamic therapy A therapy that focuses on unconscious processes as they are manifested in a person's current behavior.
Psychosomatic The constant and inseparable interaction of the psyche (mind) and the soma (body). Commonly used to refer to illnesses in which the manifestations are primarily physical with at least a partial emotional etiology.
Social phobia An anxiety disorder characterized by persistent, irrational fear and excessive self-consciousness in everyday social situations in which an individual can be observed by others.
Stigma The negative reaction of people to an individual because of some assumed inferiority or source of difference that is degraded.
Stress The pattern of specific and nonspecific response to a stimulus or events that threaten or upset equilibrium.
Tardive Dyskinesia Literally late appearing abnormal movements; a variable complex of choeiform or athetoid movements developing in patients exposed to antipsychotic drugs. Typical movements include tongue-writhing or protrusion, chewing, lip-puckering, choreiform finger movements, toe and ankle movements, leg-jiggling, or movements of neck, trunk, and pelvis.
Transference The unconscious assignment to others of feelings and attitudes that were originally associated with important figures (parents, siblings, etc.) in one's early life. The transference may be negative or positive.

Mohammad Jafferany

28 Common dermatotologic lesions

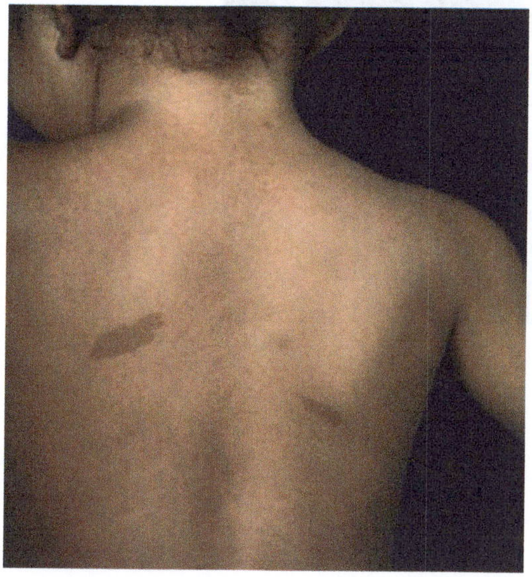

Figure 28.1: Macule

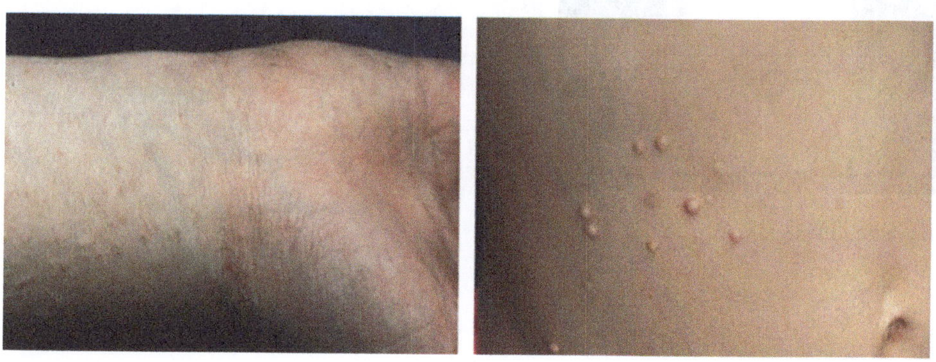

Figure 28.2: Papule

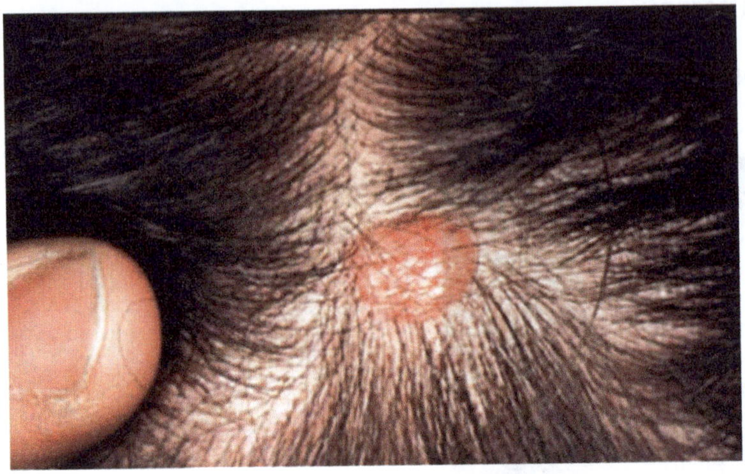

Figure 28.3: Nodule

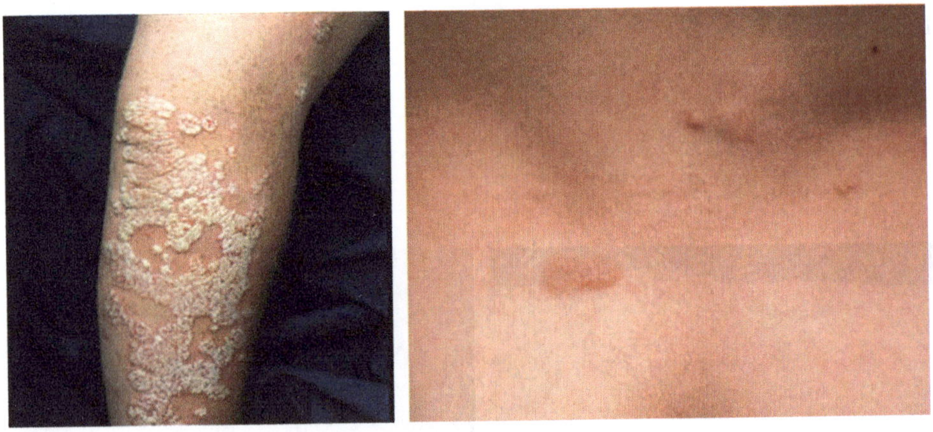

Figure 28.4: Plaque

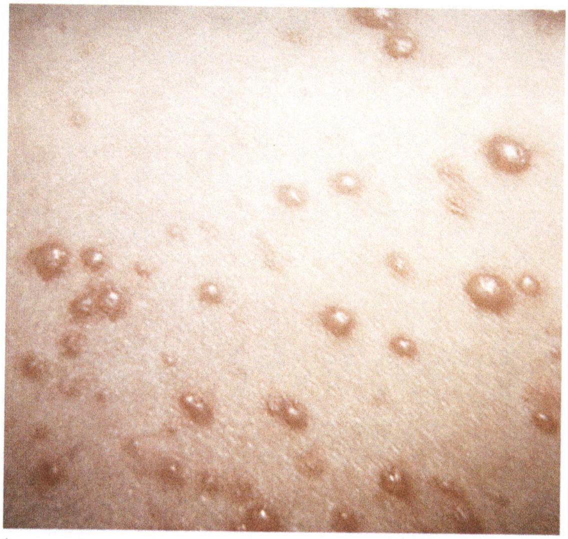

Figure 28.5: Vesicle

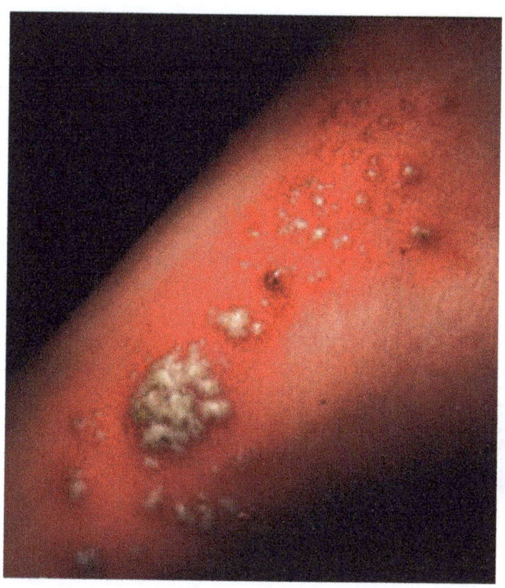

Figure 28.6: Pustule

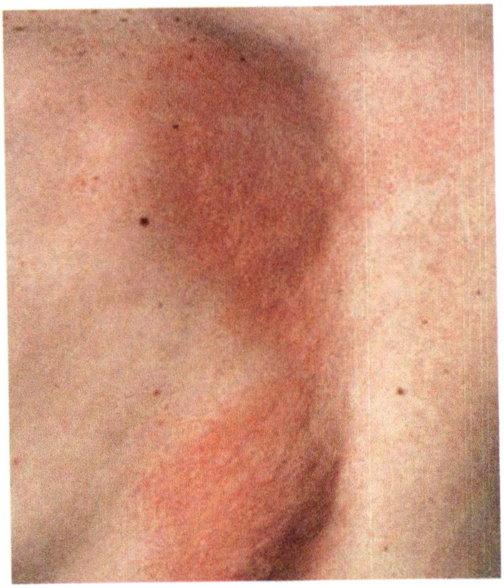

Figure 28.7: Wheal

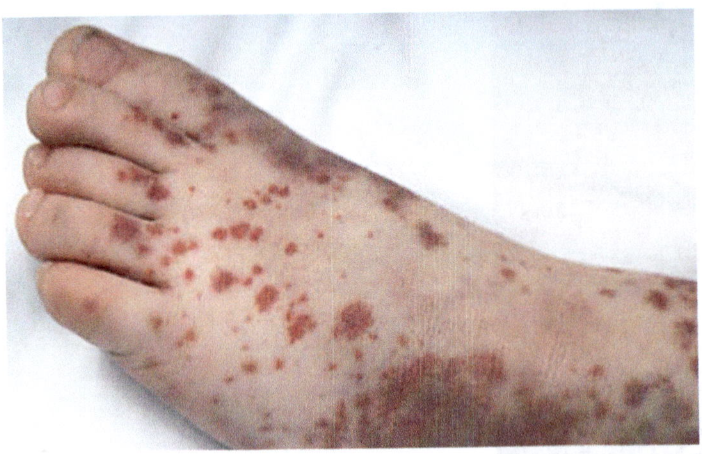

Figure 28.8: Purpura/Echymoses

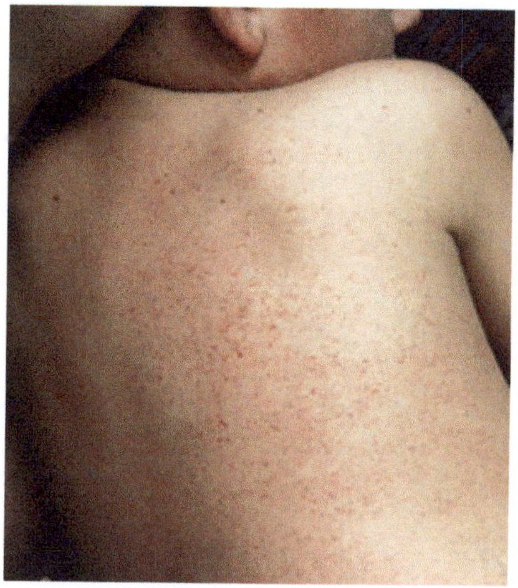

Figure 28.9: Petechiae

Index

Plate section

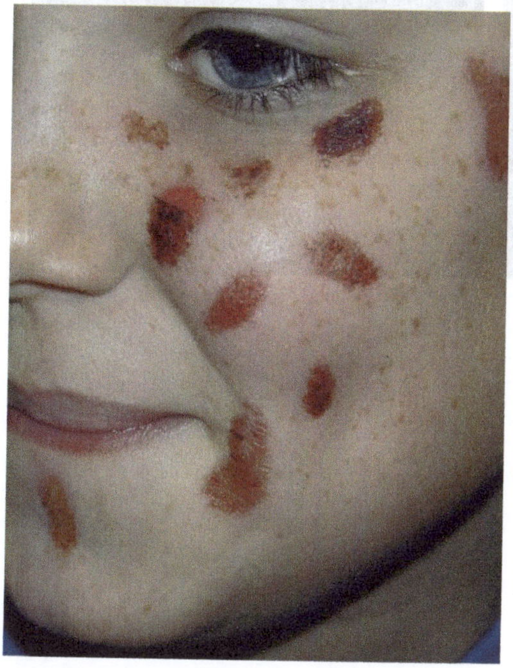

Dermatitis Artefacta

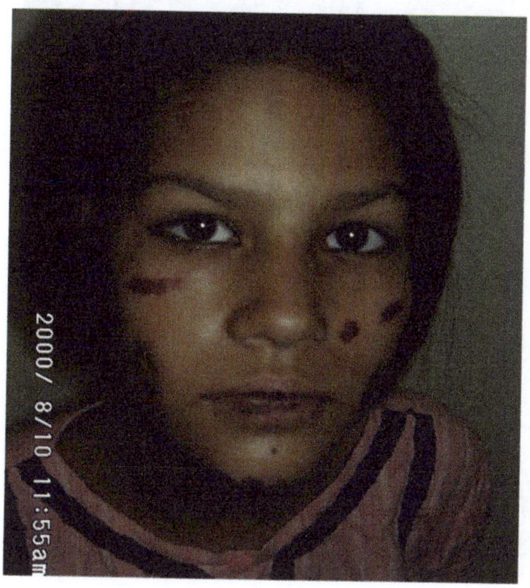

Dermatitis Artefacta

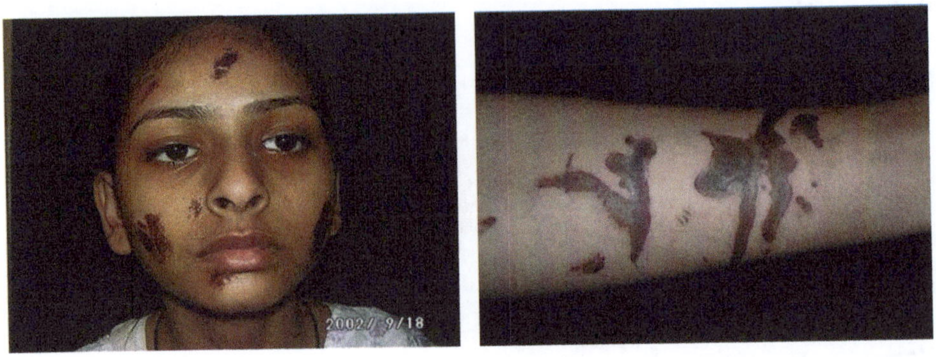

Dermatitis Artefacta

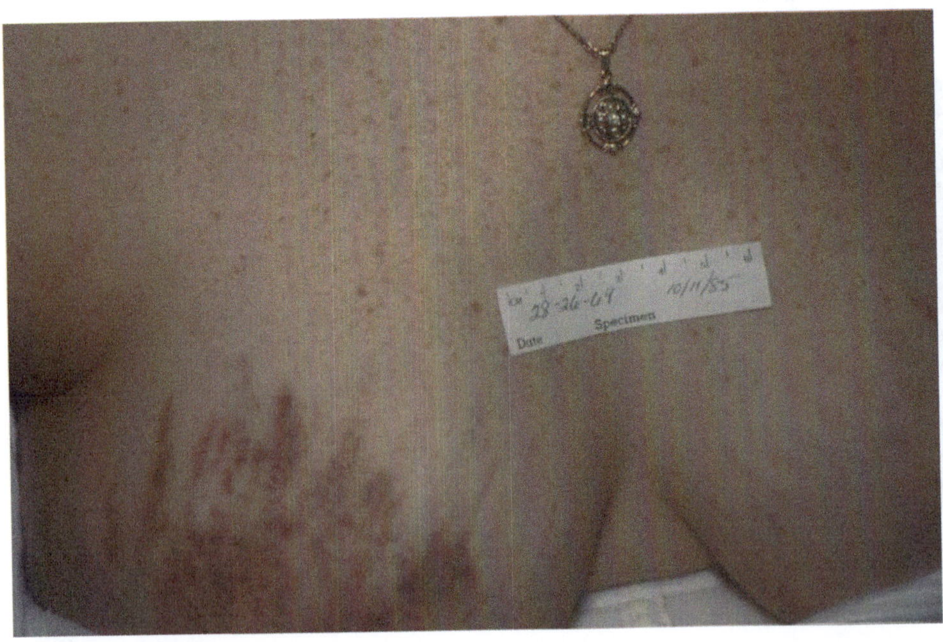

Dermatitis Artefacta

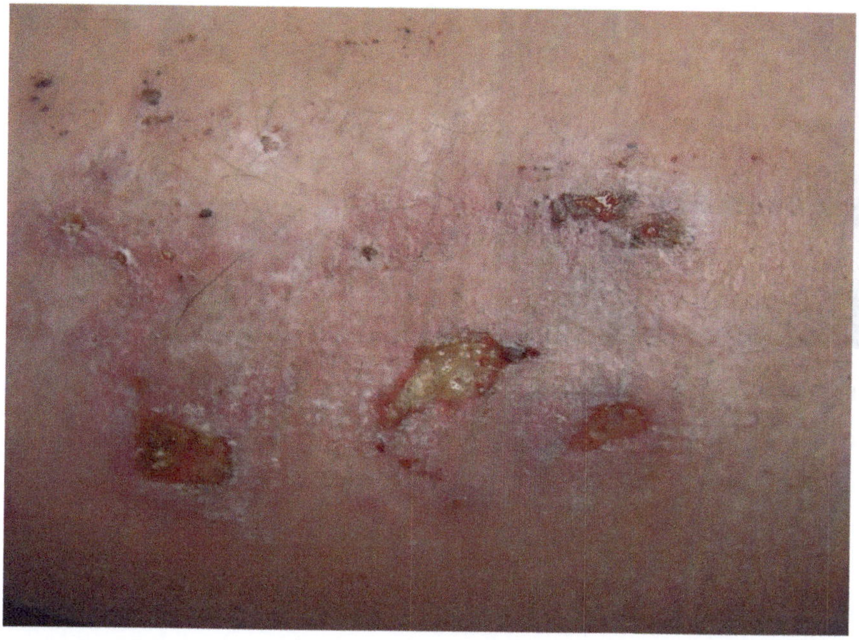

Dermatitis Artefacta

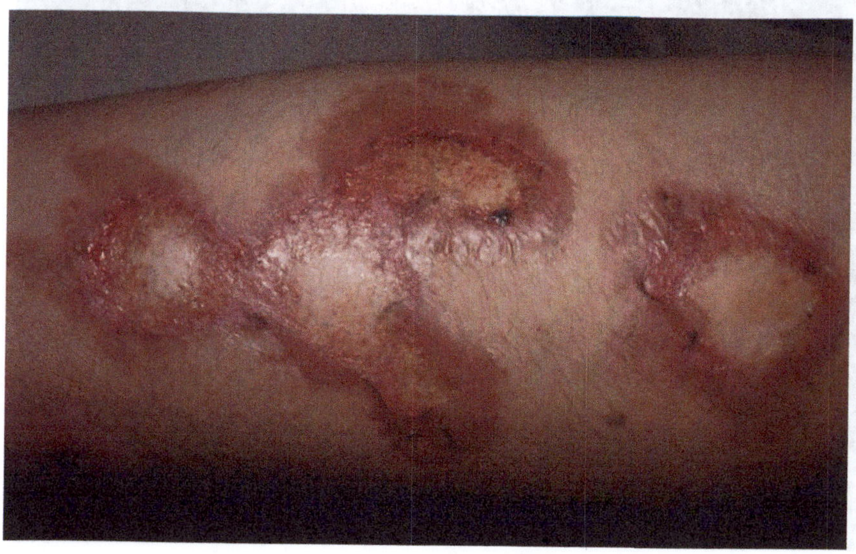

Dermatitis Artefacta

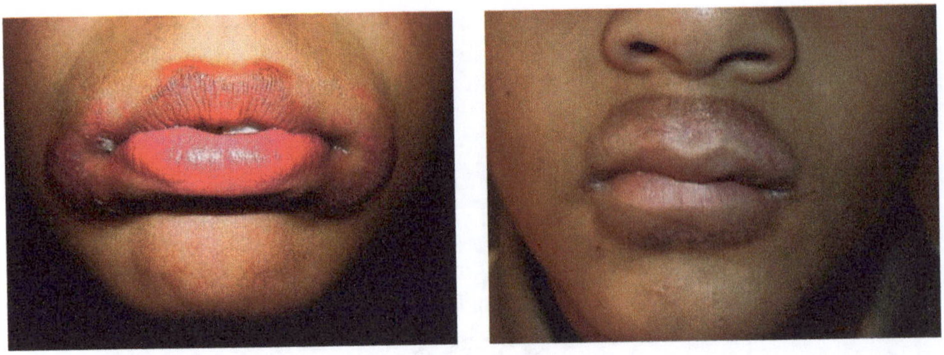

Lip Licking Dermatitis

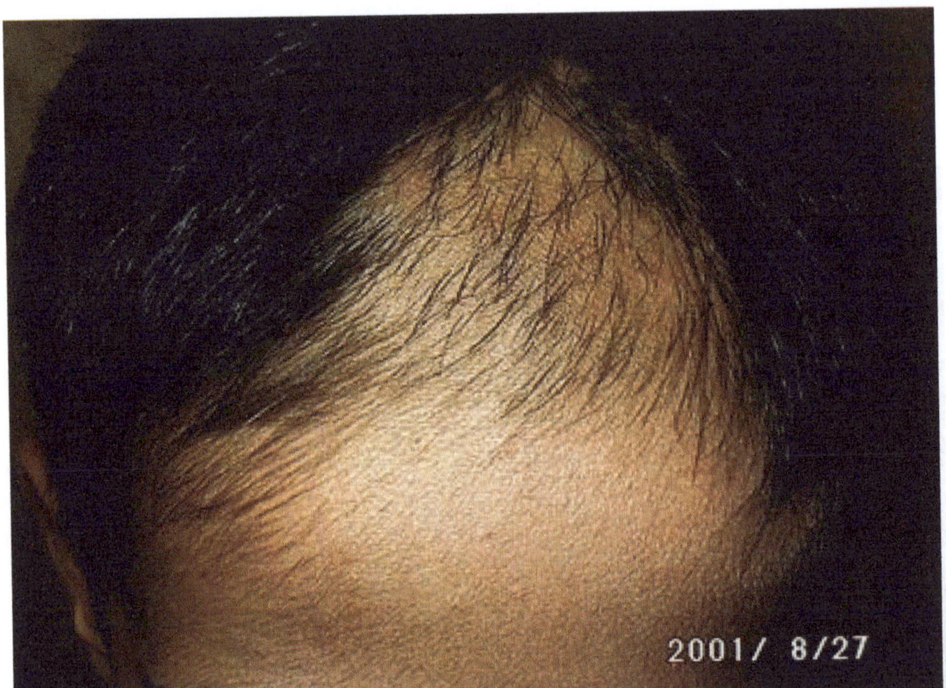

Trichotillomania

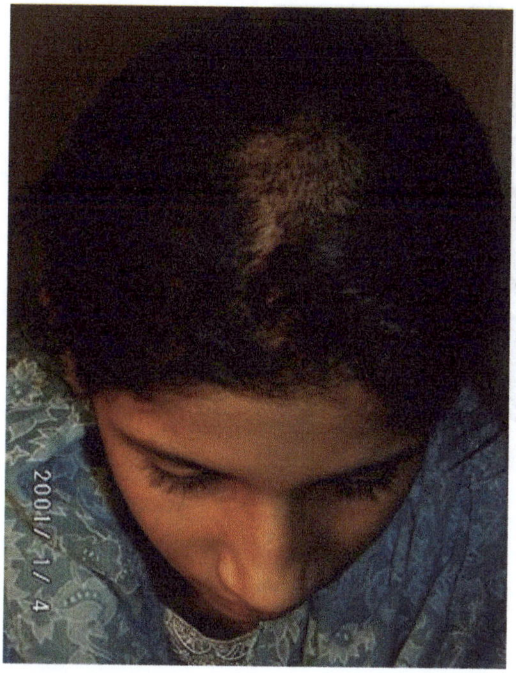

Trichotillomania

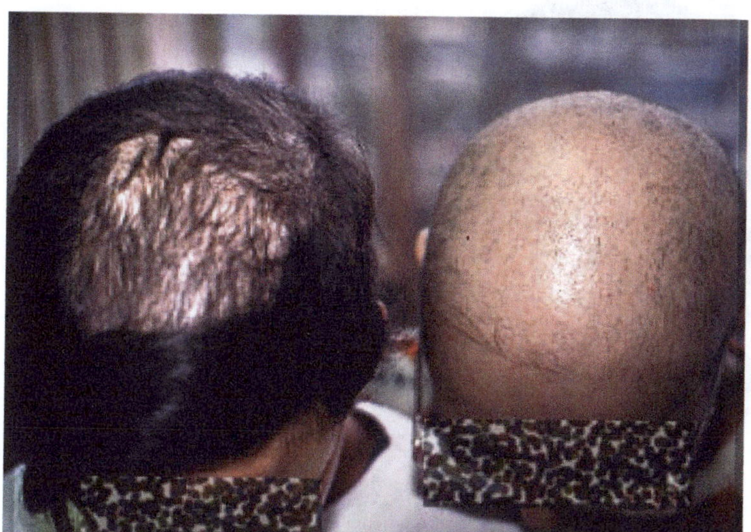

Familial Trichotillomania

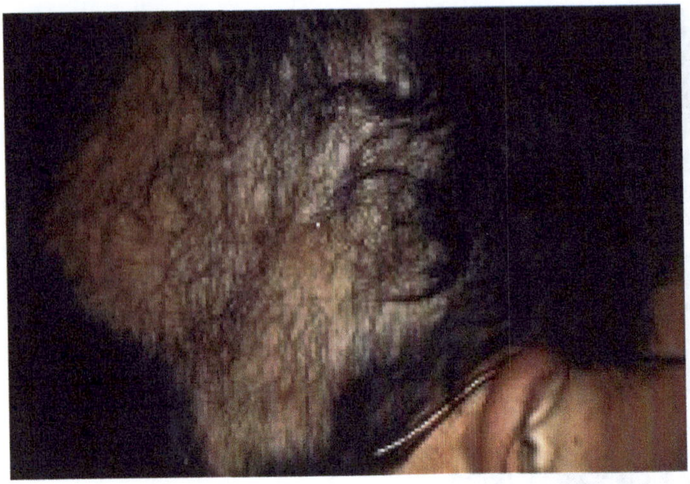

Trichotillomania

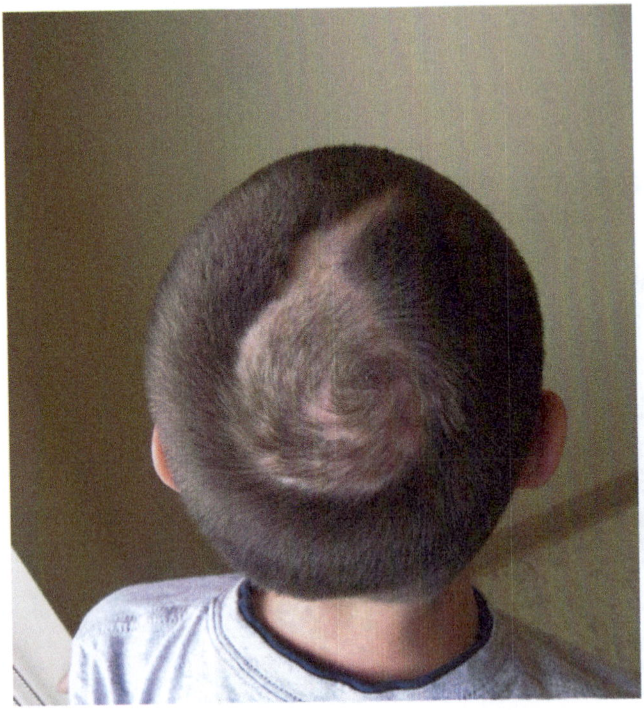

Trichotillomania

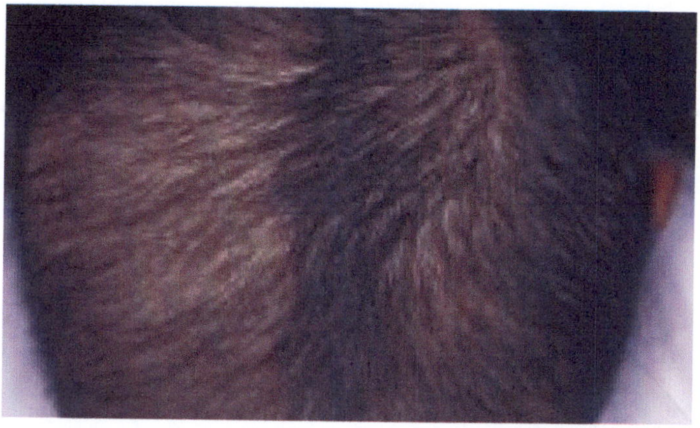

Trichotillomania

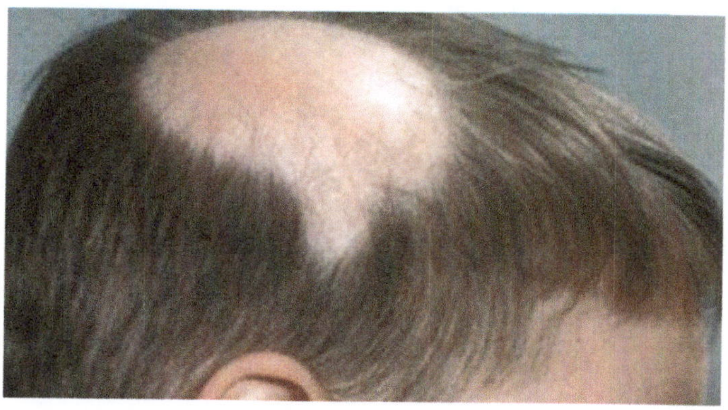

Alopecia Aereata-boy

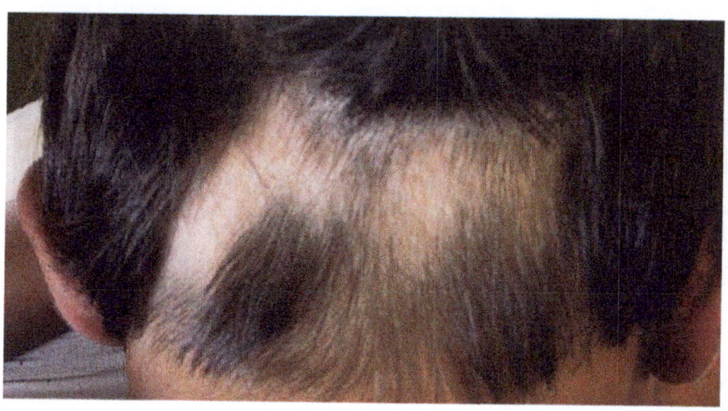

Alopecia Aereata

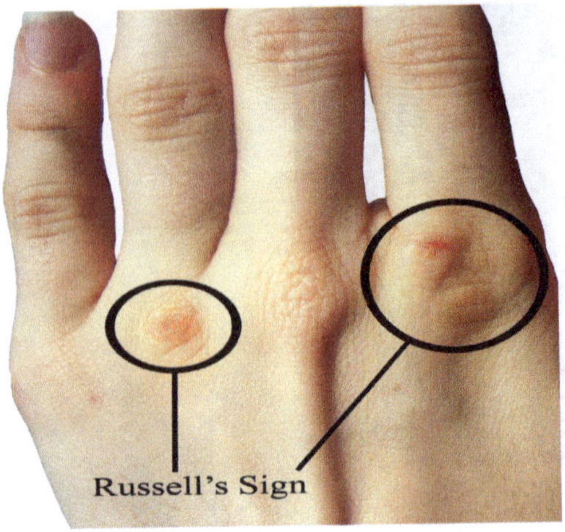

Russell's sign

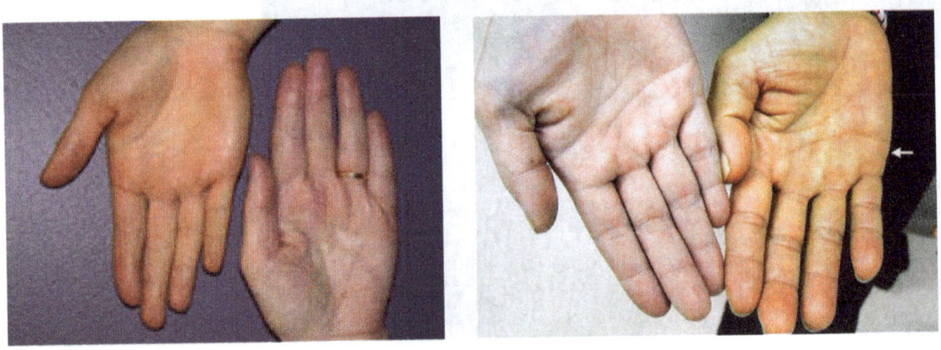

Carotenoderma

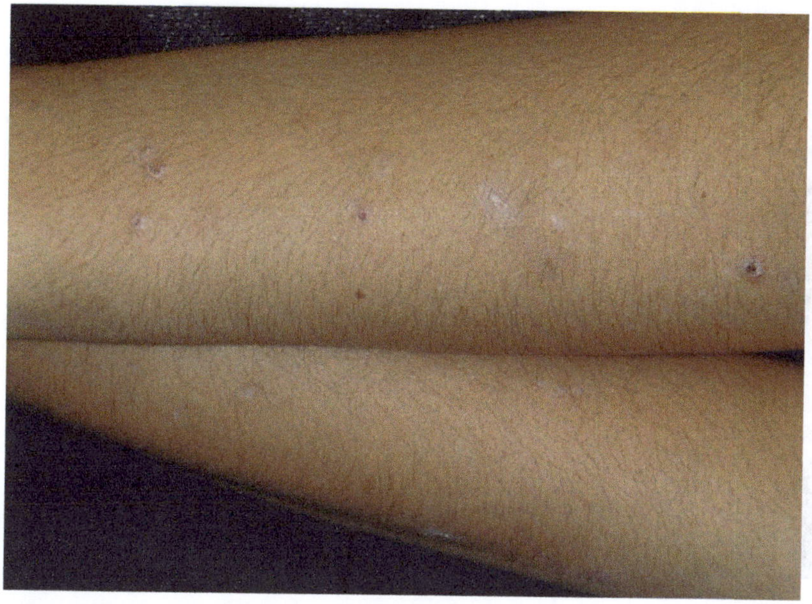

Skin Picking

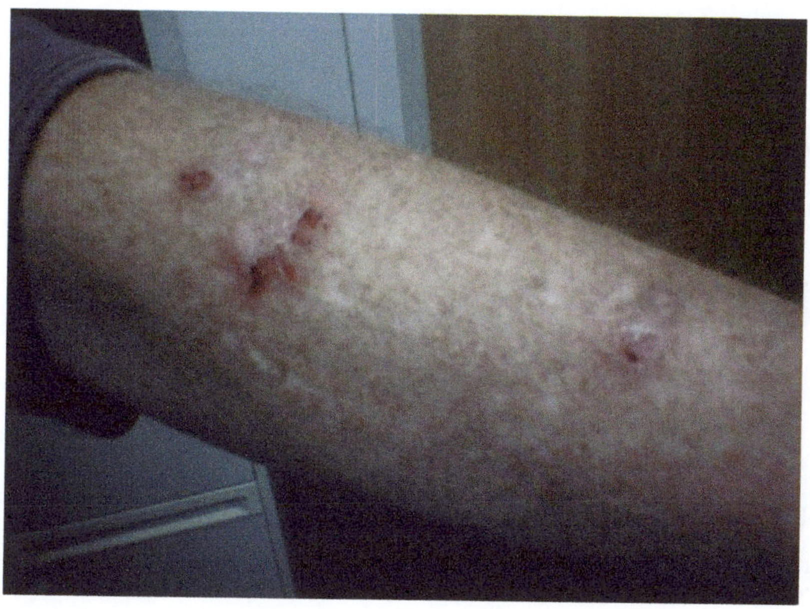

Skin Picking

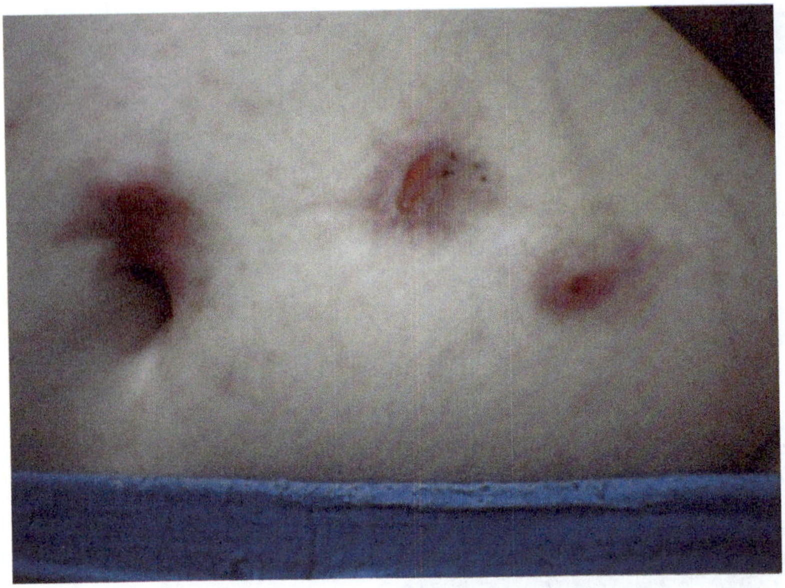

Skin Picking

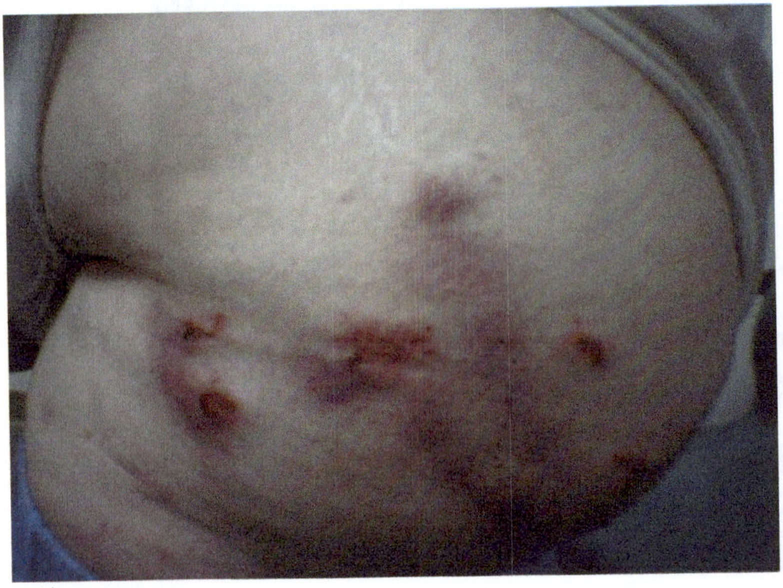

Skin Picking

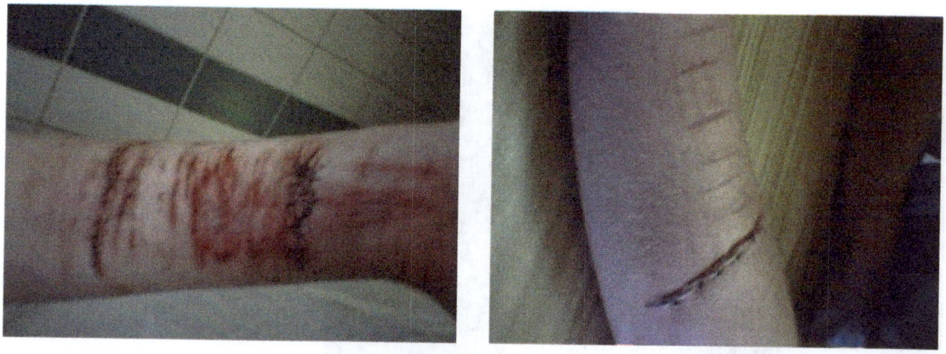

Skin Cutting

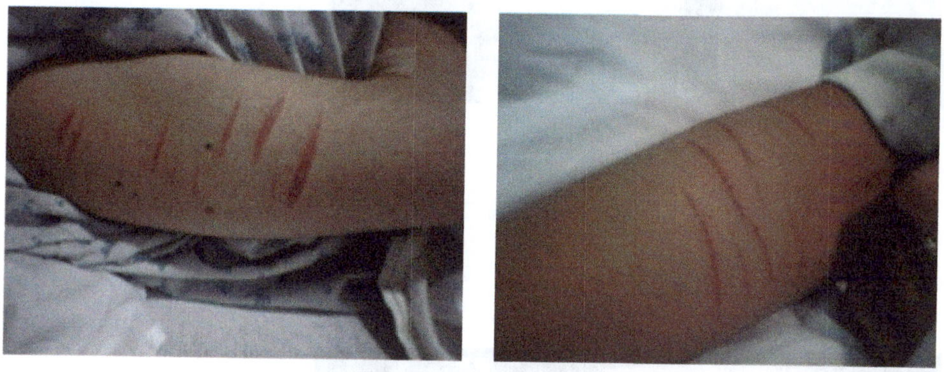

Skin Cutting

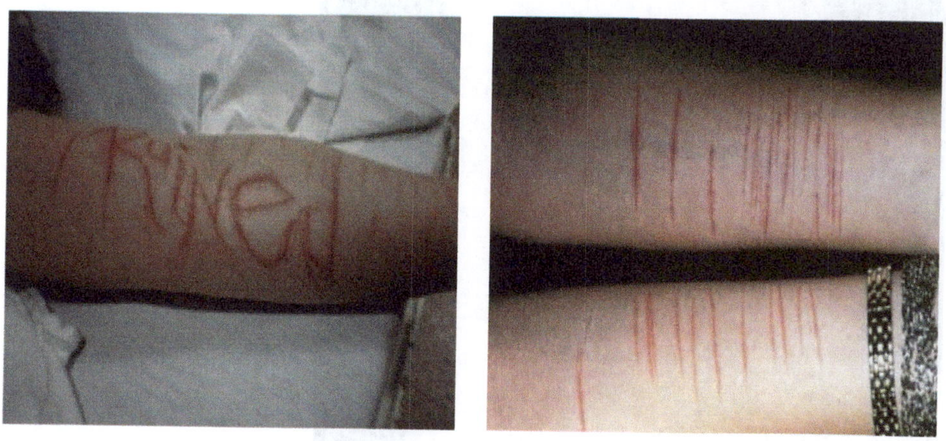

Skin Cutting

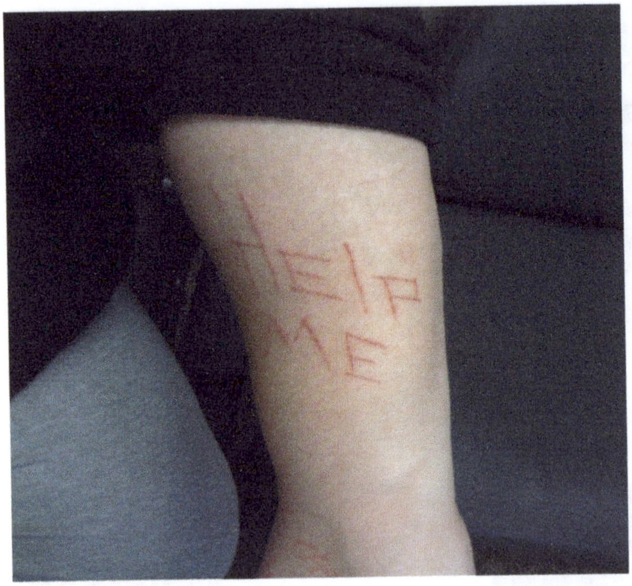
HELP
ME

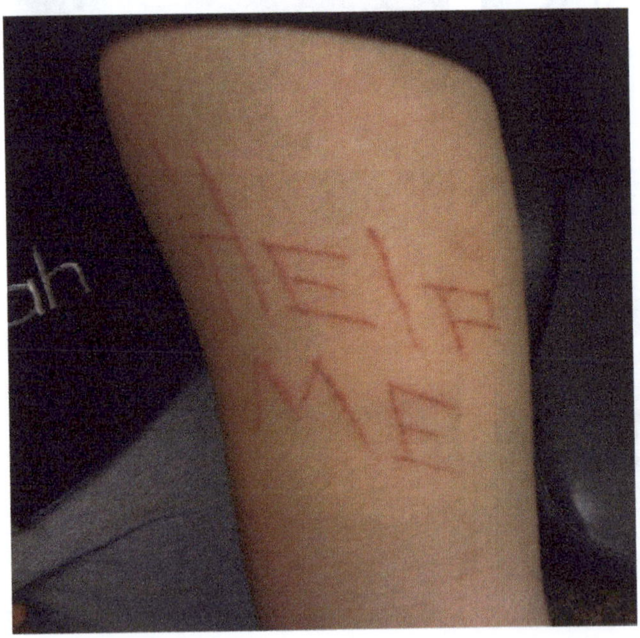
HELP
ME

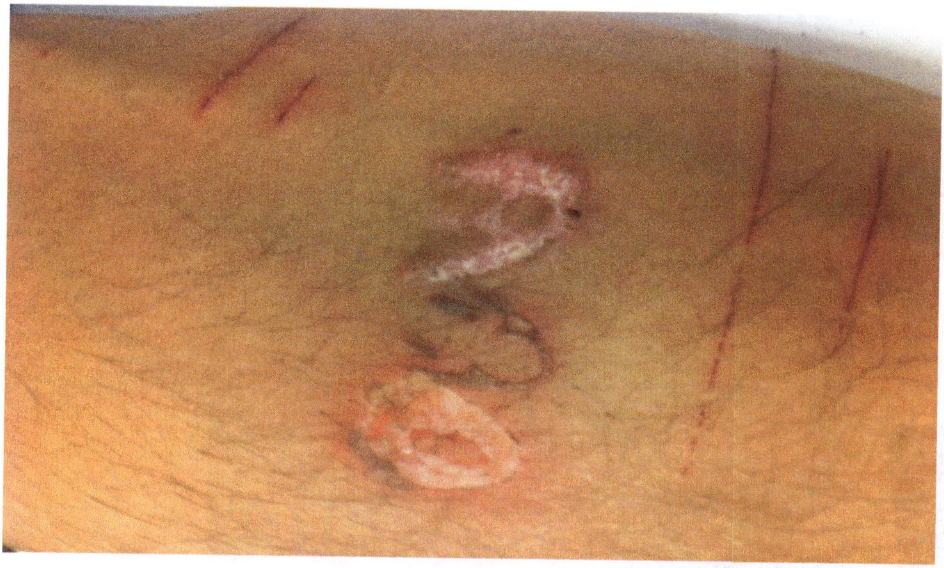

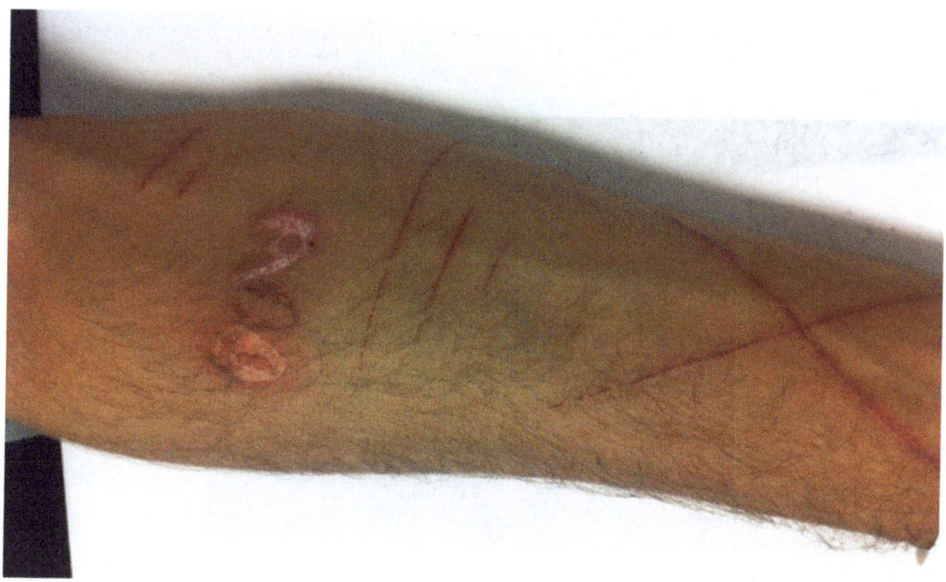

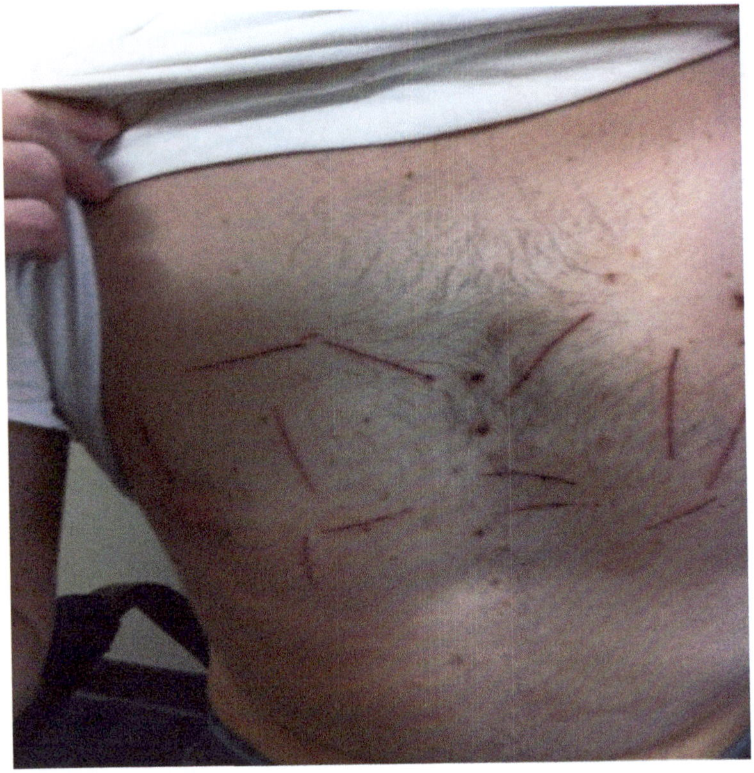

Dermatitis artefacta

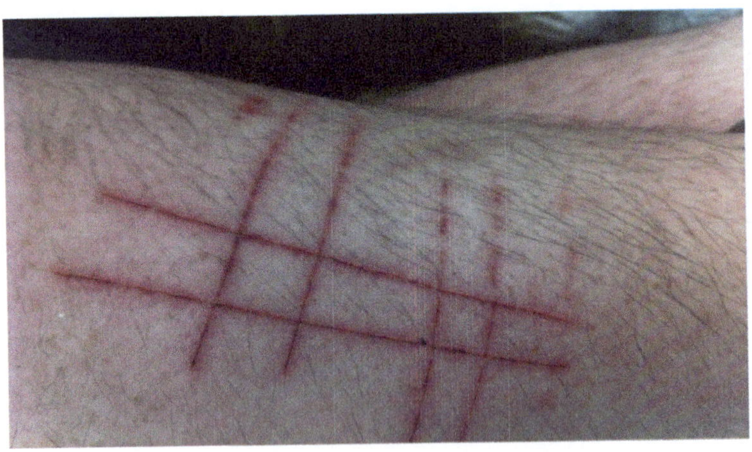

Dermatitis artefacta

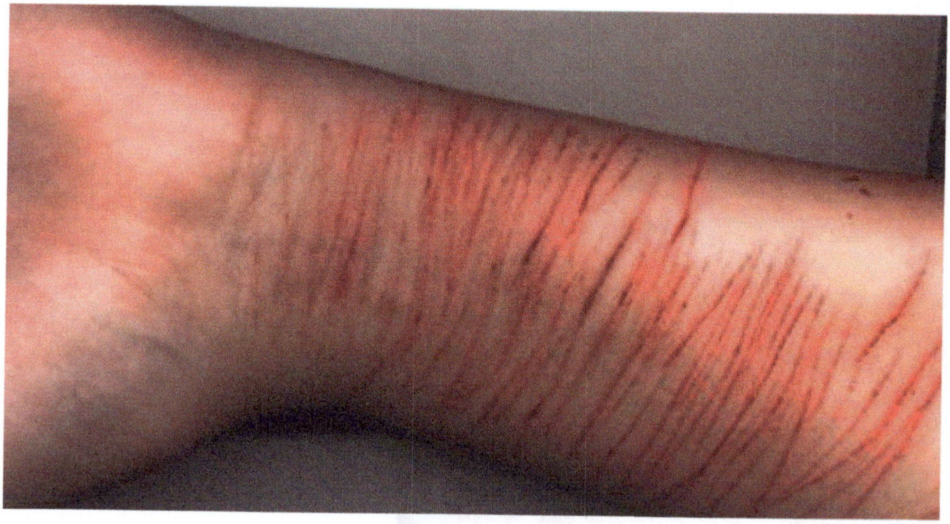

Self Cutting

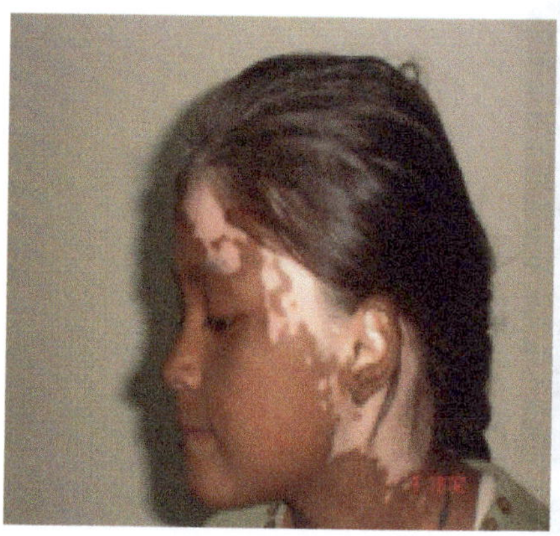

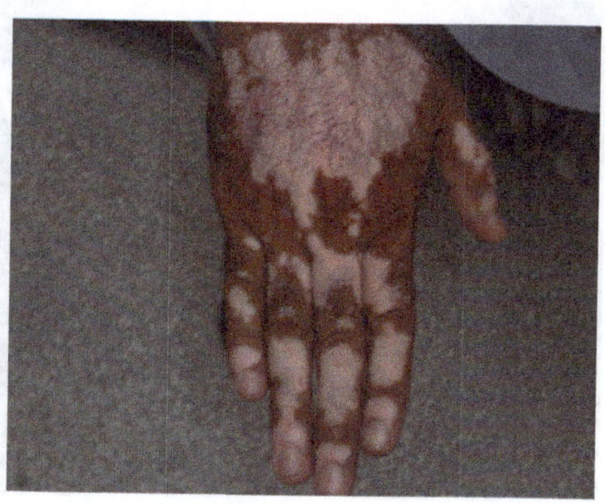

Vitiligo

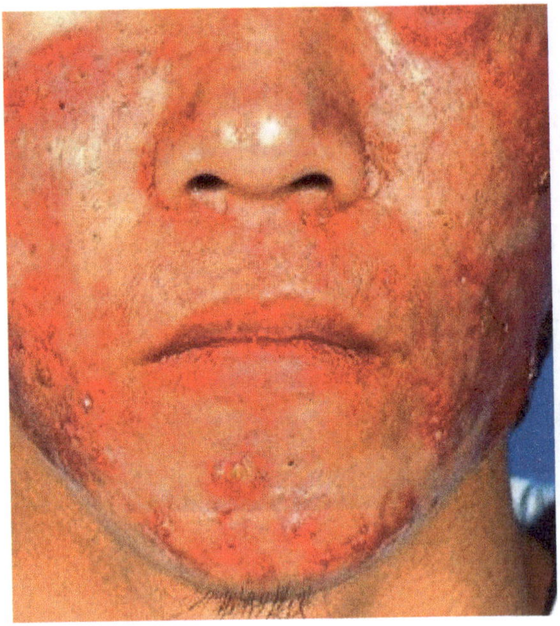

Acne excoriee

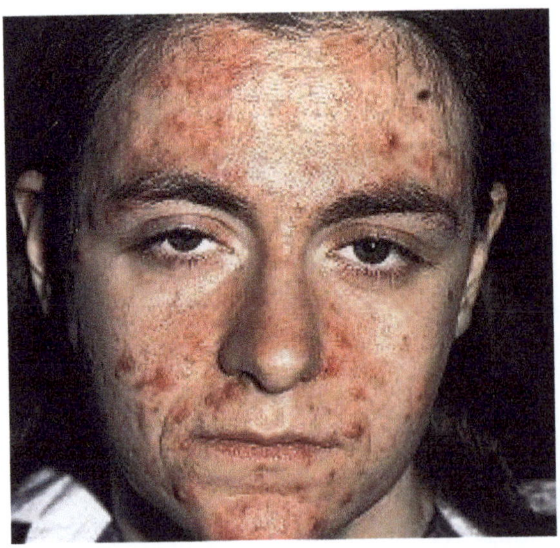

Acne excoriee

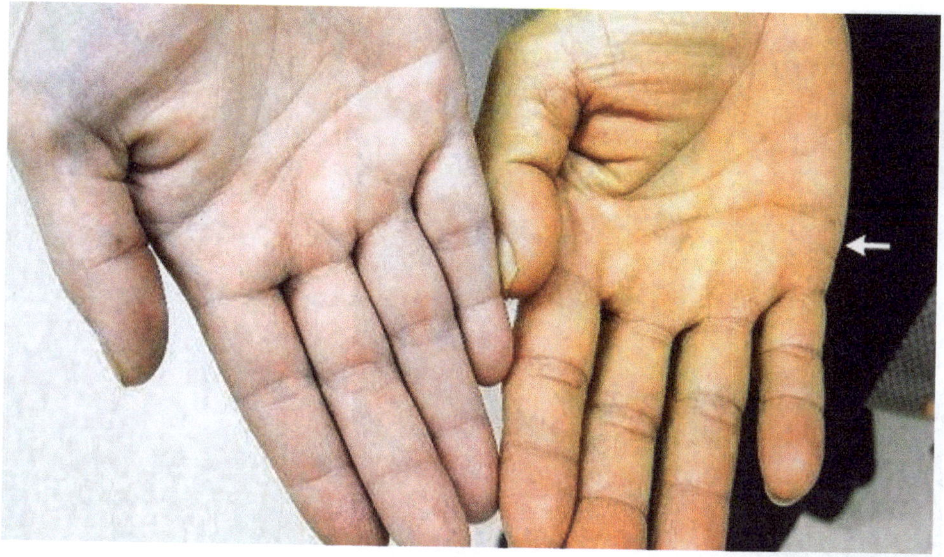

Carotenemia 2

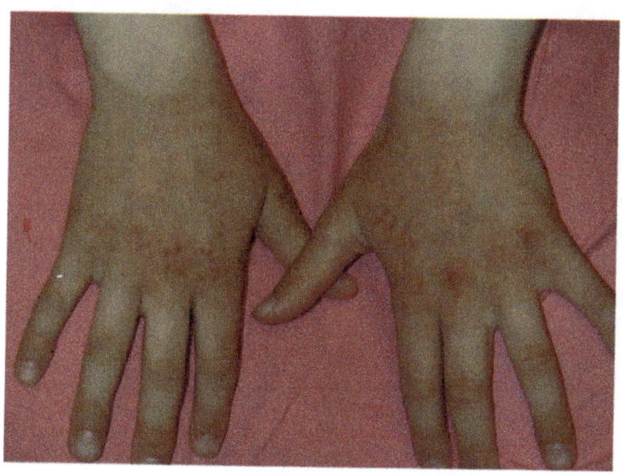

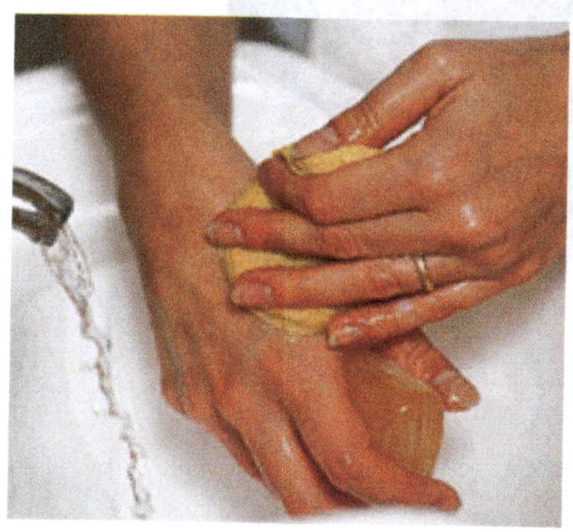

Habitual Hand Washer

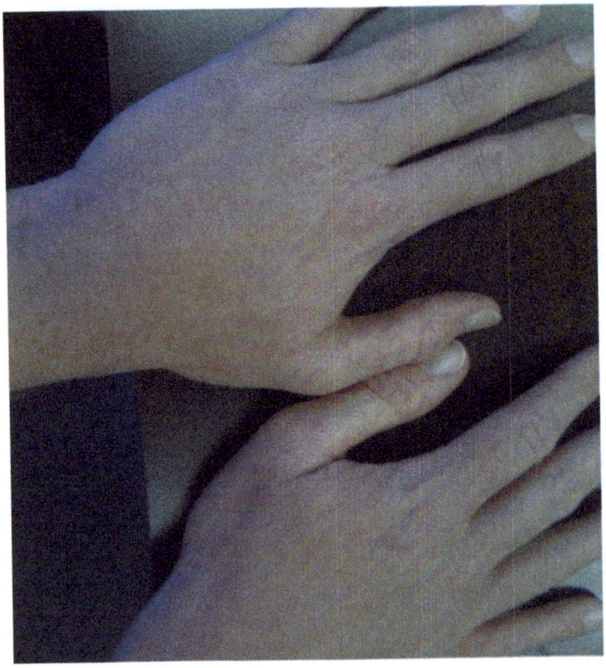

Habitual Hand washer

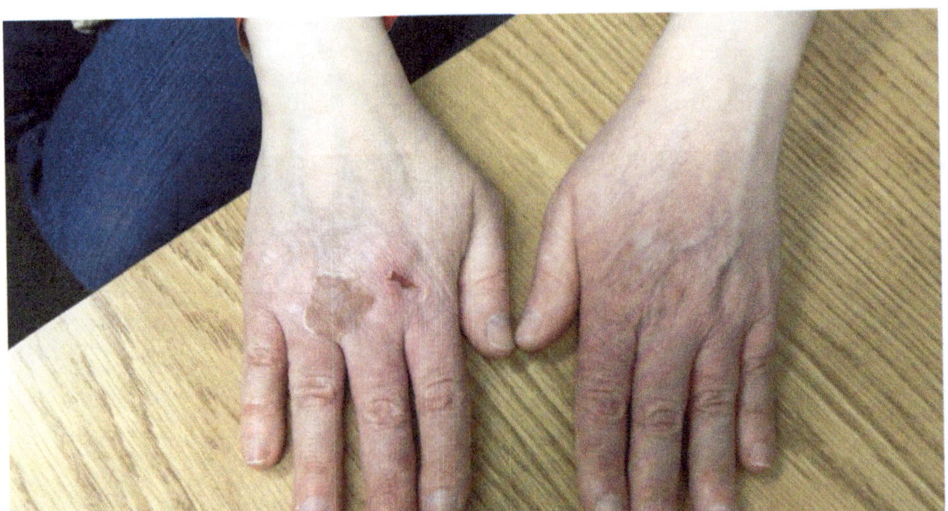

Compulsive Washing-2

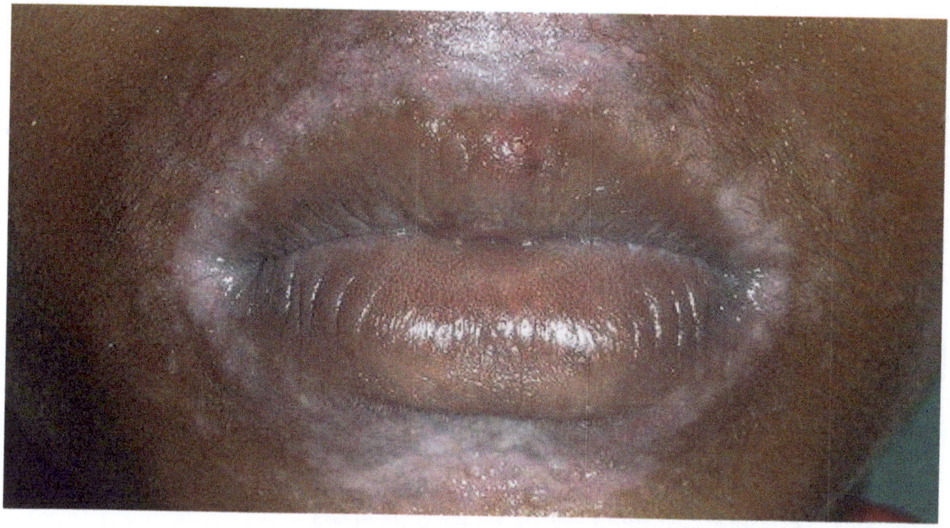

Compulsive lip licking – Cheilitis

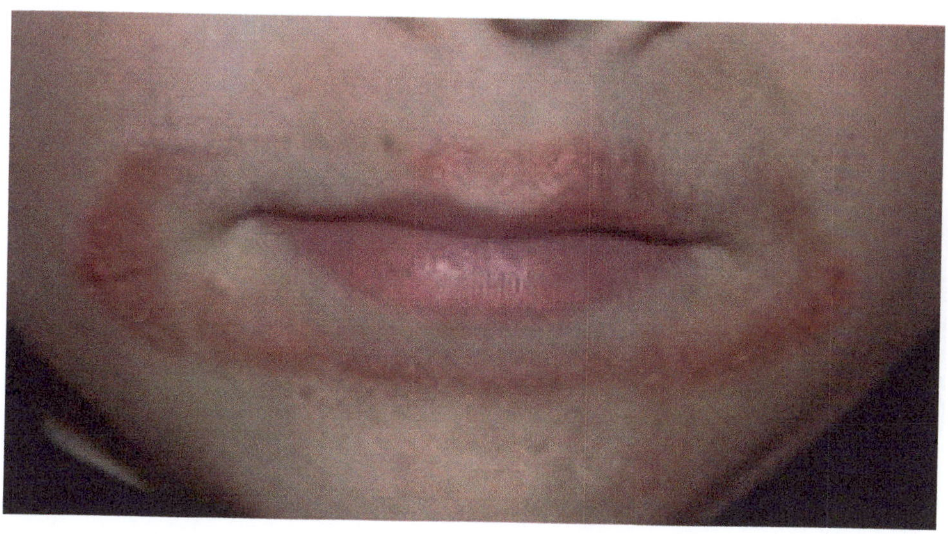

Compulsive lip licking – Cheilitis-2

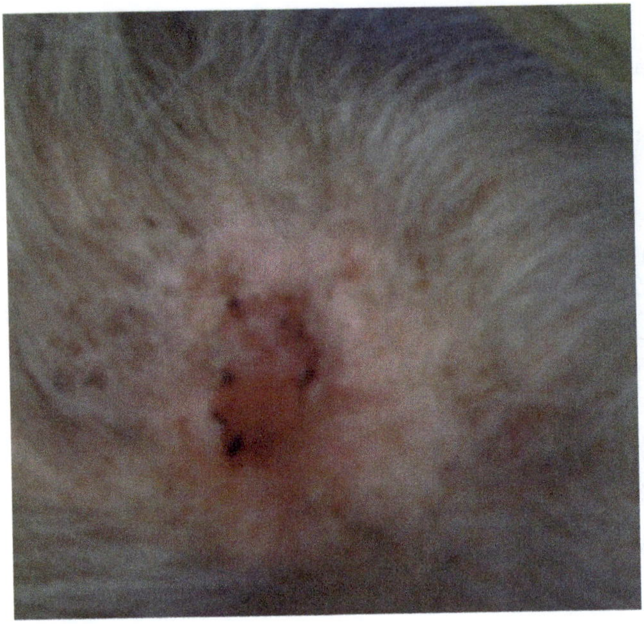

Prurigo Nodularis

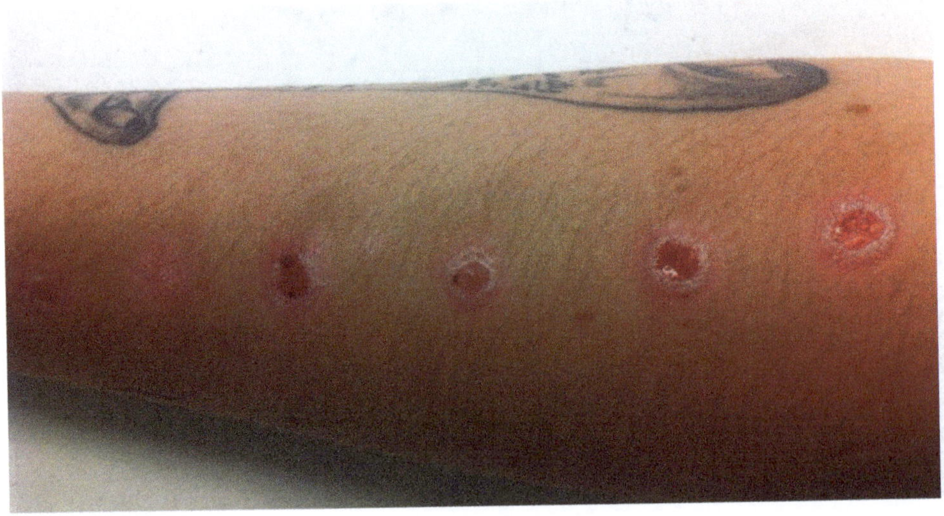

Self Induced Burns

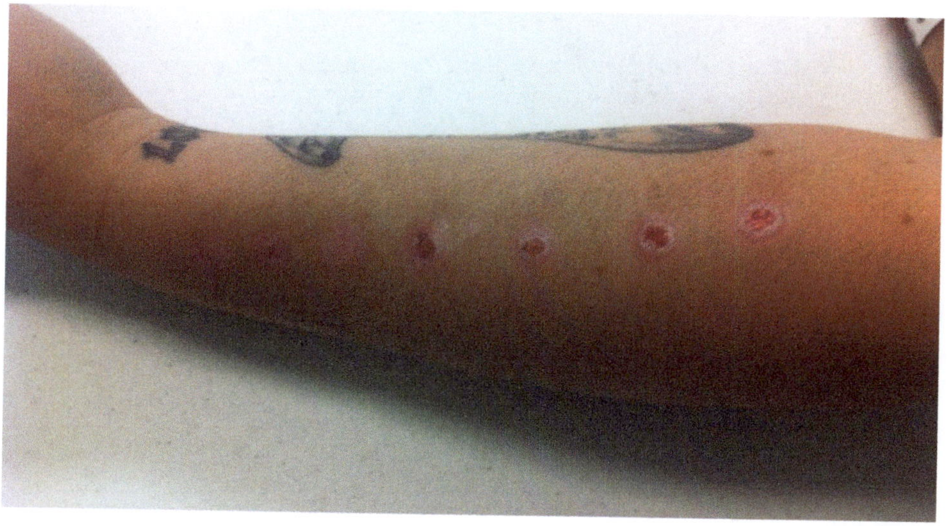

Self Induced Burns-3

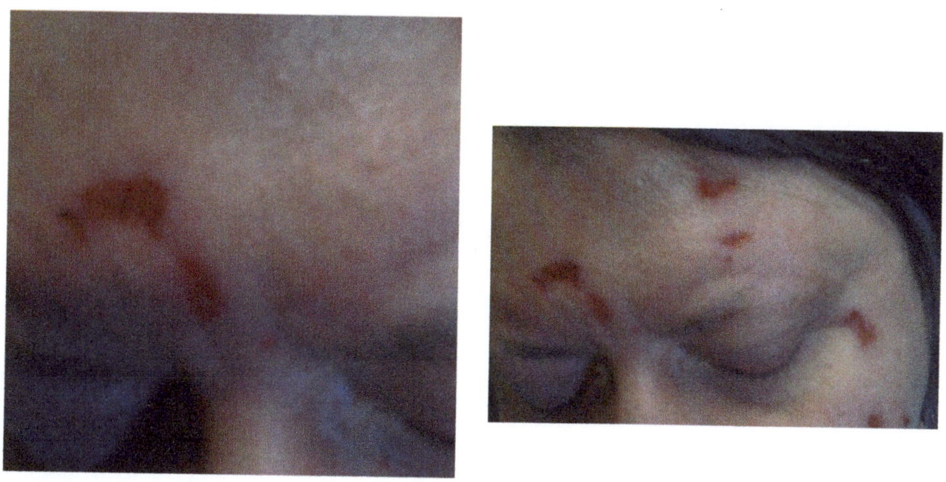

Self picking

Printed and bound by CPI Group (UK) Ltd, Croydon, CR0 4YY

16/09/2026

14963174-0001